Treatment of the
Rheumatic
Diseases

Treatment of the Rheumatic Diseases

Companion to the
Textbook of Rheumatology

MICHAEL H. WEISMAN, MD
Professor of Medicine
Division of Rheumatology
Department of Medicine
University of California at San Diego
School of Medicine
San Diego, California

MICHAEL E. WEINBLATT, MD
Associate Professor of Medicine
Harvard Medical School
Vice Chairman of Clinical Affairs
Department of Rheumatology/Immunology
Director, Robert B. Brigham Arthritis Center
Brigham and Women's Hospital
Boston, Massachusetts

W.B. SAUNDERS COMPANY
A Division of Harcourt Brace & Company
Philadelphia   London   Toronto   Montreal   Sydney   Tokyo

W.B. SAUNDERS COMPANY

A Division of Harcourt Brace & Company

The Curtis Center
Independence Square West
Philadelphia, PA 19106-3399

Library of Congress Cataloging-in-Publication Data

Treatment of the rheumatic diseases: Companion to the Textbook of Rheumatology / [edited by] Michael H. Weisman, Michael E. Weinblatt.
      p.   cm.
   ISBN 0-7216-5382-0
   1. Rheumatism--Chemotherapy. 2. Arthritis--Chemotherapy.
 I. Weisman, Michael H. II. Weinblatt, Michael E.
   [DNLM: 1. Rheumatic Diseases--drug therapy. 2. Arthritis,
Rheumatoid--drug therapy.   WE 544 D7938 1995]
RC927.D778 1995
616.7'23061--dc20
DNLM/DLC

                    94-28994

Treatment of the Rheumatic Diseases: Companion to the Textbook of Rheumatology   ISBN 0-7216-5382-0

Printed in the United States of America

Last digit is the print number: 9 8 7 6 5 4 3 2 1

To

Mary Betty Stevens,
role model and mentor for all of rheumatology

Barbara and Betsy,
who have endured

CONTRIBUTORS

CARLOS A. AGUDELO, MD

Professor of Medicine and Acting Chief, Rheumatology Section, Emory University School of Medicine; Chief of Rheumatology, Veterans Affairs Medical Center, Atlanta, Georgia
Crystal Deposition Diseases

GENE V. BALL, MD

Professor of Medicine, University of Alabama at Birmingham, Birmingham, Alabama
Uncommon Rheumatic Diseases

BRAM H. BERNSTEIN, MD, CM, FAAP, FRCP(C)

Professor of Clinical Pediatrics, University of Southern California School of Medicine; Head, Division of Rheumatology, Children's Hospital, Los Angeles, California
The Rheumatic Diseases of Childhood

HARRY G. BLUESTEIN, MD

Professor of Medicine and Director, Division of Rheumatic Diseases, School of Medicine, University of California at San Diego; Attending Physician, University of California at San Diego Medical Center and San Diego Veterans Administration Hospital, San Diego, California
The Neuropsychiatric Manifestations of Systemic Lupus Erythematosus

MARK J. BORIGINI, MD

Clinical Instructor, Division of Rheumatology, University of California at Los Angeles School of Medicine; Attending Physician, University of California at Los Angeles Center for the Health Sciences, Los Angeles, California
Rheumatoid Arthritis

DANIEL O. CLEGG, MD

Professor of Medicine, University of Utah School of Medicine; Chief, Rheumatology Section, Salt Lake City Department of Veterans Affairs Medical Center; Attending Physician, University of Utah Health Sciences Center, Salt Lake City, Utah
The Seronegative Spondyloarthropathies (Ankylosing Spondylitis, Reiter's Syndrome, Psoriatic Arthritis)

DOYT L. CONN, MD

Professor of Medicine, Mayo Medical School; Consultant, Mayo Clinic, Rochester, Minnesota
Extraarticular Manifestations of Rheumatoid Arthritis

ROBERT I. FOX, MD, PhD

Department of Immunology, The Scripps Research Institute; Division of Rheumatology, Scripps Clinic and Research Foundation, La Jolla, California
Sjögren's Syndrome

MITCHELL F. FUNG, MD

Fellow in Rheumatology, University of California at Los Angeles School of Medicine, Harbor Campus, Torrance, California
Infectious Agent Arthritis

GREGORY C. GARDNER, MD

Assistant Professor, Division of Rheumatology, and Adjunct Assistant Professor, Departments of Orthopedics and Rehabilitation Medicine, University of Washington; Attending Physician, University of Washington Medical Center, Seattle, Washington
Polymyalgia Rheumatica, Temporal (Giant Cell) Arteritis, and Takayasu's Arteritis

ELLEN M. GINZLER, MD, MPH

Professor of Medicine and Chief of Rheumatology, State University of New York Health Science Center at Brooklyn, Brooklyn, New York

Renal Disease in Systemic Lupus Erythematosus

DEIRDRE A. GRAMAS, MD, MPH

Instructor of Medicine, Department of Medicine, University of California at San Francisco, San Francisco, California

Osteoarthritis

CHRISTOPHER G. JACKSON, MD

Associate Professor of Medicine, University of Utah School of Medicine; University of Utah Health Sciences Center; Salt Lake City Department of Veterans Affairs Medical Center, Salt Lake City, Utah

The Seronegative Spondyloarthropathies (Ankylosing Spondylitis, Reiter's Syndrome, Psoriatic Arthritis)

JEFFREY N. KATZ, MD, MS

Assistant Professor of Medicine, Harvard Medical School; Co-Director, Brigham Spine Center, Department of Rheumatology/Immunology, Brigham and Women's Hospital, Boston, Massachusetts

Lumbar Spine Disease

NATHANIEL P. KATZ, MD

Instructor, Harvard Medical School; Staff Neurologist, Brigham and Women's Hospital Pain Management Center, Boston, Massachusetts

Lumbar Spine Disease

NANCY E. LANE, MD

Assistant Professor of Medicine, University of California at San Francisco; Clinical Director, Division of Rheumatology, San Francisco General Hospital, San Francisco, California

Osteoarthritis

MERYL S. LeBOFF, MD

Assistant Professor of Medicine, Harvard Medical School; Associate Physician and Director, Skeletal Health and Osteoporosis Program, Brigham and Women's Hospital, Boston, Massachusetts

Osteoporosis and Rheumatic Disorders

JAMES S. LOUIE, MD

Professor of Medicine, University of California at Los Angeles School of Medicine; Chief, Division of Rheumatology, Harbor–University of California at Los Angeles Medical Center, Torrance, California

Infectious Agent Arthritis

GARY R. MARGOLIES, MD

Associate in Medicine, Division of Clinical Immunology and Rheumatology, University of Alabama at Birmingham, Birmingham, Alabama

Uncommon Rheumatic Diseases

ALAN K. MATSUMOTO, MD

Assistant Professor, The Johns Hopkins University and The Johns Hopkins Bayview Medical Center, Baltimore, Maryland

Scleroderma and Raynaud's Phenomenon

ERIC L. MATTESON, MD, MPH

Assistant Professor of Medicine, Mayo Medical School; Attending Physician, Mayo Clinic, Rochester, Minnesota

Extraarticular Manifestations of Rheumatoid Arthritis

HAROLD E. PAULUS, MD

Professor of Medicine, Division of Rheumatology, University of California at Los Angeles School of Medicine; Attending Physician, University of California at Los Angeles Center for the Health Sciences, Los Angeles, California

Rheumatoid Arthritis

MICHELLE PETRI, MD, MPH

Associate Professor of Medicine, The Johns Hopkins University School of Medicine, Division of Rheumatology; Director, Hopkins Lupus Cohort, and Co-Director, Lupus Pregnancy Center, Johns Hopkins Hospital, Baltimore, Maryland

Systemic Lupus Erythematosus (Including Pregnancy and Antiphospholipid Antibody Syndrome)

CARLOS D. ROSÉ, MD

Assistant Professor of Pediatrics, Jefferson Medical College, Thomas Jefferson University, Philadelphia, Pennsylvania; Staff Physician, Division of Rheumatology, Alfred I. duPont Institute, Wilmington, Delaware

Juvenile Rheumatoid Arthritis and the Pediatric Spondyloarthropathies

E. WILLIAM ST. CLAIR, MD

Assistant Professor of Medicine, Duke University Medical Center, Durham, North Carolina
Vasculitis

NANCY A. SHADICK, MD, MPH

Instructor in Medicine, Harvard Medical School; Associate Rheumatologist, Robert Breck Brigham Arthritis Center, Brigham and Women's Hospital, Boston, Massachusetts
Lyme Disease

BRACHA SHAHAM, MD

Assistant Professor of Clinical Pediatrics, University of Southern California School of Medicine; Attending Physician, Division of Pediatric Rheumatology, Children's Hospital, Los Angeles, California
The Rheumatic Diseases of Childhood

ROBERT W. SIMMS, MD

Associate Professor of Medicine, Boston University School of Medicine; Director, Boston City Hospital Arthritis Clinic; Associate Visiting Physician, Boston City Hospital; Staff Physician, Boston University Medical Center, Boston, Massachusetts
Fibromyalgia Syndrome

BERNHARD H. SINGSEN, MD, MPH

Head, Section of Pediatric Rheumatology, Department of Rheumatic and Immunologic Diseases, The Cleveland Clinic Foundation, Cleveland, Ohio
Juvenile Rheumatoid Arthritis and the Pediatric Spondyloarthropathies

JOHN P. WADE, MD

Clinical Assistant Professor of Medicine, University of British Columbia; Clinical Assistant Professor of Medicine and Rheumatology, Vancouver Hospital, Vancouver, Canada
Osteoporosis and Rheumatic Disorders

FREDRICK M. WIGLEY, MD

Associate Professor of Medicine and Director, Division of Rheumatology, The Johns Hopkins University, Baltimore, Maryland
Scleroderma and *Raynaud's Phenomenon*

ROBERT L. WORTMANN, MD

Professor and Chairman, Department of Medicine, East Carolina University School of Medicine; Chief of Medical Service, Pitt County Memorial Hospital and University Medical Center of Eastern Carolina–Pitt County, Greenville, North Carolina
Idiopathic Inflammatory Diseases of Muscle

PREFACE

Although the title of this book contains the word "treatment," very few treatments in rheumatology are worthy of the name. In truth, we are talking mostly about management of the patient with rheumatic diseases. Most of the diseases that affect our patients are chronic, and sometimes the condition lasts the lifetime of the patient. Decisions are made and unmade over a period of time, often dependent on such pedestrian items as cost, individual fears and preferences, and willingness of both doctor and patient to take risks to achieve certain benefits. Many diseases change or evolve over time, and the need for aggressive therapy may not be apparent at the outset. How the patient will react to the disease or its treatment may not be clear until months or years later. The relationship of the doctor to the patient with a rheumatic disease is, therefore, by definition one of the most powerful aspects of rheumatic disease management. Probably that is why some of us chose to do this type of work on a regular basis.

The purpose of *Treatment of the Rheumatic Diseases: Companion to the Textbook of Rheumatology* is to provide the generalist as well as the specialist with accurate up-to-date information about the management of adults and children with a variety of rheumatic diseases. Currently there is considerable sharing of rheumatic disease patient care among these groups of physicians. Further changes in the health care environment that are largely beyond our control will most certainly change the mix of patients all of us see. The importance of the interchange between the primary care physician and the rheumatologist will increase with more aggressive treatment approaches to many of these illnesses. We have chosen to discuss those diseases that have an impact on society as well as on the patient. This philosophy gives the book a broad range: Low back pain, osteoporosis, and fibromyalgia are addressed as well as the complexities of managing a sick patient with systemic lupus erythematosus or systemic vasculitis. For readers seeking discussions of the diagnosis and pathogenesis of rheumatic disease or of drug metabolism, medication side effects, and drug-drug interactions, specific references are made to the appropriate chapter in the fourth edition of *Textbook of Rheumatology*, edited by W.N. Kelley, E.D. Harris, S. Ruddy, and C.B. Sledge.

Each contributing author was asked to review the available data on which to base therapeutic decisions and to give his or her specific recommendations about treatment decisions. Each chapter roughly covers the natural history of the disease without treatment, open studies, controlled clinical trials, long-term experience, the authors' approach to management, drug side effects and recommended monitoring schedules, and investigational drugs. Each chapter reflects the experience, knowledge, and creativeness of its author or group of authors. The authors have attempted to make their recommendations as specific as possible, recognizing that much of what we do as rheumatologists is highly "individualistic" and is considered an art as much as a scientific experiment. We, as editors, have tried to maintain as much of this individuality and uniqueness as possible, remaining mindful of the need for some consistency across chapters as well as in the recommendations. Therefore there is some overlap of ideas as well as technical redundancy from one chapter to the next. For example, therapeutic strategies using NSAIDs and corticosteroids may be the same or different for rheumatoid arthritis, polymyalgia rheumatica, and psoriatic arthritis, since individual authors may view the risk/benefit ratio of these agents differently.

The primary focus in management has been on the use of drugs, not because they are the only way to manage patients but because they provide us with the most options for patient management. Whenever nondrug treatments are important, we have asked the authors to describe these options and to explain how they fit into the overall management of the patient. It is hoped the very near future will bring us new, more effective tools.

We are most appreciative of the efforts of the W.B. Saunders staff and our colleague Richard Zorab. We are most grateful to Drs. Kelley, Harris, Ruddy, and Sledge, the editors of the fourth edition of *Textbook of Rheumatology*, for their support and confidence in our abilities to enhance their superb textbook with this companion volume. However, this book is clearly the result of an enormous effort by some of the most capable people in rheumatology, defined in advance by their willingness to respond to the call by the editors to produce their chapters in spite of all else they were doing at the time. We are truly grateful for their commitment.

Michael H. Weisman, MD
Michael E. Weinblatt, MD

CONTENTS

LUMBAR SPINE DISEASE

Jeffrey N. Katz
Nathaniel P. Katz

Many clinicians find the management of low back pain daunting, and perhaps for good reason. The pathophysiology of low back syndromes is poorly understood, the physical examination is seldom rewarding, diagnostic tests are frequently misleading, treatments are poorly studied and often marginally useful at best, and some patients have perverse disincentives to improve. Discouraged by these and other factors, many clinicians never develop a systematic approach to low back pain, and consequently patients with low back pain are often managed haphazardly and suboptimally.

Our goal in this chapter is to present a systematic classification system for low back disorders that will allow the clinician to place each patient within a conceptual framework. We will then discuss the management of patients within each category, including medications, rehabilitation, local injections, chronic pain management, and surgery.

CLASSIFICATION OF LOW BACK DISORDERS

In more than 80% of patients with low back disorders, the precise cause and pathogenesis of the symptoms are not known. Therefore, classification systems are necessarily phenomenologic rather than pathophysiologic. In a landmark study of the classification and management of low back disorders, the Quebec Task Force devised an 11-category classification system distin-

guished principally by clinical manifestations rather than presumed pathophysiology.[1] We have adopted an analogous but simpler system,[2] which is presented in Table 1–1. The major entities include lumbago, sciatica, neurogenic claudication, chronic low back pain, inflammatory back pain, and osseous pain syndromes including fractures, infections, and tumors. Inflammatory back pain and osteoporotic fractures are covered elsewhere in this book and will not be discussed in detail in this chapter.

LUMBAGO

Epidemiology. *Lumbago* simply indicates pain in the back and is by far the most common low back pain syndrome. More than 80% of all persons develop lumbago over the course of their lifetime. Approximately 80% of the episodes are resolved within 2 weeks, and well over 90% resolve over a period of several months.[3] Fewer than 1% of the patients with lumbago progress to a chronic pain syndrome with associated psychosocial features.

Risk factors for low back pain include obesity, alcohol use, smoking, low income, and low educational attainment.[4] In addition, occupational exposure to heavy lifting and vibration are associated with low back pain.[5] For example, workers who perform heavy industrial tasks have twice the prevalence of low back pain as bank clerks.[6] Decreased satisfaction with work is also associated with greater low back disability.[7]

Pathophysiology. The term *lumbago* is entirely descriptive and implies nothing about

Supported by NIH Grant AR36308 and an Arthritis Investigator Award from the Arthritis Foundation to Dr. Jeffrey N. Katz.

TABLE 1–1
A Simple Classification System for Select Low Back Pain Syndromes

SYNDROME	CLINICAL FEATURES	RADIOGRAPHIC FEATURES	RESOLVED AT 3 MO
Lumbago	Central low back pain Nondermatomal radiation Neurologic examination normal Ubiquitous	Nonspecific	90%
Sciatica	Dermatomal, sciatic distribution Worse with valsalva, flexion Monoradicular neuro deficit in 50% Straight leg raise in 80%–90% Peak incidence in 40s	Herniated disc	60%–80%
Neurogenic claudication	Dermatomal, nondermatomal symptoms Comfortable in flexion Polyradicular neuro deficits Peak incidence in 60s–70s	Lumbar spinal stenosis	<10%
Chronic low back pain	Duration >6 months Psychosocial features common Occurs at all ages	Varies	Nil
Osseous	Pain constant No comfortable position Systemic features	Destruction, fracture, mass	Varies
Inflammatory	Stiffness, onset before 30	Sacroiliitis	Nil

pathophysiology. In fact, lumbago likely represents a collection of diverse disorders with distinct pathologic mechanisms; the term *mechanical low back pain* is often applied to these conditions. The tissues responsible for mechanical low back pain syndromes include muscles, tendons, ligaments, discs, and facet joints. In some instances, the clinician can make an educated guess about which tissues are responsible for symptoms. For example, younger patients who develop pain while lifting a heavy object probably have simple muscle strain. Older patients with central low back pain exacerbated by leaning forward or coughing likely have symptomatic intervertebral disc degeneration. Similarly, patients with degeneration of the discs and facet joints whose pain occurs primarily with extension and is relieved with flexion may have symptomatic facet joint arthropathy. Additional theories abound implicating numerous structures, including the sacroiliac joint and vertebral subluxations.

It is useful to determine whether lumbago, or backache, occurs in the setting of degen-erative radiographic changes. Degenerative changes increase with age, are ubiquitous by the age of 70,[8] are correlated with back pain,[9] and yet may not be associated with any symptoms at all. When lumbago arises in patients with progressive degenerative change, the prognosis is generally less favorable than in patients without degenerative change.

Diagnostic Features. Lumbago is generally centered in the lower lumbar region. Radiation into the sacroiliac and coccygeal regions and the buttocks is also common. In addition, radiation into the thighs and even the calves occurs frequently and does not necessarily indicate involvement of nerve roots.[10] Stiffness for up to 30 minutes is common and suggests degenerative disc disease or facet arthropathy. Patients with lumbago have negative straight leg raising tests and normal lower extremity neurologic examination findings unless they have primary neurologic disorders, such as diabetic neuropathy. Radiographic tests are generally unrevealing in patients with lumbago and should be ordered only to rule out infections or tumors in patients with findings that raise the question of more ominous lesions, such as systemic features, abnormal laboratory findings, or known primary tumors.

SCIATICA

Epidemiology. Sciatica refers to pain radiating down the lateral thigh and calf, often into the foot, in a sciatic nerve distribution. The lifetime prevalence of sciatica is approximately 40%, with peak prevalence in the forties and fifties. Approximately 1% to 2% of Americans have had surgery for herniated lumbar discs. More than 90% of patients with sciatica due to herniated disc syndromes experience improvement by 6 months; however, up to 10% do not and must consider more invasive interventions, including lumbar disc surgery.[3,4,6,11]

Pathogenesis. Most episodes of sciatica arise from nerve root impingement from a herniated lumbar intervertebral disc. More than 90% of herniated discs occur in the L4-5 and L5-S1 interspaces, affecting the L5 and S1 nerve roots. Central disc herniations may rarely cause cauda equina syndrome, which is characterized by saddle anesthesia and bowel and bladder incontinence. Sciatica may also arise from compression of the exiting nerve root within a narrowed neural foramina (typically due to degenerative lesions); this entity is termed foraminal stenosis. The differential diagnosis of sciatic pain in the absence of structural disc herniation or foraminal stenosis includes extraspinal sciatic nerve compression and irritation of the sciatic nerve by metabolic or inflammatory processes. Finally, as mentioned above, pain that radiates in a sciatic distribution may simply arise from irritation of nonneural spinal structures.

Diagnostic Features. Sciatica due to a herniated disc results in pain and paresthesia occurring in a dermatomal distribution, usually corresponding to the L5 or S1 nerve root. Likewise, physical examination findings should be monoradicular and dermatomal. Both the sensitivity and the specificity of sensibility deficits are 0.50. The sensitivity of muscle weakness is 0.10 to 0.40, while the specificity of radicular muscle weakness is 0.50 to 0.90. The straight leg rais-

ing test, considered positive when pain radiates to the popliteal fossa or distally, has a sensitivity of 0.80 in patients with documented herniated discs with a specificity of about 0.40. The crossed straight leg raising test, in which raising the contralateral leg causes ipsilateral radiating pain, is less sensitive (0.2 to 0.3) but highly specific (0.9 to 1.0).[12]

NEUROGENIC CLAUDICATION

Epidemiology. Neurogenic claudication is most frequently due to lumbar spinal stenosis, which usually occurs in older patients as a structural complication of degenerative disease of the spine. Although there are no reliable data on the incidence or prevalence of this syndrome, approximately one in every 1000 persons over the age of 65 years undergoes decompressive laminectomy for spinal stenosis each year.[13] The natural history is much less favorable than that of lumbago and sciatica. After a follow-up period of 3 years in one study of 19 patients who did not undergo surgical treatment,[14] 32% rated their overall status as improved, 58% as unchanged, and 10% as worse. Similarly, 42% rated their walking capacity as improved, 32% as unchanged, and 26% as worse. Information on larger cohorts is needed; however, it is clear that the natural history is much less favorable for neurogenic claudication than for lumbago or sciatica.

Pathogenesis. There are numerous causes of spinal stenosis, including congenital, degenerative, postsurgical, metabolic, and inflammatory processes.[15] The most common is degenerative lumbar spinal stenosis, with or without an accompanying degenerative spondylolisthesis. Disc degeneration leads to loss of disc height and osteophytosis and sclerosis of the vertebral end plates. Loss of height anteriorly loads the facet joints posteriorly, leading to degenerative facet arthropathy with osteophytes, which can project centrally into the spinal canal. In addition, the ligamentum flavum hypertrophies. The combination of posteriorly protruding disc material, ligamentum flavum and facet joint hypertrophy, and osteophyte formation all lead to a reduction in the cross-sectional area available for the contents of the spinal canal. The stenotic process can occur centrally as well as in the neural foramina.

These degenerative changes can also lead to degenerative spondylolisthesis, which may exacerbate nerve root compression.[16]

Diagnostic Features. Neurogenic claudication consists of low back pain with radiation into the buttocks and the lower extremities, which is exacerbated by lumbar extension and improved with lumbar flexion.[17] Typical activities that make the pain worse include walking, standing, or lying flat in bed. Patients prefer to sit down and stoop forward. Loss of sensation and sense of position in the lower extremities typically causes a wide-based, pseudocerebellar gait. The pain, numbness, and tingling are usually distributed in a polyradicular pattern, as multiple nerve roots are often involved. Patients also have nonradicular back and lower extremity pain from degenerative disease. The physical examination generally reveals limitation of lumbar extension with radiation of pain into the buttocks and legs on prolonged lumbar extension and relief with flexion. The neuromuscular examination may be negative early in the course of the disorder. Findings are often bilateral and polyradicular. The most sensitive modality for detecting neuromuscular deficits is vibration sensibility, which is impaired in more than 50% of the patients in our series. Pinprick deficits occur in just under 50% of patients, whereas muscle weakness is seen generally in about one third.[18] Many of these findings are nonspecific because of associated neurologic problems in older patients. The stenotic process can be confirmed with imaging modalities, either computed tomography, myelography, or magnetic resonance imaging.

CHRONIC LOW BACK PAIN

Chronic low back pain refers to a back pain syndrome that has lasted more than about 6 months.[3] By definition, chronic low back pain occurs commonly in patients with back pain syndromes that have a poor prognosis, such as spinal stenosis. In some patients chronicity of symptoms is associated with a subtle shift in clinical phenomenology with increased prominence of psychosocial features and the dissociation of documented physiologic impairment from reported symptoms.[19] The chronic pain syndrome is multidimensional; its principal features are listed in Table 1–2. These include

---

TABLE 1–2
Features of the Chronic Pain Syndrome

Physical
Deconditioning
Muscle atrophy, stiffness, spasm
Poor posture
Inappropriate signs (e.g., nondermatomal deficits)

Cognitive
"Catastrophizing"
Exaggerated fear of activity

Affective
Depression
Anxiety
Anger, hostility

Psychodynamic
Primary or secondary gain

Social
Disrupted marital and family relationships
Sexual dysfunction
Loss of provider role
Unemployment, Worker's Compensation, legal
  difficulties

---

physical manifestations, such as muscle atrophy and deconditioning; cognitive phenomena, such as exaggerated fear of activity; affective symptoms, including depression and anxiety; the emergence of primary or secondary gain; and social dysfunction, including disruption of work, marital and family relationships, and sexual dysfunction.

The disability resulting from chronic low back pain is costly. The likelihood of return to work is about 50% for workers with 6 months of back disability, 20% after 1 year of disability, and essentially nil after 2 years of low back disability.[3,6]

The explanations for the poor prognosis and prominence of psychosocial features are complex. Deconditioning resulting from bed rest, sometimes prescribed for an inappropriate length of time, leads to rapid loss of muscle strength, flexibility, and general cardiovascular fitness.[20] The problem is compounded by "catastrophizing" about the consequences of specific activities and the exaggerated fear of physical activity. Loss of work results in loss of income, self-esteem, and role as provider in the family. This may produce anxiety, frustration, and depression, as well as a very realistic fear of the future. This is particularly true in laborers with limited resources to explore alternative employment opportunities. Some patients find that pain satisfies certain deeply hidden primary needs, such as self-punishment. Other patients derive secondary gain from work absence, compensation, and/or attention from others.

From a clinical standpoint, chronic guarding of the painful part further exacerbates muscle stiffness and spasm, as do anxiety and emotional stress. Thus there ensues a vicious cycle in which physical and psychological causes of disability potentiate each other. Insomnia and inappropriate use of narcotics and sedative medications may worsen these problems still further.

The clinical examination in patients with chronic low back pain and associated psychological features is often confounded by signs and symptoms that reflect emotional distress rather than physical impairment. For example, such symptoms as numbness or pain may be reported over an entire leg rather than in a dermatomal distribution. Sensory or motor deficits may be reported in nondermatomal locations. Straight leg raising or weakness may be inconsistently reported if the examiner attempts to distract the patient during the examination. These inappropriate signs and symptoms are a clue to psychosocial distress.[21]

OSSEOUS PAIN

The most common cause of osseous bone pain is vertebral fractures, particularly osteoporotic compression fractures, which are covered in detail in the section of this book on osteoporosis. (See Chapter 22.) Tumors and infections are rare causes of back pain, but it is extremely important to identify them. Tumors in the spine are generally metastatic, arising from common solid tumors such as prostate cancer, myeloma, and lung and breast cancer. Infections may occur in the vertebrae, disc spaces, or epidural spaces. They may be due to pyogenic infections, typically *Staphylococcus aureus,* or to chronic granulomatous processes, such as tuberculosis or fungi.

Several key historical features point to the presence of tumors and infections. Patients generally have unrelenting pain in virtually all positions. In most other types of low back pain patients can find a position that makes them relatively comfortable, or they may have relief

of pain at night. Systemic symptoms, including weight loss, generalized fatigue, fever, and sweats, are also associated with tumors and infections.[22] On physical examination, direct palpation over the spine may reveal bony tenderness. Radiographs generally reveal bony lesions; earlier on in the course, computed tomography or magnetic resonance imaging may be required.

POSTSURGICAL BACK PAIN

The existence of "failed back surgery syndrome" speaks to the frequency of unsuccessful operations on the lumbar spine and the importance of identifying preoperatively those patients who are likely to benefit. Failed back surgery syndrome has been reported most commonly after surgery for herniated lumbar discs. Inadequate decompression, postsurgical scarring, arachnoiditis, and psychosocial features have all been implicated along with poor patient selection.[23]

MANAGEMENT OF LOW BACK PAIN: LUMBAGO

This section will review treatment approaches to the major low back pain syndromes discussed in the preceding section. See Table 1–3.

Because mechanical low back pain improves within weeks to months in more than 90% of patients, therapies must be highly effective to be superior to the natural history. The clinician is well advised, above all, to do no harm.

The traditional intervention for a sore back is bed rest. Although the logic of resting injured tissues is clear, the lost productivity and reinforced sense of disability that accompany a prescription for bed rest can be more devastating than the backache itself. The therapeutic efficacy of bed rest for acute mechanical low back pain has been well established in a randomized controlled trial conducted in military recruits.[24] However, Deyo and colleagues[25] showed that a recommendation of 2 days of bed rest rather than 7 resulted in 45% fewer days of work missed and no differences in other functional or subjective outcomes. The message is that, for patients with mechanical low back pain, a brief period of bed rest is useful but prolonged bed rest (i.e., greater than a couple of days) appears to have little benefit

TABLE 1–3
Conservative Therapy for Low Back Pain

THERAPY	SYNDROME	EVIDENCE OF EFFICACY	COMMENTS
Bed rest	Lumbago, sciatica	RCT	Limit to 2–3 d
Exercises	All	RCT	Conflicting results
TENS	Chronic	Negative RCT	Untested in stenosis
Traction	Sciatica	Negative RCT	
Orthoses	All	Observational	Rational in LSS, postop
NSAIDs	All	RCT	Caution in elderly
Acetaminophen	All	NA	Safe, useful
Muscle relaxants	All	RCT	Useful if spasm, sleep disorder
Narcotics	All	Observational	Safe in select patients
Manipulation	Lumbago, sciatica	RCT	Best in early lumbago
Epidural injection	Sciatica, neurogenic claudication	RCT	Radicular pain responds best
Facet injection	Lumbago, chronic	Negative RCT	Untested in degenerative facet arthropathy

RCT = randomized control trial.

and may entail major costs, including increased work absenteeism, muscle atrophy, and deconditioning among others.[26]

Medications

The most commonly prescribed medications for patients with low back pain include nonsteroidal antiinflammatory drugs (NSAIDs), muscle relaxants, and antidepressants. Although each of these has been shown in randomized control trials to be superior to placebo,[26] the benefit from these medications is generally modest and side effects are not trivial.

Patients with prominent stiffness appear to benefit the most from NSAIDs. In general, NSAIDs appear to function primarily as analgesics. Of note, acetaminophen has been shown to be as effective as ibuprofen in the short-term treatment of osteoarthritis of the knee.[27] Although a similar study has not been performed for patients with low back pain, we have found that up to 4 g of acetaminophen daily can often be used alone or added to a NSAID for greater analgesic effect with no additional toxicity. Continued high doses of acetaminophen should be avoided in patients with liver dysfunction. In older patients we are particularly inclined to use acetaminophen rather than nonsteroidal antiinflammatory medication. When NSAIDs are used in older patients, agents with long half-lives (such as piroxicam) should be avoided.

Patients with prominent muscle spasm frequently appear to benefit most from muscle relaxants, such as cyclobenzaprine, methocarbamol, carisoprodol, and others. These medications all have the potential to cause sedation. Generalized fibromyalgia with characteristic tender points and sleep disorder may occur in association with low back pain and is an indication for a trial of tricyclic antidepressants.

Although clinicians are generally reluctant to use narcotics in patients with back pain, these agents may be quite useful. The risk of addiction in properly selected patients with no history of substance abuse is quite low.[28] The issues involved in prescribing narcotics are discussed in the section of this chapter on management of chronic back pain. An effective dose should be prescribed, as ineffective dosing may prompt medication-seeking behavior. The prescription should be made for a limited, defined period.

Perhaps the most useful point to be made about use of medication in lumbago is that the benefits are generally marginal and patients' expectations should, accordingly, be modest. The central strategy in treating patients with lumbago is to rely on the natural history and encourage patients to adapt exercise programs to try to prevent future occurrences. An overemphasis on the role of medications will encourage patient passivity, which may prolong disability.

Exercises and Modalities

A variety of exercise programs have been advocated, including Williams' flexion exercises,[40] extension exercises modeled after those of McKenzie et al., and aerobic conditioning exercises. The efficacy of exercises administered by physiotherapists has been reviewed recently.[29] Of sixteen randomized controlled trials of exercise programs for low back pain, six showed benefit from an exercise program whereas ten reported no benefit. The exercise regimens used in these various studies differed markedly and included stretching, abdominal flexion, and back extension along with a variety of modalities. Thus the role of exercises in the management of acute low back pain is controversial. Primary and secondary exercise programs and education regarding posture and back protection are also somewhat controversial but appear to be beneficial in reducing recurrences of low back pain.[30]

Rehabilitative Approach

The rehabilitative approach to low back pain often includes various modalities, including the use of heat, cold, ultrasonography, and vapocoolant. In general, these strategies have not been evaluated critically. Traction has been studied critically and appears to have no role in the management of low back pain. Lumbar corsets have received little critical study. The Quebec Task Force believed that corsets do not reduce the period of disability from low back pain. Corsets are frequently used to enhance spinal stability after spinal surgery, particularly fusion, and to discourage lumbar extension in patients with spinal stenosis.[26]

Transcutaneous Electrical Nerve Stimulation

Transcutaneous electrical nerve stimulation (TENS) is used widely in chronic pain conditions, including low back pain. TENS would appear to have essentially no role in acute mechanical low back pain because of the favorable natural history of the disorder. TENS has been studied critically in a randomized control study of patients with chronic low back pain.[31] In this study TENS was no more effective than sham TENS and offered no advantage over simple exercises alone. However, TENS has not been subjected to randomized control trials in patients with spinal stenosis, disc syndromes, or osteoporotic fractures, and its utility in these settings should be considered uncertain.

Myofascial Trigger Point Injection

Myofascial pain is thought to arise from trigger points. A trigger point is defined as a palpable nodule that, on palpation, reproduces the quality, location, and referral pattern of the patient's pain. Occasionally, palpation of a trigger point produces muscle fasciculation.[32] There are no reliable diagnostic criteria for this syndrome; thus its prevalence is unknown.[33]

Patients may experience prolonged, tender muscle spasms as a result of, rather than as a cause of, their underlying back pain problem. This phenomenon is referred to as secondary myofascial pain. A number of different treatments are used for myofascial pain,[34] including ultrasound, stretching and strengthening exercises, general aerobic conditioning, stretch and spray, and trigger point injections.

In trigger point injections, a small volume of local anesthetic is injected through a narrow-gauge needle into the trigger points. Local anesthetic is more effective than simple dry needling and is considerably more comfortable as well.[34] Therapy should be geared to the complexity of the clinical problem: simple trigger point injections for patients with isolated localized myofascial pain; incorporation of a stretching and strengthening program for patients with impaired regional function; a full reconditioning program for patients with significant disability; and multidisciplinary rehabilitation for patients with psychological and other needs.

Chiropractic Manipulation

Chiropractic manipulation involves abrupt movement of vertebrae beyond their physiologic but not their anatomic range of motion. Well-designed randomized controlled trials have shown that chiropractic manipulation leads to faster improvement in symptoms in patients who have acute low back pain without nerve root involvement.[35] Patients also appear to be more satisfied with chiropractic care than with orthodox medical treatment for low back pain.[36] Specifically, patients value the chiropractor's confidence in the accuracy of diagnosis and efficacy of prescribed treatment, even though chiropractic diagnostic findings have poor reproducibility.[37] Patients are uneasy with the orthodox medical presumption that the cause of low back pain is generally unknown and that treatment is nonspecific. Thus the positive style of chiropractic practice and the technical aspects of manipulation appear to underlie the improved outcomes of chiropractic care. These fascinating data suggest that patients appreciate a more positive and knowledgeable discussion of low back pain therapy and its likely outcomes.

Alternative Therapies

One third of Americans use some form of alternative therapy. By far the most common problem associated with the use of alternative treatment is back pain.[38] The most frequent alternative treatments include massage, relaxation, chiropractic care, and acupuncture. Chiropractic appears to be beneficial in acute lumbago, as noted above. Acupuncture is more effective than control treatments that do not include needling but has no advantage over needling of control sites, suggesting a nonspecific effect of needling. Although there is little scientific support for most alternative treatments (with the exception of chiropractic), the same can be said for many orthodox treatments, as noted in previous paragraphs.

Epidural and Facet Injections

The efficacy of epidural steroid injections in patients without nerve root involvement has not been studied critically. Epidural steroid injections are usually reserved for patients with evidence of nerve root irritation. Facet joint injections are occasionally used in patients with lumbago but usually after months to years of symptoms. Steroid injections into the epidural space and facet joints will be discussed in the sections of this chapter on management of sciatica and chronic back pain, respectively.

Surgery

Some patients with severe radiographic degenerative disc disease and central low back pain, without objective evidence of nerve root impingement or dynamic spondylolisthesis, are offered lumbar fusion. There is considerable debate within the surgical community about the appropriateness of lumbar fusion in this setting.

MANAGEMENT OF SCIATICA

As with lumbago, management of sciatica should begin with a clear explanation of the likely natural history. Resolution of symptoms is slower and less complete than in most cases of lumbago. One recent study[39] showed that 44% of patients were free of pain 1 month after an episode of sciatica and 55% were free of pain at 1 year. By 1 year, 7.5% were out of work and 45% had some restriction in work. Thus the natural history is generally favorable, and interventions must be quite effective to be superior to simple observation alone.

Conservative management of sciatica parallels that of lumbago. Bed rest is often useful. More than 48 hours of bed rest may be indicated in patients with severe pain and disability, but the potential for muscle atrophy and lost productivity must be weighed against benefits of prolonged bed rest.

Medications are prescribed in much the same manner as for mechanical low back pain. Short courses of systemic oral corticosteroids are occasionally prescribed for sciatica; given the toxicity of high-dose systemic steroids, even for a short period of time, we do not recommend this practice. Muscle relaxants can be quite useful, inasmuch as secondary muscle spasm is common in herniated disc syndromes. Pain should be treated with analgesics, including acetaminophen, NSAIDs, or both. Of note, a recent community-based study showed that piroxicam was of no benefit over placebo in the management of sciatica, raising questions about the routine use of NSAIDs.[39] Short courses of narcotics may be necessary early in the course for patients at low risk of addiction. Narcotic use is discussed in detail in the section of this chapter on management of chronic back pain.

The rehabilitative approach to patients with herniated disc syndrome generally includes a program that emphasizes the use of lumbar extension, modeled after the work of McKenzie and others.[40] Extension exercises are purported to accelerate resorption of the protruding disc material. Accordingly, symptoms "centralize," with radiating leg pain shifting to central low back pain.[40] Strengthening programs are indicated for patients with functionally limiting muscle weakness arising from radiculopathy.

Chiropractic manipulation is frequently administered to patients with sciatica due to herniated disc syndromes. There is less scientific information on the value of manipulation in this setting.

EPIDURAL STEROID INJECTIONS

Injection of a combination of local anesthetic and steroid into the epidural space of the spine is widely performed by anesthesiologists and other practitioners. Several controlled trials have been conducted in patients with radicular pain syndromes.[41] The results are conflicting, owing in part to differences in study design. We interpret the data to suggest that epidural steroid injections are beneficial for a few months in patients with radicular pain. However, it appears that by 12 months after the procedure there is no difference between epidural steroid injections and control injections. Also, it appears that acute radicular pain (less than 3 to 6 months in duration) responds better than chronic pain.[41] This may simply reflect the generally favorable natural history of sciatica. Most of the available evidence supports the use of epidural steroid injections as a relatively safe and beneficial adjunctive therapy with short- to medium-term efficacy (weeks to months), particularly in patients without chronic symptoms.[41-44]

Chronic nonradicular back pain in conditions such as degenerative disc disease without radiculopathy and spondylolisthesis rarely improves with epidural steroid injections alone. Transient responses may be seen, however; therefore epidural steroid injections may be used as an adjunct to a complete rehabilitation program, even for these less responsive conditions. Our unpublished data suggest that patients with extensive psychological overlay seldom respond to the injections. In fact, these patients may have exacerbations of pain and disability after epidural steroid injection, resulting in further prolonged dependence on the health care profession.

Epidural steroid injection is a safe outpatient procedure. Fewer than 1% of patients will have an unintentional dural puncture with the resulting possibility of spinal headache. Patients with steroid-sensitive conditions, such as diabetes or congestive heart failure, may experience brief exacerbations of their illnesses after an epidural steroid injection. Hyperglycemia may occur in diabetics, for example. Rarely, patients may experience a prolonged exacerbation of their pain after epidural steroid injection.[41,44]

Given the foregoing uncertainties in selecting patients for epidural steroid injections, a reasonable approach in the patient with acute low back pain would be to employ conservative therapy at the outset, with physical therapy and medications. If, after a few months, the patient is still experiencing significant pain or disability, enrollment in a comprehensive rehabilitation program is advisable, with epidural steroid injection as an adjunct, particularly in the patient with radicular pain. If patients do not improve with these nonoperative approaches but have surgical lesions, referral to a spine surgeon is appropriate. Patients whose pain is purely axial, or who have significant psychosocial overlay, should generally not be injected. Patients with chronic sciatica should undergo epidural steroid injections as a means of enhancing their rehabilitative potential rather than as an isolated intervention.

SURGERY

More than 200,000 lumbar discectomies are performed annually in this country, and the rate appears to be increasing about 10% per year.[13] Striking variations exist in discectomy rates across small geographic regions and also across large regions of the country, suggesting considerable uncertainty among physicians about the appropriate indications for surgery.[45] The large body of literature on failed back surgery syndrome offers sad testimony to the observation that many patients are operated on inappropriately with poor results.[23]

Cauda equina syndrome, consisting of bowel and bladder dysfunction in addition to saddle anesthesia, is an absolute indication for surgery in patients with disc herniations. Progressive muscle weakness that becomes functionally disabling is also a strong indication for lumbar disc surgery. These two indications, however, account for fewer than one fifth of the surgical procedures for disc herniations. The other discectomies must be viewed as elective.

Weber[46] performed an elegant randomized trial of discectomy versus conservative therapy on patients who did not have cauda equina syndrome or progressive neuromuscular deficits.[46] Of the patients randomized to receive conservative treatment, 33% were completely satisfied with their status after 1 year, 51% after 4 years, and 55% after 10 years of conservative therapy. Of patients initially randomized to surgical therapy, 66% were completely satisfied at 1 year, 66% at 4 years, and 58% after 10 years. Twenty-six percent of patients initially randomized to conservative therapy opted for surgery during the first year and experienced results similar to the surgical group. Thus, while surgical therapy was associated with greater patient satisfaction in the first years, there appears to be little difference in outcome between surgery and conservative care after 10 years of follow-up. These results indicate that in patients without cauda equina syndrome or rapidly progressive neurologic deficit, the decision to operate should be made on the basis of patient preferences regarding the risks and benefits of the operation.

A recent review of 81 studies of discectomy found that, on average, operative mortality was 0.15%, dural tears were reported in 3.7%, and permanent nerve root injuries in 0.8%. Thrombophlebitis was reported in 1.6%, pulmonary emboli in 0.6%, and wound infections in 2%. Reoperation rates increased with longer duration of follow-up, reaching 10% by 10 years. The review noted success rates of about 70%, on average, for standard discectomy, microdiscectomy, and percutaneous descectomy.[47]

Given the substantial proportion of patients (up to 30%) with poor outcomes, identification of prognostic factors is crucial. Twenty-six percent of the variance in the outcome of surgical discectomy is explained by psychological and social factors, while just 14% is explained by preoperative radiographic and physical examination findings.[48] Psychological and social factors associated with poor prognosis include elevated hysteria or hypochondriasis scores on the Minnesota Multiphasic Personality Inventory and the presence of litigation or Worker's Compensation claims.[48,49] The following factors are associated with favorable outcomes of discectomy for herniated disc syndrome:

- Positive straight leg raising test
- Presence of neurologic deficit attributable to involved nerve root
- Imaging test evidence of compression of involved nerve root
- Absence of litigation, Worker's Compensation

In multivariable models these factors contribute independently to the likelihood of a good outcome. Prognostic scoring systems that use these factors effectively predict the out-

come of surgery.[49] Patients with negative prognostic factors, such as Worker's Compensation, depression, or a negative physical examination, should not necessarily be denied surgery, but their expectations should be adjusted accordingly.

Several surgical alternatives to conventional discectomy, including microdiscectomy, percutaneous discectomy, and chymopapain injection, have been introduced. Microdiscectomy uses microsurgical techniques, leaving a smaller wound and leading to earlier mobilization and less postoperative disability. Surgical outcomes appear to be comparable to those of traditional discectomy.[50] Percutaneous discectomy involves suctioning disc material from the body of the herniated disc, thereby decompressing the disc and presumably relieving pressure on the nerve root. This procedure is also associated with a low complication rate and rapid rehabilitation. Randomized controlled trials have not been performed; however, open series suggest success comparable to that of traditional discectomy.[51] Chemonucleolysis involves introduction of a proteolytic enzyme, typically chymopapain, into the nucleus of the affected disc. The proteolytic enzyme digests disc material and apparently decompresses the disc in a manner analogous to percutaneous discectomy. Randomized controlled trials have found that standard discectomy is superior to chemonucleolysis.[52,53] The technique is not employed frequently in the United States because of reports of complications, including anaphylaxis, in about 0.3% of patients and rare but potentially devastating neurologic complications.

NEUROGENIC CLAUDICATION

The management of neurogenic claudication due to degenerative spinal stenosis pivots around the observation that the natural history is unfavorable. Spontaneous sustained improvement is unusual.

Conservative therapy is similar to that advocated for mechanical back pain and sciatica. The typical amelioration of symptoms with lumbar flexion provides a rationale for the use of lumbar corsets. Degenerative spinal stenosis occurs in older patients who are less tolerant of NSAIDs. We use acetaminophen and narcotics more frequently for symptomatic degenerative lumbar stenosis than for most other spinal problems. There is no critical literature on the value of an exercise program for patients with spinal stenosis.

Lumbar epidural steroid injections are used frequently in patients with spinal stenosis. Benefit occurs in about two thirds of the patients but typically lasts just a few months. Patients with numerous comorbidities who are poor surgical candidates may receive epidural steroid injections every 4 months or so on an ongoing basis as an alternative to decompressive surgery. The role of epidural injections in spinal stenosis has not been adequately studied, and recommendations are generally extrapolated from the outcome of injections in the disc-protrusion population.[41,44] Studies of epidural injection specifically in the management of symptomatic spinal stenosis are needed.

Surgical therapy consists of decompression laminectomy with medial facetectomy and occasionally spinal fusion. The indications for fusion are controversial. It appears that patients with spinal stenosis due to degenerative spondylolisthesis benefit from stabilization.[54] In patients with multilevel stenosis, or with no evidence of spondylolisthesis, the indications for fusion are controversial. Analysis of Medicare data shows that fusion is associated with a higher risk of mortality, medical complications, and subsequent reoperations and higher costs.[55] There is heated debate about the relative merits of fusion with autologous bone alone versus augmentation with pedicle screws or other instrumentation systems. Instrumentation leads to more solid fusions but is associated with greater expense and complications.

The outcome of decompressive surgery for spinal stenosis is fair. A recent literature synthesis estimated a success rate of 64%.[56] In our retrospective study, 31% of patients had severe back or buttock pain after an average of 4.5 years of follow-up and 17% required reoperation because of recurrent stenosis or symptomatic instability. Patients with medical comorbidities had worse outcomes.[57] Our most recent evaluation after 7 to 10 years of follow-up has not yet been analyzed fully but shows that about 30% of patients continue to have severe symptoms. This procedure is performed in elderly patients whose functional status is affected by nonspinal problems, including osteoarthritis of the hips or knees, cardiac and pulmonary disease, and visual problems, among others. Thus some patients may experience functional decline despite resolution of back symptoms. In our ongoing prospective study of surgery for spinal stenosis, approximately one quarter of the patients are bothered by severe pain just 6 months after surgery and about one quarter of the patients are dissatisfied with the results of operation after just 6 months. Predominance of pain in the lower extremities is associated with greater satisfaction, whereas predominance of pain in the back is associated with a less favorable result.[58] A conservative orthopedist or neurosurgeon is one who operates only for pain. The presence of greater medical comorbidity is also associated with worse outcomes. Whether depression, anxiety, and work disability (less relevant in this older population) are associated with outcome has not yet been examined.

CHRONIC PAIN SYNDROME

Management of chronic pain syndromes involves the conservative therapies listed previously, along with several specific modalities that will be discussed in detail, including multidisciplinary pain treatment centers, narcotic use, facet injections, and spinal cord stimulators.

Chronic Pain Treatment Centers

Patients with chronic pain are best managed in a multidisciplinary system in which they are typically evaluated by a psychologist or a psychiatrist, a physical therapist, and a physician, typically a neurologist or an anesthesiologist.[59] The physician will review the diagnostic workup, ensuring that no specifically treatable cause for the back pain has been overlooked. The next step typically is to optimize the use of medications. This usually involves streamlining multiple medications, weaning patients from narcotics or benzodiazepines. Insomnia, depression, and anxiety are addressed with medications as well. The psychologist will evaluate for behavioral factors, such as secondary gain in the workplace or in the family, that may be perpetuating the pain. The patient will also be assessed for psychological comorbidity, such as anxiety, posttraumatic stress, panic, or depression. The patient will then be treated with a variety of cognitive and behavioral techniques, often in combination with medications, for the psychological symptoms. Patients will be trained to manage their lives despite their pain with coping strategies, nonpharmacologic therapy for insomnia, and other approaches. The physical therapist will assess the patient's rehabilitative needs and attempt to restore functional status, usually relying on active rather than passive conditioning programs. In a full-service program the patient will be triaged into a return-to-work program, often in conjunction with employers or payors. Patients may also be screened for more sophisticated pain-management techniques such as spinal cord stimulation, implantable opiate pumps, or chronic oral narcotic therapy.

Overall success rates for interdisciplinary pain clinics vary, depending on the population studied and the outcome measure.[60] Although return-to-work rates for a chronic out-of-work population are in the range of 15% to 25%, the cost of financially supporting young injured workers for the rest of their lives is enormous. Thus even programs with an apparently low success rate may be cost-effective. Select programs report return-to-work rates of 85%.[61] Return to work may not be the sole important factor, since the ability to be functional at home, restoration of family life, and reduction of suffering are laudable goals as well.[62]

Chronic Narcotic Therapy

Long-term use of oral narcotics for patients with unrelenting pain is controversial.[28] It has traditionally been assumed that a significant percentage of patients given narcotics for pain become addicted to them. This is not true in the acute pain setting,[63] and the incidence of addiction in the chronic pain setting has been poorly studied. The following are generally regarded as risk factors for narcotic addiction: previous history of substance abuse, ongoing substance abuse, high levels of psychosocial distress, psychological symptoms that may respond to narcotics (e.g., anxiety, panic attacks), use of short-acting narcotics, and prescription on an as-needed basis rather than a fixed schedule. Our own unpublished data suggest that the risk of prescribing to patients with a history of substance abuse may be lower than previously thought.

A reasonable approach to patient selection for chronic narcotic therapy would require a mental health evaluation before initiation of therapy. Narcotics should be administered strictly on a trial basis at first, perhaps for several months, and under strictly supervised conditions, with outcomes documented. If the patient's clinical status is not improved during the trial, narcotic therapy can be justifiably stopped.

If the oral route is unavailable or impracticable, narcotics can be administered by a number of different routes, including sublingual, rectal, vaginal, subcutaneous, intravenous, or transdermal. A recent advance has been the development of the transdermal patch, which delivers fentanyl, a lipophylic narcotic. The patch is easily applied and typically lasts 3 days. There is no obvious advantage to the transdermal patch in patients who tolerate oral narcotics. The patch may be quite expensive.

Facet Injections

The lumbar facet joints are thought to give rise to clinical low back pain. Pain syndromes that emanate from the facet joints consist of a dull ache radiating into the low back, buttocks, hips or thigh, and even beyond the knee.[64] Pain is worsened by back extension or rotation, such as rolling over in bed, and can be reproduced on physical examination by prolonged back extension. Radiographic abnormalities of the facet joints are common but are only loosely correlated with clinical symptoms, suggesting that one should make this diagnosis with caution and on the basis of congruent radiographic and clinical findings.[65]

In patients with pain that seems to emanate from facet joints, facet joint injections would appear at least conceptually to have a role. Carrette et al.[66] studied the efficacy of facet joint injections in a randomized control trial. Patients were selected for participation if they had more than 50% pain relief after a facet joint injection with local anesthetic. Even in this select group enriched for presumed facet joint syndrome, facet joint injections with corticosteroids led to improvement at 6 months in only 20% versus 10% in patients injected with saline solution placebo. Thus, even in patients with back pain that appears to arise from true facet arthropathy, injection with corticosteroid was of little value in this study. It should be noted that fewer than half of the patients in the study had radiographic evidence of degenerative changes at the facet joint. Thus the role of facet injections in patients with suspected symptomatic degenerative arthropathy of the facet joints remains unproven. Data on complications of facet joint injections are sparse and would be useful in evaluation of the relative costs and benefits of the procedure.

Radiofrequency denervation of the facet joints is performed in some centers as an alternative approach to management of patients with suspected symptomatic facet arthropathy.[67] The facet joints are innervated by the medial branches of the dorsal rami of the spinal nerves. These medial branches are blocked with local anesthetic. If this rather simple procedure is successful in temporarily relieving the patient's pain, it can be followed with radiofrequency denervation wherein the medial branches are coagulated with a radiofrequency probe. This approach has not been evaluated in controlled trials.

Spinal Cord Stimulation

Spinal cord stimulation has been used since the early 1970s for treatment of chronic pain. A number of well-designed trials have demonstrated that at 20-year follow-up, spinal cord stimulation is highly effective for neuropathic pain, including radicular pain.[68,69] The technique is relatively straightforward and quite safe. All patients undergo a temporary trial with an externalized stimulating electrode. If the trial is not successful, the electrode can be easily removed. Patients who do respond become candidates for the implantable stimulator. Carefully selected patients will enjoy an average of 50% improvement in their pain or activity level, which can be maintained even during long-term follow-up. Patients with pain primarily in the extremities and with minimal axial pain are most likely to benefit. Spinal cord stimulation is probably the most effective treatment for properly selected patients with failed back surgery syndrome.[70]

Spinal Opiate Administration

Administration of spinal opiates has been recognized for several decades as a useful technique in the management of selected patients with cancer pain. Patients usually obtain analgesia that is equal or superior to that achieved with systemic opiate administration, with fewer side effects.[71] Recently, the use of this modality has been expanded to the noncancer population.[72] These patients undergo a trial with a temporary spinal catheter, and those who have a successful response may then undergo implantation of an opiate pump connected to an intrathecal catheter. The pumps must be refilled monthly. Although there is a small incidence of infection, the procedure is generally safe in experienced hands.[73] There are no large case series or controlled studies of opiate pumps for noncancer conditions; hence many questions regarding effectiveness and complications remain unanswered.

REFERENCES

1. Quebec Task Force on Spinal Disorders Report. Spine (suppl) 1987.
2. Katz JN. The assessment and management of low back pain: a critical review. Arthritis Health Care Res 1993;6:104.
3. Frymoyer JW. Back pain and sciatica. N Engl J Med 1988;318:291.
4. Deyo RA, Bass JE. Lifestyle and low back pain: the influence of smoking and obesity. Spine 1989;14:501.
5. Kelsey JL, Githens PB, O'Conner T, et al. Acute prolapsed lumbar intervertebral disc: an epidemiologic study with special reference to driving automobiles and cigarette smoking. Spine 1984;9:608.
6. Anderson GBJ. The epidemiology of spinal disorders. In: Frymoyer JW, ed. The adult spine: principles and practice. New York: Raven Press, 1991:107.
7. Bigos SJ, Battie MC, Spengler DM, et al. A prospective study of work perceptions and psychosocial factors affecting the report of back injury. Spine 1991;16:1.
8. Powell MC, Szpryt P, Wilson M, Symonds EM, Worthington BS. Prevalence of lumbar disc degeneration observed by magnetic resonance in symptomless women. Lancet 1986 (Dec. 13); 1366.
9. Lawrence JS. Disc degeneration: its frequency and relationship to symptoms. Ann Rheum Dis 1969;28:121.
10. Kellgren JH. On the distribution of pain arising from deep somatic structures with charts of segmented pain areas. Clin Sci 1939;4:35.
11. Deyo RA, Tsui-Wu YJ. Descriptive epidemiology of low back pain and its related medical care in the United States. Spine 1987;12:264.
12. Deyo RA, Rainesville J, Kent DL. What can the history and physical examination tell us about low back pain? JAMA 1992;268:760.
13. Graves EJ. National Hospital Discharge Survey. Vital Health Stat 1989;13(100):176.
14. Johnsson KE, Uden A, Rosen I. The effect of decompression on the natural course of spinal

stenosis: a comparison of surgically treated and untreated patients. Spine 1991;16:15.

15. Moreland LW, Lopez-Mendez A, Alarcon GS. Spinal stenosis: a comprehensive review of the literature. Semin Arthritis Rheum 1989;19:127.

16. Spengler DM. Degenerative stenosis of the lumbar spine. J Bone Joint Surg 1987;69A:305.

17. Katz JN, Dalgas M, Stucki GH, Lipson SJ. The diagnosis of lumbar spinal stenosis. Rheum Dis Clin North Am 1994 (in press).

18. Katz JN, Dalgas M, Bayley J, et al. Degenerative lumbar spinal stenosis: diagnostic value of the history and physical examination. Arth Rheum 1994;37(suppl):[in press].

19. Waddell G. A new clinical model for the treatment of low back pain. Spine 1987;12:632.

20. Bortz WM. The disuse syndrome. West J Med 1984;141:691.

21. Waddell G, McCulloch JA, Kummel ED, Venner RM. Nonorganic physical signs in low back pain. Spine 1980;5:117.

22. Deyo RA, Diehl AK. Cancer as a cause of back pain: frequency, clinical presentation, and diagnostic strategies. J Gen Intern Med 1988;3:230.

23. Gill K, Frymoyer JW. The management of treatment failures after decompressive surgery. In: Frymoyer JW, ed. The adult spine: principles and practice. New York: Raven Press, 1991: 1849.

24. Wiesel SW, Cuckler JM, Delucca F, Jones F, Zeide MS, Rothman RH. Acute low back pain: an objective analysis of conservative therapy. Spine 1980;5:324.

25. Deyo RA, Diehl AK, Rosenthal M. How many days of bed rest for acute low back pain? A randomized controlled clinical trial. N Engl J Med 1986;315:1064.

26. Deyo RA. Non-operative treatment of low back disorders: differentiating useful from useless therapy. In: Frymoyer JW, ed. The adult spine: principles and practice. New York: Raven Press, 1991:1567.

27. Bradley JD, Brandt KD, Katz BP, Kalasinski LA, Ryan SI. Comparison of an antiinflammatory dose of ibuprofen, an analgesic dose of ibuprofen, and acetaminophen in the treatment of patients with osteoarthritis of the knee. N Engl J Med 1991;325:87.

28. Portenoy RK. Chronic opioid therapy in nonmalignant pain. J Pain Symptom Manag 1990;5: 546.

29. Koes BW, Bouter LM, Beckerman H, van der Heijden FJ, Knipschild PG. Physiotherapy exercises and back pain: a blinded review. BMJ 1991;302:1572.

30. Schlapach P. Back school. In: Schlapach P, Gerber NJ, eds. Physiotherapy: controlled trials and facts. Vol 14. Rheumatology. Basel: Karger, 1991:25.

31. Deyo RA, Walsh NE, Martin DC, Schoenfeld LS, Ramarurthy S. A controlled trial of transcutaneous electrical nerve stimulation (TENS) and exercise for chronic low back pain. N Engl J Med 1990;322:1627.

32. Travell JG, Simons DG. Myofascial pain and dysfunction: the trigger point manual. Baltimore: Williams & Wilkins, 1983.

33. Fricton JR. Myofascial pain syndrome: characteristics and epidemiology. In: Fricton JR, Awad E, eds. Advances in pain research and therapy, Vol 17. New York: Raven Press, 1990.

34. Fricton JR. Management of myofascial pain syndrome. In Fricton JR, Awad E, eds. Advances in pain research and therapy, Vol 17. New York: Raven Press, 1990.

35. Shekelle PG, Adams AH, Chassin MR, Hurwitz EL, Brook RH. Spinal manipulation for low back pain. Ann Intern Med 1992;117:590.

36. Cherkin DC, MacCornack FA. Patient evaluations of low back pain care from family physicians and chiropractors. West J Med 1989;150: 351.

37. Haas M, Nyiendo J, Peterson C, et al. Interrater reliability of roentgenological evaluation of the lumbar spine in lateral bending. J Manip Physiol Therap 1990;13:179.

38. Eisenberg DM, Kessler RC, Foster C, Norlock FE, Calkins DR, Delbanco TL. Unconventional medicine in the United States: prevalence, costs, and patterns of use. N Engl J Med 1993;328: 246.

39. Weber H, Holme I, Amlie E. The natural course of acute sciatica with nerve root symptoms in a double blind placebo controlled trial evaluating the effect of piroxicam. Spine 1993;18:1433.

40. Donelson RG, McKenzie R. Mechanical assessment and treatment of spinal pain. In: Frymoyer JW, ed. The adult spine: principles and practice. New York: Raven Press, 1991:1627.

41. Benzon H. Epidural steroid injections for low back pain and lumbrosacral radiculopathy. Pain 1986;24:277.

42. Ridley MG, Kingsley GH, Gibson T, Grahame R. Outpatient lumbar epidural steroid injections for low back pain and lumbrosacral radiculopathy. Pain 1986;24:277.

43. Dilke TFW, Burry HC, Grahame R. Extradural corticosteroid injection in management of lumbar nerve root compression. Br Med J 1973;2: 635–7.

44. Benzon H. Epidural steroids. In: Raj PP, ed. Practical management of pain. 2nd ed. St. Louis: Mosby–Year Book, 1992.

45. Violinn E, Mayer J, Diehr P, et al. Small area analysis of surgery for low-back pain. Spine 1992;17:575.

46. Weber H. Lumbar disc herniation: a controlled prospective study with ten years of observation. Spine 1983;8:131.

47. Hoffman RM, Wheeler KJ, Deyo RA. Surgery for herniated lumbar discs: a literature synthesis. J Gen Intern Med 1993;8:487.

48. Spengler DM, Oullette EA, Battie M, Zeh J. Elective discectomy for herniation of a lumbar disc: additional experience with an objective method. J Bone Joint Surg 1990;72A:230.

49. Herron LD, Turner J. Patient selection for lumbar laminectomy and discectomy with a revised

objective rating system. Clin Orthop 1985;199: 145.

50. Williams RW. Microlumbar discectomy: a 12 year statistical review. Spine 1986;11:851.

51. Schaffer JL, Kambin P. Percutaneous posterolateral lumbar discectomy and decompression with a 6.9 millimeter cannula: analysis of operative failures and complications. J Bone Joint Surg 1991;73A:822.

52. Ejeskar A, Nachemson A, Herberts P, et al. Surgery versus chemonucleolysis for herniated lumbar disks: a prospective study with random assignment. Clin Orthop 1983;174:236.

53. Crashaw C, Frazer AM, Merriam WF, Mulholland RC, Webb JK. A comparison of surgery and chemonucleolysis in the treatment of sciatica: a prospective randomized trial. Spine 1984; 9:195.

54. Herkowitz HN, Kurz LT. Degenerative lumbar spondylolisthesis with spinal stenosis: a prospective study comparing decompression with decompression and intertransverse process arthrodesis. J Bone Joint Surg 1991;73A:802.

55. Deyo RA, Cherkin DC, Loeser JD, Bigos SJ, Ciol MA. Morbidity and mortality in association with operations on the lumbar spine. J Bone Joint Surg 1992;74A:536.

56. Turner JA, Ersek M, Herron L, Deyo R. Surgery for lumbar spinal stenosis: attempted meta-analysis of the literature. Spine 1992;17:1.

57. Katz JN, Lipson SJ, Larson MG, McInnes JM, Fossel AH, Liang MH. The outcome of decompressive laminectomy for degenerative lumbar spinal stenosis. J Bone Joint Surg 1991;73A:809.

58. Katz JN, Lipson SJ, Brick GW, et al. Clinical correlates of patient satisfaction with laminectomy for lumbar spinal stenosis. Spine 1994;[in press].

59. Ng LKY, ed. New approaches to treatment of chronic pain: a review of multidisciplinary pain clinics and pain centers. Rockville, Maryland: NIDA Research Monograph 36, 1981.

60. Aronoff FM, Evans WO, Enders PL. A review of follow-up studies of multidisciplinary pain units. Pain 1983;16:1.

61. Mayer TG, Gatchel RJ, Mayer H, Kishino ND, Keeley J, Moorly V. A prospective two-year study of functional restoration in industrial low back injury: an objective assessment procedure. JAMA 1987;258:1763.

62. Seres JL, et al. Evaluation and management of chronic pain by nonsurgical means. In: Fletcher LJ, ed. Pain management: symposium on the neurosurgical treatment of pain. Baltimore: Williams & Wilkins, 1977.

63. Porter J, Jick H. Addiction rare in patients treated with narcotics. N Engl J Med 1980; 302:123.

64. Mooney V, Robertson J. The facet syndrome. Clin Orthop 1976;115:149.

65. Destonet JM, Gilula LA, Murphy WA, et al. Lumbar facet joint injection: indication, technique, clinical correlation and preliminary results. Radiology 1982;145:321.

66. Carrette S, Marcour S, Truchon R, et al. A controlled trial of corticosteroid injections into facet joints for chronic low back pain. N Engl J Med 1991;325:1002.

67. Bogduk N. Back pain: zygapophyseal blocks and epidural steroids. In: Cousins MJ, Bridenbaugh PO, eds. Neural blockade in clinical anesthesia and management of pain. 2nd ed. Philadelphia: JB Lippincott, 1988:935.

68. North RB, Kidd DH, Zahurak M, James CS, Long DM. Spinal cord stimulation for chronic, intractable pain: experience over two decades. Neurosurgery 1993;32:384.

69. North RB, Ewend MG, Lawton MT, Kidd DH, Piantadosi S. Failed back surgery syndrome: 5 year follow-up after spinal cord stimulator implantation. Neurosurgery 1991;28:692.

70. De La Porte C, Siegfried J. Lumbosacral spinal fibrosis (spinal arachnoiditis): its diagnosis and treatment by spinal cord stimulation. Spine 1983;8:593.

71. Coombs DW, Maurer LH, Saunders RL, Gaylor M. Outcomes and complications of continuous intraspinal narcotic analgesia for cancer pain control. J Clin Oncol 1984;2:1414.

72. Magora F, Olshwang D, Eimerl D, et al. Observations on extradural morphine analgesia in various pain conditions. Br J Anaesth 1980;52: 247.

73. Waldman SP, Coombs DW. Selection of implantable narcotic delivery systems. Anesth Analg 1989;68:377.

2

FIBROMYALGIA SYNDROME

Robert W. Simms

Fibromyalgia syndrome is an increasingly recognized chronic musculoskeletal pain disorder of unknown etiology.[1] The American College of Rheumatology (ACR) has published the results of a large multicenter study to identify diagnostic criteria for the syndrome, which were shown to have high sensitivity and specificity.[2] A recently conducted community-based prevalence study estimated that approximately 2% of the adult population meets ACR criteria for the syndrome.[3] This may indicate that fibromyalgia syndrome is twice as common as rheumatoid arthritis. Fibromyalgia syndrome is predominantly a disorder of young and middle-aged women and is the second or third most common diagnosis in rheumatology practices.[1,4] The clinical presentation of fibromyalgia syndrome is generally that of chronic, diffuse musculoskeletal pain, typically accompanied by fatigue and sleep disturbance, with findings of multiple locations of tenderness, predominantly over muscle-insertion sites.[1]

Investigators have studied a variety of pathophysiologic mechanisms, including sleep disturbance, psychological dysfunction, and muscle abnormalities, although no clear understanding of etiology has yet emerged.[1] Recently much attention has focused on central mechanisms and especially on neurohormonal function. Griep et al.[5] have demonstrated that patients with fibromyalgia have enhanced pituitary adrenocorticotropic hormone (ACTH) release in response to ovine corticotropin-releasing hormone (CRH) and to insulin-induced hypoglycemia, although adrenocortical secretion after these neuroendocrine challenge tests did not differ from that in control subjects. The authors suggested that

these findings indicated adrenocortical insufficiency in patients with fibromyalgia. Crofford et al.[6] have also found evidence of low basal hypothalamic-pituitary-adrenal (HPA) function as measured by 24-hour urinary free cortisol, findings that are similar to those found in patients with chronic fatigue syndrome.[7] Thus, although patients with both fibromyalgia and chronic fatigue syndrome appear to have significantly lower basal measures of adrenal cortisol output, precise localization of the defect in the HPA axis remains uncertain. Furthermore, it is uncertain whether the observed findings with respect to the HPA axis are primary to fibromyalgia syndrome or are a function of having the disorder.

Other studies of neurohormonal function include the observation by Bennett et al.,[8] who found low serum levels of the growth hormone analog, somatomedin C, in fibromyalgia patients when compared to controls. Bennett et al.[8] suggested that reduced growth hormone secretion during disturbed Stage 4 sleep could explain the muscle pain that characterizes the disorder, since growth hormone is involved in muscle homeostasis. Russell et al.[9] recently found low cerebrospinal fluid levels of biogenic amines in patients with fibromyalgia as compared with controls, a finding that appeared consistent with earlier studies suggesting a deficiency of serotonin metabolism.[1]

The natural history of fibromyalgia syndrome has received relatively little attention. The only available studies are those that have evaluated patients receiving some form of treatment, and no studies have evaluated patients without therapy. Hawley et al.[10] found

TABLE 2–1
Placebo-Controlled Therapeutic Trials of Medication in Fibromyalgia Syndrome

MEDICATION	REFERENCE	TRIAL DURATION (wk)	DOSE (mg/day)	BETTER THAN PLACEBO?
Amitriptyline	21	9	50	Yes
Amitriptyline	22	6	25	Yes
Amitriptyline	23	2	10	Yes
Amitriptyline	27	24	30	No
Cyclobenzaprine	25	12	30	Yes
Cyclobenzaprine	26	4	30	Yes
Cyclobenzaprine	13	6	30	Yes
Alprazolam	29	6	0.5–3	No
Temazepam	30	12	15–30	Yes
Prednisone	31	2	15	No
Naproxen	22	6	1000	No
Ibuprofen	32	3	2400	No
S-Adenosylmethionine	34	3	200	Yes
Carisprodol	33	8	1200	Yes
Fluoxetine	28	6	20	No

that most patients at 1 year of follow-up had persistent pain symptoms. Felson and Goldenberg[11] conducted a telephone survey of patients who had been enrolled 3 years earlier in a clinical trial of amitriptyline. Sixty percent of the patients experienced continuing severe symptoms at follow-up. Nørregaard et al.[12] conducted a follow-up evaluation of 91 patients with fibromyalgia a median of 4 years after diagnosis. Seventy-three percent reported worsened pain, 16% reported no change, and 9% reported improvement.

Because of the lack of understanding of the basis for fibromyalgia, therapy remains empiric. Available treatments range from conventional medication therapy with tricyclic antidepressants to nonconventional interventions such as biofeedback and electroacupuncture. A substantial number of placebo-controlled trials have demonstrated that many available therapies are effective (Table 2–1). There remain, however, few long-term trials, few trials of comparative therapies, and few trials that have assessed the same outcomes and have employed the same definitions of response to therapy.[13] In this chapter we shall review published controlled and uncontrolled trials of therapy in fibromyalgia syndrome and attempt to identify avenues of future research.

CONTROLLED TRIALS OF MEDICATION THERAPY

Psychotropic Agents

Moldofsky et al.[14] first identified a sleep electroencephalographic (EEG) abnormality termed alpha/delta sleep in patients with fibromyalgia syndrome. This abnormality consisted of intrusion of the normal awake EEG pattern (alpha waves) into the deepest non–rapid eye movement (REM) sleep EEG pattern (delta waves). Moldofsky and Scarisbrick[15] were further able to show that experimentally reproducing alpha/delta sleep in normal subjects resulted in the appearance of musculoskeletal and mood symptoms identical to those of fibromyalgia syndrome. Moldofsky and Scarisbrick[15] hypothesized that fibromyalgia symptoms were the result of this disordered delta sleep and that serotonin, a neurochemical involved in modulation of both sleep and pain, may be deficient in patients with the syndrome. Moldofsky and Lue[16] then performed a clinical trial involving 15 patients with fibromyalgia syndrome who were randomized to receive 5 g of L-tryptophan or 100 mg of chlorpromazine in a 3-week, double-blinded study, with sleep EEGs performed before and after medication. L-tryptophan had no effect on the alpha/delta sleep abnormality or on the patients' symptoms. Chlorpromazine resulted in an increase in delta sleep and an improvement in patient pain rating and tender point scores, although chlorpromazine has since been judged to be too sedating.

Tricyclic Agents and Other Antidepressants

As inhibitors of serotonin reuptake, tricyclic antidepressants were of interest on the basis of Moldofsky's serotonin deficiency hypothesis.[15] At low doses, several tricyclic agents also have both hypnotic properties, causing REM suppression and prolongation of stages 3 and 4 non-REM sleep.[17] Tertiary amine tricyclics, such as amitriptyline, imipramine, and doxepin, inhibit neuronal uptake of serotonin more than the secondary amine demethylated metabolites, such as desipramine and nortriptyline.[17] Initial uncontrolled reports suggested that amitriptyline was useful in the management of fibromyalgia syndrome.[18–20]

Carrette et al.[21] performed a 9-week double-blind, placebo-controlled trial in 70 patients. Patients were recruited from three centers and met the criteria proposed by Smythe.[19] Patients assigned to the treatment arm received amitriptyline, 10 mg nightly for the first week, 25 mg for the second to the fourth week, and 50 mg for the final 5 weeks of the trial. Evaluations of efficacy at baseline and at weeks 5 and 9 included duration of morning stiffness, overall pain, sleep quality, and overall disease assessment. Patients who received amitriptyline had significant improvement in their morning stiffness and pain analog scores at 5 and 9 weeks as compared with baseline scores, although the placebo group had no changes in these measures. Forty-four percent of the amitriptyline-treated patients had ≥50% improvement in morning stiffness or pain analog, whereas 22% of the placebo patients had ≥50% improvement in these two parameters (p = NS). No change was seen in the end-of-trial myalgic scores (defined as the sum of individual tender point scores with a dolorimeter).

Goldenberg et al.[22] randomized 62 patients to receive one of four regimens in a 6-week double-blind trial: (1) 25 mg of amitriptyline at bedtime and 500 mg of naproxen twice daily, (2) amitriptyline alone with naproxen placebo, (3) naproxen alone with amitriptyline placebo, or (4) double placebo. Amitriptyline was used at doses that were believed to be low enough to have no significant effect on depression. At study entry, patients were required to have a score of at least 4 on either the initial pain or global assessment analog scale. Amitriptyline-containing regimens resulted in significant improvements in mean scores of pain, sleep, patient global assessment, and tender point score. There was no association with initial sleep difficulty or preexisting psychopathology in response to amitriptyline. Marginal additional benefit of naproxen was seen. Not determined, however, was the proportion of patients who experienced substantial improvement in one or more outcomes because of the relatively small numbers of patients in each arm of the study. Dry mouth was the principal adverse side effect attributable to amitriptyline but did not cause discontinuation in any patient. Interestingly, although the principal therapeutic effect of amitriptyline was thought to be improvement of sleep physiology, there was no association with initial sleep difficulty and response, suggesting a different mechanism of action, possibly via effects on serotonin or endogenous opioids, such as endorphins or enkephalins.

Jaeschke et al.[23] conducted 23 N-of-1 randomized controlled trials (RCTs) of amitriptyline in patients who had shown initial improvement with an open trial of amitriptyline. The N-of-1 design consists of pairs of active/placebo, high or low dose, and first drug/additive combination with the order of administration determined by random allocation. Assessments are performed in a double-blind fashion with trial duration determined by both physician and patient. Most of the treatment periods were 2 weeks in duration, with outcome assessment every 2 weeks. The mean difference in multiple symptoms favored amitriptyline over placebo in 18 versus 5 trials. Jaeschke et al. noted rapid improvement with amitriptyline, generally occurring within 1 week—a phenomenon also noted by Goldenberg et al.[22] Jaeschke et al. concluded that it is not necessary to give the standard dose of 25 to 50 mg to obtain significant improvement. Smaller doses, such as 10 mg at bedtime, may be effective in some patients and avoid the anticholinergic side effects of amitriptyline. Of 23 N-of-1 RCTs, 15 resulted in a decision to continue the drug on a long-term basis. The authors of this study concluded that, overall, 25% of patients with fibromyalgia syndrome derived clinically significant benefit from amitriptyline. In eight cases, the N-of-1 RCT was followed by a decision to stop the drug; therefore these patients were spared long-term or even lifelong therapy, even though the initial open trial suggested improvement with amitriptyline. These data indicate the importance of the N-of-1 RCT format in decisions about long-term continuation of therapy in individual patients.

Of the parallel RCTs and the N-of-1 trials published thus far, only a small proportion of patients with fibromyalgia actually appear to achieve clinically significant improvement—on the order of 25% to 30%. Uniformity in defining those patients who undergo significant clinical improvement would provide investigators conducting clinical trials in fibromyalgia with the tools to identify subsets of patients who improve substantially and eventually with predictors of response to therapy. Along these lines, Simms et al.[13] developed a set of preliminary response criteria for use in fibromyalgia clinical trials; they used data from the original Goldenberg trial[22] and determined which combination of outcome measures best distinguished patients treated with amitriptyline from those treated with placebo, using a stepwise logistic regression analysis and receiver-operating characteristic (ROC) curves. An ROC curve is a graphic depiction of the pairing of true-positive and false-positive rates that correspond to each possible cutoff for either diagnostic tests or criteria. The optimal ROC curve comparing different diagnostic tests or response criteria is that which maximizes the area under the curve. The combination of outcome measures with the greatest area under the ROC curve (i.e., that with the highest specificity and sensitivity in distinguishing treated from placebo patients) consisted of the following: (1) physician global assessment score ≤4 (0 = extremely well, 10 = extremely poorly), (2) patient sleep score ≤6 (0 = sleeping extremely well, 10 = sleeping extremely poorly), and (3) tender point score ≤14 (maximum possible tender point score = 20). Using these criteria, Simms et al.[13] analyzed a randomized, double-blind, crossover trial of cyclobenzaprine versus placebo in 24 patients conducted

by the same investigators with identical entry criteria and outcome assessment. Sensitivity was defined as the number of patients identified by the criteria as responders divided by the number of patients who received cyclobenzaprine. Specificity was defined as the number of patients not identified by criteria divided by the number who received placebo. The criteria identified 7 of 24 treated patients (sensitivity of 30%), whereas 23 of 24 untreated patients were not identified by the criteria, for a specificity of 96%. In the amitriptyline trial, 44% of the amitriptyline-treated patients were identified as responders. To determine the criterion validity of the response criteria, the investigators compared the performance of the criteria in the cyclobenzaprine trial with a composite outcome measure that consisted of a summation of change in visual analog scores of patient global assessment, patient pain assessment, physician global assessment, and tender point score. In this comparison the criteria identified 11 of 14 patients in the amitriptyline trial and 4 of 6 patients in the cyclobenzaprine trial who had high composite outcome scores, indicating that the criteria had reasonably high criterion validity. Three points can be made from this preliminary attempt to define acceptable response criteria: (1) a small percentage of patients in both analyzed trials met the criteria (44% for amitriptyline-treated patients and 30% for cyclobenzaprine-treated patients), (2) only conventional outcomes were assessed and no psychological or functional outcomes were determined, (3) interestingly, pain, a cardinal feature of fibromyalgia and a criterion of the ACR diagnostic criteria, did not discriminate as well as other outcome measures.

Cyclobenzaprine is a tricyclic agent similar in chemical structure to amitriptyline, which has been marketed as a muscle relaxant on the basis of its ability to reduce brain stem noradrenergic function and motor neuron efferent activity.[24] Several trials have used this agent in fibromyalgia syndrome. Bennett et al.[25] conducted a 12-week, double-blind, randomized, controlled trial of 120 patients. Modest efficacy was demonstrated in that patients' assessment of sleep and pain improved significantly ($p < 0.02$) in the cyclobenzaprine group compared with the placebo group from weeks 2 to 12. Fatigue improved at weeks 2 to 4 ($p < 0.02$)

but not for weeks 8 to 12. Physician assessment of global pain did not differ between the two treatment groups. Twenty-one of 61 cyclobenzaprine-treated patients and 9 of 57 placebo-treated patients had a moderate or marked overall physician-rated response. Of note, in this trial 60% of the placebo-treated patients and 35% of the cyclobenzaprine-treated patients withdrew from the study, with adverse reactions accounting for 8% in the cyclobenzaprine-treated patients and 5% in the placebo-treated patients.

Reynolds et al.[26] evaluated the effect of cyclobenzaprine on sleep physiology in 12 patients who participated in a crossover study of 4 weeks' duration. Patients were treated with 30 mg/day of cyclobenzaprine. With the exception of a decrease in afternoon sleepiness and an increase in total sleep time, no effect of cyclobenzaprine was seen on other clinical or sleep parameters. This study, however, was probably too short in duration and of inadequate power for any definite conclusions to be drawn.

Carrette et al.[27] have conducted the only long-term comparative trial of amitriptyline, cyclobenzaprine, and placebo to date in the treatment of fibromyalgia syndrome. Two hundred eight patients fulfilling the 1990 ACR criteria for the diagnosis of fibromyalgia syndrome were entered into a 6-month double-blind, multicenter trial. Patients assigned to amitriptyline received 10 mg daily at bedtime for the first week, 25 mg for the second through the twelfth week, and 50 mg at bedtime for the last 12 weeks of the trial. Cyclobenzaprine-treated patients received escalating doses beginning at 10 mg at bedtime for the first week, 20 mg at bedtime for the second through the twelfth week, and 10 mg in the morning with 20 mg at bedtime for the last 12 weeks of the trial. A variety of patient-derived assessments were performed throughout the trial and included visual analog scales evaluating pain, sleep, morning stiffness, global fibromyalgia symptoms, the McGill Pain Questionnaire, the Sickness Impact Profile, and the Health Assessment Questionnaire (HAQ). Psychological status was also assessed by the anxiety and depression scales of the Arthritis Impact Measurement Scales (AIMS) and the Minnesota Multiphasic Personality Inventory (MMPI). Physician assessments included dolorimeter scores at tender point locations. According to

the criteria of Simms et al.[13] for improvement, 21% of amitriptyline-treated patients and 12% of cyclobenzaprine-treated patients were significantly different than the placebo-treated patients at 1 month. At 3 months and at 6 months, however, the proportion of responders was not different among the three groups (19% of the placebo group were classified as responders). Only physician global assessment of treated patients was superior to that of the placebo group at 6 months. Of note, 95% of amitriptyline-treated and 98% of cyclobenzaprine-treated patients experienced side effects compared with 62% of placebo-treated patients, although only 13% of cyclobenzaprine-treated and 6% of amitriptyline-treated patients withdrew because of side effects. A normal MMPI was the strongest predictor of response to active drug treatment at 1 month.

In summary, as the best studied of the tricyclic agents, both amitriptyline and cyclobenzaprine appear to be effective in the short-term therapy of fibromyalgia syndrome. The overall or mean degree of efficacy is modest, although a subset of patients may have marked improvement on multiple outcome measures. Unfortunately, there are currently no reliable ways to identify responders to these or other tricyclic agents in advance. Although side effects attributable to these agents in both short-term and longer-term trials are relatively mild (principally dry mouth and excessive drowsiness) and resolve relatively quickly, maintenance of long-term efficacy compared to placebo remains to be demonstrated.

Other Antidepressants

Fluoxetine, a selective serotonin reuptake inhibitor, which is a potent antidepressant agent, has been recently studied in fibromyalgia syndrome.[28] Forty-two women with fibromyalgia syndrome were randomized to receive either fluoxetine at 20 mg daily or a placebo for 6 weeks. At 6 weeks, both AIMS depression scales and Beck depression scores, and sleep quality showed significant improvement in the fluoxetine-treated patients compared with those receiving placebo, although no other studied variables showed improvement.[27] Wolfe et al.[28] concluded that fluoxetine was not an effective agent in the treatment of fibromyalgia syndrome. Unfortunately, 57% of those receiving placebo dropped out of the study before the week 6 assessment (compared with 29% of fluoxetine-treated patients). It is therefore likely that this study had insufficient power to conclude that fluoxetine is an ineffective agent in the therapy of fibromyalgia syndrome, and further study of this and related compounds such as paroxetine are indicated.

Benzodiazepines

Alprazolam is a triazolobenzodiazepine approved for the treatment of anxiety and depression associated with anxiety.[17] Because its antidepressant and antianxiety effects are comparable to those of tricyclic agents, and because alprazolam may be better tolerated, several clinical trials have assessed its efficacy in fibromyalgia syndrome. Russell et al.[29] randomized 78 patients into four groups: alprazolam with or without ibuprofen, ibuprofen alone, and placebo for 6 weeks followed by 24-week open label extension for 63 patients. Dolorimeter score, tender point index, patient assessment of pain, physician global assessment, HAQ score, and assessments of depression were determined at weekly intervals during the 6-week trial. All treatment groups improved at week 6 compared with baseline. There was no significant difference in the mean change in outcome variables between the double-placebo group and the other three treatment groups at the end of the 6-week trial, although lower patient rating of disease severity and lower severity of tenderness on palpation were found in the patients who were receiving the combination of alprazolam and ibuprofen. Power calculations indicated that there was inadequate power in this study to detect improvement of at least 25% in one of the three active treatment arms. Both patient rating of pain and tenderness scores quickly worsened during a brief 2-week cessation of therapy. Among the 52 patients who completed the open label portion (all patients receiving the combination of ibuprofen and alprazolam) of the study, which was 8 weeks in duration, small but statistically significant levels of improvement were seen in several outcomes. With clinically relevant improvement defined as greater than or equal to 30% at baseline, 7 of 16 patients in the drug-coded trial combination group showed improvement compared with only 4 of 14 in the

double-placebo group. With respect to pain assessment, 6 of 15 patients in the combination group compared with only 3 of those in the double-placebo group obtained clinically relevant improvement, suggesting a benefit of the combination over the placebo, at least in a subset of patients. This trial thus illustrates the value of using response criteria to identify a subset of patients who improve, even though mean overall levels of improvement may not differ between treatment and placebo groups.

Hench et al.[30] compared the therapeutic effects of amitriptyline, temazepam, and placebo on clinical and sleep parameters in a double-blind, placebo crossover study of 10 patients for 12 weeks. Temazepam produced significant improvement in physician and patient global assessment, sleep disturbance, and morning stiffness, although paradoxically it appeared to decrease sleep duration and increase sleep latency (the time interval between going to bed and falling asleep). Amitriptyline, by contrast, produced significant improvement only in the number and severity of tender points.

Long-term use of benzodiazepines has been tempered by concern over dependence and possible withdrawal reactions, especially seizures.[17] In the Russell trial[29] there were few side effect–related dropouts attributable to alprazolam, and no information on side effects was reported in the Hench[30] trial, although it is unlikely that either trial was of sufficient duration to assess the issues of dependence and problems due to withdrawal. Alprazolam should therefore be considered as an only modestly effective agent that should probably be reserved for short-term use only in the treatment of fibromyalgia syndrome.

Antiinflammatory Agents

Both corticosteroids and nonsteroidal antiinflammatory agents have been studied in the treatment of fibromyalgia syndrome. Systemic corticosteroid therapy was evaluated by Clark et al.[31] in a 2-week double-blind, placebo-controlled crossover trial involving 20 patients. Patients were assigned to treatment with either 15 mg of prednisone per day or placebo. Mean changes in analog scores of pain, sleep, fatigue, and dolorimeter score showed no difference between the prednisone and placebo treatment periods. Several patients who had mild elevation of serum creatine phosphokinase also had no significant or consistent improvement in symptom scores during treatment with prednisone.

The apparent lack of improvement in fibromyalgia with the use of systemic corticosteroid therapy is of particular interest in light of recent studies of chronic fatigue syndrome (a condition with many clinical features similar to fibromyalgia syndrome) and fibromyalgia syndrome, which have suggested mild perturbations of the HPA axis. Demitrack et al.[7] performed a series of assessments of the HPA axis in 30 patients with chronic fatigue syndrome, including measurement of 24 urinary free cortisol, ACTH and cortisol responses to CRH, and net integrated cortisol response to ACTH. They found reduced pituitary and adrenal responses to CRH and slightly reduced plasma cortisol concentrations, as well as low 24-hour urinary free cortisol. Demitrack et al.[7] argued that the demonstrated mild glucocorticoid deficiency seen in these patients with chronic fatigue syndrome was most likely the result of a mild central adrenal insufficiency possibly secondary to mild deficiency of CRH. As noted above, Griep et al.[5] have demonstrated that patients with fibromyalgia have enhanced pituitary ACTH release in response to ovine CRH and to insulin-induced hypoglycemia, and Crofford et al.[6] have found that basal HPA function as measured by 24-hour urinary free cortisol was low when compared with that of normal subjects.

If patients with chronic fatigue syndrome/fibromyalgia syndrome have either mild central or adrenal insufficiency, as is suggested by these studies, then one would expect symptomatic improvement with the use of corticosteroids. The results of the Clark et al. study[31] are therefore at odds with these recent findings with respect to the HPA axis and are difficult to reconcile. It may be that the Clark et al. study[31] was too short in duration and involved too few patients for definite conclusions to be drawn regarding the efficacy of corticosteroids in these conditions; alternatively, additional studies of the HPA axis in fibromyalgia syndrome may fail to confirm these preliminary findings.

In the earlier trial by Goldenberg et al.[22] of amitriptyline, naproxen, and placebo, naproxen alone (1000 mg per day) was no more effective than placebo, although the combination of amitriptyline and placebo was slightly more effective than amitriptyline alone. Possible synergism of nonsteroidal antiinflammatory drugs (NSAIDs) and other "central nervous system (CNS)–active" medication was seen in Russell's[29] trial of alprazolam and ibuprofen, where there was a trend toward greater improvement in patients treated with the combination than in those treated with either agent alone.

Yunus et al.[32] studied the efficacy of ibuprofen in 46 patients with fibromyalgia syndrome in a double-blind, placebo-controlled trial of 3 weeks' duration. Patients receiving a psychotropic drug at a stable dose were allowed to remain on the drug for the duration of the study. At the end of the trial, there were no significant differences in any of the four measured variables (pain, fatigue, sleep difficulty, or total tender points). Both treatment and placebo groups experienced significant improvement compared with baseline in both fatigue and number of tender points, reinforcing the concept that placebo effects of up to 50% improvement in some variables may occur in short-term trials in fibromyalgia syndrome.

In summary, antiinflammatory agents appear to have little, if any, efficacy alone in the treatment of fibromyalgia syndrome. When combined with other "CNS-active" agents, NSAIDs may confer slight synergistic analgesic benefit, although it could be argued that the marginal additional benefit of NSAIDs (particularly when used in the long term), given their potential toxicity, is not cost-effective. Understandably, corticosteroids have received little attention in fibromyalgia syndrome, given the lack of evidence that there is an inflammatory basis for the disorder and on the basis of the controlled short term trial by Clark et al.[30] Recent data suggesting that there is hypofunction of the HPA axis, at least in some patients with fibromyalgia syndrome, may necessitate a reevaluation of corticosteroids in the disorder, although at this time there remains no indication for the routine use of corticosteroids in clinical practice.

Other CNS-Active Medications

Soma, a combination of carisprodol (1200 mg), acetaminophen, and caffeine, has also been studied in fibromyalgia syndrome and was shown to be more effective than placebo in an 8-week trial of 58 patients.[33] Improved outcome measures in the treatment group included pain, sleep quality, and general feeling of sickness. Also, pressure pain threshold increased in the treatment group but not in the placebo group, despite the fact that 43% of the patients in the placebo group but none in the active treatment group used either tricyclic antidepressants, anxiolytics, or sedatives.

S-adenosylmethionine (SAMe), an antidepressant, was studied in a short-term (3-week) placebo-controlled trial involving 25 patients with fibromyalgia syndrome.[34] Depression as assessed by the Hamilton Depression Rating Scale improved, and decreased trigger point scores were seen after SAMe administration but not after placebo. This agent has not gained acceptance, however, because it requires intramuscular administration and the investigators noted abscesses at injection sites, although the precise number was not detailed.[34]

EXERCISE THERAPY

In light of the observation by Moldofsky and Scarisbrick[15] that interference with stage IV sleep in trained athletes did not lead to an overnight increase in musculoskeletal symptoms, McCain et al.[35] performed a 20-week trial comparing the efficacy of cardiovascular fitness training (CVR) with simple flexibility and stretching (FLEX) in 42 patients with fibromyalgia syndrome (Table 2–2). The CVR program consisted of supervised aerobic fitness training for 20 minutes three times weekly and was designed to result in an increase in heart rate to 75% of the predicted maximum. The FLEX program consisted of a supervised stretching and flexibility program. At the end of the study, patients assigned to CVR exhibited increased cardiovascular fitness as determined by an aerobic fitness test, and there were significant improvements in both patient and physician global assessments and tender point pain thresholds. Also, a greater proportion of the CVR patients experienced moderate or marked improvement compared to the FLEX group, although patients assigned to the CVR group had higher pain scores at study entry and therefore may have had a greater tendency to "regress to the mean" or improve spontaneously. Despite this favorable effect of CVR, patients did experience immediate postexertional worsening of symptoms and few patients continued with long-term aerobic fitness at the conclusion of the trial. This observation tends to mirror the clinical experience with aerobic fitness programs: relatively few patients are able to comply with a long-term aerobic activity, and many patients are not able to participate at all because of immediate postexertion exacerbation of symptoms. Nevertheless, among patients who are able to participate in long-term aerobic activity, many are able to successfully wean off other medication and are able to avoid the vicious cycle of worsening pain and muscle deconditioning, which unfortunately may occur in patients with more severe symptoms.

Mengshoel and Førre[36] performed a clinical trial of low-intensity endurance training in 25 patients with fibromyalgia syndrome. Eleven patients were randomized to a modified low-impact aerobic dance program twice weekly for 20 weeks. Each session lasted 60 minutes, although the training intensity was kept at a heart rate level not exceeding 150 beats per minute. Fourteen patients randomized to the control group did not change their level of physical activity. At the end of 20 weeks there was no change in the level of pain (as assessed by the McGill Pain Questionnaire) or fatigue

---

TABLE 2–2
Non-Medication-Controlled Therapeutic Trials in Fibromyalgia Syndrome

INTERVENTION	COMPARISON INTERVENTION	REFERENCE	DURATION (wk)	INTERVENTION EFFICACY
Cardiovascular fitness training	Flexibility and stretching	35	20	Yes
EMG-biofeedback	Sham	37	24	Yes
Electroacupuncture	Sham	44	3	Yes
Hypnotherapy	Physical therapy	45	12	Yes

(as assessed by visual analog scales) in the training group from the beginning to the end of the training period; nor was there any detectable difference between the training and control groups with respect to either the pain or the fatigue variables. The small sample sizes, the uncertain level of baseline fitness in either experimental or control group (both groups may have had relatively high levels of physical fitness and therefore one would not expect the experimental group to improve significantly), and the lack of measurement of other outcomes such as sleep or overall symptom severity make it difficult to conclude that low-level physical activity is ineffective. In clinical practice, many patients experience significant benefit from low-level aerobic fitness, which can be accomplished with such simple activities as a regular walking program.

LONG-TERM EXPERIENCE

As indicated above, only one trial has been reported with significant long-term experience.[27] In this comparative placebo-controlled trial of amitriptyline and cyclobenzaprine of 6 months' duration, no difference in the proportion of responders between the two active treatments and placebo was noted at the conclusion of the trial.[27]

CONTROLLED TRIALS OF NONCONVENTIONAL THERAPY

Electromyography-Biofeedback

Electromyography (EMG)-biofeedback has been shown to be of benefit in psychosomatic disorders, such as functional diarrhea and tension headache. With this procedure, patients receive auditory feedback of ongoing muscle tension in scalp muscles determined with the use of surface electrodes placed on the forehead. Typically, the feedback is presented in the form of pulse sounds that are proportional to the level of scalp muscle tension and patients then attempt to control their muscle tension to obtain relief. Under the presumption that fibromyalgia may have a psychosomatic basis, Ferraccioli et al.[37] performed a controlled study of biofeedback in 12 patients, following an open study in 15 patients in which they reported a 50% clinical improvement in nine pa-

tients at 6 months (Table 2–2). Biofeedback therapy was conducted in 20-minute sessions twice weekly for a total of 15 sessions. In the controlled trial, patients who received biofeedback demonstrated improvement in all outcome variables which was apparently sustained for 6 months, although patients who received sham biofeedback (they were disconnected from the recording of muscle tension and therefore had no acoustic signal to determine progressive relaxation) experienced improvement only in tender point counts. Using the MMPI, Ferraccioli et al. surprisingly found no correlation between depression or "an overt psychosomatic background" and response to EMG-biofeedback. As Wolfe[38] has pointed out, the blinding status of patients in this study is uncertain and the psychiatric instrument may have been inappropriate. Therefore the role of biofeedback in fibromyalgia syndrome remains uncertain, and additional studies are required.

Acupuncture/Electroacupuncture

Despite its apparent popularity, the role of acupuncture, particularly in the therapy of chronic pain, remains controversial. Two recent meta-analyses reached opposite conclusions regarding the efficacy of acupuncture in the therapy of chronic pain. Patel et al.[39] pooled the results of 14 randomized trials and concluded that "while few individual trials had statistically significant results, pooled results of many subgroups attained statistical significance in favour of acupuncture." ter Riet et al.[40] performed a criteria-based meta-analysis of 51 controlled studies, which emphasized an assessment of study design and assigned a possible maximum of 100 points based on four main categories: (1) comparability of prognosis, (2) adequate intervention, (3) adequate effect measurement, and (4) data presentation. No study in their analysis earned more than 62% of the maximum score. The results of the better studies (>50% of the maximum score) were contradictory, and a separate subgroup analysis of studies employing sham procedures showed a comparable number of positive and negative results.[40] The authors concluded that "the efficacy of acupuncture in the treatment of chronic pain remains doubtful."[40]

Considerable research has been conducted into the possible mechanism of acupuncture.

Most recent data appear to favor a neurohumoral explanation with activation of endogenous pain control mechanisms such as via the opioid or serotoninergic pathways.[41,42] Acupuncture may work by activation of these endogenous pain-modulating systems through the noxious stimulation of heterotopic body areas at the segmental level or via the systemic release of peptides by the adrenals.[43] Electroacupuncture or application of an electric current at the site of application of the acupuncture needle has physiologic effects similar to those of traditional acupuncture.

Deluze et al.[44] have recently reported the only randomized clinical trial of electroacupuncture in the treatment of fibromyalgia (Table 2–2). In this study, 36 patients were randomized to electroacupuncture and 34 to a sham procedure for 3 weeks. Treatment consisted of six sessions of electroacupuncture spread over 3 weeks with the application of electroacupuncture at four common acupuncture points (dorsal interosseus muscle of the hand and the inferior knee bilaterally) and up to six "empirically" chosen sites, "depending on the patient's symptoms and pain pattern." The sham procedure consisted of needle insertion approximately 20 mm away from the point that would have been chosen for the real procedure with the application of a weaker electric current. Although seven of eight outcome measures showed improvement in the active treatment group, none were improved in the sham-treatment group. Pain threshold, which was considered the principal outcome measure, improved by 70% in the electroacupuncture group and 4% in the control group ($p = 0.03$). There were several limitations to this study: (1) It is unclear whether electroacupuncture is equivalent to conventional acupuncture (some acupuncturists claim that electroacupuncture provides only short-term analgesic benefit whereas conventional acupuncture may provide longer-lasting analgesia); (2) patients may not have been optimally blinded in this study, since the sham protocol involved a shallower needle insertion and a weaker electric current; (3) there was no measure of functional or psychological status; and (4) the time that assessments were performed after the treatment was not detailed. This latter point is crucial since the analgesic effect of acupuncture may be short-lived, particularly for protocols involving less than 4 weeks of treatments.

Hypnotherapy

On the basis of the utility of hypnotherapy in disorders such as asthma, peptic ulcer disease, and irritable bowel syndrome, in which psychological factors may contribute to pathogenesis, Haanen et al. performed a controlled trial of hypnotherapy in fibromyalgia (Table 2–2).[45] Forty patients were randomized to either hypnotherapy or physical therapy for 12 weeks with follow-up at 24 weeks. Patients in the hypnotherapy group experienced significantly greater improvement in pain, fatigue, and global assessment at both 12 and 24 weeks.[45] Hypnotherapy, therefore, may be a useful intervention in some patients with particularly refractory symptoms.

UNCONTROLLED THERAPIES (TABLE 2–3)

Local injection of tender points has been advocated by several authors.[46–48] In general, a local anesthetic with or without local depot corticosteroid has been advocated and may provide relief for up to 2 months.

Low-frequency transcutaneous electrical nerve stimulation (TENS) may increase skin and muscle microcirculation and also activate endogenous opioids.[49] TENS was administered to 40 patients with fibromyalgia syndrome and appeared to produce transient benefit in 70% of the patients, although the long term benefits are unknown.[50] A controlled-trial is needed, however, given the lack of benefit of TENS observed in low back pain.[51]

Cognitive-behavioral treatment (CBT) of chronic pain involves a set of interventions

TABLE 2–3

Uncontrolled Interventions in Fibromyalgia Syndrome

INTERVENTION	REFERENCE
Transcutaneous nerve stimulation	50
Local injection	46, 47, 48
Cognitive behavioral therapy	52, 55
Multidisciplinary therapy	56

which address the sensory, affective, cognitive, and behavioral components of chronic pain and has been effective in a variety of disorders such as low back pain, headache, and temporomandibular joint pain.[52] This approach has also been shown to be useful in the treatment of rheumatoid arthritis, not only demonstrating improvement in psychological outcomes, but also in measures of disease activity such as joint tenderness and swelling.[53,54] Nielson et al.[52] studied 30 patients who met American College of Rheumatology criteria for the diagnosis of fibromyalgia. Patients were excluded if they were unable to attend the daily sessions or were unwilling to stop narcotic medication for control of pain. The CBT intervention consisted of a 3-week inpatient program that combined educational techniques (including the use of a videotape in which chronic pain was portrayed as a multidimensional phenomenon that involved cognitive, affective, sensory, and behavioral components), cognitive techniques, aerobic exercises and stretching, pacing and enhancement of pain tolerance, and family education (with at least one family member). Twenty-five patients completed the program, and "target" variables such as pain severity, perceived interference with life, sense of control over pain, and emotional distress, all showed statistically significant improvement after the CBT program compared to baseline. "Nontarget" variables, such as perceived support by others, response by significant other to pain, marital adjustment, and activity level, did not change with the CBT program. Thus, in this short-term, inpatient trial, CBT appears to be effective, although precisely which components of the program were effective is uncertain. Also, the confounding effects of cardiovascular training and concomitant use of medication hinder interpretation of the results.

Other groups have used similar combination therapy approaches that employ CBT, physical therapy, and cardiovascular exercise as well as medication in outpatient settings.[55,56] It appears that these approaches demonstrate improvement in the majority of patients in uncontrolled settings, although the long-term cost-effectiveness of these intensive programs is not known.

Other commonly employed therapies, such as chiropractic manipulation and myofascial therapy (including "spray and stretch" techniques), have been advocated on the basis of anecdotal experience.[46,56]

AUTHOR'S APPROACH TO MANAGEMENT

Education is an important component of any therapeutic regimen for patients with fibromyalgia syndrome. Patients and their families should be instructed to view fibromyalgia as a disorder that is not crippling. While fibromyalgia is generally a chronic condition, effective therapy is available, although there is no specific "cure." When possible, patients should be encouraged to take an active, "self-help"–oriented approach, rather than a passive, physician- or health provider–dependent approach to the treatment of their condition. Emphasis should be placed on the positive or "well" role, as opposed to the negative or "sick" role. Enrollment in patient support groups is to be encouraged.

Amitriptyline in low doses should be the initial medication tried in patients with fibromyalgia syndrome. Starting doses of 10 mg may minimize anticholinergic and sedating side effects and yet may confer symptomatic improvement. The drug should be given 1 hour before bedtime to reduce sleep disturbance and minimize "morning-after" sedation. Occasionally, in patients who are particularly sensitive to side effects, as little as 5 mg daily may be effective. (This generally requires either breaking the scored tablets or grinding the 10 mg tablets into powder and dividing the powder in half.) If there is no response to the initial 10 mg dose after 1 week and side effects are tolerable (frequently side effects such as dry mouth or drowsiness that are mild or moderate will subside with continued therapy), the dose should be increased to 20 mg daily and increased in 10 mg increments on a weekly basis thereafter. In general, doses that exceed 50 mg daily confer little additional benefit if there is no response to lower doses. For patients who achieve significant improvement, a stable dose of amitriptyline is then continued for a period of approximately 3 months. The dose may then be tapered in 10 mg decrements monthly to the minimum effective dose. Frequently, patients may continue the minimum effective dose for years without side effects, although rebound insomnia may occur with abrupt stoppage of any of the tricyclics when used for more than several weeks. Patients should be instructed to gradually taper amitriptyline to avoid rebound insomnia.

For patients who are unable to tolerate amitriptyline or who do not attain significant improvement with the drug, nortriptyline or cyclobenzaprine could be tried, initially at the lowest possible doses. Alternatives include alprazolam, although since it is a benzodiazepine, patients should be cautioned about potential dependence and the possibility of withdrawal reactions. For patients with particularly severe pain symptoms, NSAIDs can be added, although generally on an intermittent basis only, given the potential for gastrointestinal toxicity. As with any chronic pain disorder, narcotic analgesic agents should be avoided. Despite preliminary evidence suggesting that some patients may have adrenocortical dysfunction, the weight of evidence at this time does not support the use of systemic corticosteroid therapy.

Low-level aerobic exercise, such as walking or riding a stationary cycle, on a regular basis is a useful adjunct to medication therapy and may be advised either concurrently or shortly after initiation of medication therapy. Frequently, patients who are able to engage in regular aerobic exercise may be able to eventually taper off medication. Muscle-strengthening exercises should be employed cautiously.

Judicious use of local anesthetic injections (with or without depot corticosteroid injection) may be helpful in selected patients who have local symptoms that are particularly severe at times.

For patients with concomitant depression or severe fatigue, fluoxetine or paroxetine in doses beginning at 20 mg daily may be used. Since fluoxetine may cause insomnia, occasionally it may be necessary to add a low dose of a tricyclic agent at bedtime. For patients with more severe depression or other psychiatric disturbance, referral to a psychiatrist is generally indicated. Patients with more severe or recalcitrant symptoms may benefit from referral to a multidisciplinary chronic pain management facility.

DRUG SIDE EFFECTS AND RECOMMENDED MONITORING SCHEDULES

The most common side effects experienced with drug therapy of fibromyalgia syndrome are outlined in Table 2–4. Additional side effects noted with the use of tricyclic agents in low doses include weight gain, nightmares, or vivid dreaming, and occasionally paradoxic reactions such as insomnia may occur. Tricyclic agents, even at low doses, should be used with extreme caution in patients with a history of urinary retention or narrow-angle glaucoma. As noted above, abrupt discontinuation of these agents may produce rebound insomnia. These agents should be used with extreme caution in elderly patients because of the increased potential for confusion, disorientation, and

TABLE 2–4
Side Effects of CNS Active Drugs for Fibromyalgia Syndrome

DRUG	SEDATION	INSOMNIA	ANTICHOLINERGIC EFFECTS
Amitriptyline	+++	0	+++
Desipramine	+	+	+
Doxepin	+++	0	++
Imipramine	++	0	++
Nortriptyline	++	0	+
Protriptyline	+	++	++
Fluoxetine	0	++	0
Alprazolam	+	0	0
Cyclobenzaprine	++	0	++

Zero indicates no side effect; +, a minor side effect; ++, a moderate side effect; and +++, a major side effect.
Adapted from Potter WZ, Rudorfer MV, Manji H. N Engl J Med 1993;325:633–42.

hallucinations. Routine laboratory monitoring is generally not necessary for drug therapies used in the treatment of fibromyalgia (with the possible exception of NSAIDs for which periodic monitoring of the hematocrit, liver function studies, and renal function is recommended), although it is recommended that initially patients be surveyed at least quarterly to monitor for side effects.

PERTINENT CLINICAL PHARMACOLOGY AND DRUG INTERACTIONS

Many of the antidepressant agents employed in the therapy of fibromyalgia syndrome may potentiate central nervous system (CNS) depression that may occur with alcohol, sedative-hypnotics, and other CNS-depressant drugs, and should therefore be used with extreme caution, if at all, in these settings. The tricyclics are contraindicated in the presence of monoamine-oxidase inhibitors. In conjunction with anticholinergic agents, they may cause acute glaucoma, urinary retention, and paralytic ileus. Concomitant use of the tricyclics with clonidine and guanethidine may reduce the antihypertensive effect of the latter. All of these agents have unknown effects on the fetus and are therefore contraindicated during pregnancy. Pregnancy, anecdotally in my experience, usually results in spontaneous improvement of symptoms, and withdrawal of medication during pregnancy is generally well tolerated.

SUMMARY AND CONCLUSIONS

Many different interventions have been reported in the fibromyalgia syndrome (Tables 2–1, 2–2, and 2–3). While many have been effective, in general, trials of therapy have been of short duration. Furthermore, important or substantial improvement, when it has been assessed, occurs in only small proportions of patients. Long-term comparative trials of both efficacy and toxicity are necessary, although trials such as these require large numbers of patients and therefore are expensive and difficult to accomplish. Two other approaches offer potential solutions to the problem of adequate long-term comparative trials: (1) N-of-1 trials and (2) meta-analysis. N-of-1 trials have the advantage of random assign-

ment, double-blinding, and multiple potential comparisons in the same patient. Meta-analysis involves combining the results of studies, which individually may have conflicting results and lack adequate statistical power, to reach an overall result with sufficient statistical power to make meaningful conclusions, especially with respect to comparative efficacy. Lack of uniformity in the use of outcome measures hinders the application of meta-analytic methods, and for this reason future clinical trials in the fibromyalgia syndrome should ideally employ the same outcome measures.[57]

Few trials have assessed improvement in functional status. Functional status measures such as the Health Assessment Questionnaire (HAQ),[58] the Fibromyalgia Impact Questionnaire,[59] or similar instruments should be employed in future studies of therapy in fibromyalgia.

No studies have yet assessed the comparative cost-efficacy of available treatments. Studies that address the cost-efficacy of commonly employed but unproven treatments, such as physical therapy and chiropractic manipulation, are urgently needed.

REFERENCES

1. Bennett RM. The fibromyalgia syndrome: myofascial pain and the chronic fatigue syndrome. In: Kelly WN, Harris ED, Ruddy S, Sledge CB, eds. Textbook of rheumatology. 4th ed. Philadelphia: WB Saunders, 1992:471.
2. Wolfe F, Smythe HA, Yunus MB, et al. The American College of Rheumatology 1990 criteria for the classification of fibromyalgia. Arthritis Rheum 1990;33:19.
3. Wolfe F. The prevalence and characteristics of fibromyalgia in the general population. Arthritis Rheum 1993;36:S48.
4. Goldenberg DL. Fibromyalgia syndrome: an emerging but controversial condition. JAMA 1987;257:2782.
5. Griep EN, Boersma JW, De Kloet ER. Altered reactivity of the hypothalamic-pituitary-adrenal axis in the primary fibromyalgia syndrome. J Rheumatol 1993;20:469.
6. Crofford L, Pillemer SR, Kalogeras KT, et al. Perturbations of hypothalamic-pituitary-adrenal axis function in patients with fibromyalgia [Abstract]. Arthritis Rheum 1993;36:S220.
7. Demitrack MA, Dale JK, Straus SE, et al. Evidence for impaired activation of the hypothalamic pituitary-adrenal axis in patients with chronic fatigue syndrome. J Clin Endocrinol Metab 1991;73:1224.
8. Bennett RM, Clark SR, Campbell SM, et al. Low levels of somatomedin C in patients with

the fibromyalgia syndrome: a possible link between sleep and muscle pain. Arthritis Rheum 1992;35:1113.

9. Russell IJ, Vaeroy H, Javors M, et al. Cerebrospinal fluid biogenic amine metobolites in fibromyalgia/fibrositis syndrome and rheumatoid arthritis. Arthritis Rheum 1992;35:550.

10. Hawley DJ, Wolfe F, Cathey MA. Pain, functional disability and psychological status: a 12 month study of severity in fibromyalgia. J Rheumatol 1988;15:1551.

11. Felson DT, Goldenberg DL. The natural history of fibromyalgia. Arthritis Rheum 1986;29:1522.

12. Nørregaard J, Bülow PM, Prescott E, et al. Preliminary results of a 4-year follow-up study in fibromyalgia. J Muscul Pain 1992;1:159.

13. Simms RW, Felson DT, Goldenberg DL. Development of preliminary criteria for response to treatment in fibromyalgia syndrome. J Rheumatol 1991;18:1558.

14. Moldofsky H, Scarisbrick P, England R, et al. Musculoskeletal symptoms and non-REM sleep disturbance in patients with fibrositis syndrome and healthy subjects. Psychosom Med 1975;37:341.

15. Moldofsky H, Scarisbrick P. Induction of neurasthenic musculoskeletal pain syndrome by selective sleep stage deprivation. Psychosom Med 1976;38:35.

16. Moldofsky H, Lue LA. The relationship of alpha and delta EEG frequencies and mood in "fibrositis" patients treated with chlorpromazine and L-tryptophan. Electroencephalogr Clin Neurophysiol 1980;50:71.

17. Potter WZ, Rudorfer MV, Manji H. The pharmacologic treatment of depression. N Engl J Med 1993;325:633.

18. Yunus M, Masi AT, Calabro JJ, et al. Primary fibromyalgia (fibrositis): clinical study of 50 patients with matched normal controls. Semin Arthritis Rheum 1981;11:151.

19. Smythe HA. Fibrositis and other diffuse musculoskeletal syndromes. In: Kelly WN, Harris ED, Ruddy S, Sledge CB, eds. Textbook of rheumatology. Philadelphia: WB Saunders, 1981:485.

20. Connolly RG. Treatment of fibromyositis with fluphenazine and amitriptyline: a preliminary report. Del Med 1981;53:189.

21. Carrette S, McCain GA, Bell DA, et al. Evaluation of amitriptyline in primary fibrositis: a double blind, placebo-controlled study. Arthritis Rheum 1986;29:655.

22. Goldenberg DL, Felson DT, Dinerman H. A randomized controlled trial of amitriptyline and naproxen in the treatment of fibromyalgia syndrome. Arthritis Rheum 1986;29:1371.

23. Jaeschke R, Adachi J, Guyatt G, et al. Clinical usefulness of amitriptyline in fibromyalgia: the results of 23 N-of-1 randomized controlled trials. J Rheumatol 1991;18:447.

24. Barnes CD, Fung SJ, Gintautus J. Brainstem noradrenergic system depression by cyclobenzaprine. Neuropharmacology 1980;19:221.

25. Bennett RM, Gatter RA, Campbell SM, et al. A comparison of cyclobenzaprine and placebo in the management of fibrositis: a double-blind controlled study. Arthritis Rheum 1988;31;1535.

26. Reynolds WJ, Moldofsky H, Saskin P, Lue F. The effects of cyclobenzaprine on sleep physiology and symptoms in patients with fibrositis. Arthritis Rheum 1989;B115.

27. Carrette S, Bell MJ, Reynolds WJ, et al. Comparison of amitriptyline, cyclobenzaprine and placebo in fibromyalgia: a randomized double-blind clinical trial. Arthritis Rheum 1994;37:32.

28. Wolfe F, Cathey MA, Hawley DJ. A double-blind placebo controlled trial of fluoxetine in patients with fibromyalgia. Arthritis Rheum 1993;36(suppl):S220.

29. Russell IJ, Fletcher EM, Michalek JE, et al. Treatment of primary fibrositis/fibromyalgia syndrome with ibuprofen and alprazolam: a double-blind, placebo-controlled study. Arthritis Rheum 1991;34:552.

30. Hench PK, Cohen R, Mitler MM. Fibromyalgia: effects of amitriptyline, temazepam and placebo on pain and sleep. Arthritis Rheum 1989;32 (suppl):S47.

31. Clark S, Tindall E, Bennett RM. A double blind crossover trial of prednisone versus placebo in the treatment of fibrositis. J Rheumatol 1985; 12:980.

32. Yunus MB, Masi AT, Aldag JC. Short-term effects of ibuprofen in primary fibromyalgia syndrome: a double blind, placebo controlled trial. J Rheumatol 1989;16:527.

33. Vaeroy H, Abrahamsen A, Frre O, et al. Treatment of fibromyalgia (fibrositis syndrome): a parallel double blind trial with carisprodol, paracetamol and caffeine (Somadril comp) versus placebo. Clin Rheumatol 1989;8:245.

34. Tavoni A, Vitali C, Bombardieri S, et al. Evaluation of s-adenosylmethionine in primary fibromyalgia: a double-blind crossover study. Am J Med 1987;83 (suppl 5A):107.

35. McCain GA, Bell DA, Mai FM, et al. A controlled study of the effects of a supervised cardiovascular fitness training program on the manifestations of primary fibromyalgia. Arthritis Rheum 1991;31:1135.

36. Mengshoel AM, Førre Ø. Physical fitness training in patients with fibromyalgia. J Musculoskeletal Pain 1993;1:267.

37. Ferraccioli G, Ghirelli L, Scita F, et al. EMG-biofeedback training in fibromyalgia syndrome. J Rheumatol 1987;14:820.

38. Wolfe F. Fibromyalgia: whither treatment? J Rheumatol 1988;15:1047.

39. Patel MS, Gutzwiller F, Pacaud F, et al. A metaanalysis of acupuncture for the treatment of pain: a review of evaluative research. Pain 1986; 24:15.

40. ter Riet G, Kleijnen J, Knipshild P. Acupuncture and chronic pain: a criteria-based meta-analysis. J Clin Epidemiol 1990;43:1191.

41. Han JS. Central neurotransmitters and acupuncture analgesia. In: Pomeranz B, Stux G, eds. Scientific bases of acupuncture. Berlin: Springer Verlag, 1989:7.

42. Fields HL, Basbaum A. Endogenous pain control mechanisms. In: Wall PD, Melzack R, eds. Textbook of pain. Edinburgh: Churchill Livingstone, 1989:206.
43. Ho WKK, When HL. Opioid-like activity in the cerebrospinal fluid of pain patients treated by electroacupuncture. Neuropharmacology 1991; 28:961.
44. Deluze C, Bosia L, Zirbs A, et al. Electroacupuncture in fibromyalgia: results of a controlled trial. Br Med J 1992;305:1249.
45. Haanen HCM, Hoenderdos HTW, Van Romunde LKJ, et al. Controlled trial of hypnotherapy in the treatment of refractory fibromyalgia. J Rheumatol 1991;18:72.
46. Masi AT, Yunus MB. Fibromyalgia—which is the best treatment? A personalized, comprehensive, ambulatory, patient-involved management programme. Ballière's Clin Rheumatol 1990;4: 333.
47. Sheon RP, Moskowitz RW, Goldberg VM. Intralesional soft tissue injection technique. In: Soft tissue rheumatic pain: recognition, management, prevention. 2nd ed. Philadelphia: Lea & Febiger, 1987:293.
48. Yunus MB. Diagnosis, etiology and management of fibromyalgia syndrome: an update. Compr Ther 1988;14:8.
49. McCain GA. Non-medicinal treatments in primary fibromyalgia. Rheum Dis Clin North Am 1989;15:73.
50. Kaada B. Treatment of fibromyalgia by low-frequency transcutaneous nerve stimulation. Tidsskrift Nor Laegeforen 1989;109:2992.

51. Deyo RA, Walsh NE, Martin DC, et al. A controlled trial of transcutaneous electrical nerve stimulation (TENS) and exercise for chronic low back pain. N Engl J Med 1990;322:1627.
52. Nielson WR, Walker C, McCain GA. Cognitive behavioral treatment of fibromyalgia syndrome: preliminary findings. J Rheumatol 1992;19:98.
53. Bradley LA, Young LD, Anderson KO, et al. Effects of psychological therapy on pain behaviour of rheumatoid arthritis patients: treatment outcome and six month follow-up. Arthritis Rheum 1987;30:1105.
54. Parker JC, Frank RG, Beck NC, et al. Pain management in rheumatoid arthritis patients: a cognitive-behavioural approach. Arthritis Rheum 1988;31:593.
55. Goldenberg DL, Kaplan KH, Nadeau MG. The impact of cognitive-behavioral therapy on fibromyalgia. Arthritis Rheum 1991;34(suppl):S190.
56. Bennett RM, Campbell S, Burckhardt C, et al. A multidisciplinary approach to fibromyalgia management. J Musculoskel Med 1991;8: 21.
57. Peluso P, Bombardier C, Guillemin F. A meta-analysis of controlled trials in the treatment of fibromyalgia syndrome [Abstract]. Arthritis Rheum 1993;36:S49.
58. Fries JF, Spitz PW, Kraines RG. Measurement of patient outcome in arthritis. Arthritis Rheum 1980;23:137.
59. Burckhardt CS, Clark SR, Bennett RM. The fibromyalgia impact questionnaire (FIQ): development and validation. J Rheumatol 1991;18: 728.

RHEUMATOID ARTHRITIS

Mark J. Borigini
Harold E. Paulus

NATURAL HISTORY

Rheumatoid arthritis (RA) is a chronic, systemic, inflammatory disorder of unknown etiology, affecting approximately 1% of the world's population.[1] Women are affected two to three times more often than men, but this female preponderance is less impressive when one considers only those patients who are serologically positive for rheumatoid factor and are found to have radiographic evidence of erosive changes in joints.[2] RA can occur at any age; it appears, however, to increase in incidence with advancing age.

There are occasions in which several family members are found to have RA; a greater than expected incidence occurs in monozygotic twins.[3] Studies of the class II gene products (HLA-DR, DQ, DP) of the major histocompatibility complex have shown that susceptibility to RA is determined by the immune response genes.[4] HLA-DR4 is the primary susceptibility haplotype in most ethnic groups (black Americans being an exception).[5] Although the relative risk of developing RA is several times greater in DR-4 persons, only a minority of them are affected. In fact, a significant number of patients with RA have a haplotype other than DR-4. Monoclonal antibodies have defined an epitope present on several different classes of HLA-D that confers a higher relative risk for the development of RA. As class II molecules are involved in antigen presentation to thymocytes, it is possible that further analysis will lead to identification of an infectious or chemical antigen that may be responsible for the development of RA.

Although RA is characterized largely by the manner in which it involves joints, in most patients symptoms begin as gradually increasing malaise and fatigue, likely to be accompanied by diffuse musculoskeletal pain. Joint involvement is appreciated as pain, tenderness, swelling, and redness. Symmetry is characteristic, most commonly involving the joints of the hands, wrists, elbows, and shoulders, but also involving the knees, ankles, and feet; virtually any diarthrodial joint can be affected.[6]

Inactivity, such as sleep or prolonged sitting, is often followed by stiffness. In fact, the duration of morning stiffness is one measure of the severity of RA. The stiffness—and pain—may increase as the disease progresses, often limiting the patient's ability to perform basic activities of daily living. Other systemic manifestations include weight loss, depression, and low-grade fever.[2]

In about 20% of patients the onset of RA is acute. Frequently disease activity is at first intermittent; with the passage of time, it becomes more sustained. Some patients may have no more than a few months of discomfort; others become severely disabled. Spontaneous remission is not likely, however, if disease has been continuous for 2 or more years.

Continued articular inflammation results in progressive joint destruction, deformity, and subsequent incapacitation, each to varying degrees. Extraarticular features such as rheumatoid nodules, vasculitis, neuropathy, scleritis, pericarditis, lymphadenopathy, and splenomegaly are other manifestations, which are most often associated with more aggressive, rheumatoid factor-positive disease.[7] An individual patient may manifest any or all of these clinical features at any given time.

An analysis of RA patients followed prospectively for 6 years showed that 18% had at least one remission; the remission periods comprised 35% of the follow-up period for those in remission, and the mean length of remission was 10 months.[8] Development of RA after the age of 60 or being male was found to increase the probability of remission. On the other hand, early development of erosions decreased the probability of remission.

The median life expectancy of persons with established RA is less than that of control populations. A 25-year prospective study showed that median life expectancy was shortened by 7 years in males and 3 years in females.[9] Another study showed that 48% of patients were without disability at the onset of the survey period; after 12 years this figure had declined to 17%.[10] At the study's initiation 3% were completely disabled; this increased to 16% at the end of 12 years. Disability develops most rapidly during the first 2 years of disease and progresses less rapidly in subsequent years. Factors that influenced outcome included older age, functional class, radiographic grade, and female sex. Patients with an insidious onset of disease appear to do less well than those with an acute onset.[11]

Potentially morbid complications include atlantoaxial subluxation, cricoarytenoid synovitis, and sepsis of involved joints. Those extraarticular complications that potentially may result in mortality include Felty's syndrome (possible life-threatening infection), Sjögren's syndrome, cardiopulmonary complications, systemic vasculitis, gastrointestinal complications of treatment, amyloidosis, and infection.[12] Chronic inanition and debilitation may increase the risk of death from all causes. Interestingly, the increased mortality associated with rheumatoid arthritis is equivalent to that of patients with Hodgkin's disease, diabetes mellitus, and stroke (age-adjusted).[13] Of particular note is that education level of patients is reported to be inversely proportional to mortality.[14]

Seropositivity for rheumatoid factor has been associated with a poorer prognosis in RA.[15] These patients have a greater number of involved joints and develop more erosions and ligamentous instability.[16] As rheumatoid nodules occur almost solely in patients who are seropos-

itive for rheumatoid factor, patients with such nodules have a poorer outcome and more frequent erosions.[16]

REST

Most would agree that the main objectives in the management of RA should include relief of pain, reduction of inflammation, preservation of muscle strength and joint function, and maintenance of as normal a lifestyle as possible while minimizing side effects from treatment. All patients should be taught the most basic treatment of joint inflammation: adequate rest.

Whole-body rest can decrease the general systemic inflammatory response; in addition, local rest of an inflamed joint protects the joint to permit repair. Exercise of an inflamed joint is proinflammatory; splinting of a joint is antiinflammatory (although one must use caution with this practice; initially, splints can increase the sensation of joint stiffness and its duration).[17] When a patient with RA suffers a stroke, the rheumatoid joints on the paralyzed side lose their inflammation. The prescription of rest should be accompanied by the caution that the level of physical activity should not be immediately increased as joint inflammation decreases.

Patients will often discover that fatigue that occurs in the midafternoon can be significantly reduced by a nap. This helps patients cope with the remainder of the day. A regularly disciplined afternoon nap can be an effective part of any treatment program. Acute exacerbations of disease may require longer periods of rest in bed to suppress the inflammatory process. Nevertheless, full range of motion of joints should be maintained by a graded exercise program.

McCarty[18] suggests that upper extremity joints be rested by splinting for 3 weeks after intraarticular corticosteroid injection. However, the splint should be removed and one full range of motion performed daily in each joint in the fingers and wrists. In the case of the joints of the lower extremity, he advises patients to avoid weight-bearing for 8 weeks after the injection. A controlled study showed that 88% of upper extremity joints remained free of inflammation almost 2 years after local triamcinolone injection administered in this manner.[18] Although theoretically desirable, prolonged splinting may not be practical.

DRUG THERAPY: NSAIDs

The choice of drug therapy for RA today is more often than not determined by the degree of disease activity, the apparent disease severity, and the adverse effects of the drugs. For example, explosive polyarticular disease with severe systemic symptoms, early extraarticular signs (e.g., serositis and episcleritis), and nodules suggest aggressive disease. Although in most patients the pattern of disease severity is established during the first year, activity can wax and wane over varying periods of time. Predicting a disease course or eventual outcome may be possible for groups or large numbers of subjects in an epidemiologic study; in an individual patient it may not be so easy. Therefore, careful initial and periodic follow-up assessments are necessary in administration of an appropriate drug program.

The traditional approach to the treatment of RA is to begin with symptomatic treatment of inflammation with salicylates or other nonsteroidal antiinflammatory drugs (NSAIDs) in addition to rest and corticosteroid injections (as needed). As the severity of the disease progresses, the clinician progresses up the "therapeutic pyramid" to more effective, and possibly more toxic, drugs. Much time may be spent at the "base" of the pyramid, prescribing several NSAIDs in sequence in the hope that the patient may undergo a spontaneous remission of disease activity. The assumption of the pyramid approach is that all patients will receive the "basic" therapy, with fewer patients receiving more aggressive therapy at a later date. This approach, however, is being questioned and is under review for a variety of reasons (see below).

By impairing the activity of various natural mediators of inflammation, such as bradykinins, prostaglandins, and oxygen radicals, NSAIDs partially impair the final expression of inflammation. Because they act on terminal events in the inflammatory cascade, the benefits of these drugs are quickly evident. However, since these drugs do not fully prevent tissue injury, it is not surprising that joint damage and other evidence of organ damage may progress during therapy. Sustained drug-induced remission generally is not expected with these short-acting antirheumatic agents, which act distally in the inflammatory cascade.

NSAIDs reduce but do not completely eliminate the signs and symptoms of established inflammation. The presence of drug in the blood is associated with a rapid onset of benefit, but exacerbation of signs and symptoms occurs quickly after metabolism or excretion of the drug. There is no proof that NSAIDs have a major effect on the underlying RA disease process. In addition to their antiinflammatory effects, NSAIDs decrease pain, suppress fever, and decrease platelet adhesiveness, leading to a multitude of short-term and long-term prescribed and nonprescribed uses. In the United States, available NSAIDs include aspirin, salicylsalicylate, magnesium choline salicylate, other salicylates, ibuprofen, phenylbutazone, indomethacin, sulindac, naproxen, tolmetin, fenoprofen, meclofenamate sodium, diflunisal, piroxicam, ketoprofen, diclofenac, flurbiprofen, etodolac, ketorolac, nabumetone, and oxaprozin (Table 3–1). Many others are under development or available elsewhere.[18]

Most NSAIDs are organic acids and are highly bound to plasma proteins. (Nabumetone, however, is a nonacidic pro-drug that is metabolized to an active organic acid.) These properties may enhance drug concentrations in inflamed tissues, which are more permeable to plasma proteins and tend to have a lower pH. Although their chemical structures differ somewhat, the clinical usefulness of available NSAIDs does not relate to their chemical class. It is more useful to remember their plasma half-life, which is related to the frequency of administration and in some instances to the occurrence of adverse reactions, especially in the elderly. NSAIDs have a broad range of pharmacologic activities; they are able to inhibit cyclooxygenase, the enzyme that transforms arachidonic acid via endoperoxides to prostaglandins, prostacyclin, and thromboxanes. Currently available drugs have little direct effect on lipoxygenase, which transforms arachidonic acid to leukotrienes. (Diclofenac has an indirect inhibitory effect on lipoxygenase by stimulating uptake of arachidonic acid into triglycerides.) NSAIDs also have been shown to suppress bradykinin release, alter lymphocyte responses, and limit granulocyte and monocyte migration and phagocytosis under certain laboratory conditions.[19]

Although NSAIDs are generally well tolerated, they are associated with a wide spectrum of potential clinical toxicities. Aspirin is the most difficult to use effectively, has more frequent side effects and the most complex dosing schedule, and is more dangerous if overdoses

TABLE 3–1

Nonsteroidal Antiinflammatory Drugs Used in Rheumatoid Arthritis

DRUG	DOSE RANGE (mg/d)	HALF-LIFE (h)	COMMENTS
Salicylates			
Aspirin (acetylsalicylic acid)	1000–6000	4–15	
Nonacetylated Salicylates			
Magnesium choline salicylate	1500–4000	4–15	Decreased effect on platelets, gastric mucosa,
Salsalate	1500–5000	4–15	and (to a certain extent) prostaglandin-
Sodium salicylate	3000–5000	4–15	mediated renal function
Short Serum Half-life NSAIDs			
Diclofenac sodium	75–150	1–2	Higher incidence of liver function test abnormalities
Fenoprofen calcium	1200–3200	2	Rarely associated with acute T cell–mediated interstitial nephritis with renal failure
Flurbiprofen	100–300	3–4	
Ibuprofen	1200–3200	2	
Ketoprofen	100–400	2	
Meclofenamate sodium	200–400	2–3	Associated with a higher incidence of severe diarrhea
Tolmetin sodium	800–1600	1	Because there is less hepatobiliary recircula- tion, may cause less gastrointestinal toxicity in the elderly
Long Serum Half-life NSAIDs			
Diflunisal	500–1500	7–15	Although a derivative of the salicylates, it does not break down in the body to actually form a salicylate
Indomethacin	50–200	3–11	
Nabumetone	1000–2000	24	Nonacidic prodrug with active acidic metabolite
Naproxen	750–1500	13	
Oxaprozin	600–1200	21–25	
Phenylbutazone	200–800	40–80	
Piroxicam	20	30–86	
Sulindac	300–400	16	Associated with a lower incidence of prostaglandin-mediated renal insufficiency

are taken. Side effects tend to be dose related.[20] Because NSAIDs suppress prostaglandin synthesis, gastric acid production is increased; also, the production of gastric mucus and bicarbonate is decreased, as is the rate of cellular proliferation of the gastric mucosa, impairing the normal protective mechanisms of the stomach and thus causing gastric irritation and the exacerbation of peptic ulcers. If gastrointestinal bleeding recurs, it is worsened, because NSAIDs decrease platelet adhesiveness and increase acid production in the stomach. Firmly compressed aspirin tablets may dissolve slowly in the stomach, causing irritation and superficial ulceration of the gastric mucosa directly under the undissolved tablet. Ion trapping of weak organic acids such as NSAIDs in mucosal cells leads to back-diffusion of hydrogen ions and may result in mucosal damage.

NSAIDs may produce two types of anticoagulant effects. First, NSAIDs decrease platelet adhesiveness by inhibiting a prostaglandin-initiated sequence that is necessary for platelet activation. Because platelets lack mitochondria and are unable to synthesize additional cyclooxygenase, acetylation of this enzyme by aspirin irreversibly decreases platelet aggregation in response to various stimuli; this effect persists for about 10 to 12 days until the acetylated platelets are replaced by new platelets that have not been exposed to aspirin. In contrast, cyclooxygenase inhibition by other NSAIDs is reversible, their platelet effects persisting only as long as the drug is present. The second type of anticoagulant effect occurs when protein-bound NSAIDs displace warfarin from plasma protein-binding sites, thus increasing warfarin's anticoagulant effect, a mechanism that is significant only for phenylbutazone and for salicylates in toxic concentrations. Because the nonacetylated salicylates are poor inhibitors of cyclooxygenase, they have little or no effect on platelets, and modest doses sometimes may be used when other NSAIDs are contraindicated by an excessive risk of bleeding.

Reversible hepatocellular toxicity, characterized by elevations in the level of one or more liver enzymes, has been observed in up to 15% of patients treated with NSAIDs.[21] Transaminase elevations usually revert to normal after discontinuation of the drug and sometimes become normal, even when the drug is continued. Rarely, hepatic dysfunction may be severe, requiring discontinuation of the drug. Fatal fulminant hepatitis occurs rarely; transaminase levels should be checked on a regular basis during treatment, especially after a change of NSAIDs or an increase in dose.

NSAIDs may decrease creatinine clearance and increase serum creatinine levels in some patients predisposed by hypovolemia, impaired renal function, concomitant use of diuretics, or decreased renal blood flow, probably by suppressing the vasodilatory function of renal prostaglandins. NSAIDs should be used with caution in patients with conditions that impair renal perfusion or function, in patients with decreased circulating blood volume, and in the elderly. Acute interstitial nephritis and the nephrotic syndrome rarely occur with NSAIDs; most patients recover when the drug is discontinued, but occasionally dialysis or high-dose corticosteroid therapy is needed to support patients before recovery of renal function.[22]

Other adverse effects include various skin reactions and rashes.[20] Hypersensitivity responses include an aspirin-associated syndrome of rhinitis, nasal polyposis, and asthma. Anaphylaxis has been associated with NSAID use, as have agranulocytosis and aplastic anemia—the latter two are more frequent with phenylbutazone but may also occur rarely with other NSAIDs.

Salicylates cause blood level–related tinnitus and hearing loss; overdoses can cause a variety of central nervous system manifestations, including coma. Headaches occur with indomethacin and other NSAIDs, and confusion may appear in elderly patients treated with indomethacin, naproxen, or ibuprofen. Although reported more commonly in patients with lupus, aseptic meningitis has occurred in normal subjects treated with ibuprofen, sulindac, and other NSAIDs.

Generally speaking, NSAIDs are completely absorbed shortly after oral administration, unless enteric-coated or sustained-release forms are used. Aspirin, nabumetone, and sulindac have active metabolites with longer half-lives than the parent drugs. Indomethacin, meclofenamate sodium, and sulindac display enterohepatic recirculation. As some metabolites of salicylate and diflunisal exhibit Michaelis-Menton kinetics, the plasma half-life of the drug increases as the plasma concentration increases. It follows that doses need to be given less frequently when plasma concentrations are high; toxic concentrations take much longer to clear than would be anticipated. The pro-drug, nabumetone, is a poor inhibitor of prostaglandin synthesis but is rapidly transformed by the liver to an acidic metabolite with potent inhibitory effects. Virtually all available NSAIDs are eventually converted by the liver to inactive metabolites that are excreted predominantly in urine and bile; however, sulindac may also be converted to an inactive metabolite by the kidney.[19]

It is important to individualize treatment with aspirin and the other NSAIDs. Substantial individual variability is present with respect to the pharmacology and pharmacokinetics of these drugs, which also vary in effectiveness. Patients with rheumatoid arthritis usually need prolonged treatment with maximum tolerated doses. Whereas aspirin has a long history of efficacy in the treatment of rheumatoid arthritis, side effects, with gastrointestinal distress most prominent, make it intolerable for many patients in the doses required for efficacy in rheumatoid arthritis. Enteric-coated aspirin preparations somewhat relieve these gastric symptoms. The nonacetylated salicylates have fewer of the side effects that are typically associated with NSAID-induced suppression of prostaglandin production. With salicylates, it is important to use sufficient amounts to achieve a clinical response. Doses can be adjusted by following serum salicylate levels (a therapeutic level being

20 to 30 mg/dl), which could be checked during the first 2 to 4 weeks of therapy.[23] Occasional monitoring after 1 to 2 months is also appropriate, as the increased metabolism that is caused by the salicylate itself can decrease salicylate levels by 15% to 20%.[24] The nonacetylated salicylates have a prolonged serum half-life at antiinflammatory concentrations, and have been shown to be as effective as aspirin in patients with RA.[25] Nonacetylated salicylates (except sodium salicylate) are more expensive than aspirin, but they have the advantage of being 25 to 50 times less potent than aspirin as prostaglandin synthetase inhibitors, and thus they may be useful in patients with bleeding tendencies or possibly in patients with compromised renal function.[25] They may also have an advantage in patients with a history of NSAID-induced asthma or nasal polyposis, as a correlation exists between potency as a cyclooxygenase inhibitor and induction of asthma (but the first dose should be given under close supervision).[25] Despite the availability of salicylate levels for monitoring purposes, the clinician must remain vigilant for side effects, such as hearing loss (mostly in the elderly) and the other laboratory and clinical abnormalities mentioned earlier.

Obviously the selection of a particular agent depends on the patient's medical history (e.g., history of gastrointestinal bleeding or intolerance) and on the personal preference and previous experience of the prescribing physician and the patient. If the patient has insufficient benefit from or intolerable sensitivity to a specific NSAID, another NSAID is often substituted, initially at a moderate dose to establish tolerance. (Interestingly, an average patient with rheumatoid arthritis tries more than three NSAIDs before finding the one that is most satisfactory.[26]) The dose is then carefully increased to the maximal dose recommended or tolerated and continued for at least 2 weeks.[27] The biologic effects of NSAIDs do not depend directly on serum levels but, rather, on tissue concentrations and the effect that these concentrations have on the inflammatory process. As these latter effects may require days to appear, a delay can be expected between kinetic equilibrium and maximum clinical response. There is little evidence to suggest that combinations of salicylates and NSAIDs, or of one NSAID with another, are more beneficial than single-drug therapy, whereas toxicity is probably additive.[28]

Caution is advised in prescribing NSAIDs to the elderly, to patients with peptic ulcer disease, impairment of renal or hepatic function, dehydration, congestive heart failure, or hypertension, and to those being treated with anticoagulants, oral hypoglycemics, or other drugs that may interact with the NSAID. Because these conditions are frequent in hospitalized patients, great care should be taken when NSAIDs are given to these patients. It should be recalled that any side effect related to serum concentration will be prolonged with those drugs that have a prolonged serum half-life.[20]

Patients should be followed particularly closely during introduction of an NSAID, when doses are increased, or when the patient's condition changes. Although prostaglandin-mediated or hypersensitivity-mediated renal failure is rare, and abnormal liver function test findings are uncommon as a result of using NSAIDs, it is best to check baseline serum creatinine and hemoglobin levels and liver function tests before starting a new NSAID. It is reasonable to repeat these tests every 2 to 4 weeks for the first 3 to 4 months. Renal function and liver function abnormalities are relatively rare in an uncomplicated patient after an NSAID has been used for several months.

Even optimal use of NSAIDs does not completely suppress all evidence of inflammation, particularly in chronic RA. If the patient with RA does not have a spontaneous remission within a reasonable period of time (usually months), according to the traditional pyramid approach, a slow-acting antirheumatic drug should be added to the continuing maximal NSAID therapy.

DMARDs

Disease-modifying antirheumatic drugs (DMARDs) is a term for a group of medications with diverse mechanisms of action. Other names for these drugs are (1) slow-acting antirheumatic drugs, (2) remission-inducing drugs, and (3) second-line antirheumatic agents. They have traditionally been used if the disease is not responding to NSAIDs and other conservative treatment modalities. They include gold compounds, chloroquine or hydroxychloroquine, sulfasalazine, D-penicillamine, azathioprine, and methotrexate (Table 3–2). They have been demonstrated to produce additional clinical

TABLE 3–2
DMARDs Commonly in Use in the United States

| DRUG | DOSE | EFFICACY | TOXICITY | | MONITORING (AUTHORS' RECOMMENDATIONS) |
			TREATMENT LIMITING	LIFE THREATENING	
Methotrexate	7.5–15 mg PO or IM once weekly	+++	++	Hepatic fibrosis, acute interstitial pneumonia, bone marrow suppression	Baseline chest radiograph and hepatitis B,C serologies CBC every 2–4 weeks for 4 months, then every 4 weeks Liver function tests every 4–8 weeks Creatinine levels every 4 weeks
Sulfasalazine	500–3000 mg/d PO	+++	++++	Bone marrow suppression	Baseline G6PD CBC every 2 weeks for 8 weeks, then monthly for 6 months, then every 2–3 months Liver function tests at 1 month and then every 2–3 months
Gold sodium thiomalate	Start with 10, 25, and then 50 mg/wk IM	+++	+++++	Aplastic anemia, thrombocyto-penia, pneumonitis	CBC and urinalysis before each injection Liver function tests and creatinine levels every 3 months
D-Penicillamine	250 mg/d PO for 4–6 weeks, then 500–750 mg/d	+++	++++	Aplastic anemia, thrombocytope-nia, obliterative bronchiolitis, polymyositis	CBC and urine protein levels every 1–2 weeks for 6 months, then monthly. Liver function tests and creatinine levels every 1–3 months
Hydroxy-chloroquine sulfate	400 mg/d PO	++	+	Rare	Ophthalmologic examination (baseline, then every 6 months) CBC, liver function tests, and creatinine levels every 3 months
Azathioprine	2–2.5 mg/kg/d (100–150 mg/d)	++	+++	Probable twofold increase in the relative risk of inducing non-Hodgkin's lymphoma	CBC every 1–2 weeks for 2 months, then every other week for 2–4 months, then every 2–4 weeks Liver function tests every 1–2 months
Auranofin	3 mg PO b.i.d.	+	++	Rare	CBC and urine protein levels every 2–4 weeks Liver function tests every 1–2 months

CBC, complete blood count; G6PD, glucose-6-phosphate dehydrogenase.
Efficacy and toxicity estimates based on Felson DT, Anderson JJ, Meenan RF. The comparative efficacy and toxicity of second-line drugs in rheumatoid arthritis. Arthritis Rheum 1990;33(10); and Felson DT, Anderson JJ, Meenan RF. Use of short-term efficacy/toxicity tradeoffs to select second-line drugs in rheumatoid arthritis. Arthritis Rheum 1992;35(10).

benefit when added to continuing stable background NSAID with or without concomitant low-dose corticosteroid therapy. Occasionally remissions occur during DMARD therapy, but the relationship of the remission to the DMARD therapy has been difficult to prove. DMARDs differ from NSAIDs in their delayed onset of action and lack of analgesia. They appear to act more proximally on the inflammatory process, perhaps on the immunologic initiators of tissue injury, but without actually removing the basic cause of disease. They often affect laboratory tests that measure acute-phase reactants such as C-reactive protein and erythrocyte sedimentation rate, and sometimes they affect immunoglobulins and rheumatoid factor. Probably because their proximal effects take considerable time to influence the intermediate and distal sites of inflammation, it takes weeks or months of DMARD treatment before clinical benefit is recognized. However, they most often only moderate the disease process; some level of chronic inflammation generally persists. Even if a drug-induced remission does occur, it is likely that the disease will recur—with a delay of weeks to months—when the drug is discontinued. Although the phenomenon is not well understood, the disease will be exacerbated even when the drug is being maintained at the same dose. DMARDs may slow the rate of progression of joint erosion or destruction and disability.[29]

Sulfhydryl-containing organic gold compounds were first used to treat arthritis in the 1920s, and Forestier's enthusiastic report stimulated their use.[30] Their value in RA was established in a double-blind trial that was published by the Empire Rheumatism Council in 1960.[31] Intramuscular gold has been found to be effective in about 60% to 80% of patients, with the response beginning in 3 to 6 months.[32] Aurothiomalate and aurothioglucose, water-soluble preparations given by intramuscular injection, are 50% gold by weight. Their administration requires regular office visits to monitor for toxicity and efficacy. The standard injection schedule involves respective test doses of 10 mg and 25 mg in the first 2 weeks and then a routine dosage of 25 to 50 mg weekly, assuming tolerance has been established. The orally absorbed gold preparation, auranofin, is lipid soluble, 30% gold by weight, and usually is given in a dosage of 6 mg/d.[33]

In the case of both aurothiomalate and auranofin, animal studies indicate that gold and the thiomalate or phosphine portions of the respective molecules dissociate within hours of administration and have different tissue distributions and excretion patterns, suggesting that gold is the pharmacologically effective portion of the molecule.[33] Although the exact mechanism of action has not been definitively established, studies have shown that gold compounds diminish acute and chronic inflammatory responses, acting at many points in the sequence of inflammatory events. They may reduce vascular permeability, reduce cell number at sites of inflammation, suppress phagocytosis, prevent protein denaturation, and suppress both lysosomal and nonlysosomal enzymes. Human lymphocyte responses to mitogens and antigens are inhibited by gold in culture conditions. Monocyte participation in cell-mediated in vitro responses is impaired by gold.[34] In patients, however, there is no evidence of generalized suppression either of inflammatory responses or of cellular and humoral immune responses. Still, gold treatment produces major improvement and occasional remission in some patients with RA and may reduce the progression of joint erosions.

Unfortunately, about 35% of patients discontinue gold injections because of side effects.[33] The most common side effects are rash and stomatitis, which occur in 15% to 30% of patients.[33] More serious toxic manifestations include an immune complex–mediated membranous glomerular nephritis in 3% to 7% of patients, leukopenia in 2% to 5%, thrombocytopenia in about 3% and, rarely, aplastic anemia.[33] A minor degree of proteinuria may require only interruption of the treatment, which can be resumed once the urinalysis is again normal. Nitritoid reactions (flushing, sometimes accompanied by transient hypotension) immediately after injections occurs only with aurothiomalate and can be relieved by a change to aurothioglucose.[33] Interestingly, among drug-induced causes of death in the United Kingdom, gold compounds were a major contributor.[33]

In controlled prospective studies, there were fewer withdrawals because of toxicity from auranofin than from aurothiomalate. Dose-related loose stools or diarrhea are frequent complaints with auranofin, and can usually be controlled by decreasing the dose.[33] Although stomatitis and rashes are about equally frequent with oral and injectable gold, proteinuria and hematologic toxicity are less common with the oral preparation. However, physicians generally believe that auranofin is slightly less effective than intramuscular preparations. A large double-blind study showed that, compared with placebo, intramuscular gold decreased the bony erosion rate over the course of a year, while auranofin did not.[33] Thus auranofin is a drug that might be used early in cases of potentially mild RA.

Routine monitoring of the complete blood count (CBC) and urinalysis is required with parenteral gold. At our institution it is mandatory that these studies be obtained before each injection of gold; however, it is recognized that other rheumatologists use different monitoring schedules. When major clinical benefit occurs, the frequency of injections can be reduced to alternate weeks and, if benefit persists, then to every third or fourth week. There is no maximum time limit to intramuscular gold treatment; it is continued as long as it is tolerated and beneficial. Liver function tests should be performed every 1 to 3 months. A CBC and urinalysis should be performed every 2 to 4 weeks on the patient who is taking auranofin, and liver function should be monitored every 1 to 3 months.[35]

Antimalarial agents have been used to treat some rheumatic diseases since the 1800s.[36] In 1951 Page first suggested using antimalarial agents in patients with other connective tissue diseases and described remission of "associated rheumatoid arthritis" in his series of patients.[36] Efficacy in RA was shown in the 1950s and 1960s in several double-blind, placebo-controlled trials that used chloroquine hydrochloride.[37] Many controlled and uncontrolled trials of hydroxychloroquine have been conducted, with varying results. Some have suggested that hydroxychloroquine is as effective as gold, D-penicillamine, and azathioprine.[37] In fact, the recent meta-analyses by Felson et al.[38] suggest that antimalarial drugs have a better risk/benefit ratio than do azathioprine and auranofin.[38]

Hydroxychloroquine is probably the least toxic DMARD. A member of the quinolone group of drugs, the dosage is generally 400 mg/d orally.[36] It is well absorbed and extensively distributed into the tissues, with high concentrations in liver, lung, kidney, heart, and pigmented tissue. Excretion is slow and may continue for as long as 5 years after the drug is discontinued. As the antimalarial compounds are weak bases that lack protons at the neutral pH of serum, they can diffuse into acidic vacuoles, where they become protonated. The more polar protonated molecules are unable to diffuse out of the vacuoles, and the pH within the vacuole becomes elevated by 1 to 2 pH units. The elevation of intracytoplasmic pH, in turn, alters the molecular assembly of α-β-peptide complexes. This may interfere with antigenic processing and lead to a reduced stimulation of autoimmune CD4[+] T cells, resulting in a downregulation of autoimmune responses.[39] Chloroquine has been shown to decrease antigen processing and presentation by both macrophages and lymphoid dendritic cells.[40]

Hydroxychloroquine has a delayed onset of action; response is seen in 40% to 60% of patients by 3 to 6 months, but it may take 9 to 12 months for maximum response to occur.[41] Nevertheless, this drug has relatively few serious side effects.[36] The high concentrations found in the pigment layers of the retina may lead to retinal damage with destruction of rods and cones; however, the frequency of significant retinopathy is no more than 0.5% with current dosing regimens.[42] Early changes can be detected on an electroretinogram or by changes in color vision or visual fields; abnormal results in a sensitive ophthalmologic examination occur in 0.5% to 10% of patients without symptoms. If clinical symptoms of visual impairment occur, the damage may be irreversible; therefore a patient should undergo an ophthalmologic examination for retinopathy before starting hydroxychloroquine therapy and every 6 months thereafter.[42] The drug should be stopped at the first sign of retinal toxicity. Other side effects include dermatitis (including phototonic and photosensitivity reactions), nausea and epigastric pain, insomnia, myopathy, headache, blurred vision, hemolytic anemia, and rarely leukopenia. Blurred vision is noted frequently with hydroxychloroquine. It is not due to retinal damage; it is reversible; and it may be eliminated by dosage reduction in some patients. All side effects, however, are extremely infrequent. Life-table analysis has shown less toxicity with hydroxychloroquine than with intramuscular gold and D-penicillamine.[43] Most clinicians would agree that the place of hydroxychloroquine in the sequence of DMARD use is in early mild disease, and they often continue it as a background therapy when another DMARD is started.[44]

D-Penicillamine is an established DMARD. In well-controlled studies comparing gold, D-penicillamine, and azathioprine, no statistically significant differences in clinical response were found.[45] In most well-controlled 6- to 12-month trials, however, between 30% and 50% of the patients taking D-penicillamine stopped the drug because of side effects such as leukopenia, rash, thrombocytopenia, and proteinuria.[46] It can also cause rare "autoimmune" side effects, such as conditions resembling systemic lupus erythematosus, polymyositis, myasthenia gravis, and Goodpasture's syndrome. Many physicians believe that it is more toxic than either gold or azathioprine, and this fact limits its usefulness. In addition, it must be taken on an empty stomach without other medications or food to avoid wide swings in intestinal absorption.

The mechanism of action of D-penicillamine on rheumatoid arthritis is unknown. Some studies demonstrate a suppressant effect of the drug on cellular immune responsiveness; in other situations, immune enhancement was found. It has been reported to selectively inhibit human helper T cell function.[47]

D-Penicillamine is usually started in a single daily dose of 250 mg, but therapy may be started at 125 mg/d to determine early tolerance. Inasmuch as the clinical response is slow, increments in dosage are usually not made in less than 8-week intervals up to a maximum dose of 750 to 1000 mg/d, as this is the time period required to assess the effectiveness of the newer dosage level.[48] With lower doses, the incidence of adverse reactions is reduced, but 125 mg/d may be too low a dose.[49] In fact, it has been suggested that intermittent therapy can sustain a successful response, at the same time reducing the total dose of drug taken by 75%[50]; although it has a half-life of less than 24 hours, it does bind strongly to both cellular and serum proteins. Recently it has been shown that the half-life of a D-penicillamine albumin complex is between 14 and 21 days, which could have a bearing on the effectiveness of intermittent therapy.[51]

It may take more than 12 weeks before there is evidence of a response to the drug. The dura-

tion of treatment in a patient who has shown a good response is variable. Some suggest a gradual reduction in decrements of 125 mg/d at approximately 8-week intervals. Some patients can be completely withdrawn and remain in a condition of relative remission for years. However, one study showed a relapse rate of 80% in the first year with gradual withdrawal of the drug, compared with 17 of 19 who remained in remission when no change in dosage was made.[52] Further study is needed to evaluate the utility of intermittent therapy. CBC, platelet count, and urinalysis should be monitored every 2 weeks for 6 months. This interval may be gradually lengthened thereafter.

The earliest use of an antifolate for the treatment of nonmalignant diseases was reported by Gubner et al.,[53] who, in 1951, successfully treated patients with RA and psoriatic arthritis with aminopterin. The introduction of steroids in the early 1950s diverted attention away from the use of antifolates in RA. At that timer, however, aminopterin's less toxic replacement—methotrexate—was used for the treatment of psoriasis. Interestingly, in a subset of patients with psoriasis, improvement in both skin and joints was observed, but it was not until the 1980s that methotrexate became an acceptable option in the treatment of rheumatoid arthritis.[54]

A number of clinical trials have provided evidence that methotrexate is effective in RA. It has a significant antiinflammatory effect within 3 to 4 weeks after start of therapy; it is taken 1 day a week in doses of 5 to 20 mg, depending on efficacy and toxic reactions.[55] Weinblatt et al.[56] showed that after 84 months of treatment methotrexate remained effective.

In RA patients treated with low doses of methotrexate once a week, inhibition of dihydrofolate reductase is incomplete and perhaps is not essential for efficacy.[57] As polyglutamates of methotrexate are direct inhibitors of thymidylate synthase and folate-dependent enzymes of purine biosynthesis, efficacy of methotrexate may involve blockage of these pathways. It has been hypothesized that one such blockade alters purine biosynthesis, producing immunosuppression by secondary inhibition of crucial enzymes and perhaps also by decreasing leukotriene production and interleukin-1 expression.[58,59] The actual mechanism of action of the drug has not yet been clarified.

Methotrexate is cleared through the kidneys. Thus one must decrease the dosage in patients with mild renal insufficiency to offset the higher risk of adverse effects. The drug should not be used in patients with renal failure or in patients on dialysis. Reported adverse effects include stomatitis, nausea, vomiting, diarrhea, usually reversible bone marrow suppression, teratogenesis, pulmonary symptoms, and, rarely, liver fibrosis and cirrhosis.[55] Rare pulmonary hypersensitivity reactions (cough, progressive dyspnea, and markedly decreased oxygenation) usually will improve with prompt discontinuance of the drug and corticosteroid therapy.[55] Methotrexate may be associated with occasional systemic fungal infections and other unusual infections.

The frequent side effects led one group to conclude that toxicity, rather than lack of efficacy, is the major factor limiting the clinical usefulness of methotrexate. However, 1 mg of folate per day reduced the toxicity experienced with a median weekly methotrexate dose of 7.5 mg without altering the efficacy of methotrexate.[57] Risk factors for methotrexate-induced hepatic cirrhosis include long duration of treatment with methotrexate, age, and possibly ethanol abuse. Coadministration of an NSAID has been rarely associated with leukopenia and thrombocytopenia, perhaps because of an NSAID-induced decrease in glomerular filtration and inhibition of renal tubular secretion of methotrexate, both of which cause a reduction in methotrexate clearance.[55] Methotrexate toxicity may be diminished by giving folic acid (1 mg daily) or folinic acid (leucovorin), 5 mg, 8 to 12 hours after the weekly dose of methotrexate.[55]

Many physicians use the weaker antifolate, sulfasalazine, for patients with mild RA; it is one of the few drugs originally developed to treat RA.[60] It has been postulated that its mechanism of action may be similar to that of methotrexate. Although several studies have indicated that sulfasalazine is effective for RA, one study was unable to separate sulfasalazine from placebo because of an unusually high placebo response.[60]

Sulfasalazine is a chemical combination of a salicylate and a sulfa moiety and is thus contraindicated in patients with sulfa or salicylate allergies. Side effects include gastrointestinal upset, rash, hemolytic disease, agranulocytosis, drug-induced hepatitis, and rare instances of lupuslike illness.[60] A number of studies have indicated that the rate of discontinuation of sulfasalazine is comparable to (or better than) that of other DMARDs. One recent study showed a continuation rate at 5 years of 22%.[61] (By way of contrast, the continuation rate of gold injections at 5 years was 8%.) The usual starting dose of sulfasalazine is 500 mg or 1000 mg/d, slowly raised to 2 or 3 g/d over a 4- to 6-week period—an approach that may decrease the incidence of adverse reactions.[61]

Azathioprine is an immunosuppressive drug. Used in concert with steroids, it has been standard therapy for inhibition of organ transplant rejection. Its use is suggested in patients with rheumatoid arthritis who have not responded to conventional therapy. Dosage usually is begun at 1.0 mg/kg/d and gradually increased to no more than 2.5 mg/kg/d. The white blood cell count should be monitored and should not be allowed to fall below 3000 cells/mm^3. Dosage should be increased as tolerated, if necessary, to control the arthritis. Improvement may begin by 12 weeks, but studies have suggested that improvement often does not plateau until 6 months or longer.[62]

The undesirable adverse effect of greatest concern when azathioprine is used over a long period is the potential for lymphoreticular cancer.[63] However, there is no proof that this drug is associated with a risk beyond the risk associated with the disease itself. Other adverse effects include hepatotoxicity, leukopenia (more often than thrombocytopenia or anemia), superimposed opportunistic infections, nausea, and a macrocytic anemia.[64] The clinician may decide to forego the use of azathioprine in a patient with a strong family history of non-Hodgkin's lymphoma or a personal history of malignant disease. Full discussion of the potential risks is mandatory before one prescribes azathioprine as well as other DMARDs.

CORTICOSTEROIDS

Therapeutic administration of corticosteroids produces rapid, potent, and reliable suppression of inflammation, the extent and duration of which depend on the dose, the dosing schedule, and the length of treatment. Their unsurpassed short-term efficacy and versatility have made corticosteroids a key element in the treatment of many rheumatic diseases.

Corticosteroids enter target cells and couple with a specific cytoplasmic receptor before transfer to the nucleus, where the corticosteroid-receptor complex binds to chromatin and modulates protein synthesis.[65] Corticosteroids decrease collagen synthesis and impair wound healing, augment gluconeogenesis and glycogen deposition while inhibiting the action of insulin, impair lipogenesis and stimulate lipolysis in adipose tissue, and increase liver synthesis of protein while enhancing its peripheral catabolism. They have a profound effect on bone metabolism through interference with intestinal absorption of calcium, inhibition of osteoblast collagen synthesis, elevation of parathyroid hormone levels resulting in amplification of osteoclast bone resorption, and enhanced renal calcium excretion.[66]

Corticosteroids have a short-term effect on inflammation, probably mediated by interfering with the inflammatory and immune cascade at the following levels:

- Impairment of antigen opsonization
- Interference with inflammatory cell adhesion and migration through vascular endothelium
- Interruption of cell-cell communication by altering the release or antagonizing the action of cytokines
- Impairment of leukotriene and prostaglandin synthesis
- Inhibition of neutrophil superoxide production.[66]

Corticosteroids decrease immunoglobulin generation, inhibit immune clearance of sensitized erythrocytes, and impair the transit of immune complexes across basement membranes.[67]

Cortisol is the prototype for the available synthetic corticosteroids. Minor structural modifications of this parent hormone have led to the creation of a panel of drugs with a wide spectrum of plasma half-lives, antiinflammatory potency, and mineralocorticoid effect (Table 3–3). Corticosteroids have biologic half-lives that are 2 to 36 times longer than their plasma half-lives, but the onset of biologic effect lags behind peak plasma levels. Corticosteroids are widely and rapidly distributed in tissues.

In general, increasing doses and dosing frequencies of corticosteroids correspond to enhanced inflammatory suppression, more rapid onset of therapeutic benefits, and increased side effects. Thus doses given several times a day are more potent than once-a-day dosing. When disease control is required in a timely but nonurgent manner, once-daily oral dosing, given in the morning to minimize adrenal suppression, is adequate. Prednisone is most frequently used for RA, the usual dose being 5 mg to 15 mg daily, a dose often used for long periods. Tapering should be gradual to avoid disease flares; serial reductions of 0.5 mg to 1.0 mg per day every few weeks to months should be tried when daily doses are below 10 to 15 mg/d. Dose reduction should not be more frequent than the time required to detect a steroid dose–related exacerbation of disease activity, which in rheumatoid arthritis can be as short as a few days. In the case of doses below 10 mg/d, the reduction interval must be long enough to

TABLE 3–3
Glucocorticoid Preparations

DRUG	RELATIVE ANTI-INFLAMMATORY POTENCY	SODIUM-RETAINING POTENCY	EQUIVALENT DOSE (mg)	BIOLOGIC HALF-LIFE (h)
Short-acting				
Hydrocortisone	1	2+	20	8–12
Cortisone	0.8	2+	25	8–12
Prednisone	4	1+	5	12–36
Prednisolone	4	1+	5	12–36
Methylprednisolone	5	0	4	12–36
Triamcinolone	5	0	4	12–36
Long-acting				
Betamethasone	20–30	0	0.6	36–54
Dexamethasone	20–30	0	0.75	36–54

allow incremental recovery of adrenal function; the interval increases with the duration of corticosteroid therapy. Alternate-day administration of short-acting preparations such as prednisone usually avoids the adverse cushingoid and adrenal suppressive effects seen with more frequent doses, but it is of limited usefulness in RA because symptoms usually exacerbate during the day without steroids.

In the situation in which rapid amelioration of damaging inflammation is desired, treatment can be initiated with a short course or even a single dose of high-dose corticosteroid. Pulsed doses of methylprednisolone, 1 g intravenously daily for 1 to 3 days, has been proven to show efficacy in the treatment of RA.[68] Profound effects on lymphocyte function may occur, leading to a prolonged effect on disease activity. Interestingly, 100 mg and 300 mg doses given intravenously also have been shown to be as effective, or nearly as effective, as 1 g doses.[69] Intravenous therapy appears to relieve symptoms for about 3 to 6 weeks, but there is no evidence that it changes the underlying course of the disease.[69]

Prolonged administration of corticosteroids leads to generalized adrenal suppression and the development of unwanted side effects. The severity of these side effects depends on the maximum dose, the dosage schedule, the duration of treatment or the cumulative dose, and the type of corticosteroid used. Accelerated osteoporosis with pathologic fractures may occur. Supplemental calcium and vitamin D may slow this process.[68] See Chapter 22 for guidelines in this area.

Exogenous administration of corticosteroids can stop native adrenal corticosteroid production through effects on the pituitary-adrenal axis; in the face of stressors, addisonian crisis and shock may develop. The chances of developing adrenal suppression increase as:

- Doses exceed the average daily equivalent output of the adrenal glands of 5.0 to 7.5 mg prednisone
- Therapy continues for more than a few weeks or months
- Doses are given late in the day or in split doses
- Long-acting corticosteroid preparations are used.

Adrenal suppression can sometimes develop with short courses and low doses of corticosteroid. If doubt exists, an adrenocorticotropic hormone stimulation test or a metyrapone test may be performed to determine whether pituitary and adrenal functions are preserved before discontinuation of corticosteroid treatment. A recent study of factors related to corticosteroid therapy and recovery of the hypothalamic-pituitary-adrenal (HPA) axis in patients receiving 10 mg or less of prednisone was performed with a single injection of synthetic ACTH and measurement of cortisol levels; current steroid therapy was the only significant factor determining HPA axis integrity. Subjects receiving 5 mg or more had varied responses to ACTH, whereas patients receiving less than 5 mg of prednisone daily displayed a normal stimulation response. The investigators speculated that spontaneous recovery of the HPA axis is expected for rheumatic disease patients taking 5 mg or less of prednisone daily.[70] However, normalization of the adrenal response to stress may be markedly delayed, and intravenous administration of hydrocortisone during general anesthesia is prudent for at least 1 year after the last dose of corticosteroids.

The inhibitory effect of corticosteroids on inflammatory and immune responses results in increased risk of bacterial and opportunistic infections, such as tuberculosis, *Pneumocystis carinii,* and fungi. Effects on glucose and protein metabolism may cause hyperglycemia, centripetal fat deposition leading to rounded facies and a cervical fat pad, and hyperlipidemia. They can cause hypokalemia, fluid retention, edema, and hypertension. Cutaneous problems include capillary fragility with petechiae and easy bruising, acne, hirsutism, impaired wound healing, hyperhidrosis, and striae. Glaucoma and cataract formation are further complications, as are myopathy, possible ulcerogenicity, pancreatitis, premature atherosclerosis, avascular necrosis of bone, psychiatric disturbances, and bowel or diverticular perforations. High-dose steroids can mask the symptoms of other inflammatory processes, making diagnosis difficult. One-gram pulses may induce cardiac arrhythmia in hypokalemic patients and may result in the hematogenous dissemination of previously localized infections. Concomitant illnesses or previous adverse reactions may guide the physician in prescribing corticosteroids. For example, a patient with known hypertension may better tolerate a corticosteroid that has a lower mineralocorticoid effect.

An alternative to (long-term) oral therapy is the occasional use of intraarticular injections.[68] It has been noted that injection of the equivalent of 10 to 20 mg of prednisone sometimes gives relief in the injected joint for up to 10 weeks.[68] Because the drug diffuses systemically, there may be systemic effects, including a generalized improvement (albeit short-term) in the patient's arthritis. However, there are no specific side effects. Hollander documented crystal-induced synovitis in about 1% of patients; 0.01% may have intraarticular infections (although the figure is undoubtedly lower today with modern disposable equipment), and a small number of patients may have ligamentous rupture.[68] Apparently, crystal-induced synovitis occurs less often with triamcinolone hexacetonide and other modern intraarticular preparations.[68] The danger here is to avoid chronic therapy with repeated, regular monthly intraarticular injections (albeit into different joints). This form of treatment often brings the patient back into the office because of the "wearing off" of systemic effects of glucocorticoids in the weeks following the joint injection. However, the use of repeated injections in this manner is equivalent to monthly intramuscular corticosteroid administration and should be recognized for what it is and avoided for chronic, long-term therapy because other alternatives are available (see below).

TREATMENT STRATEGIES FOR RHEUMATOID ARTHRITIS

The traditional pyramid approach to RA therapy has been challenged; earlier use of DMARDs has been suggested. The concept of "waiting" months or years for a natural remission while the patient takes NSAIDs alone is thought today to be counterproductive; disability and functional loss appear early in RA and the delay of aggressive management is thought by most rheumatologists to be inappropriate. Although proof for this approach is lacking, rheumatologists today will institute a DMARD or DMARDs once the diagnosis of rheumatoid arthritis is secure. Of course, the ideal drug should provide maximal efficacy with minimal toxicity (in both the short and long terms). Felson et al.[43] found, in a recent meta-analysis of published clinical trials, that antimalarial drugs and methotrexate had the best balance of efficacy and toxicity in the treatment of RA. Azathioprine scored in the intermediate range in terms of both efficacy and toxicity. Injectable gold was the most toxic drug, and auranofin was among the weakest. Long-term observational studies using drug termination as the measure of overall drug appeal indicate that methotrexate and antimalarial drugs are the drugs that patients are the most likely to continue taking for several years. The strong DMARDs were found to be injectable gold, D-penicillamine, methotrexate, and sulfasalazine.

Patients with aggressive synovitis develop radiographically evident joint damage in the first 2 years of disease; nearly 50% become disabled within 5 years after onset of disease,[71] 90% by 30 years.[72] Life expectancy may be shortened by 10 to 15 years, particularly in patients with severe disease or extraarticular complications.[14] An emerging school of thought believes that, to prevent such morbidity, early control of inflammation and the disease itself is critical; this conflicts with the 5 to 8 years usually required to traverse the therapeutic pyramid.[73] Thus, as patient and physician work their way up the pyramid, considerable delay occurs and there is irreversible joint damage leading to severe functional impairment and likely premature death.

In addition, the perceived success of the traditional pyramid approach is based on the assumption that short-term clinical responsiveness to drugs (demonstrated in clinical trials) is equivalent to long-term control. The paradox of short-term success and long-term failure is based on factors inherent in clinical trial methods, including exclusion criteria in drug studies, emphasis on marginal benefits with large numbers of patients, and failure to adjust for patient dropout in drug studies.[74] Aside from corticosteroids and methotrexate, fewer than 20% of patients remain on single-agent therapy longer than 3 years because of lack of effectiveness, toxicity, or "escape from control."[75] Clinical trials demonstrating efficacy usually run for 1 year or less, whereas more protracted observational studies show increasing morbidity after most drugs have been discontinued by patients or have lost their effect.[72] Remission in aggressive RA is unusual, and sustained control of inflammation is rare.[76] Not surprisingly, many gains in patient function over the past 15 years can be attributed to joint replacement.[77]

A number of paradigms have been brought forward to replace the therapeutic pyramid. Some prospective and retrospective studies have suggested that combinations of DMARDs are adequately tolerated and may be more efficacious than high doses of a single agent.[78] If the combination therapy is introduced within the first year or two after diagnosis, it is thought to be even more effective. Methotrexate, azathioprine, and hydroxychloroquine in combination were found to be well tolerated and more effective than any one agent alone in uncontrolled studies. Other studies have suggested that methotrexate and auranofin, methotrexate and sulfasalazine, sulfasalazine and D-penicillamine, and methotrexate and injectable gold are useful combinations.[79] However, in randomized, double-blind, controlled trials, the superiority of combination therapy over monotherapy has been difficult to prove.[79]

Another proposed substitute for the traditional pyramid is Wilske and Healey's "step-down bridge" approach.[73] Patients are screened with a medium (10 to 20 mg/d) dose of prednisone. Patients in whom disease is not promptly suppressed or patients in whom prednisone cannot be tapered to lower dosages after 1 month are given a combination that includes methotrexate, azathioprine, gold, auranofin, and hydroxychloroquine. As disease is controlled, the most potentially toxic drugs are sequentially withdrawn; it is thus hoped that long-term maintenance control of disease can be achieved with less toxic drugs, such as hydroxychloroquine or auranofin. Approximately 60 patients have been entered into this paradigm; those with disease duration of less than 2 years have done well, although reduction to monotherapy has not been possible.[79]

The graduated-step approach stages RA as mild, moderate, or severe.[80] Mild disease is treated with hydroxychloroquine plus an NSAID. Moderate disease is treated with the same, plus auranofin, sulfasalazine, or methotrexate; these patients may also be given low doses of prednisone. Patients with severe disease may be given up to three DMARDs, including the three given to those with moderate disease, plus D-penicillamine, injectable gold, or azathioprine. This approach, although not explicitly stated or described, is probably what many rheumatologists use today. The goal is to limit the number of swollen, tender joints to four or less. Others have suggested "debulking" severe synovitis with a short course of nitrogen mustard or pulses of methylprednisone as an adjunct to other therapies. This latter approach is less accepted today.

It is doubtful that one treatment strategy or a single treatment modality will be the best therapy for all patients with RA. However, the consensus is growing that all therapeutic regimens should emphasize early control of disease, with the hope of a resultant sustained improved function. Interestingly, most patients favor a more aggressive approach; one study reported that patients would accept a 21% risk of death in exchange for a cure and a 17% risk of death for relief of pain.[81] However, the willingness to accept risk decreases with decreased disease duration and with functional improvement as measured by self-assessment questionnaires. It should be emphasized that patient acceptance of risk may be heavily influenced by the way it is presented by the physician.

Many believe that RA is more or less fully explained by the so-called immunopathogenic model: the inheritance of certain motifs in the major histocompatibility complex (either by their effect on the T cell repertoire or through their capacity to present specific environmentally derived antigens or antigens localized in the joint) results in an abnormal immune response and cytokine cascade, which uses infiltrating chronic inflammatory cells and normal synovial cells to cause chronic inflammation and thus tissue damage in RA. In this situation, the "biologicals," such as cytokines and their inhibitors, antibodies to T cell subsets and adhesion molecules, oral antigen ingestion, substitute peptides for major histocompatibility complex presentation, etc., should allow interference in immune response and cytokine activities so that disease might be controlled.[82]

Of course, the immunopathogenic theory may not be completely accurate. Others believe that the immune disturbance and "inflammation" actually follow the onset of cartilage destruction.[83] For example, oncogenes activated by retroviruses may switch on catalytic enzymes within cartilage and synovial cells; the product of this reaction then stimulates an immune response, which promotes chronicity. Interestingly, there are patients with little apparent histologic inflammation who exhibit progressive

TABLE 3–4
Some New and Novel Therapies for Rheumatoid Arthritis

I. Biological Response Modifiers
  A. Noncytotoxic
    1. Cytokine modifiers: interferon gamma
    2. Growth factors: GMCSF, GCSF, EPO
    3. Cytokines
      a. IL1 (receptor antagonist, soluble receptor)
      b. TNF (murine MAB, soluble receptor)
    4. Activation antigens
    5. Adhesion molecules (murine MAB)
    6. T cell vaccination
    7. Oral tolerance
  B. Cytotoxic
    1. IL2R (fusion toxins, murine MAB)
    2. T cell
      a. CD4 (murine and chimeric MAB)
      b. CD5 (immunoconjugate MAB)
      c. CD7 (murine MAB)
      d. CDw52 (humanized MAB)
II. Immunosuppressors
  A. Noncytotoxic
    1. Cyclosporin A
    2. FK 506
    3. Rapamycin
    4. Immunoglobulin therapy (IV Ig)
    5. Extracorporeal protein immunoadsorption
    6. Extracorporeal photochemotherapy
  B. Cytotoxic
    1. Mycophenolate Mofitil
III. Immunomodulators
  A. Levamisole
IV. Arachidonic Acid Metabolite Modifiers
  A. Tenidap
  B. 5-Lipoxygenase inhibitors
    1. Zileuton
V. Antioxidants
  A. Vitamin E
  B. Fish oil
VI. Inhibitors of Cartilage Catabolism
  A. Metalloproteinase inhibitors
VII. Antibiotic
  A. Minocycline

Ziff M. Rheumatoid arthritis—its present and future. J Rheumatol 1990;17(2).

Miller-Blair DJ, Robbins DL. Rheumatoid arthritis: new science, new treatment. Geriatrics 1993;48(6).

joint destruction. The aforementioned "biologicals" would not necessarily be of benefit in such a senario.[83]

At least in the immediate future, management of RA will be focused on control as opposed to cure.[84] The therapeutic repertoire will be larger, allowing one to combine older therapies with newer experimental agents.

One newer therapy is cyclosporin A, a noncytotoxic, immunomodulating agent that primarily inhibits the activation of T helper-inducer lymphocytes by blocking IL-2 production; it also inhibits production of γ-interferon and IL-3. It has been shown to be effective in open and randomized short-term trials; patients experience disease flare on withdrawal.[85–87] Side effects include acute and chronic nephrotoxicity, neurotoxicity (hyperesthesia, tingling, nervousness, tinnitus, and tremor), hypertension, and hypertrichosis. The dose probably should not exceed 5 mg/kg/d; once a stable dose is established, laboratory monitoring should be done monthly. The role for cyclosporin A in RA has not been defined, and the drug is not yet approved for this indication by the U.S. Food and Drug Administration.

Other newer treatment modalities are undergoing clinical trials, and are listed in Table 3–4.

AUTHORS' APPROACHES TO MANAGEMENT OF RHEUMATOID ARTHRITIS PATIENTS

Our personal approach to the management of RA is illustrated in the following hypothetical cases. It is risky to describe a "cookbook" approach because RA management blends the art of medicine with a thorough understanding of the scientific basis of the pharmaceutical and physical interventions available for its treatment. Optimal management requires that both the physician and the patient understand the character of the disease in that particular patient, its interactions with the patient's life situation, the vagaries of the disease course, and its response to treatment. It is essential that the physician and the patient are honest with and trust each other. If this feeling of confidence and trust has not developed after the first few visits, the patient should find a more compatible physician; no single physician can be "right" for all patients.

We will assume that each of the hypothetical patients is coming to us for the first time, although some have had much previous therapy. As discussed earlier in this chapter, whole-body rest is one of the most important and least understood components of RA treatment. For all RA patients, we spend most of the first several visits determining how their life situation affects their ability to obtain adequate rest and to deal with the disease. This includes *prescribing* specific additional hours of bed rest to demonstrate its value to the patient. Splinting of appropriate inflamed joints, joint protection, and range-of-motion exercises are initiated at the same time. NSAID doses are optimized; the NSAID is changed and adjunctive therapy to improve gastric tolerance is added if indicated. DMARDs are discussed but are not added or changed until we are satisfied that the patient has mastered the basic program.

HYPOTHETICAL CASE 1: New-onset RA, seropositive, functional, and working. This patient is cautioned to avoid overcommitment that may lead to physical exhaustion and exacerbation of the RA. Additional rest is scheduled, but the patient can continue to work. With relatively mild synovitis and no joint erosions, if spontaneous remission does not occur after 1 to 3 months of basic therapy, we would add a relatively low-risk DMARD such as hydroxychloroquine or sulfasalazine. In this seropositive patient without joint erosions, x-ray films of hands and feet may be obtained every 6 months until the first definite erosion is found. The appearance of the first erosion in a well functioning patient or an otherwise unacceptable level of pain, stiffness, or diminished function are indications for a more aggressive approach. At this point we usually will add injectable gold or oral methotrexate to the first DMARD in an attempt to produce a drug-induced remission.

HYPOTHETICAL CASE 2: New-onset RA, nonfunctional, devastated by the illness, many systemic features such as marked fatigue and weight loss. The explosive onset of severe, disabling, polyarticular synovitis does not necessarily imply a poor prognosis, particularly if the rheumatoid factor is negative and no joint erosions are present. Ideally, this patient should receive 10 days to 2 weeks of inpatient treatment with intensive bed rest (up to 16 or 18 hours per day), education, passive and active physical and occupational therapy, and pharmaceutical therapy. However, hospitalization is ideal but rarely practical or affordable. Full-dose NSAID therapy will probably control the fever and help to cool the joints. Corticosteroid injections of several joints, a 1- to 3-day course of intravenous minipulse corticosteroid therapy, or both, could be used and will sup-

press the synovitis and expedite physical therapy. If the patient is seropositive or if erosions or nodules are present, methotrexate is started immediately, with rapid increase to a maximum tolerated dose of 15 to 25 mg/wk—intramuscularly if necessary. Plaquenil could be added to the methotrexate regimen. Folic acid, 1 mg daily, or leucovorin (folinic acid), 5 mg, is added 8 to 12 hours after the methotrexate dose if needed to improve tolerance. If the patient is seronegative and nonerosive, hydroxychloroquine is started, with methotrexate held in reserve to use if a lot of improvement is not seen after 3 or 4 months. Joint injections (or intravenous corticosteroid pulses) are given as needed (but cautiously) for the first 3 or 4 months, but we try to avoid daily oral prednisone. Most patients will be markedly improved in 3 or 4 months, and some will be in remission by the end of the first year.

HYPOTHETICAL CASE 3: Active RA after failure of one or two second-line drugs. This is a very common situation among patients with RA who are referred to us, and our response depends on the details of the prior "failed" treatment program. Many patients abandon a DMARD if they have not had dramatic improvement in 3 or 4 months or if they experience relatively minor side effects. Generally we do not consider a DMARD to have failed until adequate doses have been used for 1 year or a major adverse effect has occurred, so we sometimes continue the "failed" treatment with adjustments in dosage, concomitant therapies, and insistence on the basic program of increased rest and physical therapy. Many patients have a gratifying response to this program. If the RA is particularly active, with rapidly progressing erosions, we would try to control it with higher-dose weekly parenteral methotrexate (20 to 35 mg intramuscularly per week) and, on rare occasions, monthly 1 g pulses of intravenous methylprednisolone. Azathioprine or injectable gold or sulfasalazine may be added to the regimen at this time.

HYPOTHETICAL CASE 4: Long-standing RA, all drugs failed, many steroid side effects. The general approach is similar to that with Case 3, except that we have the additional debilitation of prolonged poorly controlled RA and long-term steroid use. The patient must be considered to have active disease with progressing erosions, even if the steroids are suppressing the usual signs of joint inflammation. (Serial joint x-rays will document the progression of joint damage in these patients.) We start with the basic program of increased bed rest balanced with exercise. In this patient, exercise of some sort is particularly important; we find that pool therapy three times a week is most helpful if it can be arranged. The degree of osteoporosis is documented and appropriate therapy is initiated (see Chapter 22). For such patients, the benefits of daily prednisone are vanishingly small and the adverse effects are obvious, even to the patient, but attempts to decrease the dose cause immediate flare-ups of discomfort and synovitis. However, if the patient can tolerate it, the withdrawal-induced flare-up will subside after a variable time that depends on the magnitude of the dosage decrement. We explain this to the patient and then try to find a dosage decrement that causes a flare-up for only 3 to 7 days. This decrease in dosage can then be repeated every 2 to 4 weeks without causing any deterioration in the basic control of the RA. If the flare-up has not subsided after 2 to 4 weeks, the next decrease in dose is delayed, but we ask the patients not to increase the prednisone dosage. When the flare-up eventually subsides, the dosage decrease schedule is resumed. The size of the decrements depends partly on the patient's tolerance, the starting dosage, and the duration of prior steroid therapy. Usually we can decrease prednisone by 1 mg at a time if the daily dose is more than 12 mg and by 0.5 mg if it is between 5 mg and 12 mg. Below 5 mg daily doses, one must allow time for adrenal recovery after each dose reduction, and we often use more gradual dose-reduction programs, sometimes reducing by 0.5 mg on one additional day each week, taking 7 weeks to decrease the daily dose by 0.5 mg. Patients who have taken daily steroids for more than 10 years may have permanently suppressed adrenal glands, in which case they will need 3.5 mg to 4.5 mg of prednisone daily forever. The steroid-reduction program will not be successful if the disease activity cannot be controlled with other agents.

We review the reasons for failure of the previously tried DMARDs and usually find one or two agents that can be tried again and continued for a longer time at a higher or lower dosage, or with adjunctive therapy such as leucovorin with high-dose methotrexate. Sometimes a patient will respond to low-dose cyclosporin or will be entered in a protocol to evaluate a new investigational therapy. Treating a Case 4 patient takes several years and requires a major commitment by both the physician and the patient. The results are usually incomplete, as the patient will continue to have substantial disability from the cumulative RA damage, but the patient generally is grateful to have gotten off the slippery slope of ever-increasing steroid side effects and is a much better candidate for reconstructive surgical procedures.

HYPOTHETICAL CASE 5: Older male patient with acute seronegative polyarthritis. In this case, rheumatologists in Europe have found sulfasalazine to be a powerful tool in the treatment of the elderly patient with active rheumatoid arthritis. Some in the United States consider this to be a variant of polymyalgia rheumatica (PMR) and use prednisone to treat it, avoiding NSAIDs because of their increased gastrointestinal toxicity in the elderly. If the major complaints are of shoulder and/or hip girdle pain, associated with a very high erythrocyte sedimentation rate and only mild small-joint synovitis, we would treat the condition like PMR with corticosteroids, beginning with doses at the 10 to 15 mg/d level and then tapering (see Chapter 11). If small-joint synovitis is prominent and symmetrical, we would treat it like RA, using sulfasalazine first and adding small doses of methotrexate if the response is poor. It may be necessary to use small doses of prednisone (5 mg for women, 7.5 mg for men) in a patient at high risk for NSAID use or who is intolerant of NSAIDs. If predominantly large joints are involved, particularly if involvement is asymmetrical, we would search diligently for chronic calcium crystal deposition disease and treat with NSAIDs and prophylactic colchicine, 0.6 mg once or twice a day.

SUMMARY

In all cases, we see patients more frequently than the long intervals recommended by managed-care algorithms. Frequent hands-on personal interactions between the patient and the physician are essential to maintain the patient's confidence and commitment to the difficult treatment regimens and to permit timely adjustments to deal with changing circumstances. In the long run, these frequent brief outpatient visits are much more cost-effective than the increased probability of disability and hospitalizations associated with inadequate care.

REFERENCES

1. Hochberg MC. Adult and juvenile rheumatoid arthritis: current epidemiologic concepts. Epidemiol Rev 1981;3:27.
2. Harris ED. The clinical features of rheumatoid arthritis. In: Kelley WN, Harris ED Jr, Ruddy S, Sledge CB, eds. Textbook of rheumatology. 4th ed. Philadelphia: WB Saunders, 1993:874.
3. Harvald B, Hauge M. In Genetics and the epidemiology of chronic diseases. Washington, DC: US Government Printing Office, 1965:61.
4. Nunez G, Moore SE, Ball GV, et al. Study of HLA antigens in ten multiple-case rheumatoid arthritis families. J Rheumatol 1984;11:129.
5. Christiansen FT, Kelly H, Dawkins RL. Rheumatoid arthritis. In: Albert ED, Baur MP, Mayr WR, eds. Histocompatibility testing. Berlin: Springer-Verlag, 1984:378.
6. Fleming A, Benn RT, Corbett M, Wood PHN. Early rheumatoid disease. II. Patterns of joint involvement. Ann Rheum Dis 1976;35:361.
7. Hurd ER. Extra-articular manifestations of rheumatoid arthritis. Semin Rheum Dis 1979; 8:151.
8. Wolfe F, Hawley DJ. Remission in rheumatoid arthritis. J Rheumatol 1985;12:245.
9. Van der Grouche JP, Hazevoct HM, Cats A. Survival and cause of death in rheumatoid arthritis: a 25-year prospective follow-up. J Rheumatol 1984;11:158.
10. Sherrer YS, Block DA, Mitchell DM, et al. The development of disability in rheumatoid arthritis. Arthritis Rheum 1986;29:494.
11. Luukkainen R, Isumaki H, Kajander A. Prognostic value of the type of onset of rheumatoid arthritis. Ann Rheum Dis 1983;42:274.
12. Sharp JT, Calkins E, Cohen AS, et al. Observations on the clinical, chemical, and serologic manifestations of rheumatoid arthritis, based on the course of 154 cases. Medicine 1964;43:41.
13. Mitchell DM, Spitz PW, Young DY, et al. Survival, prognosis, and causes of death in rheumatoid arthritis. Arthritis Rheum 1986;29:706.
14. Pincus T, Callahan LF. Taking mortality in rheumatoid arthritis seriously—predictive markers, socioeconomic status and comorbidity. J Rheumatol 1986;13:841.
15. Kellgren JH, O'Brien WM. On the natural history of rheumatoid arthritis in relation to the sheep cell agglutination test. Arthritis Rheum 1962;5:115.
16. Jacoby RK, Jayson MIV, Cosh JA. Onset, early stages and prognosis of rheumatoid arthritis: a clinical study of 100 patients with 11-year follow-up. Br Med J 1973;2:96.
17. Gault SJ, Spyker JM. Beneficial effect of immobilization of joints in rheumatoid arthritis and related arthritides: a splint study using sequential analysis. Arthritis Rheum 1969;12:34.
18. McCarty DJ. Treatment of rheumatoid joint inflammation with triamcinolone hexacetomide. Arthritis Rheum 1972;15:157.
19. Clements PJ, Paulus HE. Non-steroidal anti-inflammatory drugs. In: Kelley WN, Harris ED Jr, Ruddy S, Sledge CB, eds. Textbook of rheumatology. 4th ed. Philadelphia: WB Saunders, 1993:700.
20. Schlegel SI, Paulus HE. NSAIDs—use in rheumatic disease, side effects and interactions. Bull Rheum Dis 1986;36:1.
21. Katz LM, Love PY. NSAIDs and the liver. In: Famaey JP, Paulus HE, eds. Clinical applications of NSAIDs, subpopulation therapy and new formulations. New York: Marcel Dekker, 1992: 247.
22. Blackshear JL, Napier JS, Davidman M, et al. Renal complications of NSAIDs. Arch Intern Med 1985;143:1130.
23. Furst DE, Blocka K, Cassell S, et al. A strategy for reaching therapeutic salicylate levels in patients with rheumatoid arthritis using standardized dosing regimens. J Rheumatol 1987;14: 342.
24. Day RO, Furst DE, Dromgoole SH, et al. Changes in salicylate serum concentration and metabolism during chronic dosing in normal volunteers. Biopharm Drug Dispos 1988;9:273.
25. Paulus HE. Aspirin versus nonacetylated salicylates [Editorial]. J Rheumatol 1989;16:264.
26. Cooperating Clinics of the New York Chapter of the Arthritis Foundation. A retrospective look at prescribing practice of NSAIDs in rheumatoid arthritis [Abstract]. Proceedings of Eighth Pan-American Congress of Rheumatology, San Francisco, June 7, 1982.
27. Broader RN, Heel RL, Speight TM, et al. Tolmetin: a review of its pharmacological properties and therapeutic efficacy in rheumatic diseases. Drugs 1978;15:429.
28. Furst DE, Blocka K, Cassell S, et al. A controlled study of concurrent therapy with a nonacetylated salicylate and naproxen in rheumatoid arthritis. Arthritis Rheum 1987;30:146.
29. Iannuzzi L, Dawson N, Zein N, et al. Does drug therapy slow radiographic deterioration in rheumatoid arthritis? N Engl J Med 1983;309: 1023.
30. Forestier J. Rheumatoid arthritis and its treatment with gold salts. J Lab Clin Med 1935;20: 827.
31. Research Subcommittee of the Empire Rheumatism Council. Gold therapy in rheumatoid arthritis. Ann Rheum Dis 1960;19:95.
32. Blocka K, Paulus HE. The clinical pharmacology of the gold compounds. In: Paulus HE, Furst DE, Dromgoole SH, eds. Drugs for rheumatic disease. New York: Churchill Livingstone, 1987:49.
33. Gordon DA. Gold compounds in the rheumatic diseases. In: Kelley WN, Harris ED Jr, Ruddy S,

Sledge CB, eds. Textbook of rheumatology. 4th ed. Philadelphia: WB Saunders, 1993:743.

34. Lipsky PE, Ugai K, Ziff M. Alterations in human monocyte structure and function induced by incubation with gold sodium thiomalate. J Rheumatol 1979;6(suppl 5):130.

35. Paulus HE. Government affairs: FDA Arthritis Advisory Committee meeting: Auranofin. Arthritis Rheum 1985;28:450.

36. Wickens S, Paulus HE. Antimalarial drugs. In: Paulus HE, Furst DE, and Dromgoole SH, eds. Drugs for rheumatic disease. New York: Churchill Livingstone, 1987:113.

37. Rynes RI. Antimalarial drugs. In: Kelley WN, Harris ED Jr, Ruddy S, Sledge CB, eds. Textbook of rheumatology. 4th ed. Philadelphia: WB Saunders, 1993:731.

38. Felson DT, Anderson JJ, Meenan RF. Use of short-term efficacy/toxicity trade-offs to select second-line drugs in rheumatoid arthritis. Arthritis Rheum 1992;35:1117.

39. Fox RI, Kang H. Mechanism of action of antimalarial drugs: inhibition of antigen processing and presentation. Lupus 1993;2(suppl 1):S-9.

40. Guidos C, Wong M, Lee KC. A comparison of the stimulatory activities of lymphoid dendritic cells and macrophages in T proliferative responses to various antigens. J Immunol 1984; 133:1179.

41. Runge LA. Risk/benefit analysis of hydroxychloroquine sulfate treatment in rheumatoid arthritis. Am J Med 1983;75(1A):52.

42. Bernstein HN. Ophthalmologic considerations and testing in patients receiving long-term antimalarial therapy. Am J Med 1983;75(1A):25.

43. Felson DT, Anderson JJ, Meenan RF. The comparative efficacy and toxicity of second-line drugs in rheumatoid arthritis. Arthritis Rheum 1990;33:1449.

44. Davis MJ, Dawes PT, Fowler PD, Clarke S, Fisher J, Shadforth MF. Should disease-modifying agents be used in mild rheumatoid arthritis? Br J Rheumatol 1991;30:451.

45. Day RO, Paulus HE. D-Penicillamine. In: Paulus HE, Furst DE, and Dromgoole SH, eds. Drugs for rheumatic disease. New York: Churchill Livingstone, 1987:85.

46. Jaffe IA. Penicillamine. In: Kelley WN, Harris ED Jr, Ruddy S, Sledge CB, eds. Textbook of rheumatology. 4th ed. Philadelphia: WB Saunders, 1993:760.

47. Lipsky PE. Immunosuppression by D-penicillamine in vitro: inhibition of human T lymphocyte proliferation by copper- or ceruloplasmin-dependent generation of hydrogen peroxide and protection by monocytes. J Clin Invest 1984; 73:53.

48. Scott DL, Williams JD, Greenwood A, et al. Assessing the outcome of penicillamine therapy. Br J Rheumatol 1986;25(suppl 21):114.

49. Williams HJ, Ward JR, Reading JC, et al. Low dose D-penicillamine therapy in rheumatoid arthritis: a controlled double-blind clinical trial. Arthritis Rheum 1983;26:581.

50. Doyle DV, Perrett D, Foster OJF, Ensor M, Scott DL. The long-term use of D-penicillamine for treating rheumatoid arthritis: is continuous therapy necessary? Br J Rheumatol 1993;32:614.

51. Joyce DA, Day RO, Murphy BR. The pharmacokinetics of albumin conjugates of D-penicillamine in humans. Drug Metab Disp 1991;19:309.

52. Ahern MJ, Hall ND, Case K, et al. d-Penicillamine withdrawal in rheumatoid arthritis. Ann Rheum Dis 1984;43:213.

53. Gubner R, August S, Ginsburg V. Therapeutic suppression of tissue reactivity. II. Effect of aminopterin in rheumatoid arthritis and psoriasis. Am J Med Sci 1951;221:176.

54. Weinblatt ME, Coblyn JS, Fox DA, et al. Efficacy of low-dose methotrexate in rheumatoid arthritis. N Engl J Med 1985;312:818.

55. Weinblatt ME. Methotrexate. In: Kelley WN, Harris ED Jr, Ruddy S, Sledge CB, eds. Textbook of rheumatology. 4th ed. Philadelphia: WB Saunders, 1993:767.

56. Weinblatt ME, Weissman BN, Holdsworth DE. Long-term prospective study of methotrexate in the treatment of rheumatoid arthritis. Arthritis Rheum 1992;35:129.

57. Morgan SL, Baggott JE, Vaughn WH, et al. The effect of folic acid supplementation on the toxicity of low-dose methotrexate treatment of rheumatoid arthritis. Arthritis Rheum 1990;30:9.

58. Sperling RI, Benincaso AI, Anderson RJ. Acute and chronic suppression of leukotriene B4 synthesis ex vivo in neutrophils from patients with rheumatoid arthritis beginning treatment with methotrexate. Arthritis Rheum 1992;35:376.

59. Connolly KM, Stecher VJ, Davis E. Alteration of interleukin-1 production and the acute phase response following medication of adjuvant arthritic rats with cyclosporin-A or methotrexate. Int J Immunopharmacol 1988;10:717.

60. Day RO. Sulfasalazine. In: Kelley WN, Harris ED Jr, Ruddy S, Sledge CB, eds. Textbook of rheumatology. 4th ed. Philadelphia: WB Saunders, 1993:692.

61. Skosey JL. Comparison of responses to and adverse effects of graded doses of sulfasalazine in the treatment of rheumatoid arthritis. J Rheumatol 1988;16(suppl):5.

62. Fauci AS, Young KR Jr. Immunoregulatory agents. In: Kelley WN, Harris ED Jr, Ruddy S, Sledge CB, eds. Textbook of rheumatology. 4th ed. Philadelphia: WB Saunders, 1993:797.

63. Kinlen LJ. Incidence of cancer in rheumatoid arthritis and other disorders after immunosuppressive treatment. Am J Med 1985;78(1A):44.

64. Singh G, Fries JF, Spitz P, et al. Toxic effects of azathioprine in rheumatoid arthritis: a national post-marketing perspective. Arthritis Rheum 1989;32:837.

65. Chen L, O'Malley BW. Steroid hormone action: recent advances. Ann Intern Med 1978;89:694.

66. Weiss MM. Corticosteroids in rheumatoid arthritis. Semin Arthritis Rheum 1989;19:9.

67. Parrillo JE, Faucci AS. Mechanisms of glucocorticoid action on immune processes. Ann Rev Pharmacol Toxicol 1979;19:179.

68. Garber EK, Targoff C, Paulus HE. Corticosteroids in the rheumatic diseases: chronic low doses, chronic high doses, "pulses," intra-articular. In: Paulus HE, Furst DE, Dromgoole SH, eds. Drugs for rheumatic disease. New York: Churchill Livingstone, 1987:443.

69. Radia M, Furst DE. Comparison of three pulse methylprednisolone regimens in the treatment of rheumatoid arthritis. J Rheumatol 1988;15:24.

70. La Rochelle GE, La Rochelle AG, Ratner RE, et al. Recovery of the hypothalamic-pituitary-adrenal (HPA) axis in patients with rheumatic disease receiving low dose prednisone. Am J Med 1993;95:258.

71. Caruso I, Santandrea S, Sarzi Puttini P, et al. Clinical, laboratory and radiographic features of early rheumatoid arthritis. J Rheumatol 1990; 17:1268.

72. Scott DL, Symmons DPM, Coulton BL, et al. Long-term outcome of treating rheumatoid arthritis: results after 20 years. Lancet 1987;1: 1108.

73. Wilske KR, Healey LA. Remodelling the pyramid: a concept whose time has come. J Rheumatol 1989;16:565.

74. Gabriel SE, Luthra HS. Rheumatoid arthritis: can the long-term outcome be altered? Mayo Clin Proc 1988; 63:58.

75. Pincus T. Rheumatoid arthritis: disappointing long-term outcomes despite successful short-term clinical trials. J Clin Epidemiol 1988;41: 1037.

76. Thompson PW, Kirwan JR, Barnes CG. Practical results of treatment with disease-modifying anti-rheumatoid drugs. Br J Rheumatol 1985; 24:167.

77. Wolfe F, Hawley DF. Remission in rheumatoid arthritis. J Rheumatol 1985;12:245.

78. Kushner I. Does aggressive therapy of rheumatoid arthritis affect outcome? [Editorial]. J Rheumatol 1989;16:1.

79. Paulus HE. Current controversies in rheumatology: the use of combinations of disease-modifying anti-rheumatic agents in rheumatoid arthritis . Arthritis Rheum 1990;33;113.

80. Wilke WS, Clough JD. Therapy for rheumatoid arthritis: combinations of disease-modifying drugs and new paradigms of treatment. Semin Arthritis Rheum 1991;21(suppl):21.

81. O'Brien BJ, Elswood J, Calin A. Willingness to accept risk in the treatment of rheumatic disease. J Epidemiol 1990;44:249.

82. Skeith KJ, David P. New horizons in the medical treatment of rheumatoid arthritis. Curr Opinion Rheum 1992;4:365.

83. Gay S, Gay RE. Cellular and molecular basis of joint destruction: oncogene expression and retroviral sequences in rheumatoid arthritis. In: Hedqvist P, Kalder JR, Muller-Peddinghaus R, Robinson DR, eds. Trends in RA research: advances in rheumatology and inflammation. Vol 1. Basel: Eular Publishers, 1991:19.

84. Edmonds J: Better guidelines to rheumatoid arthritis therapy. Aust N Z J Med 1993;23:143.

85. Yocum DE, Klippel JH, Wilder RL, et al. Cyclosporin A in severe, treatment-refractory rheumatoid arthritis. Ann Intern Med 1988; 109:863.

86. Dougados M, Awada H, Amor B. Cyclosporin in rheumatoid arthritis: a double-blind, placebo controlled study in 52 patients. Ann Rheum Dis 1988;47:127.

87. Tugwell P, Bombardier C, Gent M, et al. Low-dose cyclosporin versus placebo in patients with rheumatoid arthritis. Lancet 1990;335:1051.

EXTRAARTICULAR MANIFESTATIONS OF RHEUMATOID ARTHRITIS

Eric L. Matteson
Doyt L. Conn

Extraarticular features of rheumatoid arthritis may occur at any time in the course of the disease and may even overshadow the joint disease. An understanding of the systemic nature of rheumatoid arthritis is essential to its successful treatment. The systemic or extraarticular manifestations will sometimes be the major manifestations requiring treatment, and at other times they may be in the background, apparent only because of constitutional symptoms such as weight loss, low-grade fever, malaise, and generalized weakness. When systemic features dominate, they may be life-threatening and may constitute true emergencies. These complications must be recognized and treated appropriately, because systemic features of rheumatoid arthritis are major predictors of overall morbidity and mortality.[1]

GENERAL PRINCIPLES

The treatment of extraarticular manifestations of rheumatoid arthritis is guided by the specific organ system involved and by the severity of involvement. In general, therapeutic strategies designed to control the joint involvement are often effective in treating systemic disease. They include the use of nonsteroidal antiinflammatory drugs (NSAIDs), slow-acting antirheumatic drugs such as gold, penicillamine, hydroxychloroquine, methotrexate, sulfasalazine, azathioprine, and glucocorticosteroids, and rarely other cytotoxic agents such as cyclophosphamide and chlorambucil. In our view, the use of glucocorticosteroids is the mainstay for managing systemic inflammatory features of rheuma-

toid arthritis. The initial dose of glucocorticosteroid is commensurate with the organ involved and the degree of involvement; it is given orally as a daily divided dose and is tapered according to the response of the organ system involved. At the same time, baseline therapy with NSAIDs and slow-acting antirheumatic drugs is usually continued. Frequently, the tapering of glucocorticosteroid dosage or its termination after 1 or 2 weeks is undertaken too rapidly, resulting in relapse of the disease manifestation being treated and an unnecessary cycle of "burst and taper" therapy. The role of high-dose "pulse" glucocorticosteroid therapy ($\geq$1 g IV methylprednisolone [Solu-Medrol]) is not established, but in our experience it is rarely, if ever, required for treating any disease manifestation. Many of the manifestations of extraarticular disease require 2 or more months of glucocorticoid therapy and frequently maintenance therapy with low doses of glucocorticoids.[1] In some cases, it is necessary to add cytotoxic agents as adjunctive therapy. It is our opinion that cytotoxic drugs are rarely necessary and that their use should not be routine but, rather, extraordinary and adapted on a case-by-case basis. Surgical management of specific target organ involvement is sometimes necessary (for example, cervical spine fusion for C-1/C-2 instability or pericardiectomy for restrictive pericarditis).

PULMONARY DISEASE

Pulmonary involvement in rheumatoid arthritis is frequent, although often not clinically significant. Pulmonary fibrosis may occur in up to 28% of patients.[2] Interstitial pulmonary fibrosis is strongly related to smoking.[3] Because smoking can accelerate the development of pulmonary fibrosis, an important therapeutic intervention in these patients is cessation of smoking.

The treatment of pulmonary fibrosis has traditionally focused on the use of glucocorticosteroids.[4,5] It is unclear whether or how glucocorticosteroids affect the fibrotic disease process. Short-term high doses of glucocorticosteroids (generally between 20 and 40 mg per day for periods of 1 to 2 months and then tapering slowly over a 6-month period) may have a beneficial effect in improving exercise tolerance.[6,7] In general, the use of protracted high-dose glucocorticosteroids in patients with interstitial fibrosis does not appear to be justified as long-term therapy if there is no beneficial response in the initial 2 to 4 months. Penicillamine has been used in some patients with interstitial lung disease, cardiovascular diseases, and rheumatoid arthritis with variable and uncertain success.[8]

Cytotoxic agents are sometimes used in patients with rheumatoid arthritis to control aggressive pulmonary fibrosis. Numerous case series and case reports of patients treated suggest potential improvement with methotrexate, penicillamine, azathioprine, cyclophosphamide, and cyclosporine.[8–13] As with glucocorticosteroids, there are no controlled studies demonstrating the benefit of this approach.

Autopsy studies have shown that pleural involvement occurs in up to 50% of patients with rheumatoid arthritis. Male patients with active seropositive nodular disease are often affected. Pleurisy and pleural effusions may improve spontaneously or require treatment, particularly when the pleuritic pain or shortness of breath become intolerable. It is important to rule out other causes of pleurisy and pleural effusion, most notably infection. Pleurisy without large pleural effusions frequently responds to the use of NSAIDs for 2 to 4 weeks or modest doses of prednisone (less than 15 mg per day) for 1 to 2 months, with doses tapered thereafter. Large effusions, particularly those that cause respiratory compromise, may be treated with higher doses of glucocorticosteroids. Prednisone, 40 to 60 mg per day in divided doses, may be given over a 2- to 4-week period, with the dose tapered as the symptoms resolve and the chest roentgenogram clears.

Patients who experience marked shortness of breath may require thoracentesis or continuous suction drainage to evacuate the pleural effusion. Pleurectomy may be necessary if persistent effusions lead to pleural fibrosis limiting lung expansion. Care must be taken in the evacuation of these effusions because of the risk of lung puncture and infection.[14]

Parenchymal pulmonary nodules are usually asymptomatic and occur in patients with seropositive rheumatoid arthritis who have widespread synovitis and who usually have nodules elsewhere. These nodules tend to be peripheral in location and are from less than 1 cm to 6 to 8 cm in diameter.[15] Pulmonary nodules can persist unchanged for years, or they may resolve spontaneously. These nodules may present a dilemma that is more diagnostic than therapeutic, as it is necessary to consider the possibility of neoplasia, tuberculosis, and fungal infections in the differential diagnosis. In general, rheumatoid pulmonary nodulosis does not require specific therapeutic intervention if asymptomatic; the treatment of the underlying rheumatoid disease frequently results in improvement of the nodules. Cavitation may occur and can be associated with hemoptysis or infection, requiring more specific therapy. The occurrence of a bronchopulmonary fistula may be life-threatening and require surgical repair. Pneumothorax may occur; this can resolve spontaneously or may also require surgical intervention.[15,16]

Caplan's syndrome, defined as pneumoconiosis in patients with rheumatoid arthritis, is characterized by multiple nodules greater than 1 cm in diameter scattered throughout the peripheral lung field.[16] This condition is seen in patients with rheumatoid arthritis associated with extensive exposure to silica. Some patients with Caplan's syndrome have exacerbations of their rheumatoid arthritis in association with the development of pneumoconiosis.[16] In addition to treatment of the underlying disease, avoidance of the offending exposure would seem to be the best treatment course.

Obliterative bronchiolitis has been reported in patients with rheumatoid arthritis.[17] It is not known whether this pulmonary manifestation is a consequence of the rheumatoid inflammatory process, another concomitant process, or medications. Bronchiolitis obliterans can be obstructive or associated with organizing pneumonia.[18,19] It frequently leads to rapidly progressive respiratory insufficiency.[20,21] Bronchiolitis obliterans–organizing pneumonia (BOOP) may respond rapidly to high-dose glucocorticosteroid treatment (60 to 80 mg per day for 2 to 4 weeks), reducing the dose by about 10% every 1 to 2 weeks according to patient response.[22] The duration of therapy required is not known but may exceed 3 to 6 months, and protracted low-dose glucocorticoid therapy may be necessary. Anecdotal experience with cytotoxic agents is also reported. Cyclophosphamide has been successfully used orally and intravenously in patients with bronchiolitis obliterans and interstitial fibrosis refractory to glucocorticoid therapy. The duration of cytotoxic therapy required has not been established, but conventional use is generally over the course of several months and up to 1 year.[23,24]

The long-term outcome in patients in whom bronchiolitis obliterans develops is unclear; it has been suggested that the disease does not respond to glucocorticosteroids and has an invariably poor, if not fatal, outcome within a few months of diagnosis.[17] It is our view and experience that outcome is often good with treatment, and often there is improvement if causative drugs such as penicillamine or gold can be identified and removed and the patient is given vigorous respiratory support and treated with glucocorticosteroids in high doses.

Pulmonary arteritis is an uncommon complication of rheumatoid arthritis. Although it may be the sole manifestation of lung disease, it is usually associated with other manifestations of rheumatoid lung disease, such as interstitial fibrosis and nodulosis.[25] The literature reveals virtually no experience with treatment of this disease complication. As an arteritis that may be associated with acrocyanosis and digital infarction, pulmonary arteritis may respond to glucocorticosteroid treatment as well as vasodilatory agents, including calcium channel blockers.

Rheumatoid arthritis involving the larynx may lead to upper airway obstruction and dyspnea. As many as 26% of patients with rheumatoid arthritis may have cricoarytenoid involvement.[26] Moderate obstruction may cause no symptoms, although if laryngeal edema is present the obstruction may interfere with normal tidal breathing.[27] Upper airway obstruction may be of acute onset and constitute an emergency. This is especially true of patients who develop an ordinary upper respiratory tract infection and experience sudden respiratory decompensation.[28] Patients with symptoms of hoarseness, shortness of breath, and possibly laryngeal discomfort or dysphagia should undergo direct laryngoscopy. This may show decreased mobility of the true vocal cords and erythema of the arytenoid mucosa.[26] Initial management should be prompt and should include prednisone, 20 mg three times daily for 1 week and tapered thereafter according to symptoms. Injection of the cricoarytenoid joints with triamcinolone acetonide may greatly accelerate the resolution of inflammation.[29,30] It must be emphasized that for patients who have a compromised airway, a trial of systemic glucocorticosteroids and close observation in the hospital is warranted. In some cases tracheostomy is necessary. Patients in whom cricoarytenoid ankylosis develops may have stable upper airway disease that may not even be symptomatic because of relatively sedentary lifestyles.[27] After the diagnosis of ankylosis is established, the degree of laryngeal obstruction should be determined by spirometry and flow volume loops and bilateral paralysis of the recurrent laryngeal nerves should be excluded. Surgical interventions to relieve airway obstruction may include lateral fixation.[27,31,32] Arytenoidectomy is regarded as definitive therapy and is usually performed unilaterally.[33]

CARDIAC DISEASE

Cardiac involvement in patients with rheumatoid arthritis reflects the systemic nature of the underlying disease. Patients may have pericarditis as a form of serositis, nodulosis of the myocardium or valves and conduction pathways, or vasculitis of the coronary arteries. Pericarditis is the most common of these manifestations, occurring in up to 50% of patients.[34]

Pericarditis may be associated with chest pain and dyspnea, usually in the context of active rheumatoid arthritis, although it may occur in patients with otherwise quiescent disease.[35] In contrast to the high incidence found by electrocardiographic, echocardiographic, or postmortem studies, clinically symptomatic pericarditis is relatively unusual, occurring in approximately 3% of patients.[36,37] In one large series, three fourths of the patients had acute pericarditis and the remainder had recurrent acute pericarditis and chronic pericarditis with effusion or chronic constrictive carditis.[38] Uncomplicated clinical pericarditis may respond to medical management, including the use of NSAIDs, glucocorticosteroids, or both.[37] In general, we favor the use of glucocorticosteroids in low doses (10 to 15 mg per day tapering as symptoms tolerate) for the treatment of chest discomfort associated with pericarditis in patients with small nonconstricting effusions or no effusion. Patients with tamponade and constrictive pericarditis require pericardiectomy.[38] Emergency pericardiocentesis may be lifesaving. This may be followed by intracardiac injections of glucocorticosteroids.[39] These procedures should be regarded as emergency procedures. Patients who have tamponade or impending tamponade require surgical intervention because of the high mortality (approaching 100%) of this condition.[39–41]

Although pericardial resection appears to be the treatment of choice, one study failed to find any beneficial effect of pericardiectomy on the survival of patients with rheumatoid arthritis.[38] Even when it is performed, 2-year mortality may be high if cardiac compression has occurred. This may be because of the generally debilitated condition of these patients. The pericardiectomy should be as extensive as possible.[40,42] A pericardial window is usually inadequate in preventing reaccumulation and should be reserved for ill patients who are unable to tolerate a thoracotomy.[39,43] It cannot be emphasized enough that glucocorticosteroid treatment of cardiac tamponade neither prevents its development nor effects its regression. Symptom-free patients without evidence of tamponade in whom small pericardial effusions are found on incidental echocardiographic examinations may not require treatment. Glucocorticosteroid therapy usually reverses the symptoms and signs of rheumatoid pericarditis in 2 to 4 weeks.[44] Reaccumulation of pericardial fluid should be considered a strong indication for consideration of pericardiectomy.[44] It has been estimated that roughly one third of patients with pericarditis eventually require pericardiectomy.[45]

Myocardial disease may be focal or diffuse and may lead to frank muscle necrosis.[45] Nonspecific myocarditis is thought to be asymptomatic and rarely affects cardiac size or function.

Hence it is rarely recognized, and the natural history and treatment are uncertain. Postmortem examination has revealed nonspecific myocarditis in as many as 19% of autopsy cases.[45]

Myocardial and endocardial disease associated with rheumatoid arthritis is usually a result of vasculitis with or without nodule formation. Small vessel vasculitis may be seen in up to 20% of cases.[46] Rheumatoid vasculitis in the form of coronary arteritis is also reported. How often this leads to myocardial infarction is not known. One study of 90 patients with rheumatoid vasculitis revealed evidence of myocardial infarction in five patients, in one of whom angiitis was seen at autopsy.[47] Vasculitis of the small vessels of the myocardium leading to congestive heart failure has been seen on percutaneous catheter-directed endomyocardial biopsy. A high degree of clinical suspicion is necessary to recognize vasculitis and to institute therapy promptly, as patients may respond well to glucocorticosteroid therapy.[48]

Rheumatoid granuloma in or near the atrioventricular node or bundle of His may result in arrhythmias, including complete heart block and syncope. The effect of medications, including glucocorticosteroids, on arrhythmias and their role in preventing complete heart block is unclear. Some patients with minor degrees of heart block later develop complete heart block, which is usually discovered only after syncope or on physical examination and electrocardiogram of an otherwise symptom-free patient.[49] Patients with complete heart block generally have established erosive nodular disease and test positive for rheumatoid factor. Typically, patients are already undergoing disease-modifying antirheumatic drug therapy with nonsteroidals, antiinflammatory agents, and even glucocorticosteroids when heart block appears. The role of medications, including glucocorticosteroids, in the treatment of arrhythmias in patients with rheumatoid arthritis is uncertain; cardiac pacemakers are the treatment of choice for complete heart block. Chloroquine has been associated with prolongation of the PR interval[50] and may be a cause of heart block. Rarely would this complication appear to be a clinically significant problem in patients with rheumatoid arthritis.[51,52]

Valvular disease is well recognized in patients with rheumatoid arthritis. The aortic valve appears to be most often affected, with abnormalities in up to 20% of cases at autopsy.[53] Nodules and cusp thickening may be present. Perforation of the cusps can result in valve incompetence.[54] Patients with endocardial disease who have other active extraarticular features of rheumatoid arthritis, including pleurisy and cutaneous vasculitis, may respond to high doses of glucocorticosteroids (between 40 and 60 mg per day initially). In the absence of these features, the role of glucocorticosteroids in the treatment of endocardial lesions is uncertain. The heart disease should be managed in conjunction with the cardiologist and the cardiac surgeon.

Inflammatory aortic root disease may be symptomatic or asymptomatic at the time of diagnosis, with a typical murmur of aortic regurgitation.[55] Clinically evident aortic incompetence probably affects fewer than 1% of patients who have rheumatoid arthritis.[56] In cases of active aortitis and dilatation, immunosuppressive therapy may be useful at the outset, including oral prednisone at 60 mg per day and azathioprine or cyclophosphamide.[55] The treatment response can be followed according to clinical status, echocardiographic findings, and the erythrocyte sedimentation rate. Some authors have also found factor VIII–related antigen levels to be useful in following these patients.[55] If surgery is required, it is likely to be more successful if aortic root inflammation is suppressed.[56,57]

OCULAR DISEASE

Keratoconjunctivitis sicca affects between 10% and 35% of patients with rheumatoid arthritis.[58] Symptoms may be pain, visual disturbance, foreign body sensation, and mucoid discharge. Treatment of keratoconjunctivitis sicca remains symptomatic. It is important to emphasize that the treatment of keratoconjunctivitis sicca also has the purpose of preventing scarring because of dryness as well as infection, and even patients with asymptomatic dry eyes should be treated with artificial tears, including methylcellulose-containing products. Several different preparations are available, including Liquifilm, Liquifilm Forte, Tears Plus, Tears Naturale, and others. In some cases the preservatives contained in these artificial tears may cause topical irritation.[59] Ointments such as Lacri-Lube or Duolube may be used at bedtime.

Humidifiers, wraparound glasses, and goggles may be useful, especially during flares.[60] In patients who have refractory dryness of the eyes, obliteration of the puncta and canaliculi may be considered. On rare occasions a partial tarsorrhaphy may become necessary. Unless inflammation is present, topical steroids should be avoided because of the potential for corneal perforation. Please see Chapter 5 for a detailed discussion of Sjögren's syndrome.

Episcleritis often correlates with the activity of the rheumatoid arthritis disease. Episcleritis may be nodular or diffuse and may cause eye redness and pain but only rarely causes changes in visual acuity.[58] Improved control of the rheumatoid arthritis itself may or may not improve the episcleritis. In general, episcleritis is self-limited and usually does not require treatment. When it is recurring or uncomfortable, topical glucocorticosteroids may be employed under the supervision of an ophthalmologist.

Like other extraarticular manifestations of rheumatoid arthritis, scleritis usually occurs in patients with longer-standing and more widespread systemic disease. Scleritis may result in severe ocular pain, erythema, and even eventually perforation. Approximately one third of the patients will develop iridocyclitis or choroiditis.[61] In cooperation with an ophthalmologist, glucocorticosteroid therapy in doses from 40 to 100 mg per day may be initiated.[62] Systemic and topical cyclosporine A may also be effective in the treatment of necrotizing scleritis.[63] Other cytotoxic agents, including nitrogen mustard and duazomycin, have also been used.[61] In advanced cases scleral grafting may be necessary.[61] It has been thought that corneal and scleral disease in rheumatoid arthritis may be accelerated by cataract extraction.[64,65] A recent study demonstrates that these problems are no more frequent in patients with rheumatoid arthritis who undergo cataract surgery than in the general population.[66] However, patients with keratoconjunctivitis sicca should be carefully managed perioperatively because of increased risk of corneal surface disease, including superficial puntate keratopathy.[66]

Tenosynovitis of the superior oblique tendon sheath may lead to mechanical obstruction when the patient attempts to raise the eye in adduction (Brown's syndrome). Patients may have diplopia and pain on attempted upward and inward gaze.[67,68] This manifestation may improve with oral glucocorticosteroids, although local injection of the tendon sheath or even nodule removal may be necessary.

It has been suggested that the eye is a sensitive indicator of occult systemic vasculitis in patients with rheumatoid arthritis in whom peripheral ulcerative keratitis or necrotizing scleritis develops. A nonrandomized trial compared cytotoxic immunosuppression with steroid plus nonsteroidal inflammatory therapy for 34 patients with rheumatoid arthritis who developed peripheral ulcerative keratitis or necrotizing scleritis; 9 of 17 patients on conventional therapy died of a vasculitis-related event during the 10-year follow-up. In 13 of these 17 patients the ocular inflammatory lesions progressed, and in 5 patients extraocular but nonlethal vasculitic lesions developed. Only 1 of 17 patients treated with long-term immunosuppression died, and this death occurred after cytotoxic therapy was withdrawn. None of the patients on immunosuppressive regimens developed extraocular vasculitis while taking cytotoxics and then had progression of the ocular destructive lesions.[69]

NEUROLOGIC DISEASE

Nerve compression is a common cause of neurologic impairment in rheumatoid arthritis. Peripheral entrapment neuropathies are not related to the duration, degree of activity, or severity of extraarticular manifestations of rheumatoid arthritis, although they do tend to correlate with the degree and severity of local synovitis. The median, ulnar, posterior tibial, and posterior interosseous branch of the radial nerves are the most commonly involved nerves.[70–72] Although no formal studies have evaluated this question, it has been our experience that when active synovitis is present, relief can be afforded by local steroid injection as well as by resting of the adjacent joint and splinting. The use of NSAIDs is also necessary. If unsuccessful, and especially in instances in which there is compression without active synovitis, surgical nerve release can be effective.

It has been estimated that 35% to 40% of patients with rheumatoid arthritis have peripheral neuropathy that is manifested as paresthesias, dysesthesias, and burning.[73] In addition to treatment of the underlying inflammatory process, the use of thiamine (50 mg per day), diphenylhydantoin (100 mg three times a day),

carbamazepin (100 to 800 mg per day), or amitriptyline (50 to 150 mg per day) may be beneficial.[73]

Mononeuritis multiplex and related conditions are discussed in the section on vasculitis.

Atlantoaxial subluxation caused by erosion of the odontoid process and/or the transverse ligament of C-1 may allow the odontoid process to slip posteriorly and lead to cervical myelopathy.[74] Basilar invagination may also occur, leading to upward impingement of the odontoid process on the foramen magnum and resulting in cord compression.[75] Signs and symptoms of cord compression include hyperreflexia, motor weakness of the extremities, a positive Babinski sign, Lhermitte sign, and posterior neck pain. If the posterior cerebral circulation is affected, visual disturbances, vertigo, paresthesias, and paresis may occur. Most patients with cervical subluxation have extensive erosive joint disease and nodulosis with positive rheumatoid factor.[76]

Neck instability and pain can usually be managed conservatively with a collar to immobilize the neck, with the patient instructed to use the collar particularly while riding in motor vehicles and to take care to avoid whiplash injuries and falls. Unfortunately, these collars are often quite burdensome and are frequently rejected by the patient.[77] Patients with progressing spinal cord signs should be considered for surgical cervical immobilization and traction.[78,79]

Several operative techniques have been employed to relieve posterior cervical pain and stabilize neurologic defects. Surgical decompression of the cervical medullary junction is considered for patients with irreducible encroachment.[80] A transoral-transpalatine approach may be used to resect irreducible invaginated odontoid granulation tissue.[81] Stabilization is most frequently attempted by means of posterior occipital cervical fusion with bone grafting, acrylics, and wire. Preoperative halo traction may help reduce cervical subluxation.[82] Occipital cervical fusion is recommended after any of these procedures.[75] These patients must be managed in conjunction with a surgery team skilled in the treatment of rheumatoid arthritis and these surgical techniques. Such procedures usually lead to excellent fusion rates approaching 100%, although tissue healing may be slowed in patients with rheumatoid arthritis, and pseudarthrosis may occur.[83]

AMYLOIDOSIS

Rarely, amyloidosis may complicate rheumatoid arthritis in patients with long-standing disease.[84] Secondary amyloidosis in rheumatoid arthritis may occur in 5% to 15% of patients.[84,85] The average survival time after the diagnosis of secondary amyloidosis-associated rheumatoid arthritis is estimated to be about 4 to 5 years.[84,86] Amyloidosis has been the attributed cause of death in about 8% of patients with rheumatoid arthritis at autopsy.[87] Renal amyloidosis in particular has been associated with diminished survival.[86,88] There are no controlled studies that address the treatment of amyloidosis in rheumatoid arthritis. Chlorambucil, cyclophosphamide, and azathioprine are among the drugs whose use has been advocated.[89]

FELTY'S SYNDROME

Felty's syndrome is defined as the presence of leukopenia and splenomegaly in rheumatoid arthritis. It occurs in 1% to 3% of patients with rheumatoid arthritis. It develops in that subset of patients with long-standing (over 10 years), seropositive, nodular, and destructive joint disease. These patients usually display extraarticular features of disease, including rheumatoid nodules, skin lesions of nail fold infarcts and leg ulcers, peripheral neuropathy, and sicca syndrome.[90] In addition to Felty's syndrome, they usually have a high-titer rheumatoid factor, antinuclear antibody, cryoglobulins, and a diminished serum complement.[91] There is frequently a family history of rheumatoid arthritis, and most of the patients will have the genetic type HLA-DR4 and an increased frequency of the DQW3 variant, 3b.[92] These patients, like patients with rheumatoid vasculitis, have homozygosity for the HLA-DRB1 allele 0401.[93] Patients with rheumatoid arthritis and neutropenia without splenomegaly have the same clinical features as the defined Felty's syndrome, including the development of the extraarticular features and an increased susceptibility to infections.[94]

The neutropenia of Felty's syndrome predisposes the patient to infections, and 60% to 95% of the patients will develop a superficial or deep infection (i.e., pneumonia or joint infection).[95] It is uncertain whether there is a correlation between the neutrophil count and the incidence of infections.[96]

Large granular lymphocyte syndrome (LGL syndrome) is a condition that may accompany rheumatoid arthritis and simulate Felty's syndrome.[97] Affected patients have lymphocytosis and sometimes neutropenia. They have a subset of lymphocytes that are large with abundant pale blue cytoplasm. The patients commonly have polyarthritis, splenomegaly, and recurrent infections. Usually the total white blood cell count is normal, with lymphocytosis. The patients also will commonly have rheumatoid factor and antinuclear antibodies.[94] The patients with the primary LGL syndrome usually do not have destructive joint disease or extraarticular features of disease that characterize patients with rheumatoid arthritis. Typing of the lymphocytes in these patients shows that there is a predominance of CD3, CD16, and CD57.[98] The lymphocytes have a T cell receptor gene rearrangement. It is not known whether this occurs because of a reactive change to an unknown antigen or a neoplastic change. Most patients have a nonprogressive course. This syndrome occurs one half as commonly as Felty's syndrome.

There are patients who have Felty's syndrome with neutropenia for many years without infections. Likewise, there are case reports of patients with neutropenia due to Felty's syndrome who improve spontaneously.[99] There are likely to be several mechanisms responsible for the clinical finding of Felty's syndrome; spontaneous regression may occur depending on the specific pathogenetic process involved. There are no prospective-controlled treatment studies of Felty's syndrome. In one case-controlled study, the outcome was poor, with an increasing mortality with time as compared with rheumatoid controls without Felty's syndrome.[92] In another study that compared the outcome in patients with Felty's syndrome and in matched controls with rheumatoid arthritis, there was no difference in the incidence of infections or in death rates.[100] Death rates were increased in both groups.

There is no ideal therapy for Felty's syndrome. The reason for the lack of an effective approach to management is an incomplete understanding of the cause of Felty's syndrome, which may vary from patient to patient. A major mechanism present in Felty's syndrome is the presence of immune complex disease. Polymorphonuclear leukocytes phagocytize

TABLE 4–1
Changes in Laboratory Data After Parenteral Gold Therapy

	BEFORE TREATMENT		AFTER TREATMENT (MOST RECENT VALUE)	
	MEAN	RANGE	MEAN	RANGE
Hemoglobin (g/dl)	11.0	8.1–14.2	12.5	9.2–15.8
Total leukocytes (No./mm³)	1970	400–7000	4720	800–9300
Granulocytes (No./mm³)	464	13–1496	2853	496–6004
Lymphocytes (No./mm³)	1107	288–5496	1374	128–6231
Erythrocyte sedimentation rate (Westergren) (mm in 1 h)	75	30–141	31	10–77

From Dillon AM, Luthra HS, Conn DL, Ferguson RH. Parenteral gold therapy in the Felty syndrome: experience with 20 patients. Medicine 1986;65:107–12. Copyright 1986 Williams & Wilkins Company.

immune complexes, and these engorged PMNs are removed by the reticuloendothelial system. In addition, there may be decreased cytokine production, humoral inhibition of marrow responsiveness to colony-stimulating activity and T-cell-mediated immune suppression of granulopoiesis.[94]

Glucocorticoids in higher doses may stimulate neutrophilia, but low doses may not maintain this improvement. Parenteral testosterone may stimulate granulopoiesis but is too toxic, particularly for long-term use in women.[101] Lithium carbonate stimulates granulopoiesis; it is a short-term measure but has no lasting benefit and any benefit disappears after treatment is discontinued.[102] Intravenous γ-globulin is not effective.[103]

Retrospective studies suggest that the best treatment for Felty's syndrome is the use of disease-modifying drugs. When this was examined in the early 1980s, most patients with Felty's syndrome either had not been given a disease-modifying agent or had been inadequately treated, sometimes because of adverse reactions to this type of drug.[104] This observation raises the possibility that early treatment of rheumatoid arthritis with disease-modifying drugs may prevent the development of Felty's syndrome.

Parenteral gold is the agent most widely reported in retrospective studies of treatment of Felty's syndrome. In one study, 80% of patients with Felty's syndrome had improvement of neutropenia and a diminution of infections[105] (Tables 4–1 and 4–2). Penicillamine has not been as effective, partly because of frequent side effects in these patients.

Methotrexate is probably as effective as parenteral gold for the treatment of Felty's syndrome.[105] Cyclophosphamide has been shown to be effective but, because of the side effects, should be used only in selected cases in which other disease-modifying agents have not been effective.

Granulocyte colony-stimulating factor (CSF) has been used to correct neutropenia in Felty's syndrome.[94] The results have been mixed. The neutrophil count can be stimulated acutely but declines with time. In one case study, however, the neutrophil count was maintained over 1 year with weekly injections of granulocyte CSF.[106] With the increase in the neutrophil count, the arthritis may worsen. It has been shown that, despite an increase in the peripheral neutrophil count, the bone marrow shows persistent maturation arrest.

TABLE 4–2
Clinical Responses to Parenteral Gold Therapy

CRITERION	NO.*	%
Decrease ≥50% in recurrent infections:		
Superficial	14/17	82
Deep	11/17	65
Cessation of recurrent fevers	10/12	83
Decrease ≥50% in cutaneous ulcers	7/10	70
Resolution of hemolytic anemia	2/2	100
Vasculitis improved	5/6	83
Splenomegaly decreased	13/16	81

*Responding/number at risk.
From Dillon AM, Luthra HS, Conn DL, Ferguson RH. Parenteral gold therapy in the Felty syndrome: experience with 20 patients. Medicine 1986;65:107–12. Copyright 1986 Williams & Wilkins Company.

A reasonable management approach in Felty's syndrome is as follows:

1. Rheumatoid arthritis must be appropriately managed with timely initiation of disease-modifying antirheumatic drug (DMARD) therapy, use of NSAIDs and, when needed, low doses of prednisone. This approach may prevent the development of Felty's syndrome.
2. If Felty's syndrome develops despite the use of a disease-modifying agent, then another disease-modifying agent should be tried.
3. If the patient has Felty's syndrome but no associated infection, then the current management approach should be continued with a disease-modifying agent. The neutropenia does not require treatment if there is no apparent increased susceptibility to infections.
4. Patients with properly treated Felty's syndrome and persistent neutropenia who develop infections should be treated with the appropriate antibiotics.
5. Patients with properly treated Felty's syndrome who have neutropenia and uncontrolled recurrent infections should be considered for granulocytic CSF therapy.

RHEUMATOID VASCULITIS

Rheumatoid vasculitis occurs when small blood vessels, small and medium-sized arteries outside the joints, become inflamed and result in clinical features of disease. Organs that are usually involved in rheumatoid vasculitis are the skin and peripheral nerves and, less commonly, the viscera, heart, and central nervous system. A small-vessel vasculitis is an early event in the development of rheumatoid nodules.[107] Rheumatoid vasculitis may occur in early rheumatoid arthritis but more commonly occurs later in the course of the disease.[108] The clinical features resulting from rheumatoid vasculitis include nail fold infarcts, leg ulcers, digital gangrene, and a peripheral neuropathy. The peripheral nerve involvement may be a sensory neuropathy or a sensory-motor neuropathy.[109] Less commonly the vasculitis may extend to involve the mesentery, coronary, and cerebral arteries. These manifestations of rheumatoid vasculitis may occur singly or in combination.

Rheumatoid vasculitis occurs in a setting of long-standing rheumatoid arthritis. Most patients have had their disease 10 years or more.

Men are involved as commonly as women. Patients who develop rheumatoid vasculitis have had more severe joint disease with destructive changes, rheumatoid nodules, and high titers of rheumatoid factor.[110] Patients with Felty's syndrome are more likely to develop vasculitic complications. There is a genetic predisposition to the development of extraarticular features of rheumatoid arthritis, particularly rheumatoid vasculitis.[111] Homozygosity for the HLA-DRB1 0401 allele is common in patients with rheumatoid vasculitis.[112]

The initial vascular injury in rheumatoid vasculitis is probably immunologically induced. Indirect evidence of immunologic involvement includes high-titer rheumatoid factor, circulating immune complexes, and a diminished serum complement.[113] Antiendothelial antibodies may be present.[114] The finding of immunoglobulins, complement, and fibrin in acute arterial lesions provides direct evidence of immune-induced injury in rheumatoid vasculitis. In the chronic lesions of arterial intimal proliferation and occlusion, only fibrin was found.[115] This suggests that the immune deposits initiated the injury and then were removed, leaving the fibrin which must be resistant to normal clearing mechanisms.

Rheumatoid vasculitis comprises a spectrum of clinical features. Some clinical manifestations are benign and probably do not influence outcome. Clinical experience suggests that localized skin lesions and a distal sensory neuropathy are not indicators of a poor outcome.[109] Multiple organ involvement and visceral involvement are major predictors of increased morbidity and decreased survival. There are no studies in rheumatoid arthritis that analyze the influence of individual disease manifestations on outcome. Actuarial survival is decreased in patients with clinical rheumatoid vasculitis, similar to survival in classic rheumatoid arthritis (Table 4–3). One retrospective study showed that increased age at diagnosis was the best predictor of decreased survival.[116] This study also demonstrated a decrease in actuarial survival in those patients who had not been taking NSAIDs at the time of diagnosis of vasculitis and who had previously taken cytotoxic drugs or glucocorticoids.

Randomized controlled treatment trials for rheumatoid vasculitis are not available. The management of rheumatoid arthritis is based on retrospective studies, the clinical experience of

TABLE 4–3
Relative Survival* of 52 Patients With Rheumatoid Arthritis and Rheumatoid Vasculitis

TYPE	YEARS AFTER DIAGNOSIS				
	1	2	3	4	5
Rheumatoid Arthritis (%)					
Definite	101	100	102	103	100
Classic	96	95	85	85	85
Rheumatoid Vasculitis (%)					
All patients	82	77	76	72	67
Corrected for referral bias†	95	90	92	93	87

*Each relative survival is expressed as a percentage of expected survival in comparison with survival of an age- and sex-matched upper Middle Western control from the general population.

†When corrected for referral distance, the survival with vasculitis is similar to that of classic rheumatoid arthritis without vasculitis.

From Vollertsen RS, Conn DL, Ballard DJ, Ilstrup DM, Kazmar RE, Silverfield JC. Rheumatoid vasculitis: survival and associated risk factors. Medicine 1986;65:365–75. Copyright 1986 Williams & Wilkins Company.

the clinician, and the collective experience of the clinician's institution. Since 1950 glucocorticoids have been used to manage rheumatoid vasculitis. It was observed in the 1950s that rheumatoid vasculitis appeared to be found more commonly in patients who had received glucocorticoids.[117] This observation likely represents a selection bias, because patients with more severe rheumatoid arthritis and rheumatoid vasculitis are likely to be taking glucocorticoids. Nevertheless, wide fluctuations in glucocorticoid doses, particularly a rapid tapering or switching to an alternate-day dose, may allow the suppressed vasculitis to explode and progress very rapidly. It is also possible that glucocorticoids may control inflammation but allow an occlusive vasculopathy to develop and progress.[118]

Patients who develop rheumatoid vasculitis frequently have never taken disease-modifying agents or have been unable to tolerate them.[116] This raises the possibility that patients with rheumatoid arthritis treated early in their disease with appropriate disease-modifying drugs may not develop rheumatoid vasculitis. Consequently, patients who have manifestations of rheumatoid vasculitis should be given an appropriate disease-modifying agent. Additional treatment will depend on the particular disease manifestations, extent of disease, tempo of disease, clinical or laboratory evidence of inflammation, and coexisting disease states. Coexisting diseases or factors that influence the final vascular outcome include smoking, hypertension, and diabetes mellitus.

The clinician should attempt to determine whether the vascular lesion is inflammatory. Biopsy of involved tissue is a good way to determine the degree of inflammation if accessible tissue is available. Involved accessible tissue may include the skin or the sural nerve.[119] An estimate of the inflammatory nature of the vascular process can sometimes be made from clinical and laboratory examinations. Certain skin lesions, such as palpable purpura, an expanding ulcer, or progressive mononeuritis multiplex, would all indicate an active, progressive, inflammatory process. Systemic evidence of inflammation would be reflected in the following laboratory abnormalities: an elevated erythrocyte sedimentation rate, anemia, thrombocytosis, cryoglobulinemia, diminished serum complement, and elevation of cytokines such as tumor necrosis factor and interleukin 6.[120,121]

A patient with digital-tip infarcts but no other features of disease and no laboratory evidence of inflammation probably should not be treated with high doses of steroids or cytotoxic drugs. The pathology of this lesion is probably an intimal proliferative process.[122] Treatment should be directed toward reducing vasospasm, inhibiting platelet aggregation, and promoting revascularization. This patient should be given an appropriate disease-modifying agent, a vasodilating agent, antiplatelet drugs, and possible low doses of prednisone.

In patients who have had a stable mononeuritis multiplex for several months with no other systemic vasculitic manifestations, treatment with disease-modifying drugs, NSAIDs, and low divided doses of prednisone may be sufficient.

It is important to recognize that factors in addition to the vasculitis may influence a final vascular outcome. In patients with leg ulcers there may be an initial underlying vasculitis, but the extent and chronicity may be influenced by other factors, including venous insufficiency, arterial insufficiency, dependent edema, trauma, and chronic glucocorticoid use. In patients with digital infarcts other factors that affect the blood vessels, including atherosclerosis, hypertension, diabetes mellitus, and smoking, may be as important as the vasculitic component.

Over the past two decades, the treatment of rheumatoid vasculitis has focused on the use of D-penicillamine, glucocorticoids, cytotoxic drugs, and plasmapheresis. Retrospective studies have not determined the influence of the extent of the disease, the tempo of the disease, or inflammatory features of the disease on outcome. In addition the concept of relapse, long-term toxicity, and maintenance of disease control with these agents needs to be addressed.[122a]

D-Penicillamine has been used in a number of studies for the management of rheumatoid vasculitis.[123] A significant benefit of D-penicillamine on actuarial survival remains to be demonstrated.[116] D-Penicillamine is no more effective than any of the other disease-modifying drugs for this condition.

There are small, uncontrolled series demonstrating the effectiveness of cyclophosphamide in the management of rheumatoid vasculitis.[124,125] Chlorambucil may be equally effective. Methotrexate has been reported to be beneficial in rheumatoid vasculitis.[126] Methotrexate has also been associated with the development of cutaneous vasculitis and rheumatoid nodules in rheumatoid arthritis.[127] Azathioprine is the only disease-modifying drug that has been tested in a randomized trial for rheumatoid vasculitis.[128] This study failed to demonstrate any benefit but was of brief duration and low power. A more recent study shows improvement in persons with rheumatoid vasculitis treated with high-dose prednisone and azathioprine.[129]

Pulsed, high-dose intravenous glucocorticoids, usually 1 g methylprednisolone per day for 1 to 5 days, is used empirically in the treatment of severe rheumatoid vasculitis. There is no established rationale for this therapy and no documentation showing that this dose is more efficacious than a dose in the range of 100 mg prednisone per day. Plasmapheresis used alone is not helpful. When used with prednisone and an aklylating agent, there may be improvement, but it is impossible to show any benefit attributable to the plasmaparesis.[130] Plasmapheresis cannot be recommended because of the lack of effectiveness and the expense. Intravenous immunoglobulin has been used to treat rheumatoid vasculitis and shows promise.[131] More experience with this therapy is needed.

A reasonable treatment strategy for the patient with rheumatoid vasculitis is outlined in Table 4–4. Patients with rheumatoid vasculi-

---

TABLE 4–4
Treatment of Rheumatoid Vasculitis

1. General measures	Stop smoking
	Control hypertension and diabetes mellitus
2. In all cases manage rheumatoid arthritis and constitutional features	NSAIDs
	Low-dose prednisone
	Disease-modifying drugs
3. Localized vasculitis manifestations	
a. Nail fold infarcts	Manage the rheumatoid arthritis as in (2)
b. Distal sensory neuropathy	Local care for leg ulcers, possibly skin graft
c. Leg ulcers	Antiplatelet drugs
d. Digital tip gangrene without other manifestations and no clinical evidence of inflammation	Vasodilating agents
4. Systemic vasculitis	
a. Progressive manifestations with clinical evidence of inflammation, mononeuritis multiplex, digital tip infarcts, CNS, and/or visceral involvement	High-divided-dose prednisone, azathioprine, chlorambucil, or cyclophosphamide, antiplatelet drugs
b. Resistant progressive inflammatory multisystem disease	Addition of IV immunoglobulin

tis should be given a disease-modifying drug, including parenteral gold, methotrexate, or sulfasalazine (Azulfidine), as tolerated. Sufficient doses of NSAIDs providing antiinflammatory and antiplatelet action effects are necessary. Low doses of prednisone also may be necessary to help control active vascular or joint inflammation.

Other nonvasculitic influences on the vascular system should be managed as effectively as possible. Blood pressure should be normalized, diabetes mellitus should be controlled, and smoking should be stopped.

Leg ulcers without any other vasculitic manifestations should be managed with local care. In some cases a skin graft may be necessary. Isolated digital vasculopathy should be treated with disease-modifying agents, NSAIDs, vasodilators, and an appropriate antiplatelet regimen. Rheumatoid vasculitis manifested by distal sensory neuropathy, nail fold infarcts, or both requires optimal management for rheumatoid arthritis, including methotrexate. It is not necessary to use such treatments as high doses of prednisone or cytotoxic agents to treat the nail fold infarcts or sensory neuropathy.

The treatment for patients with more extensive progressive disease and evidence of inflammation should be more aggressive. These patients would include those with progressive mononeuritis multiplex, coronary angiitis, cerebral vasculitis, and visceral ischemia. These patients should be given high doses of prednisone (between 60 and 80 mg in three or four daily doses). These patients should also be given an immunosuppressive agent. If they have been taking methotrexate or another disease-modifying agent without any benefit, then azathioprine, cyclophosphamide, or chlorambucil can be considered. If they have not been taking methotrexate, it can be considered, but there is no experience to suggest its efficacy in severe vasculitis.

Cyclophosphamide and chlorambucil may have a beneficial effect within weeks, whereas azathioprine requires several months to take effect but can generally be administered for a longer period of time. Although there is more published experience with cyclophosphamide than with chlorambucil in the treatment of rheumatoid vasculitis, the efficacy and side effects of these two drugs are probably comparable, whereas cyclophosphamide is also toxic to the bladder.

The toxic effects of cyclophosphamide may be lessened by administration in a pulse fashion over one to several days a month. There is little convincing evidence to suggest that intravenous (IV) pulsed cyclophosphamide is any more efficacious than oral cyclophosphamide in the management of rheumatoid vasculitis, although it is less toxic to the bladder.[125] Other strategies for minimizing toxic effects, especially to the bone marrow, have not been studied. Other strategies of drug administration may be as safe, less expensive, and easier to manage than the IV pulse cyclophosphamide regimen. For example, oral administration of this cytotoxic agent daily for 4 to 5 days each week and "resting" the bone marrow for the remaining 2 or 3 days of each week may be as efficacious and safe.

The usual oral doses of these cytotoxic agents in adult patients are as follows: cyclophosphamide, 125 to 150 mg a day given in a single morning dose with liberal fluids (3 to 4 L a day); chlorambucil, 4 to 6 mg a day given in either a single daily dose or a split dose. The hematology group, when cyclophosphamide is used, and the urinalysis should be monitored weekly for the first 1 to 2 months and then monthly. If azathioprine is selected, it can be given orally in a single or divided dose of between 100 and 150 mg a day total, with the hematology group and SGOT monitored monthly. Usually the initial IV pulsed cyclophosphamide is given in doses of 500 to 1000 mg in a vehicle of 5% dextrose and water over 30 to 60 minutes. Initially, it is given 1 day a month for 4 to 6 months and then less frequently, depending on response and toxicity. For an in-depth discussion of the mechanism of action of cytotoxic drugs and immunoregulatory agents, see Kelley Chapter 49.[132]

As the manifestations of vasculitis are controlled, the prednisone dose can be tapered. As prednisone is tapered, the cytotoxic drug dose may also need to be lowered. This is because the cytotoxic drug may become more suppressive of the bone marrow as the prednisone dose is reduced.

Once the disease is controlled, prednisone can be tapered, as long as disease control is maintained during the taper. In our experience, flares of the vasculitis are less likely with daily doses of prednisone than with an alternate-day regimen.

When the dose of prednisone used to control the disease is 60 mg a day or greater, tapering can be accomplished by decrements of 10 mg a day each week to a dose of 40 mg a day. Thereafter, the taper is slowed to decrements of 5 mg a day each week to a total dose of 25 mg a day. The dose should be tapered by decrements of 2.5 mg each week thereafter to a total of 15 mg a day. At this point, the taper is slowed to 1 mg per day every 2 to 3 weeks in an attempt to achieve the lowest possible prednisone dose. Some patients will require a low dose of prednisone indefinitely. The pace of the prednisone taper depends on the clinical and laboratory status of the patient.

If the disease flares during the prednisone taper, the dose of prednisone should be increased to the level that allows control of the disease. If the patient is on a single daily dose of prednisone and experiences worsening of the inflammatory features later in the day, the prednisone should be given in divided doses, usually twice daily or three times a day.

Assuming that the prednisone has been tapered to under 10 mg a day while the cytotoxic agent is continued with control of the disease, the regimen should be maintained for approximately 1 year. Thereafter, if the disease remains under control, the cytotoxic agent can be gradually tapered further and stopped altogether. If the cytotoxic agent can be tapered off and the disease remains under control, then a slow prednisone taper is undertaken by decrements of 1 mg a day each month in an attempt to reach the lowest dose of prednisone that will continue to control the disease.

REFERENCES

1. Rasker JJ, Cosh JA. Cause and age of death in a prospective study of 100 patients with rheumatoid arthritis. Ann Rheum Dis 1981;40:115.
2. Walker WC, Wright V. Diffuse interstitial pulmonary fibrosis and rheumatoid arthritis. Ann Rhemn Dis 1969;28:252.
3. Geddes DM, Webley M, Emerson PA. Airways obstruction in rheumatoid arthritis. Ann Rheum Dis 1979;38:222.
4. Walker WC, Wright V. Pulmonary lesions and rheumatoid arthritis. Medicine 1968;47:501.
5. Roschmann RA, Rothenberg RJ. Pulmonary fibrosis in rheumatoid arthritis: a review of clinical features and therapy. Semin Arthritis Rheum 1987;16:174.
6. Turner-Warwick M, Evans RC. Pulmonary manifestations of rheumatoid disease. Clin Rheum Dis 1977;3:549.
7. Wallaert B, Hatron PY, Grosbois JM, et al. Subclinical pulmonary involvement in collagen vascular diseases assessed by bronchoalveolar lavage. Am Rev Respir Dis 1986;133:574.
8. Goodman M, Knight RK, Turner-Warwick M: Pilot study of penicillamine therapy in steroid failure patients with interstitial lung disease. In: Maini RN, Berry H, eds. Modulation of autoimmunity and disease. Clinical Pharmacology and Therapeutics Series. New York: Praeger, 1981:41.
9. Scott DGI, Bacon PA. Response to methotrexate in fibrosing alveolitis associated with connective tissue disease. Thorax 1980;35:725.
10. Lorber A. Penicillamine therapy for rheumatoid lung disease: effects on protein sulphydryl groups. Nature 1966;210:1235.
11. Cohen JM, Miller A, Spiera H. Interstitial pneumonitics complicating rheumatoid arthritis. Chest 1977;72:521.
12. Brown CH, Turner-Warwick M. The treatment of cryptogenic fibrosing alveolitis with immunosuppressant drugs. Q J Med 1971;158:289.
13. Alegre J, Teran J, Alverez B, Viejo JL. Successful use of cyclosporine for the treatment of aggressive pulmonary fibrosis in a patient with rheumatoid arthritis. Arthritis Rheum 1990;33:1594.
14. Dieppe PA. Empyema in rheumatoid arthritis. Ann Rheum Dis 1975;34:181.
15. Portner MM, Gracie WA. Rheumatoid lung disease with cavitary nodules, pneumothorax, and eosinophilia. N Engl J Med 1966;275:697.
16. Caplan A. Certain unusual radiological appearances in the chest of coal-miners suffering from rheumatoid arthritis. Thorax 1953;8:29.
17. Penny WJ, Knight RK, Rees AM, Thomas AL, Smith AP. Obliterative bronchiolitis in rheumatoid arthritis. Ann Rheum Dis 1982;41:469.
18. Epler RG, Colby TV, McCloud TC, Carrington CB, Gaensler EA. Bronchiolitis obliterans organizing pneumonia. N Engl J Med 1985;312:152.
19. Gosink BB, Friedman PJ, Liebow AA. Bronchiolitis obliterans: roentgenologic-pathologic correlation. Am J Roentgenol Radium Ther Nucl Med 1973;117:816.
20. Geddes DM, Corrin B, Brewerton DA, Davies RJ, Turner-Warwick M. Progressive airway obliteration in adults and its association with rheumatoid disease. Q J Med 1977;46:427.
21. Jansen HM, Elema JD, Hylkema BS, et al. Progressive obliterative bronchiolitis in a patient with rheumatoid arthritis. Eur J Respir Dis 1982;63:43.
22. van Thiel RJ, van der Burg S, Groote AD, Nossent GD, Wills SH. Bronchiolitis obliterans organizing pneumonia and rheumatoid arthritis. Eur Respir J 1991;4:905.
23. Fort JG, Scovern H, Abruzzo JL. Intravenous cyclophosphamide and methylprednisolone for the treatment of bronchiolitis obliterans and interstitial fibrosis associated with cryotherapy. J Rheumatol 1988;15:850.
24. Van De Laar MAFJ, Westerman CJJ, Wagenaar SS, Dinant HJ. Beneficial effect of intraveous

cyclophosphamide and oral prednisone in d-penicillamine-associated bronchiolitis obliterans. Arthritis Rheum 1985;28:93.

25. Gardner DL, Duthie JR, MacLeod J, et al. Pulmonary hypertension in RA: report of a case with intimal sclerosis of pulmonary and digital arteries. Scott Med J 1957;2:183.

26. Löfgren R, Montgomery W. Incidence of laryngeal involvement in rheumatoid arthritis. N Engl J Med 1962;267:193.

27. Geterud A, Ejnell H, Mansson I, Sandberg N, Bake B, Bjelle A. Severe airway obstruction caused by laryngeal rheumatoid arthritis. J Rheumatol 1986;13:948.

28. Phellps J. Laryngeal obstruction due to cricoarytenoid arthritis. Anesthesiology 1966;27:518.

29. Dockery KM, Sismanis A, Abedi E. Rheumatoid arthritis of the larynx: the importance of early diagnosis and corticosteroid therapy. South Med J 1991;84:95.

30. Habib MA. Intra-articular steroid injection in acute rheumatoid arthritis of the larynx. J Laryngol Otol 1977;91:909.

31. Montgomery W. Cricoarytenoid arthritis. Laryngoscope 1963;73:801.

32. Kleinsasser O. Microlaryngoscopy and endolaryngeal microsurgery. Philadelphia: WB Saunders, 1968:120.

33. Simpson GT II, Javaheri A, JanFaza P. Acute cricoarytenoid arthritis: local periarticular steroid injection. Ann Otol Rhinol Laryngol 1980;89:558.

34. Bonfiglio T, Atwater EC. Heart disease in patients with seropositive rheumatoid arthritis. Arch Intern Med 1969;124:714.

35. Sigal LH, Friedman HD. Rheumatoid pancarditis in a patient with well-controlled rheumatoid arthritis. J Rheumatol 1989;16:368.

36. Gordon DA, Stein JL, Broder I. The extra-articular features of rheumatoid arthritis: a systematic analysis of 127 cases. Am J Med 1973; 54:445.

37. Wilkinson M. Rheumatoid pericarditis: a report of four cases. Br Med J 1962;2:1723.

38. Hara KS, Ballard DJ, Ilstrup DM, Connolly DC, Vollertsen RS. Rheumatoid pericarditis: clinical features and survival. Medicine 1990; 69:81.

39. Escalante A, Kaufman RL, Quismorio FP Jr, Beardmore TD. Cardiac compression in rheumatoid pericarditis. Semin Arthritis Rheum 1990; 20:148.

40. Thadani U, Iveson JMI, Wright V. Cardiac tamponade, constrictive pericarditis and pericardial resection in rheumatoid arthritis. Medicine 1975;54:261.

41. Thould AK. Constrictive pericarditis in rheumatoid arthritis. Ann Rheum Dis 1986;45:89.

42 Blake S, Bonar S, O'Neill H, et al. Etiology of chronic constrictive pericarditis. Br Heart J 1983;50:273.

43. Cameron J, Oesterle SN, Baldwin JC, et al. The etiologic spectrum of constrictive pericarditis. Am Heart J 1987;113:354.

44. Franco AE, Levine HD, Hall AP. Rheumatoid pericarditis: report of 17 cases diagnosed clinically. Ann Intern Med 1972;77:837.

45. Lebowitz WB. The heart in rheumatoid arthritis (rheumatoid disease): a clinical and pathological study of 62 cases. Ann Intern Med 1963;58:102.

46. Lebowitz WB. The heart in rheumatoid disease. Geriatrics 1966;21:194.

47. Bacon PA, Scott DGI: La vascularite rhumatoide. In: Sany J, ed. Polyarthrite rhumatoide. Paris: Medecine-Sciences, Flammarion, 1987.

48. Slack JD, Waller B. Acute congestive heart failure due to the arteritis of rheumatoid arthritis: early diagnosis by endomyocardial biopsy: a case report. Angiology 1986;37:477.

49. Ahern M, Lever JV, Cosh J. Complete heart block in rheumatoid arthritis. Ann Rheum Dis 1983;42:389.

50. Hess ME. Effect of antimalarial drugs on cardiac muscle. Fed Proc 1954;13:365.

51. Jurik AG, Moller P. Atrioventricular conduction time in rheumatoid arthritis. Rheumatol Int 1985;5:205.

52. Whisnant JP, Espinosa RE, Kierland RR, Lambert EH. Chloroquine neuromyopathy. Mayo Clin Proc 1963;38:501.

53. Iveson JMI, Pomerance A. Cardiac involvement in rheumatic disease. Clin Rheum Dis 1977;3:467.

54. Liew M, et al. Successful valve replacement for aortic incompetence in rheumatoid arthritis with vasculitis. Ann Rheum Dis 1979;38:483.

55. Townend JN, Emery P, Davies MK, Littler WA. Acute aortitis and aortic incompetence due to systemic rheumatological disorders. Int J Cardiol 1991;33:253.

56. Cosh JA, Lever JV. The aortic valve. In: Ansell BM, Simkin PA, ed. The heart and rheumatic disease. Cornwall; Butterworths International Medical Reviews-Rheumatology 2, 1984:83.

57. Isomur T, Hisatomi K, Yanagi I, et al. The surgical treatment of aortic incompetence secondary to aortitis. Ann Thorac Surg 1988;45:181.

58. Duke-Elder S, Soley RE. Summary of systemic ophthalmology. In: Duke-Elder S. ed. System of ophthalmology. St. Louis: CV Mosby, 1976:139.

59. Wilson F. Adverse external ocular effects of topical ophthalmic medications. Surv Ophthalmol 1979;24:57.

60. Fox RI, Howell FV, Bone RC, Michelson P. Primary Sjögren's syndrome: clinical and immunopathologic features. Semin Arthritis Rheum 1984;14:77.

61. Ferry AP. The eye and rheumatic disease. In: Kelley WN, et al, eds. Textbook of rheumatology. 4th ed. Philadelphia: WB Saunders, 1993:507.

62. Watson PG, Hayreh SS. Scleritis and episcleritis. Br J Opthalmol 1976;60:163.

63. Hoffman F, Wiederholt M. Local treatment of necrotizing scleritis with cyclosporin A. Cornea 1985/1986;4:3.

64. Insler MS, Boutros G, Boulware O. Corneal ulceration following cataract surgery in patients

with rheumatoid arthritis. J Am Intraocul Implant Soc 1985;11:594.

65. Maffett MJ, Johns KJ, Parrish CM, Elliott JH, Glick AD, O'Day DM. Sterile corneal ulceration after cataract extraction in patients with collagen vascular disease. Cornea 1990;9:279.

66. Jones RR, Maguire LJ. Corneal complications after cataract surgery in patients with rheumatoid arthritis. Cornea 1992;11:148.

67. Killian PJ, McClain B, Lawless OJ. Brown's syndrome: an unusual manifestation of rheumatoid arthritis. Arthritis Rheum 1977;20:1080.

68. Cooper C, Kirwan JR, McGill NW, Dieppe PA. Brown's syndrome: an unusual ocular complication of rheumatoid arthritis. Ann Rheum Dis 1990;49:188.

69. Foster CS, Forstot SL, Wilson LA. Mortality rate in rheumatoid arthritis patients developing necrotizing scleritis or peripheral ulcerative keratitis: effects of systemic immunosuppression. Ophthalmology 1984;91:1253.

70. Chang LW, Gowans JDC, Granger CV, Millender LH. Entrapment neuropathy of the posterior interosseous nerve: a complication of rheumatoid arthritis. Arthritis Rheum 1972; 15:350.

71. Baylan SP, Paik SW, Barnert AL, Ko KH, Yu J, Persellin RH. Prevalence of the tarsal tunnel syndrome in rheumatoid arthritis. Rheumatol Rehabil 1981;20:148.

72. Chamberlain MA, Bruckner FE. Rheumatoid neuropathy: clinical and electrophysiological features. Ann Rheum Dis 1970;29:609.

73. Nakano KK. Neurologic complications of rheumatoid arthritis. Orthop Clin North Am 1975;6:861.

74. Lipson SJ. Rheumatoid arthritis of the cervical spine. Clin Orthop 1984;182:143.

75. Menezes AH, VanGilder JC, Clark CR, El-Khoury G. Odontoid upward migration in rheumatoid arthritis: an analysis of 45 patients with "cranial settling." J Neurosurg 1985;63: 500.

76. Conlon PW, Isdale IC, Rose BS. Rheumatoid arthritis of the cervical spine: an analysis of 33 cases. Ann Rheum Dis 1966;25:120.

77. Smith PH, Benn RT, Sharp J. Natural history of rheumatoid cervical luxations. Ann Rheum Dis 1972;31:431.

78. Santavirta S, Kankaanpää U, Sandelin J, Laasonen E, Kottinen YT, Slätis P. Evaluation of patients with rheumatoid cervical spine. Scand J Rheumatol 1987;16:9.

79. Crellin RQ, MacCabe JJ, Hamilton EBD. Severe subluxation of the cervical spine in rheumatoid arthritis. J Bone Joint Surg 1970;52B: 244.

80. Menezes AH, VanGilder JC, Graf CJ, et al. Craniocervical abnormalities: a comprehensive surgical approach. J Neurosurg 1980;53:444.

81. Apuzzo MLJ, Weiss MH, Heiden JS. Transoral exposure of the atlantoaxial region. Neurosurgery 1978;3:201.

82. Cabonela ME. Personal communication. Mayo Clinic, Rochester, MN.

83. Weiland DJ, McAfee PC. Posterior cervical fusion with triple-wire strut graft technique: one hundred consecutive patients. J Spinal Disord 1991;4:15.

84. Husby G. Amyloidosis in rheumatoid arthritis. Ann Clin Res 1975;7:154.

85. Lender M, Wolf E. Incidence of amyloidosis in rheumatoid arthritis. Scand J Rheumatol 1972;1:109.

86. Wegelius O, Wafin F, Falck H, Tørnroth T. Follow-up study of amyloidosis secondary to rheumatic disease. In: Glenner GG, Costa PP, Falcao de Freitas A, eds. Amyloid and amyloidosis. Amsterdam: Excerpta Medica, 1980:337.

87. Koota K, Isomäki HA, Mutru O. Death rate and causes of death in patients with rheumatoid arthritis. Scand J Rheumatol 4:205,197.

88. Husby G. Amyloidsis and rheumatoid arthritis. Clin Exp Rheumatol 1985;3:173.

89. Ahlmen M, Ahlmen J, Svalander C, Bucht H. Cytotoxic drug treatment of reactive amyloidosis in rheumatoid arthritis with special reference to renal insufficiency. Clin Rheumatol 1987;6:27.

90. Thorne C, Urowitz MB. Long-term outcome in Felty's syndrome. Ann Rheum Dis 1982;41:486.

91. Weisman M, Zvaifler NJ. Cryoimmunoglobulinemia in Felty's syndrome. Arthritis Rheum 1976;19:103.

92. Campion G, Maddison PJ, Goulding N, et al. The Felty syndrome: a case-matched study of clinical manifestations and outcome, serologic features, and immunogenetic associations. Medicine 1990;69:69.

93. Weyand CM, Xie C, Goronzy JJ. Homozygosity for the HLA-DRB1 allele selects for extra-articular manifestations in rheumatoid arthritis. J Clin Invest 1992;89:2033.

94. Rosenstein ED, Kramer N. Felty's and pseudo-Felty's syndromes. Semin Arthritis Rheum 1991;21:129.

95. Dillon AM, Luthra HS, Conn DL, Ferguson RH. Parenteral gold therapy in the Felty syndrome: experience with 20 patients. Medicine 1986;65:107.

96. Breedveld FC, Fibbe WE, Hermans J, van der Meer JWM, Cats A. Factors influencing the incidence of infections in Felty's syndrome. Arch Intern Med 1987;147:915.

97. Barton JC, Prasthofer EF, Egan ML, Heck LW, Koopman WJ, Grossi CE. Rheumatoid arthritis associated with expanded populations of granular lymphocytes. Ann Intern Med 1986;014:314.

98. Loughran TP Jr. Clonal diseases of large granular lymphocytes. Blood 1993;82:1.

99. Luthra HS, Hunder GG. Spontaneous remission of Felty's syndrome. Arthritis Rheum 1975;18:515.

100. Sibley JT, Haga M, Visram DA, Mitchell DM. The clinical course of Felty's syndrome com-

pared to matched controls. J. Rheumatol 1991;18:1163.

101. Wimer BM, Sloan MW. Remission of Felty's syndrome with long-term testosterone therapy. JAMA 1973;223:671.

102. Mant MJ, Akabutu JJ, Herbert FA. Lithium carbonate therapy in severe Felty's syndrome: benefits, toxicity, and granulocyte function. Arch Intern Med 1984;14:277.

103. Breedveld FC, Brand A, Van Aken WG. High dose intravenous gamma globulin for Felty's syndrome. J Rheumatol 1985;12:700.

104. Luthra HS, Conn DL, Ferguson RH. Felty's syndrome: response to parenteral gold. J Rheumatol 1981;8:902.

105. Fiechtner JJ, Miller DR, Starkebaum G. Reversal of neutropenic with methotrexate treatment in patients with Felty's syndrome. Arthritis Rheum 1989;32:194.

106. Wandt H, Seifert M, Falge C, Gallmeier WM. Long-term correction of neutropenia in Felty's syndrome with granulocyte colony-stimulating factor. Ann Hematol 1993;66:265.

107. Sokoloff L, Bunim JJ. Vascular lesions in rheumatoid arthritis. J Cronic Dis 1957;5:668.

108. Lakhanpal S, Conn DL, Lie JT. Clinical and prognostic significance of vasculitis as an early manifestation of connective tissue disease syndromes. Ann Intern Med 1984;101:743.

109. Conn DL. Rheumatoid neuropathy. In: Utsinger PD, Zvalifer NJ, eds. Rheumatoid arthritis. Philadelphia: JB Lippincott, 1985.

110. Vollertsen RS, Conn DL. Vasculitis associated with rheumatoid arthritis. Rheum Dis Clin North Am 1990;16:445.

111. Scott DGI, Bacon PA, Tribe CR. Systemic rheumatoid vasculitis: a clinical and laboratory study of 50 cases. Medicine 1981;60:288.

112. Weyand CM, Hicok KC, Conn DL, Goronzy JJ. The influence of HLA-DRB1 genes on disease severity in rheumatoid arthritis. Ann Intern Med 1992;117:801.

113. Luthra HS, McDuffie FC, Hunder GG, Samayoa EA. Immune complexes in sera and synovial fluid of patients with rheumatoid arthritis: radioimmunoassay with monoclonal rheumatoid factor. J Clin Invest 1975;56:458.

114. Heurkens AHN, Hiemstra PS, Lafeber GJM, Daha MR, Breedveld FC. Anti-endothelial cells antibodies in patients with rheumatoid arthritis complicated by vasculitis. Clin Exp Immunol 1989;78:7.

115. Conn DL, McDuffie FC, Dyck PJ. Immunopathologic study of sural nerves in rheumatoid arthritis. Arthritis Rheum 1972;15:135.

116. Vollertsen RS, Conn DL, Ballard DJ, Ilstrup DM, Kazmar RE, Silverfield JC. Rheumatoid vasculitis: survival and associated risk factors. Medicine 1986;65:365.

117. Kemper JW, Baggenstoss AH, Slocumb CH. The relationship of therapy with cortisone to the incidence of vascular lesions in rheumatoid arthritis. Ann Intern Med 1957;46:831.

118. Conn DL, Tompkins RB, Nichols WL. Glucocorticosteroids in the management of vasculitis—a double-edged sword? J Rheumatol 1988;15:1181.

119. Dyck PJ, Conn DL, Okazaki H. Necrotizing angiopathic neuropathy: three-dimensional morphology of fiber degeneration related to sites of occluded vessels. Mayo Clin Proc 1972;47:461.

120. Deguchi Y, Shibata N, Kishimoto S. Enhanced expression of the tumor necrosis factor/cachectin gene in peripheral blood mononuclear cells from patients with systemic vasculitis. Clin Exp Immunol 1990;81:311.

121. Dasgupta B, Panayi GS. Interleukin-6 in serum of patients with polymyalgia rheumatica and giant cell arteritis. Br J Rheumatol 1990;29:456.

122. Bywaters EGL. Peripheral vascular obstruction in rheumatoid arthritis and its relationship to other vascular lesions. Ann Rheum Dis 1957;16:84.

122a. Gordon M, Luqmani RA, Adu D, et al. Relapses in patients with a systemic vasculitis. Q J Med 1993;86:779.

123. Jaffe IA. The treatment of rheumatoid arthritis and necrotizing vasculitis with penicillamine. Arthritis Rheum 1970;13:436.

124. Abel T, Andrews BS, Cunningham PH, Brunner CM, Davis JS, Horwitz DA. Rheumatoid vasculitis: effect of cyclophosphamide on the clinical course and levels of circulating immune complexes. Ann Intern Med 1980;93:407.

125. Scott DGI, Bacon PA. Intravenous cyclophosphamide plus methylprednisolone in treatment of systemic rheumatoid vasculitis. Am J Med 1984;76:377.

126. Upchurch KS, Heller K, Bress NM. Low-dose methotrexate therapy for cutaneous vasculitis and rheumatoid arthritis. J Am Acad Dermatol 1987;17:355.

127. Segal R, Caspi D, Tishler M, Fishel B, Yaron M. Accelerated nodulosis and vasculitis during methotrexate therapy for rheumatoid arthritis. Arthritis Rheum 1988;31:1182.

128. Nicholls A, Snaith ML, Maini RN, Scott JT. Controlled trial of azathioprine in rheumatoid vasculitis. Ann Rheum Dis 1973;32:589.

129. Heurkens AH, Westedt ML, Breedveld FC. Prednisone plus azathioprine treatment in patients with rheumatoid arthritis complicated by vasculitis. Arch Intern Med 1991;151:2249.

130. Scott DGI, Bacon PA, Bothamley JE, Allen C, Elson CJ, Wallington TB. Plasma exchange in rheumatoid vasculitis. J Rheumatol 1981;8:433.

131. Jayne DRW, Davies MJ, Fox CJV, Black CM, Lockwood CM. Treatment of systemic vasculitis with pooled intravenous immunoglobulin. Lancet 1991;337:1137.

132. Kelly WN, Harris ED, Ruddy S, Sledge CB, eds. Textbook of rheumatology. Philadelphia: WB Saunders, 1993.

SJÖGREN'S SYNDROME

Robert I. Fox

Sjögren's syndrome (SS) is a combination of dry eyes (keratoconjunctivitis sicca [KCS]) and dry mouth (xerostomia). Sjögren's syndrome is divided into two forms: a primary (1°) SS, and a secondary (2°) SS in which the sicca symptoms are associated with other well-defined autoimmune diseases, such as rheumatoid arthritis, systemic lupus erythematosus (SLE), or progressive systemic sclerosis.[1] Since many patients with SS increasingly receive their "primary" care from their rheumatologist, it is important that rheumatologists, as well as other physicians, be familiar with the treatments used by ophthalmologists, otolaryngologists, and oral medicine specialists. For an in-depth discussion of the etiopathogenesis and diagnostic features of SS, please see Kelley et al., Chapter 55 (reference 42).

Although the ophthalmic component (i.e., KCS) is well defined, the criteria for classifying the oral component remains controversial, and thus no uniform classification system for SS exists. On the one hand, the San Diego criteria (described below) require objective evidence of KCS, xerostomia, characteristic lymphocytic infiltrate on minor salivary gland biopsy, and the presence of autoantibodies.[2] On the other hand, European criteria for SS can be fulfilled in the absence of biopsy or autoantibodies.[3] This lack of uniform classification criteria has led to confusion in clinical practice and in the research literature. For example, the incidence of a particular disease association (e.g., dementia or lymphoma) or the response to a particular medicine (e.g., hydroxychloroquine) is directly affected by the inclusion criteria for the study group.

The treatment for SS can be separated into conservative therapy (i.e., moisture replacement), treatment of systemic autoimmune features such as vasculitis, and management of nonspecific symptoms such as fatigue or sleep disorders. In addition, these patients have particular needs at the time of surgery to prevent complications related to their dry eyes, mouth, and upper airways. This chapter will concentrate on the conservative management of dryness complaints in the patients with SS, since this information is not easily accessible in the rheumatology literature.

EVALUATION AND TREATMENT OF THE PATIENT WITH DRY EYES

The mainstay of treatment for the patient with dry eyes is the regular use of artificial tears.[4] However, it is important to identify environmental factors and medications that contribute to dry-eye symptoms (Table 5–1). For example, symptoms of dry eyes will be exacerbated by low-humidity environments, such as airplanes, highly air-conditioned offices or department stores, and outdoor areas with strong, dry winds. The increased use of tears *before* the onset of symptoms will be symptomatically helpful and will prevent corneal abrasions. The use of cool-mist humidifiers at night (or even in the office) and wraparound sunglasses outdoors will help retard evaporation of tears. In patients who wear glasses, moisture shields can be added to the frames by the optometrist. Contact lenses, especially the soft gas-permeable type, can contribute to corneal abrasions since adequate tear film may not be available to wash out foreign substances trapped under the lens. In patients who like or need to be outdoors, ski goggles can provide a local "moisture chamber."

TABLE 5–1

Evaluation of Patient with Dry Eyes and Mouth

I. Identify cofactors such as:
   A. Low-humidity environment
   B. Exposure to cigarette smoke and other irritants
   C. Medications with anticholinergic side effects
II. Basic tests of tear and saliva volume:
   A. Schirmer's I (without anesthetic)
   B. Schirmer's II (with nasolacrimal reflex stimulation)
   C. Sialometry (measure of saliva production)
   D. Scintigraphy (excretion rate of technetium)
   E. Sialograms (to be avoided because of risk of complications)
III. Tests of tear film integrity:
   A. Rose bengal
   B. Fluorescein staining of conjunctiva
   C. Tear-breakup time (von Bijerfeld score)
IV. If eye symptoms are out of proportion to the objective findings:
   A. Rule out blepharitis (inflammation of lids)
   B. Rule out uveitis or retinitis (requires slit-lamp examination)
   C. Rule out blepharospasm (uncontrolled blink reflex)
   D. Rule out anxiety or depression

Unstimulated tear flow is referred to as "basal" flow. A decrease in basal tear flow, especially at night, often is the initial symptom. These symptoms of eye discomfort occur even though the patients can generate tears when they cry or are exposed to certain stimuli, such as onions. Tear volume is generally measured by insertion of paper strips under the lower lid in the absence of topical anesthesia for 5 minutes (Schirmer's I test). Maximally stimulated tear flow (Schirmer's II test) is measured by gentle insertion of a Q-tip into the nose to stimulate the nasolacrimal reflex.[5] The Schirmer's II test provides a rapid way to assess stimulated volume of tear flow. However, a wide range of tear volume flow occurs in normal eyes and is poorly correlated with signs and symptoms of KCS. Similarly, the volume of saliva produced as basal secretion or after stimulation correlates poorly with symptoms of dry mouth and objective signs of severe periodontal problems.[6] This suggests that the qualitative content of tears and saliva (i.e., specific glycoproteins and mucins) plays an important role in the maintenance of ocular and oral mucosal integrity and that decreases in tear volume are not the sole cause of problems. An important implication of these findings is that the next "generation" of artificial tears, artificial salivas, and toothpastes may contain bioengineered products that provide these important functions that are lacking in the currently available products.

When evaluating the patient with a complaint of dry eyes, it is important to determine whether the objective signs of dry eyes are commensurate with the patient's symptoms. The integrity of the corneal surface and tear film can be measured by means of rose bengal, fluorescein staining, or the tear-breakup time[7,8] (Table 5–1). For example, the absence of a significantly abnormal examination with rose bengal (a test that is easily performed by the rheumatologist) should suggest a search for additional causes to explain the patient's ocular complaints. These may include eye strain (poor refraction), blepharitis (irritation of the lids), blepharospasm (uncontrolled blinking due to an increased local neural reflex circuit), uveitis, retinitis, or symptoms caused by anxiety or depression.

When evaluating a particular artificial tear preparation (Tables 5–2 and 5–3), the patient must carefully determine whether (1) the tear gives benefit but the effect does not last long enough or (2) the tear causes the eye to burn immediately upon instillation. Artificial tears can be considered to have at least two distinct components: the moisturizing component and the preservative. If the tear is helpful but the

TABLE 5–2

Guidelines for Evaluation and Use of Artificial Tears

I. Do the artificial tears last long enough? If not:
   A. Use a more viscous tear
   B. Try a tear with different osmolality
   C. Use a tear with a different vehicle
      1. Hydroxymethylcellulose
      2. Dextran polymer
   D. Ophthalmologist can perform punctal occlusion to make instilled tears last longer
      1. Temporary (collagen plugs)
      2. Permanent (cautery or laser)
II. Do the tears burn after installation? If so:
   A. Choose tear with different preservative
   B. Use a nonpreserved tear
III. Anticipate low-humidity environments and start increased use of tears in advance

TABLE 5–3
Artificial Tears and Ointments

	PRESERVATIVE
Tears	
Cellufresh	None
Liquifilm	Chlorobutanol
Tears Plus	Chlorobutanol
Liquifilm Forte	Thimerosal
Hypotears	Benzalkonium chloride
Hypotears PF	None
Tears Naturale II	Polyquad
Adsorbotear	Thimerosal
Murocel	Methylparaben
Biontears	None
Aquasite	None
Ocular Ointments	
Refresh PM	None
HypoTears	None
Duolube	None
Duratears	Methylparaben
Lacri-Lube	Chlorobutanol
Lacrisert	None

benefit does not last long enough, then a more viscous tear (such as a higher concentration of hydroxymethylcellulose) or a different vehicle to concentrate the moisturizing element (such as a polymer-like dextran) is indicated.

If the eye burns soon after instillation, then an irritant reaction to a preservative in the tear must be considered.[9] These reactions were much more frequent in the past, when benzalkonium chloride and thimerosal were commonly used in artificial tears. However, it should be remembered that these preservatives are still widely used in other ophthalmologic preparations (particularly topical antibiotics) and may contribute to ocular irritation. Irritation of the eyelids in some patients with blepharitis may be related to the preservatives present in some ocular lubricants (used at night) as well as the nighttime use of excessive amounts of lubricant that plug the meibomian glands.

If the particular artificial tear seems helpful but the benefit does not last long enough, punctal occlusion may be performed on a temporary or permanent basis.[4] The puncta are the tiny openings at the medial aspects of the lids. Blockage with collagen plugs (i.e., temporary occlusion that lasts several days) will allow determination of potential symptomatic benefit and make sure that reflex tearing in the patient

does not cause tears to run down the cheeks. If helpful, "permanent" punctal occlusion can be done by electrocautery in the ophthalmologist's office, a quick procedure that is done with topical anesthesia.

Adjuncts to therapy have included acetylcysteine 10% drops to break up mucous strands, but these drops have the smell of rotten eggs and are thus objectionable to most patients.[10] Vitamin A and related preparations have a theoretical role in the treatment of dry eye, since vitamin A–deficient patients have increased keratinization of the corneal surface[11]; however, more recent studies have not supported the initial enthusiasm for this form of treatment.[4] Bromhexine, a cough syrup, has been reported to stimulate tear production.[12] Subsequent clinical trials have not been convincing, although some patients report considerable benefit.[4] Topical cyclosporin has been used to increase lacrimal flow rates in dogs with dry eyes; interestingly, it may be that these effects are not related to immune suppressive effects of cyclosporin but result from stimulation of prolactin receptors on the cell surface of corneal and lacrimal gland acinar cells.[13] However, the diluents required to dissolve cyclosporin have thus far proved too irritating to use in patients with SS.

EVALUATION AND TREATMENT OF DRY MOUTH

The principal oral symptom of SS is mouth dryness with a broad range of severity. Not all patients complain of dryness specifically; many describe difficulty in swallowing food, problems in wearing dentures, changes in their sense of taste, increased incidence of dental caries, chronic burning symptoms, intolerance to acidic or spicy foods, and inability to eat dry food or to speak continuously for more than a few minutes.[14] Nutrition may be compromised and patterns of sleep disturbed.

Examination of the mouth shows that the patient with SS lacks the normal salivary pooling under the tongue and may have rapidly progressive caries. The mouth frequently exhibits petechial lesions on the hard palate and lichen planus–like lesions (fine white lacy strands) on the buccal mucosa. These lesions result from chronic oral candidiasis in the patient with SS; it is uncommon for a patient's mouth to exhibit the "plaque"-like appearance (thrush) found in

TABLE 5–4
Guidelines for Dry Mouth

I. A dry mouth is not necessarily a painful mouth.
   A. Look for oral yeast (especially under dentures) and angular cheilitis. Common after antibiotics or steroids.
   B. Look for nasal congestion that contributes to mouth breathing.
II. Use of fluorides, toothpastes, and salivary stimulants.
   A. Fluorides
     1. Topical applications with toothbrush
     2. Direct application with dental trays
   B. Toothpastes
     1. Biotene
     2. Dental Care
     3. Retardex
   C. Prevention of decay
     1. Regular oral hygiene by trained specialist
     2. Anti-infective
       a. Peridex
       b. Retardex
III. Saliva stimulation and artificial saliva
   A. Iodines (SSKI), Organidin
   B. Chewing gum, electric stimulators
   C. Pilocarpine
   D. Bromhexine
   E. Oral balance gel
   F. Biotene mouth rinse
IV. Saliva substitutes
   A. MouthKote
   B. Salivart
   C. Saliment
   D. Xero-Lube
   E. Saliva substitute

severely immunocompromised patients. Another manifestation of oral candidiasis in the patient with SS is angular cheilitis, a condition that must be treated at the same time as the candidiasis of the buccal mucosa.

Patients with residual salivary gland function may benefit from either local or systemic methods to stimulate flow (Table 5–4). Gustatory stimulation with sugarless mints is often effective, as is chewing sugarless gum. One caution is that even sugarless gum may contain carbohydrates that have cariogenic potential in the presence of reduced salivary function.[15] Some patients find that chewing on paraffin or a fruit pit provides adequate masticatory stimulation without increasing cariogenic potential.

Systemic sialagogues have been used to increase salivation. Three agents have been studied in controlled trials. Bromhexine, a muco-lytic agent, was not found to increase salivary flow rate, but patients described subjective benefit.[16] Anethole trithione (Sialor) showed significant effects on saliva output in one study of patients with SS who had mild secretory hypofunction[17]; however, a later study failed to find a significant response in patients with severe hypofunction.[18] A series of controlled studies have indicated that pilocarpine has stimulatory properties in SS and postradiation therapy patients.[19,20,21] The drug acts primarily as a muscarinic-cholinergic agonist with mild β-adrenergic activity. In these studies, pilocarpine, 5 mg three times a day, increased salivary flow for several hours in comparison with placebo. Side effects were common and included sweating, flushing, and increased urination. Iodides (SSKI or Organidin) are thought to increase bronchial secretions and thus enhance the breakdown of tenacious mucus. Although considered helpful by some patients, there is no objective evidence of clinical efficacy in SS, although these agents can be shown at high doses to increase fluid transport in the rat trachea model.[22]

A dry mouth is not necessarily a painful mouth. It is common for a Sjögren's patient to develop a low-grade oral yeast infection.[14] Predisposing factors include recent use of antibiotics and/or corticosteroids. Treatment of this problem is particularly difficult in the patient with dentures, since continued excoriation of the mucosal surface occurs. Many topical antifungal drugs are available, but some oral preparations suffer from a low content of antifungal agent and a high concentration of glucose (to improve the taste) and thus contribute to dental decay if used for an extended period.[14] Nystatin (available as oral troches and as vaginal suppositories that can be sucked) is helpful but must be sucked for about 20 minutes twice daily for at least 6 weeks to prevent recurrence.[23] Patients with very dry mouth will require periodic sips of water to help dissolve the troches. Chlortrimazole (also available in the form of troches) may be used in the same manner. For angular cheilitis, topical antifungal creams (Lotrisone, Spectazole) are used two to three times a day for several weeks. To permit drug access to all intraoral mucosal sites, patients must remove their dentures while antifungal tablets are dissolving. The dentures also must be treated to remove traces of *Candida*, and the method of disinfectant must be discussed with the dentist. However, it is usually sufficient to soak the complete denture overnight in benzalkonium chloride (e.g., a 1/700 dilution of the surgical scrub solution, Zephiran). The dentures must be carefully cleaned with a toothbrush, and often mystatin powder must be applied to the fitting surfaces of the upper denture before reinsertion of the dentures. In extreme cases, a short course of oral antifungal therapy (such as ketoconazole or fluconazole) may be required to control oral candidiasis.

Progressive dental disease in patients with SS leads to increased need for dental restorations, particularly because of caries at the gum line and incisor surfaces. The loss of teeth and the requirement for dentures at any age, but particularly in the younger patient, may have significant emotional and economic consequences. Patients with dentures may change their social patterns of interpersonal interactions. For example, social life frequently involves eating meals with friends, and the patient may feel uncomfortable about not being able to eat the same foods. Further, the patient's diet may be shifted over to "preprocessed" foods that are often higher in sugars and thus further accelerate the rate of periodontal problems.

The use of topical fluorides may help protect dental enamel. In some patients, a neutral fluoride drop may be applied by toothbrush or by the oral hygienist. In other patients, direct contact of the dental surfaces and the fluoride gel can be achieved by using "dental plates" at night to apply the fluoride. These "plates" are made specifically for each patient by the periodontist.

The use of a correct toothbrush technique to massage the gums and remove debris is important, since this normal function of saliva is diminished in patients with SS. In some patients, a rotating toothbrush (such as Oratek) is useful, together with regular oral hygiene by a technician experienced in the care of dry mouth.

Several different types of toothpaste especially designed for periodontal problems are available for the patient with dry mouth. In the past, Peridex (a fluorine-based product) was popular but occasionally stained the dental enamel. More recently, a chlorine-based toothpaste (Retardex) is being tested and lacks this problem. An additional type of toothpaste based on the principle of generating low levels of antibacterial peroxides (i.e., Biotene) has been used.

A variety of saliva substitutes is available. They differ in their flavoring agents and preservatives. MouthKote and Salivart sprays contain mucins, which are glycoproteins that help lubricate the mouth and thus provide relief for a longer time than simply rinsing with water.[24] After administration of these sprays, parotid flow rates are increased for 7 to 8 minutes in patients with SS; however, the sense of "oral well-being" may last for several hours. Electrical (vibrating) stimulation was used to stimulate saliva in some patients with mildly decreased flow rates,[25] although the cost of the apparatus has precluded wide usage.

NASAL DRYNESS AND SINUSITIS

Many patients with SS complain of nasal dryness and have symptoms of sinusitis with postnasal drip. It is common for a simple upper respiratory tract or sinus infection to linger for months in SS patients. This probably develops because of decreased secretion of glands that line the nasopharynx, leading to crusting of mucous secretions that block drainage and predispose to subsequent bacterial infection. Our initial approach is to provide increased moisture to this region by use of normal saline sprays and humidifiers at night.

It is frequently beneficial for the patient to learn to "lavage" the sinuses to remove the dry, crusted secretions. For patients with persistent sinus symptoms, it is useful to obtain a "nasal smear" to determine whether allergic factors (indicated by the presence of eosinophils on the smear) are playing a factor. Topical nasal sprays (such as beclomethasone [Beconase AQ Nasal] or flunisolide [Nasalide]) may be helpful in these patients.

In the setting of sinusitis, it is always important to notice whether the secretions change from clear to yellow or green; the latter situation may indicate the occurrence of bacterial infection and necessitate treatment with antibiotics. Treatment of acute sinusitis often requires a temporary course of corticosteroids (prednisone, 20 mg, twice a day for 2 days with rapid taper over 1 week) plus antibiotics (especially trimethoprim-sulfamethoxazole [Bactrim DS] twice a day or amoxicillin [Augmentin], 250 mg, three times a day) for 1 week; however, this combination of medications is likely to predispose the patient to oral *Candida* infection. We frequently have patients who are taking antibiotics use antifungal oral troches or yogurt to help prevent oral candidiasis. In patients with recurrent sinusitis, "limited" computed tomography scans of the sinuses can help determine the presence of significant obstruction requiring surgical intervention by sinus endoscopy. In our experience, the use of "suppressive" or "preventive" antibiotics for patients with SS has not been as helpful as a diligent preventive program of daily sinus lavage by the patients.

SKIN AND RENAL MANIFESTATIONS

Several types of skin manifestations occur in SS patients, ranging from simple dryness to vasculitis. Increased dryness has been attributed to decreased exocrine function of the sebaceous glands in the skin. Creams are distinguished from lotions by being "greasier" than lotions, which often contain oil/water mixtures. Creams and ointments are preferred because they better "seal" in necessary moisture. In general, we suggest applying the creams after a shower or bath while the skin is still moist. Alternatively, the cream can be applied to dry skin directly after moistening with a damp cloth. Cosmetics such as lipstick can be applied 5 to 10 minutes later. Topical creams such as Eucerin, Aquaderm, and Complex 15 are available as over-the-counter preparations. In some patients, additional moisturizing compounds may be necessary. We have found that Aquaphor plus 1% hydrocortisone (mixed by a pharmacist) or Aquaphor AB (containing an antibiotic as a commercially available mixture) further aids the healing of dry skin with associated fissures.

Hyperpigmentation, termed "hyperglobulinemic purpura of Waldenström" (HGPW), occurs in the lower extremities and is characterized by a nonpalpable purpura.[8,26] Additional skin manifestations in patients with SS include leukocytoclastic vasculitis (palpable purpura) and eczematous rashes such as "subacute SLE." In some cases a lymphocytic angiitis has been reported in association with a higher incidence of visceral vasculitis.[27] In addition to symptomatic skin care as described above, my treatment of the underlying disease process can include antimalarial drugs such as hydroxychloroquine (6 to 7 mg/kg/day), chloroquine (250 to 500 mg/day), or quinacrine (100 mg/day). A course

of corticosteroids (prednisone, 10 to 20 mg) may be required for several weeks because of the slow onset of effectiveness of the antimalarial medications. The lower extremity lesions of HGPW are quite position dependent; avoiding prolonged standing and weight bearing and wearing support hose are helpful.

The most common functional renal abnormality noted in patients with SS is the inability to acidify the urine in response to an administered acid load, such as ammonium chloride. This is generally thought to be due to dysfunction of the distal nephron and may be present in a latent form in 20% to 40% of SS patients.[10] This is not generally a clinical problem in caucasoid patients but is more frequent among Chinese patients with SS, probably because of the side effects of various plant alkaloids frequently taken as herbal medications.[28,29] Among caucasoid patients, the use of particular medications such as nonsteroidal antiinflammatory drugs (NSAIDs), antibiotics such as aminoglycosides, and, increasingly, herbal medicines (at least in Southern California) may contribute to interstitial nephritis. Discontinuation of the offending agent is usually sufficient, but some patients may require bicarbonate supplementation (1 to 2 g/day), corticosteroids (prednisone, 5 to 15 mg/day), or azathioprine (50 to 100 mg/day).

Proteinuria and glomerulonephritis are unusual in primary SS and suggest an associated disease process such as SLE, amyloidosis, or mixed cryoglobulinemia. Membranoproliferative and membranous forms of glomerulonephritis have been described, and immunopathologic studies suggest that the glomerular lesions are associated with accumulation of immune complex material.[30,31]

GYNECOLOGIC ISSUES

Vaginal dryness often leads to painful intercourse (dyspareunia). It is important to reassure the patient that this does not occur in all patients with SS, even those with severe mouth and eye dryness. A gynecologic examination is important to rule out other causes of painful intercourse and other causes of vaginal dryness. When it does occur as part of SS, the patient's spouse needs to be reassured that this is a "physiologic" problem and not related to a failure of sexual arousal. Sterile lubricants such as K-Y jelly or Surgilube are helpful. The patient with

SS currently has multiple options for safe and effective vaginal lubrication. Such lubricants as Maxilube and Astroglide have slightly different physical characteristics than K-Y jelly or Surgilube and yet share the common characteristics of being water-soluble and nonirritating. This also holds true for the new nonhormonal vaginal moisturizer Replens, which may be used unassociated with intercourse. For those patients who do not like the gel-type lubricant, Lubrin (vaginal inserts) is now available. Add to this a new once-a-week vaginal lubricant called Vagikote (in clinical trials). Finding the right preparation for a specific person is often a matter of trial and error, inasmuch as satisfaction with each lubricant is a matter of personal preference. Patients should be frank with their physicians regarding satisfaction or dissatisfaction with a particular preparation. The internal use of preparations containing petrolatum or oils that "seal in" moisture, such as Vaseline or cocoa butter, may lead to maceration of the vaginal lining and are to be avoided.

Vaginal dryness in perimenopausal or postmenopausal women is often related to mucosal atrophy because of declining estrogen levels and therefore responds to vaginal estrogen creams. Cortisone creams are not beneficial in this situation. If vaginal yeast infection occurs, prompt treatment with clotrimazole cream or suppositories (Gyne-Lotrimin) is effective and safe. On the external vulvar surface, dryness may be treated with lubricating creams that are used on other skin surfaces. Several anecdotal reports note satisfaction with the use of a thin film of vitamin E oil applied to the vulva once or twice a day.

An issue of concern to female patients with SS has been whether estrogen replacement therapy is harmful to their condition. With regard to estrogen replacement in general, there is now convincing clinical evidence that estrogen treatment helps retard osteoporosis, reduces cardiovascular mortality, and improves quality of life by eliminating hot flashes and hormone-related vaginal dryness. In light of animal studies, earlier investigators were concerned that estrogen might have a negative influence on SS and may be contraindicated. At our clinic, however, we have not seen any deterioration related either to estrogen replacement therapy or to oral contraceptives in patients with SS. Because of this, we encourage adequate estrogen replacement for the properly screened postmenopausal patient with SS.

FATIGUE

Fatigue is a common complaint of patients with SS. The problem may have many causes and may be related directly or indirectly to SS. Two types of fatigue should be considered. The first type is late morning or early afternoon fatigue. In this case, the patient arises with adequate energy but simply "runs out of gas" in the early afternoon. This type of fatigue suggests an inflammatory or metabolic process. Patients describe this type of fatigue as having "flu-like" symptoms, and it is probably due to liberation by the active immune system of specific cytokines such as interleukin-1 and tumor necrosis factor. Fatigue due to active inflammation is often associated with elevated "sedimentation rate," "C-reactive protein," and polyclonal increase in immunoglobulins. An increased frequency of hypothyroidism is associated with SS, and thus periodic laboratory evaluation should be done to rule out this cause of fatigue.

A second type of fatigue is "morning fatigue," wherein the patient arises in the morning feeling that he/she has not obtained an adequate night's sleep. This type of fatigue is also quite common in SS and may exist in addition to "inflammatory" fatigue. For example, patients may have inadequate sleep because of joint or muscle pain. Also, patients with SS often drink a great deal of liquid during the day because of dry mouth and throat. Then at night they may awaken three or four times to urinate. This disrupts the sleep pattern and leads to morning fatigue. When this is the case, it is best to treat the symptoms directly, and better sleep should follow. In the treatment of sleep disorders, tricyclic drugs (such as amitriptyline, nortriptyline, and doxepin) should be avoided if possible because they increase dryness through their anticholinergic side effects (Table 5–5). Benzodiazepine agents, particularly clonazepan (Klonopin) in patients with nocturnal myoclonus, have proven helpful in patients with SS. In patients with sleep disorders related to nocturia, the use of saliva substitutes (rather than fluid ingestion) after dinner and at night may prove helpful.

Sometimes following good sleep habits is not enough to improve the sense of daytime fatigue and poor sleep. If this is the case, a specific evaluation for sleep disorders can be done. Certain persons may have a higher risk of physiologic sleep disorders, such as sleep apnea. Persons over 55 years of age who snore loudly and who

TABLE 5–5
Drugs Associated with Increased Dryness

I. Blood pressure medications
  A. α-blockers (clonidine)
  B. β-blockers (propranolol [Inderal])
  C. Combined α- and β-blockers (labetalol)
II. Antidepressants
  A. Amitriptyline (Elavil)
  B. Nortriptyline (Pamelor)
III. Muscle spasm
  A. Cyclobenzaprine (Flexeril)
  B. Methocarbamol (Robaxin)
IV. Urologic drugs
  A. Bethanechol (Urecholine)
  B. Yohimbine
V. Cardiac
  A. Disopyramide (Norpace)
VI. Parkinson's
  A. Levodopa and carbidopa (Sinemet)
VII. Decongestants
  A. Chlor-Trimeton
  B. Sudafed
  C. Other OTC preparations

have had substantial weight gain (often because of taking steroids) may be particularly prone to sleep apnea and will require C-pap.

DEPRESSION IN SJÖGREN'S SYNDROME

Depression can appear in many clinical forms, including difficulty in concentrating, poor appetite, or sleep disorder. The precise role of inflammation and hormone imbalances associated with SS as factors contributing to depression remains unclear, but certainly depression is caused in part by chemical alterations in the brain. Stress, poor sleep, and chronic illness can all contribute to depression. When antidepressant medications are used to help regulate sleep patterns and treat fatigue, drugs that have no anticholinergic side effects (such as trazodone, paroxetine [Paxil], and fluoxetine [Prozac], which interfere with serotonin uptake) are preferred.

SYSTEMIC MEDICATIONS IN PATIENTS WITH SJÖGREN'S SYNDROME

The overall approach to systemic therapy in the patient with SS is similar to that in the patient with SLE. Disease manifestations are subdivided into nonvisceral (arthralgias, myalgias, skin, fatigue) and visceral (lung, heart, kidney, brain, peripheral nervous system). Nonvisceral manifestations are generally treated with salicylates, nonsteroidal agents, and often hydroxychloroquine. Particular attention must be given to the SS patient's difficulty in swallowing pills since the decreased salivary content can lead to pills becoming stuck in the midesophagus with resultant erosions of the mucosa. Little improvement in salivary or lacrimal flow rates have been noted with NSAIDs, although some increase in tearing and salivation may occur after systemic corticosteroids. In terms of NSAIDs for patients with SS, indomethacin is the only agent readily available as a suppository for the patient with difficulty in swallowing tablets. Flurbiprofen has been shown in a pilot study to decrease periodontal inflammation and resultant gum disease.

Among the "slow-acting" drugs, antimalarials (chloroquine and hydroxychloroquine) have proven useful in decreasing arthralgias, myalgias, and lymphadenopathy in patients with SS,[32] similar to their benefit in some patients with SLE. We have given hydroxychloroquine (6 to 7 mg/kg/day) to SS patients with an elevated erythrocyte sedimentation rate (ESR) and polyclonal hyperglobulinemia, since these laboratory abnormalities suggest that symptoms of arthralgia and myalgia may have an "inflammatory" cause. We found a decrease in symptoms (arthralgias, myalgias), signs (lymphadenopathy and frequency of glandular swelling), and laboratory findings (ESR, polyclonal IgG, and frequency of circulating paraprotein) in SS patients treated at least 6 months with hydroxychloroquine (6 to 7 mg/kg/day).[32] A double-blind, 2-year study of hydroxychloroquine[33] indicated improved tear and salivary flow rates. In a European study,[33] hydroxychloroquine improved ESR but did not increase tear flow volumes. Comparison of drug benefit in SS patients in European and U.S. studies is strongly influenced by the very different inclusion criteria for diagnosis of SS (described above). When taken at the proper dose (6 to 7 mg/kg/day), hydroxychloroquine has a very good safety record, although there remains a remote possibility (probably less than 1/1,000)[34] of significant buildup in the eye. For this reason, periodic eye checks (generally every 6 to 12 months) are recommended in the United States so that the medicine can be discontinued if there is any significant buildup. In the United Kingdom, periodic eye checks are no longer recommended (or reimbursed by National Health Service) because the risk of toxicity is so low.[35]

For visceral involvement including vasculitic skin lesions, pneumonitis, neuropathy and nephritis, corticosteroids are used much as they are in patients with SLE. Initial high doses of corticosteroids (prednisone, 40 to 60 mg/day) for 1 to 2 weeks are generally followed by a tapering dose that decreases by about 10% per week.

Such drugs as hydroxychloroquine (discussed above), azathioprine, and methotrexate are used to help taper the corticosteroids. No published studies are available about the doses for either azathioprine or methotrexate in patients with SS; thus, doses similar to those given in other rheumatic disorders are generally used (i.e., azathioprine 2 to 3 mg/kg/day and methotrexate 7.5 to 15 mg per week). Cyclosporin may be used in some patients with SS,[36] but the tendency toward interstitial nephritis in many patients with SS limits the usefulness of the drug.

For life-threatening illness, cyclophosphamide is occasionally required. However, the increased frequency of lymphoma in patients with SS[37] requires caution in the use of cyclophosphamide and has suggested that it be given as a "pulse therapy" rather than by daily administration. The data relating to cyclophosphamide indicates an increased risk of leukemia and bladder cancer when the drug is used on a daily basis[38,39] and an increased risk of lymphoma in animal models of autoimmunity.[40] However, an increased incidence of tumors when cyclophosphamide is used in a monthly "pulse" regimen has not been demonstrated.[41]

SPECIAL THERAPEUTIC CONSIDERATION IN THE PATIENT WITH DRY EYES

Anesthesia and Surgery

Patients with SS have particular problems during the preoperative, perioperative, and postoperative periods. The normal preoperative instruction is "no fluids by mouth" after dinner or midnight on the day before surgery. In the absence of normal saliva flow, these patients have great discomfort that can be reduced by the use of artificial salivas.

Operating rooms and postoperative recovery areas have extremely low humidity, particularly when nonhumidified oxygen blows over a face mask. Therefore, patients with SS are at increased risk of developing corneal abrasions during surgery and in the postoperative setting. The decreased blink reflex of the patient during anesthesia also contributes to this problem. The administration of ocular lubricants before surgery and in the postoperative recovery suite will reduce the chance of this complication.

Upper airway dryness in the patient with SS may lead to mucous plug inspissation during the postoperative period, followed by obstructive pneumonias. The use of humidified oxygen and avoidance of medications that excessively dry the upper airways (i.e., used by anesthetists to control secretions) will help prevent this problem. Also, adequate hydration and respiratory therapy to keep airways clear are important.

An additional problem for the anesthesiologist is the poor state of teeth in the patient with SS. Thus a higher risk of damage to teeth during intubation must be considered. Not only can this lead to loss of the teeth and their subsequent aspiration, but these patients incur great expense in the addition of dentures to their remaining teeth that will be greatly affected by any further tooth loss.

In RA patients with secondary SS, the anesthesiologist must be informed about arthritic involvement of the neck (especially C1–C2 level). Attempts to hyperextend the neck to intubate the patient may result in transection of the cervical spinal cord and paraplegia. When cervical involvement due to RA is suspected, extreme caution during nasotracheal intubation must be taken; often intubation of the patient in a soft cervical collar may avoid this problem.

In many surgical procedures, antibiotics are routinely given. In the patient with sicca symptoms, the risk of associated oral candidiasis is greatly increased. The use of topical oral antifungal drugs, such as nystatin, will help prevent this complication. Precautions regarding steroid coverage are important since relative adrenal insufficiency remains after an extended period of taking glucocorticoids.

Finally, assessment of the "fluid status" of the SS patient in the postoperative period may be relatively difficult. Normal clinical clues such as the moisture in the ocular and oral membranes may be quite misleading. Further, some patients with SS have a tendency toward interstitial nephritis, which prevents adequate urine concentration and fluid balance. This problem may be exacerbated by antibiotics such as aminoglycosides.

ACKNOWLEDGEMENTS

The author greatly appreciates the help of Drs. M. Friedlaender (Ophthalmology), J. Willems (Gynecology), G. Izumo (Dermatology), R. Simon (Allergy), R. Stewart (Periodontal Medicine), F. Howell and T. Daniels (Oral Pathology), and K. Pischel (Rheumatology). Supported in part by NIH Grant MO1RR00833.

REFERENCES

1. Bloch KJ, Buchanan WW, Wohl MJ, Bunim JJ. Sjögren's syndrome: a clinical, pathological and serological study of 62 cases. Medicine (Baltimore) 1956;44:187.
2. Fox RI, Robinson C, Curd J, Michelson P, Bone R, Howell FV. First international symposium on Sjögren's syndrome: suggested criteria for classification. Scand J Rheumatol 1986;562:28.
3. Vitali C, Bombardieri S, Moutsopoulos HM, et al. Preliminary criteria for the classification of Sjögren's syndrome. Arthritis Rheum 1993;36:340.
4. Friedlaender M. Ocular manifestations of Sjögren's syndrome. Rheum Dis Clin North Am 1992;18:591.
5. Tsubota K. The importance of Schirmer test with nasal stimulation. Am J Ophthalmol 1991;11:106.
6. Atkinson J, Travis WD, Pillemer S, Bermudez D, Wolff A, Fox PC. Major salivary gland function in primary Sjögren's syndrome and its relationship to clinical features. J Rheumatol 1990;17:318.
7. Prause U. Clinical ophthalmological tests for the diagnosis of keratoconjunctivitis sicca. Clin Exp Rheumatol 1989;7:141.
8. van Bijsterveld OP. Diagnostic tests in the sicca syndrome. Arch Ophthalmol 1969;82:10.
9. Wilson F. Adverse external ocular effects of topical ophthalmic medications. Surv Ophthalmol 1979;24:57.
10. Lemp M. General measures in management of the dry eye. Int Ophthalmol Clin 1988;27:36.
11. Tseng S. Topical tretinoin treatment for dry-eye disorders. Int Ophthalmol Clin 1987;27:47.
12. Frost-Larsen K, Isager H, Manthorpe R. Sjögren's syndrome treated with bromhexine: a randomized clinical study. Br Med J 1978;1[6127]:1579.
13. Kaswan R, Salisbury MA. Effects of cyclosporin in treatment of keratoconjunctivitis sicca. Proc III Int Symp Sjögren's Syndrome 1991;1:47.
14. Daniels T, Fox P. Salivary and oral components of Sjögren's syndrome. Rheum Dis Clin North Am 1992;18:571.
15. Bowen W, Young DA, Peason SK. The effects of sucralose on coronal and root surface caries. J Dent Res 1990;69:1485.
16. Fox P. Systemic therapy of salivary gland hypofunction. J Am Dent Assoc 1987;115:581.
17. Epstein J, Decoteau WE, Wilkinson A. Effect of sialor in the treatment of xerostomia in Sjögren's syndrome. Oral Surg 1983;56:495.
18. Schiodt M, Oxholme P, Jacobsen A. Treatment of xerostomia in patients with primary Sjögren's syndrome with sulfarlem. Scand J Rheumatol 1986;61:250.
19. Fox P, van der Ven PF, Baum BJ. Pilocarpine for the treatment of xerostomia associated with salivary gland dysfunction. Oral Surg Oral Med Oral Pathol 1986;61:243.
20. Fox P, Atkinson JC, Macynski AA. Pilocarpine treatment of salivary gland hypofunction and dry mouth. Arch Intern Med 1991;151:1149.
21. Greenspan D, Daniels T. Effectiveness of pilocarpine in postirradiation xerostomia. Cancer 1987;59:1123.
22. Chand N, Harrison JE, Rooney S, Diamantis W, Sofia RD. Mucolytic activity of azelastine in mice and rats. Agents Actions 1993;38:165.
23. Hernandez Y, Daniels T. Oral candidiasis in Sjögren's syndrome: prevalence, clinical correlations and treatment. Oral Surg Oral Med Oral Pathol 1989;68:324.
24. Rhodus N, Schuh M. Effectiveness of three artificial salivas as assessed by mucoprotective relativity. J Dent Res 1991;70:407.
25. Steller M, Chou L, Daniels T. Electrical stimulation of salivary flow in patients with Sjögren's syndrome. J Dent Res 1988;67:1334.
26. Kyle R, Gleich G, Baynd E. Benign hyperglobulinemic purpura of Waldenström. Medicine (Baltimore) 1971;50:113.
27. Alexander EL, Provost TT. Cutaneous manifestations of primary Sjögren's syndrome: a reflection of vasculitis and association with anti-Ro (SSA) antibodies. J Invest Dermatol 1983;80:386.
28. Pun K-K, Wong C-K, Tsui E, Tam S, Kung A, Wang C. Hypokalemic periodic paralysis due to the Sjögren's syndrome in Chinese patients. Ann Intern Med 1989;110:405.
29. Abraham GN, Podell DN, Wistar R, Johnston SL, Welch EH. Immunological and structural properties of human monoclonal IgG cryoglobulins. Clin Exp Immunol 1979;36:63.
30. Siamopoulos KC, Mavridis AK, Elisaf M, Drosos AA, Moutsopoulos HM. Kidney involvement in primary Sjögren's syndrome. Scand J Rheumatol 1986;Suppl 43:156.
31. Fox RI, Baum S. Synthesis of viral RNA during restricted adenovirus infection. J Virol 1972;10:221.
32. Fox RI, Howell F, Bone R, Michelson P. Primary Sjögren's syndrome: clinical and immunopathologic features. Semin Arthritis Rheum 1984;14:77.
33. Kruize AA, Henre RJ, Kallenberg CG, et al. Hydroxychloroquine treatment for primary Sjögren's syndrome: a two-year, double-blind crossover trial. Ann Rheum Dis 1993;52:360.
34. Bernstein HN. Ocular safety of hydroxychloroquine. Ann Ophthalmol 1991;23:292.

35. Wallace D. Antimalarial agents and lupus. Rheum Dis Clin North Am 1994;20:243.

36. Dalavanga YA, Detrick B, Hooks JJ, Drosos AA, Moustopoulos HM. Effect of cyclosporin A (CyA) on the immunopathological lesion of the minor salivary glands from patients with Sjögren's syndrome. Ann Rheum Dis 1990;46:89.

37. Fox RI, Adamson TC III, Fong S, et al. Lymphocyte phenotype and function of pseudolymphomas associated with Sjögren's syndrome. J Clin Invest 1983;72:52.

38. Castor CW, Bull FE. Review of the United States data on neoplasms in rheumatoid arthritis. Am J Med 1985;78:33.

39. Rieche K. Carcinogenicity of antineoplastic agents in man. Cancer Treat Rev 1984;11:39.

40. Walker SE, Anver MR. Accelerated appearance of neoplasms in female NZB/NZW mice treated with high-dose cyclophosphamide. Arthritis Rheum 1979;22:1338.

41. Michels SD, McKenna RW, Arthur DC, Brunning RD. Therapy-related acute myeloid leukemia and myelodysplastic syndrome: a clinical and morphologic study of 65 cases. Blood 1985;65:1364.

42. Kelley WN, Harris ED, Ruddy S, Sledge CB, eds. Textbook of rheumatology. 4th ed. Philadelphia: WB Saunders, 1993.

THE SERONEGATIVE SPONDYLOARTHROPATHIES (ANKYLOSING SPONDYLITIS, REITER'S SYNDROME, PSORIATIC ARTHRITIS)

Christopher G. Jackson
Daniel O. Clegg

The seronegative spondyloarthropathies are a group of rheumatic diseases that share clinical, radiologic, and genetic similarities. Included in this group of diseases are ankylosing spondylitis, Reiter's syndrome, psoriatic arthritis, and arthritis associated with inflammatory bowel disease. These diseases are characterized by the absence of serum autoantibodies, including rheumatoid factor. It is important to distinguish them from rheumatoid arthritis because, as will be seen, treatment of the two disorders is significantly different. Some common features that the seronegative spondyloarthropathies share include:

- An association with the Class I antigen HLA-B27
- A strong predilection for symptomatic disease in young adult males
- Radiographic evidence of sacroiliitis and spondylitis
- Oligoarticular peripheral joint involvement
- Enthesopathy (inflammation at the sites of tendinous insertions)
- Extraarticular manifestations including oral ulcers, specific dermatologic lesions, uveitis, aortitis, etc.

In this chapter we will address the treatment of ankylosing spondylitis, Reiter's syndrome, and psoriatic arthritis. In general, there is a dearth of controlled clinical trials that address these issues. Where such information exists, we provide an objective summary of the material.

In addition, we present published, uncontrolled data in a balanced manner with the caveat that, as a rule, mostly positive uncontrolled reports appear in the literature.

ANKYLOSING SPONDYLITIS

Definition and Natural History

Ankylosing spondylitis is a disease that is characterized by sacroiliitis and spondylitis, commonly involving the lumbar spine and less commonly involving the thoracic and cervical spines. A number of criteria have been suggested to aid in the diagnosis of ankylosing spondylitis. Most involve assessment of the patient for inflammatory low back pain and stiffness, limitation of lumbar spine motion, limitation of chest expansion, and the presence of radiographic sacroiliitis. There is a strong association with the Class I antigen HLA-B27. In most series, well over 80% of white patients with ankylosing spondylitis are HLA-B27-positive compared with 8% of the general white population. There is also a strong association between onset of disease symptoms and males in their second and third decades. For a complete discussion of diagnosis, pathogenesis, and prognosis, see Kelley et al., Chapter 56 (reference 68).

The natural history of ankylosing spondylitis is somewhat controversial. Cheret et al.[1] described a population of 150 war veterans who were followed prospectively for more than 30 years. In this group, the mean age at onset of symptoms was 24 years, the duration of symptoms was 38 years, and the average age at follow-up was 62 years. At follow-up one third of the patients denied having any pain. Thirty-eight percent described their axial pain as mild, 28% as moderate, and 4% as severe. More than 70% of the patients stated that their symptoms had not changed in the preceding 10 years. Spinal restriction was graded as mild (41%), moderate (18%), or severe (41%); peripheral joint involvement believed to be related to ankylosing spondylitis was present in 36% of this group of patients. Peripheral joints involved, in order of decreasing frequency, were the shoulders, hips, knees, ankles, metatarsal, and interphalangeal joints. Eighty-nine percent of patients who were tested were HLA-B27-positive. Sixty-one deaths occurred in this population. Eight of these deaths were considered to be disease related: two were due to cervical subluxations, three patients died of aortic insufficiency, two of respiratory failure due to severe spinal involvement, and one of amyloidosis. Six of the eight patients who died had peripheral joint disease at onset, and six were believed to have severe spinal restriction or deformity. The conclusions of these authors include:

1. Ankylosing spondylitis can have a benign course.
2. In most patients a predictable pattern of disease emerges within the first 10 years.

Radford et al.[2] investigated age-specific mortality rates of 836 patients with ankylosing spondylitis who did not receive x-ray therapy and found that there was excess mortality due to ulcerative colitis, nephritis, and tuberculosis. In addition, mortality risks relative to the general population were increased for all gastrointestinal and circulatory diseases. Finally, Smith et al.[3] reported a mortality study of more than 14,000 patients with ankylosing spondylitis who had received x-ray therapy; they found excess risks of leukemia and other malignancies that became apparent 9 or more years after the radiation exposure.

Nonarticular Manifestations of Disease

Acute Anterior Uveitis.
Up to 40% of patients with ankylosing spondylitis will have one or more episodes of acute anterior uveitis. Eye pain, photophobia, injection, excess tearing, and impaired vision are common presenting manifestations. Early symptoms may be ignored if patients with ankylosing spondylitis are not specifically warned to expect them. Prompt diagnosis and management with the help of an ophthalmologist are important for a good outcome. Therapy is directed at topical pupillary dilation and instillation of steroid solutions.

Pulmonary Manifestations of Ankylosing Spondylitis.
Mechanical problems, such as severe thoracic kyphosis, can lead to ventilation/perfusion mismatching and restrictive pulmonary disease, but this is usually of minimal clinical significance. Apical pulmonary fibrosis is a specific but uncommon pulmonary process associated with ankylosing spondylitis. Coexistent pulmonary tuberculosis must be excluded. Patients with ankylosing spondylitis should be strongly counseled against smoking in order to avoid obstructive lung disease complicating possible restrictive disease.

Mechanical Spine Disease.
The rigid spine seen in patients with advanced, aggressive, ankylosing spondylitis can present a number of clinically challenging complications. Minor trauma can result in spinal fracture. The most common site of fracture is the C5–6 region, and instability can lead to paraplegia. Fracture can be seen in the thoracic and lumbar spine as well. Nondisplaced fractures generally do well with external fixation, whereas spinal instability generally requires internal fixation and surgical fusion.

There have been numerous reports of cauda equina syndrome in patients with advanced ankylosing spondylitis. The onset is generally insidious, making diagnosis very challenging. A high index of suspicion is necessary in patients with lower extremity symptoms. Evaluation with magnetic resonance imaging (MRI) is often necessary to document the diagnosis.

Spinal surgery in patients with ankylosing spondylitis is problematic. Patients are often osteoporotic, making fixation difficult. Prolonged bed rest and inactivity are often difficult; as is rehabilitation when movement can be reinstituted. Thus surgery should be given thoughtful, deliberate consideration by the patient, his rheumatologist, his therapist, and an experienced orthopedic surgeon.

Treatment

Although the majority of this section details the medical treatment of ankylosing spondylitis, it should be noted that before medications are instituted, patient education about the disease process and course, as well as physical therapy intervention and instruction, should be an integral part of the management of patients with ankylosing spondylitis as well as the other spondyloarthropathies. The goals of patient education should include instructions about the natural history of the disease, the prognosis, and the importance of maintaining an upright posture that will also allow function in the patient's chosen vocation. Patients should be counseled to avoid smoking and other activities that may impair pulmonary function and be additive to either the restrictive pulmonary diseases that can be seen secondary to fusion of the thoracic spine or the less common interstitial pulmonary fibrosis. Other extraarticular complications, including iritis/iridocyclitis, aortitis, and cardiac involvement, should be discussed with the patient and regularly reviewed on follow-up visits.

Physical therapy should address maintenance of good posture, spine mobility and function, muscle strengthening, general conditioning, and exercise. Kraag et al.[4] reported a randomized controlled trial of 53 patients with ankylosing spondylitis. Twenty-six patients received "extensive" education about their disease and instruction in physical therapy, while the remaining 27 patients received neither of these interventions. The results of the study showed significant improvement in fingertip-to-floor distance, the primary outcome measure of this study, as well as a functional assessment. O'Driscoll et al.[5] have shown improvement in cervical spine mobility with physical therapy.

Nonsteroidal Antiinflammatory Drugs.

Nonsteroidal antiinflammatory drugs (NSAIDs) are used almost universally in the medical treatment of ankylosing spondylitis. More than 80% of ankylosing spondylitis patients[6] in the United Kingdom take one of the NSAIDs for control of the symptoms related to the disease. Numerous comparative studies have been undertaken to evaluate the efficacy and safety of NSAIDs in ankylosing spondylitis. Table 6–1 summarizes some of the larger trials.[7] The methods of these trials are so variable that it is difficult to con-

TABLE 6–1

Some Double-blind Trials of NSAIDs in Ankylosing Spondylitis

STUDY DRUG	COMPARATOR DRUG	NO. OF PATIENTS	RESULTS
Dic	Sul	62	Dic > Sul
Eto	Indo	99	Eto = Indo
	Nap/Pl	128	Eto > Pl
Fen	Pbz	30	Fen < Pbz
	Indo	19	Fen = Indo
Flu	Indo	57	Flu = Indo
	Indo	26	Flu = Indo
	Pbz		Flu = Pbz
Ibu	Open study	65	Effective
Indo	Pl		Indo > Pl
	Nap	27	Indo > Nap
	Dic	262	Indo > Dic
Keto	Pl	13	Keto > Pl
	Pbz		Keto = Pbz
Nap	Indo	35	Nap = Indo
	Flu	30	Nap = Flu
Pbz	Nap	20	Pbz = Nap
	Nap	25	Pbz = Nap
	Keto	25	Pbz > Keto
Pir	Indo	55	Pir = Indo
	Indo	87	Pir = Indo
Sul	Pbz	120	Sul < Pbz
	Pbz	24	Sul = Pbz
	Pl	83	Sul > Pl
	Indo	23	Sul < Indo
Ten	Dic	57	Ten = Dic
Tol	Indo	60	Tol = Indo
	Nap	34	Tol = Nap

Abbreviations and symbols: Dic = diclofenac; Eto = etodolac; Fen = fenoprofen; Flu = flurbiprofen; Ibu = ibuprofen; Indo = indomethacin; Keto = Ketoprofen; Nap = naproxen; Pbz = phenylbutazone; Pir = piroxicam; Sul = sulindac; Ten = tenoxicam; Tol = tolmetin; Pl = placebo; > indicates superior efficacy; < indicates inferior efficacy; = indicates equivalent efficacy.
From Gran JT, Husby G. Ankylosing spondylitis: current drug treatment. Drugs 1992;44(4):585.

clude that any single nonsteroidal agent is either more efficacious or less toxic than any other, and thus it is difficult to establish clear preferences. Standard textbooks state that indomethacin may offer increased efficacy in these diseases,[8] and that is our clinical experience. In the United States, the following NSAIDs have received approval from the Food and Drug Administration for use in ankylosing spondylitis: indomethacin, sulindac, naproxen, diclofenac, and phenylbutazone. Because of the potential for bone marrow suppression as an adverse drug reaction, phenylbutazone should not be used unless other non-steroidal agents have failed.

Patients with ankylosing spondylitis are no more susceptible than any other group of rheumatology patients to the adverse drug effects associated with NSAIDs. Patients should be carefully interviewed concerning any evidence of previous gastrointestinal problems or potential renal insufficiency so that appropriate accommodations can be made for those at increased risk of adverse drug reactions. Otherwise, it is recommended that patients in whom NSAIDs are newly instituted have a complete blood cell count, urinalysis, and determination of creatinine, potassium, and serum transaminase levels every 1 to 3 months. Similar monitoring in patients who are stable on these medications is recommended every 3 to 12 months.[9]

In summary, NSAIDs are effective in ameliorating many of the clinical symptoms associated with ankylosing spondylitis. None has documented superiority in terms of efficacy or safety, except that phenylbutazone has more potential for bone marrow suppression. Selection of the most appropriate agent in any given patient often requires balancing between more clinical benefit and less toxicity. Patients on these regimens should be monitored for adverse reactions, be followed clinically for disease progression, receive continued education about their disease process, and receive physical therapy instruction with the objectives of maintaining function and quality of life. For a more comprehensive discussion of the individual agents, see Kelley et al., Chapter 43 (reference 68).

Other Antirheumatic Drugs

D-Penicillamine. D-Penicillamine has been used in ankylosing spondylitis in a number of open trials. The largest series was reported in a letter detailing clinical experience with D-penicillamine in 49 patients with ankylosing spondylitis.[10] The D-penicillamine was titrated to a total dose of 500 mg per day. Tytman et al.[10] noted an improvement in Schober's test and the fingertip-to-floor test within the first 4 weeks of therapy. This improvement was at a time when the patients were taking a very low dose of D-penicillamine, and improvement was seen much earlier than an antirheumatic effect from D-penicillamine would be anticipated. Steven et al.[11] report a double-blind placebo-controlled trial of D-penicillamine in 17 patients over a 6-month period in which no clinical improvement was seen.

Auranofin. Grasedyck et al.[12] reported a series of patients in whom auranofin produced no improvement in the disease manifestations of ankylosing spondylitis.

Sulfasalazine. In 1984, Amor et al.[13] suggested in a letter that sulfasalazine may be effective, particularly in ankylosing spondylitis patients with peripheral arthritis. Since that time, at least eight[14-21] other double-blind placebo-controlled trials with mixed results have been published. It appears likely that sulfasalazine has a beneficial effect on lowering erythrocyte sedimentation rates and C-reactive protein levels. Data regarding the potential benefit of sulfasalazine on clinical symptoms or signs of disease are less clear. For example, morning stiffness was improved in two of the studies with no effect in four and was not reported in two; night pain was improved in one, no effect was seen in four, and night pain was not reported in three; chest expansion was improved in three, no effect was seen in three, and this was not reported in two; spinal mobility was not improved in six and not reported in two. Ferraz et al.[22] reported a metanalysis of five randomized controlled trials. The results of this analysis indicated that sulfasalazine had clinical benefit over placebo in duration of morning stiffness, severity of morning stiffness, severity of pain, and general well-being, erythrocyte sedimentation rate, and serum IgA values.

Conceptually, it is possible that the most beneficial effect associated with sulfasalazine in ankylosing spondylitis might be seen in those patients who have peripheral arthritis in association with axial disease. Mielants and Veys[23] discuss the increased incidence of histologic changes suggestive of subclinical inflammatory bowel disease in patients with ankylosing spondylitis and peripheral arthritis. Anecdotally, those patients seem particularly responsive to sulfasalazine therapy. This may represent a subgroup of patients with subclinical inflammatory bowel disease, sacroiliitis, and peripheral arthritis rather than "true ankylosing spondylitis." The published controlled clinical trials were not analyzed specifically for potentially beneficial effects of sulfasalazine in the peripheral arthritis associated with ankylosing spondylitis.

Although the efficacy data on sulfasalazine in ankylosing spondylitis are unclear, the medication is well tolerated. Mild gastrointestinal intolerance, including nausea and anorexia, is the most commonly reported symptom. In addition, minor skin rashes are reported with some frequency. Much less frequently reported abnormalities include liver function aberrations, hematologic abnormalities, such as agranulocytosis, hemolytic anemia, and thrombocytopenia, and neurologic effects, including dizziness, headache, and vertigo. Sulfasalazine has been studied in divided doses of 2 to 3 g per day. Blood counts and chemistries should initially be monitored at twice monthly intervals to detect cytopenias; however, once a patient is successfully tolerating the medications, toxicity surveillance can be modified after several months.

In summary, sulfasalazine may have a place in the treatment of ankylosing spondylitis. There have been no studies to evaluate its long-term potential as a "disease-modifying" agent. If sulfasalazine does have a beneficial effect on ankylosing spondylitis, its effect most likely will be seen in patients with "active" disease (elevated sedimentation rate, C-reactive protein, presence of peripheral arthritis) or newly diagnosed disease. The recommended daily dose is 30 to 40 mg/kg/day. Sulfasalazine is discussed in detail in Kelley et al., Chapter 42 (reference 68).

There are anecdotal reports about methotrexate and ankylosing spondylitis involving fewer than five patients. However, to the best of our knowledge, there are no controlled trials evaluating methotrexate, antimalarials, parenteral gold, or cyclosporine in ankylosing spondylitis.

Radiotherapy. Radiotherapy was used empirically in treating the symptoms of ankylosing spondylitis in the 1940s. A sham-controlled trial using varying radiation dosages suggested improvement in ankylosing spondylitis patients who underwent radiation compared with rheumatoid arthritis controls.[24]

The use of radiotherapy declined with the introduction of effective therapy with the NSAIDs, initially phenylbutazone and then others. Subsequently, toxicity studies demonstrated an increased incidence of leukemia and other neoplasms in irradiated patients. Although studies have not been done with radiation approaches that employ smaller, well-localized fields and lower total radiation dosages, any patient considered for radiotherapy would be exceptional.

Approach to Management

After a careful diagnostic evaluation, the patient with ankylosing spondylitis should first receive education about the disease and the importance of a physical therapy program aimed at good posture and maintenance of motion and muscle strength. NSAIDs should be used for symptomatic relief of the discomfort associated with inflammatory musculoskeletal complaints. Indomethacin may be more effective than other NSAIDs; however, there are little controlled data to support this position. If sulfasalazine is beneficial, the effect is not great and most likely occurs in patients with early active disease or peripheral joint involvement. If the drug is used, it is not at all clear how long it should be maintained. There is little published clinical evidence to suggest that any of the other second-line agents have any beneficial activity in the management of ankylosing spondylitis.

REITER'S SYNDROME

Definition and Natural History

Hans Reiter first reported the association of arthritis, nongonococcal urethritis, and conjunctivitis in 1916.[25] In the early 1970s the association between Reiter's syndrome and HLA-B27 positivity was made, and from that association arose the concept of "incomplete" Reiter's syndrome,[26] which consisted of a group of patients with asymmetric oligoarthritis and HLA-B27 positivity. Because of the frequent association between venereal and enteric infections and the subsequent development of Reiter's syndrome, the term *reactive arthritis*[27] was proposed in 1969. It now seems clear that fully manifest Reiter's syndrome is seen in a subset of patients with reactive arthritis. Thus the term *reactive arthritis* seems more appropriate to describe the condition in this unique group of patients whose main clinical manifestations include asymmetric oligoarthritis, an increased prevalence of HLA-B27 positivity, nongonococcal urethritis, conjunctivitis, distinct rashes (including circinate balanitis and keratoderma blennorrhagicum), oral ulcers, uveitis, subclinical enterocolitis, carditis, and nephritis.[28] Aspects of differential diagnosis, pathogenesis, and clinical features are discussed in Kelley et al., Chapter 57 (reference 68).

The natural history of reactive arthritis is extremely variable; most patients experience exacerbations and remissions, which can last from several weeks to several months.[29] Although a few patients will have but a single episode of the disease, the rule would be to have multiple flares of disease activity. Fox et al.[30] reported that 83% of 122 patients with reactive arthritis had persistent disease at 5.6 years. Approximately one fourth of those patients were unable to work or had changed their vocation because of their disease. Inman's series of postenteric infection–reactive arthritis patients at 1 year follow-up found that 7 of 15 patients continued to have persistent joint symptoms.[31]

Reactive Arthritis and HIV Disease.   There have been several reports of reactive arthritis in association with human immunodeficiency virus (HIV) infection. Although reactive arthritis can occur after the patient becomes seropositive for HIV, clinical features of reactive arthritis frequently precede the recognition of clinical HIV-associated diseases. Therefore, a high index of suspicion is warranted.[32] HIV infection does not appear to alter the course of the reactive arthritis per se; however, there have been reports in which the use of immunosuppressive medications in this patient population resulted in abrupt clinical deterioration and the onset of other manifestations of the acquired immunodeficiency syndrome.[33]

Treatment

Patients with reactive arthritis are, in general, relatively young and geographically mobile. As has already been mentioned, reactive arthritis has a highly variable course that is punctuated by remissions and exacerbations. These factors, combined with the relatively low incidence of the disease, make it extremely difficult to conduct controlled trials with a follow-up period that is adequate to assess response and with sufficient numbers of patients to obtain clinical and statistical meaning. Therefore,

rather than report on uncontrolled and controlled experience, this section will be subdivided by drug class.

Nonsteroidal Antiinflammatory Drugs.   The NSAIDs are widely used in treating the musculoskeletal manifestations of reactive arthritis. Indomethacin has, perhaps, had the most extensive use,[34] but there are no published data to suggest that any nonsteroidal agent is either more effective or less toxic in reactive arthritis patients. To our knowledge, there are no studies to suggest that patients with reactive arthritis have any unique susceptibility or resistance to the adverse drug reactions that are commonly associated with NSAIDs. As with other inflammatory arthropathies, NSAIDs seem to improve the articular complaints associated with reactive arthritis. Choice of any given agent often requires balancing clinical response against the potential for medication toxicity.

Sulfasalazine.   Sulfasalazine is reported to have benefit in open studies.[35] Controlled trials comparing the efficacy of sulfasalazine and placebo in reactive arthritis are currently under way. The toxicity of sulfasalazine in reactive arthritis appears comparable to the toxicity seen in other spondyloarthropathy patients. Efficacy findings have not yet been published.

As has been seen with ankylosing spondylitis patients, some patients with reactive arthritis appear to have histologic enterocolitis that also improves with sulfasalazine therapy. The causal association of these findings with a clinical response to sulfasalazine remains unclear.[36]

Immunosuppressive Drugs.   Methotrexate, azathioprine, and cyclosporine have been used empirically to treat patients with recalcitrant reactive arthritis. Some improvement has been reported, although the results are not striking and published anecdotal reports are obviously biased in favor of positive results. Use of either methotrexate or azathioprine in patients with reactive arthritis and HIV seropositivity may hasten the manifestations of acquired immunodeficiency syndrome.[37] Thus the use of these medicines should be carefully considered in patients at risk of HIV positivity.

Antibiotics.   The demonstration of bacterial cell wall components in the synovium of patients with reactive arthritis[38,39] makes the idea of long-term antibiotic therapy intriguing. In an early report,[40] 10 patients with peripheral arthritis after *Chlamydia trachomatis* infection were treated for 3 months with methacycline and showed improvement in morning stiffness and number of active joints. Subsequently, a controlled trial of 40 patients who received either 2 weeks of antibiotics appropriate for their cultured infections (*Salmonella, Yersinia,* or *Campylobacter*) or placebo did not reveal a difference between the two groups.[41] Finally, in a double-blind placebo-controlled trial of 3 months of treatment with the tetracycline derivative, a group of patients with primarily post-chlamydia arthritis showed some improvement compared with the placebo group.[42] These data would suggest that short-term antibiotics do not seem to affect the course of established reactive arthritis. Longer-term antibiotics may have some role, although additional studies will be necessary to better define such a role if one exists. The mechanism responsible for a response to antibiotics remains to be elucidated.

Approach to Management

Recommendations for treatment of reactive arthritis are difficult to base on clinical data alone. Patient education and physical therapy goals as outlined in the section on ankylosing spondylitis are important in patients with chronic disease. Conventional medical therapy would be to use an NSAID or corticosteroid injection in an attempt to control the articular manifestations. Sulfasalazine may be effective in controlling chronic peripheral arthritis, and data specifically addressing that question should soon be available. Sulfasalazine is safe, well tolerated, and effective in anecdotal reports. It should probably be tried before either methotrexate or azathioprine is considered. Therapy with antibiotics for articular complaints remains controversial. If antibiotic therapy is useful, it would appear that prolonged (3 months or longer) oral tetracycline would be the medication of choice. Immunosuppressive drugs such as methotrexate or azathioprine may produce some benefit in chronic, unrelenting articular disease, but they should be used with caution in patients at risk of HIV infection. The data on treatment of established chronic Reiter's syndrome with either metho-

trexate or azathioprine are empiric. Rationale for recommending one over the other cannot be substantiated. The experience and comfort level of the treating physician with the use of these agents and with the necessary monitoring for potential toxicity play an important role in agent choice. Drug side effects and recommended monitoring have been covered in previous sections of this chapter. Except for the caveat that HIV-positive patients may have untoward reactions to immunosuppressive medications, no unique drug interactions are seen in patients with reactive arthritis.

Future Directions

The reactive arthritides comprise a spectrum of fascinating rheumatologic disorders with a genetic basis (HLA-B27) and an environmental component (postenteric or postvenereal infections). Basic research aimed at further elucidating the complex interactions between these factors is ongoing and will likely provide answers to the pathophysiology of not only the reactive arthritides but also the other seronegative spondyloarthropathies and, perhaps, other rheumatologic disorders in the future. Clinical research in reactive arthritis is problematic because new cases seem to be diminishing both in the United States and abroad. This may be the result of changes in sexual practices related to the HIV epidemic as well as improved safety of the world's food supply. Thus controlled clinical trials in the reactive arthritides are difficult because of the low incidence and diminishing prevalence of the disease, its variable natural history, and the young, mobile population that it most frequently affects. Thus current therapy is empiric and anecdotal and must be highly individualized.

PSORIATIC ARTHRITIS

Definition and Natural History

The term *psoriatic arthritis* describes a spectrum of inflammatory joint disease that occurs in association with psoriasis. Musculoskeletal complaints are not uncommon in the psoriatic population; however, the prevalence of actual inflammatory disease is about 5%. The skin disease is usually, but not uniformly, present before the development of arthritis, but neither the pattern nor the extent of skin disease predicts the eventual development or severity of the arthritis. Genetics, pathogenesis, and clinical features of psoriatic arthritis are discussed in Kelley et al., Chapter 58 (reference 68).

Psoriatic arthritis may involve both appendicular and axial skeletons, with five characteristic clinical presentations having been described: (1) asymmetric oligoarticular, (2) predominantly distal interphalangeal, (3) arthritis mutilans, (4) symmetric polyarticular, and (5) spondylitis. The asymmetric oligoarticular pattern is most common and is seen in 50% to 60% of patients, whereas the predominantly distal interphalangeal presentation occurs in 5% to 10%, arthritis mutilans in 5%, and the symmetric polyarticular pattern in approximately 25%. The activity of peripheral psoriatic arthritis is typically episodic in that relatively asymptomatic periods are usually followed by periods of flare; synchronous skin/arthritis flares may occur, but asynchronous flares appear to be more common. Spondylitis without peripheral arthritis accounts for approximately 5% of psoriatic arthritis; however, radiographic changes of sacroiliitis and spondylitis may be seen in up to 40% of the psoriatic arthritis population. Sacroiliac involvement is usually seen in HLA-B27-positive patients.

These presentations are not always distinct, and many patients will exhibit features of two or more patterns at a given time or may evolve from one pattern to another over the course of time. This heterogeneity has made it difficult to establish specific prognoses for each subtype; however, the oligoarticular presentation seems to be the least aggressive. Although the course of psoriatic arthritis is, in general, more favorable than that of rheumatoid arthritis, the destructive potential of psoriatic arthritis has been adequately demonstrated by a prospective study showing that the number of patients with psoriatic arthritis who had five or more damaged joints doubled (from 19% to 41%) over a 5-year period despite treatment that produced improvement in both the erythrocyte sedimentation rate and the number of tender/swollen joints.[43]

Evaluation of the efficacy of therapeutic interventions in psoriatic arthritis is made difficult by (1) the wide spectrum and variable activity of the arthritis, (2) the uncertain correlation between present measures of response and eventual functional outcome, and (3) the uncertain contribution of concurrent therapy directed at the skin disease. The importance of well-designed prospective studies that are carefully controlled, have an adequate number of patients and an adequate period of observation, and employ appropriate efficacy and toxicity measures cannot be overemphasized.

Treatment

In that the cause of psoriasis and psoriatic arthritis is unknown and pathologic mechanisms are only partially understood, treatment remains empiric. Most of the agents and therapeutic regimens presently in use or under investigation are (1) those that have been used with demonstrated benefit in the treatment of other inflammatory arthropathies and (2) those that have been used in the treatment of cutaneous psoriasis and have possible articular benefit.[44] The efficacy of nearly all treatment regimens in psoriatic arthritis has yet to be unequivocally established.

NSAIDs. NSAIDs are widely believed to be efficacious in psoriatic arthritis and are the most common initial therapy prescribed by most clinicians for both peripheral and axial disease. However, no controlled studies exist to document their efficacy, and no NSAID at present has formal FDA approval for use in psoriatic arthritis. Many rheumatologists prefer to use nonsalicylate NSAIDs on the basis of a clinical impression of better efficacy; no controlled data exist to either refute or substantiate that position. Arachidonic acid metabolites are known to influence the activity of cutaneous psoriasis, and worsening of the skin disease with initiation of NSAID therapy has been observed, perhaps resulting from cyclooxygenase blockade with increased use of the lipooxygenase pathway. No other unusual toxicity associated with the use of NSAIDs in psoriatic arthritis has been reported. A complete blood cell count (CBC) and chemistry profile (including transaminases) is recommended every 3 to 12 months.[45]

Glucocorticoids. Intraarticular injection of glucocorticoids can produce marked improvement in joint pain and swelling. Periodic injections can be of particular value in the management of patients with oligoarticular disease or those with controlled polyarticular disease but one or two persistently active joints. In general, systemic use of glucocorticoids should be avoided because of the possibility of provoking a pustular flare in the skin disease on withdrawal.

Other Antirheumatic Drugs. If a patient does not respond to an adequate NSAID trial or has evidence of destructive disease, the institution of additional therapy should be considered. As in other inflammatory arthropathies, these agents are sometimes referred to as "disease-modifying." However, because no true disease modification in either the peripheral arthritis or the spondylitis has yet been shown, *second-line* agents may be a preferable term.

Oral and Parenteral Gold. A beneficial response with both oral and parenteral gold in psoriatic arthritis has been observed. In a 6-month double-blind placebo-controlled study of auranofin (6 mg/day) involving 238 patients, the auranofin-treated group showed a modest but significant improvement in physician's global assessment and occupational/daily function scores compared with the placebo group, but no significant difference in morning stiffness or joint tenderness/swelling scores was seen.[46] The rate of withdrawal from auranofin because of adverse drug reactions was 10%. An uncontrolled study involving 14 patients treated with injectable gold showed either remission or improvement (50% reduction in number of inflamed joints) in 71% of the patients.[47] Toxicity was similar to that observed with parenteral gold in rheumatoid arthritis. A double-blind comparison of auranofin (6 mg/day), intramuscular gold sodium thiomalate (50 mg/wk), and placebo showed significant improvement in the Ritchie articular index, the visual analog pain score, and the erythrocyte sedimentation rate (ESR) over 24 weeks in the parenteral gold group but no significant difference in the auranofin group as compared with the placebo group.[48] Neither significant flare nor improvement in cutaneous psoriasis with oral or parenteral gold has been observed. Appropriate monitoring consists of a CBC and a urinalysis before each injection for parenteral gold and a CBC and urinalysis every 4 weeks for oral gold.

Methotrexate. The efficacy of methotrexate in psoriatic arthritis was first demonstrated in 1964 with a double-blind placebo-controlled study of 21 patients who had active skin disease and peripheral arthritis.[49] This study design compared parenteral methotrexate (1 to 3 mg/kg × 3 doses at 10-day intervals) versus placebo with an observation period of approximately 3 months. Significant improvement in joint tenderness and joint range of motion, extent of skin involvement, and erythrocyte sedimentation rate was seen. After completion of therapy, however, the majority of patients experienced a recurrence of skin and joint disease within 1 to 4 months. Although adverse effects were common (anorexia/nausea, 62%; paresthesias, 48%; transient leukopenia, 33%; oral ulcerations, 10%; and alopecia, 5%), they did not require cessation of therapy in any patient. This study and additional experience with similar doses (25 mg/week) documented the beneficial effect of methotrexate for both cutaneous and synovial disease; however, the transient nature of the response and the frequency of adverse reactions suggested that more sustained therapy with lower doses might be of greater benefit. A randomized, double-blind, placebo-controlled trial comparing oral low-dose pulse methotrexate 7.5 to 15 mg/week with placebo over 12 weeks did show better patient tolerance; however, efficacy of this regimen was not established, as the only response measure to attain statistical significance was the physician assessment of arthritis activity.[50] A larger study of longer duration might have shown greater benefit, and the clinical experience of some is consistent with this possibility. In a retrospective report of 40 patients over 12 years of treatment with a mean methotrexate dose of 11.2 mg/week, 38 patients had an excellent or good articular response, 36 had cutaneous resolution, and only two patients withdrew because of toxicity (leukopenia and stomatitis).[51] In seven patients who underwent 11 liver biopsies during the study, one patient was found to have micronodular cirrhosis at a cumulative methotrexate dose of 400 mg (with an unchanged biopsy at a cumulative dose of 1080 mg). Otherwise, no inflammation or disruption of hepatic architecture was seen on initial or serial biopsy specimens.

Appropriately, methotrexate-induced liver disease and bone marrow suppression continue to be major clinical concerns. Whether the use of methotrexate in psoriasis and psoriatic arthritis is associated with more frequent or severe adverse drug effects than with its use in rheumatoid arthritis is unknown. Less methotrexate toxicity has been observed with its present use in rheumatoid arthritis than would have been predicted from the early experience in psoriasis and psoriatic arthritis. However, this apparent decrease in toxicity may be better explained by improved patient selection, administration of smaller doses in pulse fashion, and more careful monitoring rather than postulating that psoriatic patients have a predilection to toxicity. Adverse events involving methotrexate in the two above studies were similar to the present experience in rheumatoid arthritis. Recommended monitoring consists of a monthly CBC and liver enzyme studies. Drug withdrawal should be considered if frequent, persistent, or severe transaminase elevations are seen. No consensus exists as to the indications for liver biopsy either pretreatment or at specified intervals during treatment. However, most rheumatologists would agree that a biopsy should be considered if transaminase abnormalities are recurrent or persist after drug withdrawal; discontinuation of therapy is mandatory if any clinical evidence of hepatic dysfunction appears.

Azathioprine and 6-Mercaptopurine.   Both 6-mercaptopurine and its derivative, azathioprine, are purine analogs that have been used in the treatment of psoriasis and psoriatic arthritis. Although favorable results have been reported, the study populations are very small and no placebo-controlled data are available. Eleven of 13 patients treated with 6-mercaptopurine (20 to 50 mg/kg/day) showed improvement in both joint and skin disease within 3 weeks of initiation of therapy and maintenance of this improvement on a dose of 1 mg/kg/day with minimal adverse effects.[52] A 12-month double-blind crossover study of azathioprine (3 mg/kg/day) in six patients reported moderate or marked joint improvement in all six patients and cutaneous improvement in four; however, the dose of azathioprine had to be reduced in five patients because of leukopenia.[53] In view of the known toxicity of these agents, most rheumatologists reserve their use for severe and refractory disease. Regular laboratory monitoring with a monthly CBC and hepatic transaminase determinations is imperative.

Sulfasalazine.   The effectiveness of sulfasalazine in rheumatoid arthritis and other seroneg-

ative arthritides has led to trials in psoriatic arthritis as well. Apparent efficacy was suggested in pilot studies and was subsequently confirmed in a 24-week double-blind placebo-controlled study of 30 patients using a dose of 2 g/day.[54] There was significant improvement in morning stiffness, number of painful joints, articular index, clinical score, and pain score, with the favorable response being more pronounced in the polyarticular group. The drug was well tolerated, and no exacerbation or remission of cutaneous psoriasis was seen.

Cyclosporine A.   Cyclosporine A has been used with success in cutaneous psoriasis, and preliminary experience also suggests a beneficial effect in psoriatic arthritis. Representative of this preliminary experience is a 6-month open study of eight patients (seven of whom were refractory to methotrexate) with a starting dose of 3.5 mg/day, which produced marked improvement in joint and skin disease in seven of the eight patients after 2 months.[55] There was one withdrawal from the study because of lack of efficacy, and three patients required a 25% reduction in the cyclosporine A dose because of a 50% increase in serum creatinine. Further controlled study is warranted to confirm efficacy and determine the extent to which renal toxicity will limit long-term therapy.

Antimalarial Agents.   The use of antimalarial agents in the treatment of psoriatic arthritis has been controversial. Reports of favorable response to both chloroquine (250 mg/day) and hydroxychloroquine (200 to 400 mg/day) in approximately 75% of patients have been offset by concerns that antimalarial drugs may have an adverse effect on the skin disease. The spectrum of suspected cutaneous toxicity includes exacerbation of plaques, photosensitivity, generalized erythroderma, evolution to pustular psoriasis, and the development of an exfoliative dermatitis. Although the reported incidence of these reactions ranges from 0% to 100%, it is important to note that more frequent reactions were observed in early trials that had few patients and primarily used regimens with quinacrine; much less toxicity has been seen in the more recent experience involving larger numbers of patients and using chloroquine or hydroxychloroquine.[56] Further experience would suggest that hydroxychloroquine may be safer than chloroquine. Appropriate monitoring of antimalarial agents requires baseline and periodic ophthalmologic examinations to include visual acuity, slit-lamp, funduscopic, and visual field testing. The package insert for hydroxychloroquine stipulates that such examinations should be performed every 3 months, whereas a more recent recommendation has suggested that examinations every 6 months are adequate.[44] In addition, a CBC should be obtained every six months. A prospective, controlled trial is needed to establish the efficacy and safety of these agents in the treatment of psoriatic arthritis.

D-Penicillamine. A favorable effect on psoriatic arthritis has been observed with the use of D-penicillamine, but the available information is anecdotal and very limited. Eleven patients (two with spondylitis, four with asymmetric oligoarthritis, and five with symmetric polyarthritis) were randomized to an initial phase consisting of treatment with either D-penicillamine or placebo for 4 months,[57] followed by 4 months of treatment with D-penicillamine for all patients. The maximum dose of D-penicillamine was 750 mg/day, and no unusual toxicity was observed. Clinical benefit was seen only during D-penicillamine treatment; however, no efficacy measure attained statistically significant improvement.

Colchicine. Colchicine is an alkaloid that is known to attenuate the inflammatory response by interfering with intracellular microtubule formation which, in turn, causes impaired neutrophil chemotaxis. The presence of neutrophils in early psoriatic lesions suggested that colchicine might have a beneficial effect. A pilot study showed that 11 of 22 patients treated with colchicine (0.02 mg/kg/day) had significant cutaneous clearing, while four of eight patients with arthralgias were symptomatically improved.[58] A subsequent 16-week double-blind crossover study of 15 patients compared colchicine, 1.5 mg/day, with placebo.[59] With the patient global assessment as the primary efficacy measure, colchicine was judged more effective than placebo by 10 of the 12 patients (83%) who completed the study, and significant improvement was seen in grip strength, Ritchie index, joint pain, and joint swelling during colchicine treatment. Gastrointestinal symptoms required

the withdrawal of two patients from the study and a temporary dose reduction in five other patients. No unanticipated clinical or laboratory toxicity was seen. Larger studies of longer duration are needed to establish the role of colchicine in the management of psoriatic arthritis.

Retinoids. Etretinate, a vitamin A derivative, is the most commonly used retinoid in the treatment of psoriasis, and initial experience with this agent in psoriatic arthritis suggests a beneficial effect. In one recent pilot study, 40 patients treated with etretinate (50 mg/day) for a mean of 21.9 weeks experienced significant improvement in the number of tender joints, the duration of morning stiffness, and the erythrocyte sedimentation rate.[60] Maximal improvement for most efficacy measurements was seen at between 12 and 16 weeks. Mucocutaneous reactions consisting of dried and cracked lips, mouth soreness, and nosebleeds were seen in the preponderance of patients (39 of 40) and required cessation of treatment in nine patients. Other relatively frequent adverse effects were alopecia, hyperlipidemia, myalgias, and elevated transaminase levels. Etretinate is a teratogen and should not be used in women of child-bearing potential.

Photochemotherapy. The most commonly used form of photochemotherapy involves the oral administration of 8-methoxypsoralen followed by exposure to long-wave ultraviolet-A light (PUVA). A prospective study of 27 patients treated with PUVA found a favorable response in 49% of patients with peripheral arthritis, whereas no benefit was seen in patients with spondylitis.[61] In responders, improvement in the peripheral arthritis seemed to correlate with clearing of the skin disease, whereas no such relationship was observed in patients with axial disease. Extracorporeal photochemotherapy, also known as photopheresis, has been shown to diminish the in vitro viability, proliferation, and mitogen response of lymphocytes, but clinical improvement in arthritis symptoms appears modest and no effect on skin lesions has been observed.[62]

Somatostatin. Somatostatin may benefit some psoriatic arthritis patients but requires prolonged intravenous infusion (48 hours) and is poorly tolerated because of nausea. In one study, patients with extensive skin lesions and polyarticular involvement seemed more responsive.[63]

Interferon Gamma. A placebo-controlled double-blind trial of recombinant interferon gamma in 24 patients over a period of 4 weeks showed a modest improvement in arthritis activity; however, the effect may be transient inasmuch as, over a 6-month period of observation, improvement present at 1 month was not sustained despite continued treatment.[64] The putative efficacy of interferon gamma is further clouded by reports from trials of interferon in cutaneous psoriasis where arthritis developed during interferon treatment and subsided after termination of therapy.[65]

Dietary Supplements. In a small 6-month open label trial of oral 1,25-hydroxyvitamin D_3, seven of ten patients with active arthritis experienced either substantial or moderate improvement. Hypercalciuria precluded the use of therapeutic doses in two patients.[66] Dietary supplementation with polyunsaturated ethyl ester lipids resulted in subjective articular benefit for 18 of 34 patients in an uncontrolled study.[67] Controlled trials of these agents are needed to confirm efficacy.

Miscellaneous. Other agents that have been reported to have activity in psoriatic arthritis include bromocriptine, cimetidine, fumaric acid, parenteral nitrogen mustard, peptide T, radiation synovectomy with yttrium 90, and total lymph node irradiation. Further study is needed to define what role, if any, these regimens might have in patient management.

Approach to Management

The selection of an appropriate therapeutic regimen can be made only after a careful clinical, laboratory, and, in most cases, radiographic evaluation. This evaluation should (1) determine the activity and extent of the skin disease, (2) ascertain whether joint symptoms are due to structural damage, inflammatory disease, both, or neither, (3) identify, in the case of inflammatory disease, whether peripheral and/or axial involvement is present, and (4) document the presence of any coexisting condition or disease that could either contribute to the patient's symptoms or affect the selection of therapy. Concurrent dermatologic care is strongly recommended in nearly all cases, and some patients may experience marked improvement in their joint symptoms with treatment and control of their skin disease. As is true with all inflammatory arthropathies, both patient education and the involvement of physical and occupational therapists can have a significant impact on functional capacity, especially for the spondylitic subgroup.

Although occasional patients with oligoarticular disease will benefit from intraarticular steroid injection, NSAIDs should be the initial therapeutic agent. An adequate trial of a particular NSAID should be at least 2 to 3 weeks in duration and should use maximal dosage; the efficacy of the trial is established on clinical grounds. Patients unresponsive to one NSAID may well benefit from another; the initial and subsequent selection of the particular NSAID is empiric, but in our experience indomethacin may be more efficacious for spondylitic patients.

For most patients with asymmetric oligoarticular disease, treatment with NSAIDs is usually sufficient. In unresponsive patients, particularly those with a symmetric polyarthritis or evidence of destructive disease, a second-line agent should be considered. The selection of the particular second-line agent is empiric. Nonetheless, regimens with more predictable efficacy and relatively less toxicity should be considered before those that are more experimental and potentially more toxic. Of the treatment regimens reviewed, it has been our experience that low-dose pulse methotrexate is the most consistently useful second-line agent presently available for NSAID-refractory psoriatic arthritis. If methotrexate is not effective or tolerated, a trial of gold salt therapy or sulfasalazine should be initiated in most patients. Azathioprine, with controlled data documenting its efficacy, might next be considered in patients in whom methotrexate and gold have failed. However, azathioprine toxicity is such that, at present, we most often would first favor a trial of sulfasalazine over azathioprine. It is important to note that no single regimen will be efficacious or suitable for every patient; even ideal clinical trials cannot predict individual response or toxicity, making optimal treatment for each patient dependent on thoughtful evaluation, careful monitoring, and sound clinical judgment.

REFERENCES

1. Cheret S, Graham D, Little H, et al. The natural disease course of ankylosing spondylitis. Arthritis Rheum 1983;26:186.
2. Radford EP, Doll R, Smith PG. Mortality among patients with ankylosing spondylitis not given x-ray therapy. N Engl J Med 1977;297:572.
3. Smith PG, Doll R. Mortality among patients with ankylosing spondylitis after a single treatment course with x-rays. Br Med J 1982;284:449.
4. Kraag G, Stokes B, Groh J, et al. The effects of comprehensive home physiotherapy and supervision on patients with ankylosing spondylitis. J Rheumatol 1990;17:228.
5. O'Driscoll SL, Hayson MIV, Baddeley H. Neck movements in ankylosing spondylitis and their responses to physiotherapy. Ann Rheum Dis 1978;37:64.
6. Clain A, Elswood J. A prospective nationwide cross-sectional study of NSAID usage in 1331 patients with ankylosing spondylitis. J Rheumatol 1990;17:801.
7. Gran JT, Husby G. Ankylosing spondylitis. Drugs 1992;44:585.
8. Harrison TR, Wilson JD. Ankylosing spondylitis and reactive arthritis. In: Jeffers HD, Boynton SD, eds. Principles of internal medicine. 12th ed. New York: McGraw-Hill, 1991:1453.
9. Campbell PM, Wilske K. Drug monitoring schedules. In: Weaver AL, ed. Guidelines for reviewers of rheumatic disease care. 2nd ed. The American Rheumatism Association:24.
10. Tytman K, Bernacka K, Sierakowski S. D-Penicillamine in the therapy of ankylosing spondylitis. Clin Rheumatol 1989;8:419.
11. Steven MM, Morrison M, Sturrock R. Penicillamine in ankylosing spondylitis: a double blind placebo controlled trial. J Rheumatol 1985;12:735.
12. Grasedyck K, Schattenkirchner M, Bandilla K. Treatment of ankylosing spondylitis with auranofin. J Rheumatol 1990;49:98.
13. Amor B, Kahan A, Dougados M, et al. Sulfasalazine and ankylosing spondylitis. Ann Intern Med 1984;101:878.
14. Dougados M, Boumier P, Amor B. Sulphasalazine in ankylosing spondylitis: a double blind controlled study in 60 patients. Br Med J 1986;293:911.
15. Felteluis N, Hallgren R. Sulphasalazine in ankylosing spondylitis. Ann Rheum Dis 1986;45:396.
16. Nissila M, Lehtinen K, Leirisalo-Repo M, et al. Sulfasalazine in the treatment of ankylosing spondylitis. Arthritis Rheum 1988;31(9):1111.
17. Davis MJ, Dawes PT, Beswick E, et al: Sulphasalazine therapy in ankylosing spondylitis: its effect on disease activity. Br J Rheumatol 1989;28:410.
18. Corkhill MM, Jobanputra P, Gibson T, et al. A controlled study of sulphasalazine treatment of chronic ankylosing spondylitis: failure to demonstrate a clinical effect. Br J Rheumatol 1990;29:41.
19. Fraser SM, Sturrock RD. Evaluations of sulphasalazine in ankylosing spondylitis—an interventional study. Br J Rheumatol 1990;29:37.
20. Taylor HG, Beswick EJ, Dawes PT. Sulphasalazine in ankylosing spondylitis: a radiological, clinical, and laboratory assessment. Clin Rheumatol 1991;10(1):43.
21. Clegg DO, Reda DJ. Comparison of sulfasalazine and placebo for treatment of ankylosing spondylitis. For the Department of Veteran's Affairs Cooperative Studies Program 341, Salt Lake City, UT 84132, and Hines, IL 60141.
22. Ferraz MB, Tugwell P, Goldsmith CH, et al. Meta-analysis of sulfasalazine in ankylosing spondylitis. J Rheumatol 1990;17:1482.
23. Meilants H, Veys EM. The gut in the spondyloarthropathies. J Rheumatol 1990;17(1):7.
24. Des Maris HCL. Radiotherapy in arthritis. Ann Rheum Dis 1953;12:25–8.
25. Reiter H. Über eine bisher unerkannte Spirochanteninfektion (spirochaetosis arthritica). Dtsch Med Wochenschr 1916;42:1535.
26. Arnett FC, McClusky OE, Schacter BZ, et al. Incomplete Reiter's syndrome: discriminating features and HL-A W27 in diagnosis. Ann Intern Med 1976;84(1):8.
27. Ahvonen P, Sievers K, Aho K. Arthritis associated with yersinia enterocolitica infection. Acta Rheum Scand 1969;15:232.
28. Lahesmanaa-Rantala R, Toivanen A. Clinical spectrum of reactive arthritis. In: Toivanen A, Toivanen P, eds. Reactive arthritis. Boca Raton, Florida: CRC Press, 1988:1.
29. Keat A. Reiter's syndrome and reactive arthritis in perspective. N Engl J Med 1983;309:1606.
30. Fox R, Calin A, Gerber RC, et al. The chronicity of symptoms and disability in Reiter's syndrome. Ann Intern Med 1979;91:190.
31. Inman RD, Johnston MAE, Hodge M, et al. Postdysenteric reactive arthritis. Arthritis Rheum 1988;31(11):1377.
32. Keat A, Rowe I. Reiter's syndrome and associated arthritides. Rheum Dis Clin North Am 1991;17(1):25.
33. Winchester R, Bernstein DH, Fischer HD, et al. The co-occurrence of Reiter's syndrome and acquired immunodeficiency. Ann Intern Med 1987;106:19.
34. Thim Fan P, Yu DTY. Reiter's syndrome. In: Kelley WN, Harris ED, Ruddy S, Sledge CB, eds. Textbook of rheumatology. vol I, 4th ed. Philadelphia: WB Saunders, 1993:961.
35. Zwillich SH, Comer SS, Lee E, et al. Treatment of the seronegative spondyloarthropathies with sulfasalazine. J Rheumatol 1988;15:33.
36. Meilants H, Veys EM. The gut in the spondyloarthropathies. J Rheumatol 1990;17(1):7.
37. Winchester R, Bernstein DH, Fischer HD, et al. The co-occurrence of Reiter's syndrome and ac-

quired immunodeficiency. Ann Intern Med 1987;106:19.

38. Granfors K, Jalkanen S, von Essen R, et al. Yersinia antigens in synovial fluids cells from patients with reactive arthritis. N Engl J Med 1989;320:216.

39. Granfors K, Jalkanen S, Lindberg AA, et al. Salmonella lipopolysaccharide in synovial cells from patients with reactive arthritis. Lancet 1990;335:685.

40. Panayi GS, Clark B. Minocycline in the treatment of patients with Reiter's syndrome. Clin Exp Rheumatol 1989;7:100.

41. Foyden A, Bengtsson A, Foberg U, et al. Early antibiotic treatment of reactive arthritis associated with enteric infection, clinical and serological study. Br Med J 1990;301:1299.

42. Lauhio A, Leirisalo-Repo M, Lahdevirta J, et al. Double-blind, placebo-controlled study of three-month treatment with lymecycline in reactive arthritis, with special reference to chlamydia arthritis. Arthritis Rheum 1991;34:6.

43. Gladman DD, Stafford-Brady F, Chang C, et al. Longitudinal study of clinical and radiological progression in psoriatic arthritis. J Rheumatol 1990;17:809.

44. Goupille P, Soutif D, Valat J. Treatment of psoriatic arthropathy. Semin Arthritis Rheum 1992;21:355.

45. Campbell RM, Wilske K. Drug monitoring schedules. In: Weaver AL, ed. Guidelines for reviewers of rheumatic disease care, 2nd ed. The American Rheumatism Association:24.

46. Carette S, Calin A, McCafferty JP, et al. A double-blind placebo-controlled study of auranofin in patients with psoriatic arthritis. Arthritis Rheum 1989;32:158.

47. Dorwart BB, Gall EP, Schumacher HR, et al. Chrysotherapy in psoriatic arthritis. Arthritis Rheum 1978;21:513.

48. Palit J, Hill J, Capell HA, et al. A multicentre double-blind comparison of auranofin, intramuscular gold thiomalate and placebo in patients with psoriatic arthritis. Br J Rheumatol 1990;29:280.

49. Black RL, O'Brien WM, Van Scott EJ, et al. Methotrexate therapy in psoriatic arthritis. JAMA 1964;189(10):141.

50. Willkens RF, Williams HJ, Ward JR, et al. Randomized, double-blind placebo-controlled trial of low-dose pulse methotrexate in psoriatic arthritis. Arthritis Rheum 1984;27:376.

51. Espinoza LR, Zakraqui L, Espinoza CG, et al. Psoriatic arthritis: clinical response and side effects to methotrexate therapy. J Rheumatol 1992;19:872.

52. Baum J, Hurd E, Lewis D, et al. Treatment of psoriatic arthritis with 6-mercaptopurine. Arthritis Rheum 1973;16:139.

53. Levy J, Paulus HE, Barnett EV, et al. A double-blind controlled evaluation of azathioprine treatment in rheumatoid arthritis and psoriatic arthritis. Arthritis Rheum 1972;15:116.

54. Farr M, Kitas GD, Waterhouse L, et al. Sulphasalazine in psoriatic arthritis: a double-blind placebo-controlled study. Br J Rheumatol 1990;29:46.

55. Steinsson K, Jonsdottir I, Valdimarsson H. Cyclosporin A in psoriatic arthritis: an open study. Ann Rheum Dis 1990;49:603.

56. Gladman DD, Blake R, Brubacher B, et al. Chloroquine therapy in psoriatic arthritis. J Rheumatol 1992;19:1724.

57. Price R, Gibson T. D-Penicillamine and psoriatic arthritis. Br J Rheumatol 1986;25:228 (Letter).

58. Wahba A, Cohen H. Therapeutic trials with oral colchicine in psoriasis. Acta Derm Venereol (Stockh) 1980;60:515.

59. Seideman P, Fjellner B, Johannesson A. Psoriatic arthritis treated with oral colchicine. J Rheumatol 1987;14:777.

60. Klinkhoff AV, Gertner E, Chalmers A, et al. Pilot study of etretinate in psoriatic arthritis. J Rheumatol 1989;16:789.

61. Goupille P, Soutif D, Valat J. Treatment of psoriatic arthropathy. Semin Arthritis Rheum 1992;21(6):109.

62. Wilfert J, Honigsmann H, Steiner G. Treatment of psoriatic arthritis by extracorporeal photochemotherapy. Br J Dermatol 1990;122:225.

63. Matucci-Cerinic M, Lotti T, Cappugi P, et al. Somatostatin treatment of psoriatic arthritis. Int J Dermatol 1988;27:56.

64. Fierlbeck G, Rassner G. Treatment of psoriasis and psoriatic arthritis with interferon gamma. J Invest Dermatol 1990;95:138S.

65. O'Connell PG, Gerber LH, Digiovanna JJ, et al. Arthritis in patients with psoriasis treated with gamma-interferon. J Rheumatol 1992;19:80.

66. Huckins D, Felson DT, Holick M. Treatment of psoriatic arthritis with oral 1,25-dihydroxyvitamin D_3: a pilot study. Arthritis Rheum 1990;33:1723.

67. Lassus A, Dahlgren AL, Halpern MJ, et al. Effects of dietary supplementation with polyunsaturated ethyl ester lipids (angiosan) in patients with psoriasis and psoriatic arthritis. J Int Med Res 1990;18:68.

68. Kelley WN, Harris ED, Ruddy S, Sledge CB, eds. Textbook of rheumatology. 4th ed. Philadelphia: WB Saunders, 1993.

SYSTEMIC LUPUS ERYTHEMATOSUS (INCLUDING PREGNANCY AND ANTIPHOSPHOLIPID ANTIBODY SYNDROME)

Michelle Petri

NATURAL HISTORY OF THE DISEASE WITHOUT TREATMENT

The prognosis of systemic lupus erythematosus (SLE) has improved dramatically in the last 40 years. Of 55 patients followed by Bywaters and Bauer, 52% died within 2 years of onset.[1] A similar poor outcome with a mean survival of 2 years without treatment was reported by Posnick.[2] Jessar et al.[3] reported the prognosis of 103 patients (44 of their own patients from the 15 years before 1952 and 59 from 279 gathered from the literature in the years 1948 to 1952). Only 38% survived 4 years after onset.[3]

Harvey et al.[4] reported the outcome of 99 cases diagnosed from 1949 to 1953. This case series, which included both outpatients and inpatients, reflected two major clinical advances: the evolution of the lupus erythematosus (LE) cell test and the use of ACTH and cortisone in treatment. The LE test was positive in 29 of 33 "clinically doubtful" cases that were then included in the series. ACTH or cortisone was used in the treatment of 75 of the 99 patients. The steepest decline in survivorship occurred in the first 3 months after diagnosis, with 13% of the patients dying in this period. One-year survival was 78%, and 4-year survival was 52%. Of the survivors to any year, about 10% died in the following year. This much more favorable experience probably represented both the inclusion of milder or earlier cases confirmed by the LE cell test and the beneficial effect of ACTH and corticosteroid therapy.

Some improvement in survival was due to factors other than better diagnosis and corticosteroid treatment. Ropes[5] reported a 4-year survival rate of 24% for the years 1932 to 1944, increasing to 55% for the years 1945 to 1963. She attributed much of this improved survival to antibiotic therapy.

Recent studies have continued to show improved 5- and 10-year survival. Among middle-class, privately insured SLE patients, 97% 5-year and 93% 10-year survival have been reported.[6] Inner-city academic centers in the United States report lower but still greatly improved 10-year survival.[7]

In the years before widespread use of corticosteroid therapy, it was recognized that some disease flares improved spontaneously or with bed rest.[8] The evolution of the disease over time could not be ascertained in these early studies because of the high mortality rate. We have recently shown that new disease manifestations of lupus continue to evolve more than 5 years after diagnosis.[9] Flares of lupus occur with a median time of 12 months in patients under observation and treatment.[10] Thus the understanding of treated SLE continues to expand. A general discussion of the management of SLE can be found in Kelley et al., Chapter 62. Clinical features of the disease are dis-

cussed in Kelley et al., Chapter 61, and pathogenesis in Chapter 60 (reference 112).

OPEN TRIALS

Nonsteroidal Antiinflammatory Drugs

Surprisingly, aspirin is the best-studied NSAID
in open trials of large numbers of lupus patients (Table 7–1).[4,8] Both ibuprofen and indomethacin have been effective in open trials,
especially for arthritis and pleurisy[11] and in
combination with corticosteroids and antimalarials.[12] Long-term efficacy was demonstrated for indomethacin in a 9-month trial.[12]
Open trials differ, however, in whether
NSAIDs have a corticosteroid-sparing effect;
indomethacin, for example, was corticosteroid-sparing in one trial[13] but ibuprofen was
steroid-sparing in only 18% in another.[11] In an

open trial of ibuprofen, the median time to improvement was 14 days.[11]

Antimalarials

Important open trials of the two antimalarial
drugs in common use, chloroquine and hydroxychloroquine, are summarized in Table 7–2.
Clinical manifestations of patients in these open
trials included predominantly discoid lupus, although a few trials contained patients with
other forms of cutaneous lupus.[14-16] The early
open trials used higher doses of chloroquine, up
to 750 mg a day,[8] and hydroxychloroquine, up
to 1600 mg daily in one study[17] and up to 2000
mg daily in another,[15] than are used today. Not
surprisingly, side effects were more common in
the trials that used higher doses[8,17] and included
side effects rarely seen today, such as graying of
the skin or bleaching of hair pigment.

Corticosteroids

Topical Corticosteroids.   Open trials of topical corticosteroids for cutaneous lupus (usually discoid) have reached conflicting results. In
one study of 59 patients with discoid lupus,
73% were controlled with topical fluocin-
olone.[18] In contrast, only 26% of patients with
discoid lupus had a good or better response to
topical corticosteroids in a second study.[19]

Intralesional Corticosteroids.   In two large
open trials of intralesional corticosteroids for
the treatment of chronic discoid lesions, 93%
of 28 patients treated[20] and 88% of 40 patients
treated,[19] have responded.

TABLE 7–1
**Nonsteroidal Anti-inflammatory Drugs:
Open Trials**

NSAID	STUDY, YEAR	N	OUTCOME
Aspirin	Harvey et al., 1955[4]	19	Overall: 58% improved
	Dubois, 1956[6]	163	
Ibuprofen	Dubois, 1975[11]	17	Arthritis: 69% improved
Indomethacin	Marmont et al., 1965[13]	10	
	Dubois, 1966[12]	22	Overall: 82% improved

TABLE 7–2
Antimalarial Agents: Open Trials

DRUG	STUDY, YEAR	N	OUTCOME
Chloroquine	Dubois, 1956[8]	14	86% improved
		28 (with corticosteroids)	53% improved
	Goldman et al., 1953[14]	21	76% improved
	Rogers and Finn, 1954[103]	43	91% improved
	Pillsbury and Jacobson, 1954[104]	16	94% improved
	Ziff et al., 1958[16]	4	50% improved
		12 (with corticosteroids)	92% reduced corticosteroids
Hydroxychloroquine	Cornbleet, 1956[105]	7	100% improved
	Callen, 1982[19]	34	88% improved
	Lewis and Frumess, 1956[17]	22	77% improved
	Mullins et al, 1956[15]	40	88% improved

Oral Corticosteroids. Early open trials of corticosteroids demonstrated their effectiveness in the critically ill lupus patient. For example, of 119 patients who received corticosteroids (or ACTH) for at least 48 hours, 90% achieved benefit.[8] Doses of cortisone ranged from 200 mg/day up to 4000 mg/day. In an early study, 20 of 22 patients treated with prednisone and 13 of 18 treated with prednisolone, were well controlled.[21] Fever responded in 24 to 48 hours, arthritis within several days, and pleural effusions and cutaneous lupus in 1 to 2 weeks.

Of 62 patients treated with ACTH or cortisone in another early series, 39 had an excellent immediate response, 5 had a slower but satisfactory response, 8 eventually responded to escalating doses, 6 patients had little or no response, and 4 patients were withdrawn from the study because of hypertension.[4] In later follow-up, 17 of the 42 living patients still required maintenance corticosteroid treatment.

In a series of 82 patients seen in 1949 or later, 72% at some point required corticosteroid therapy. The importance of slow reduction of dose was recognized; 2 patients in the series died within 2 weeks of rapid withdrawal.[22]

Alternate-Day Corticosteroids. A prospective study of intravenous methylprednisolone therapy, followed by alternate-day corticosteroid therapy, was prematurely terminated because only 4 of 11 patients could be maintained on alternate-day corticosteroids.[23] Three patients had worsening of presenting nonrenal symptoms, and four had worsening renal disease. However, the benefit of alternate-day administration in reducing undesirable catabolic effects of corticosteroids remains an impetus for this dosing regimen.[24]

Intravenous "Pulse" Methylprednisolone. Many case reports have demonstrated the utility of intravenous "pulse" methylprednisolone therapy in severe cases of neurologic lupus,[25] thrombocytopenia,[26] and life-threatening multisystem disease,[27] refractory to previous treatments, including high-dose oral corticosteroids, azathioprine, and cyclophosphamide. Multiple open trials (Table 7–3) have confirmed improvement, usually rapid, in extrarenal manifestations of lupus. However, the response of thrombocytopenia can be variable.[28]

Azathioprine

Azathioprine has been widely used in the control of lupus nephritis.[29–33] Its use has been beneficial for refractory discoid lupus.[34,35]

Cyclophosphamide

The majority of trials of cyclophosphamide have been for the treatment of lupus nephritis. However, cyclophosphamide has been successfully used for the treatment of autoimmune thrombocytopenia refractory to high-dose corticosteroids,[36] discoid and subacute cutaneous lupus refractory to corticosteroids and antimalarials,[37] neuropsychiatric lupus,[38] and myositis.[39]

TABLE 7–3
Intravenous Methylprednisolone "Pulse" Therapy: Open Trials

STUDY, YEAR	N	NONRENAL MANIFESTATIONS	OUTCOME
Ponticelli et al., 1977[106]	6	Fever, arthritis, rash	Improvement: fever, arthritis, rash
Dosa et al., 1978[107]	4	Leukopenia, thrombocytopenia, rash	Improvement
Eyanson et al., 1980[108]	2	Neurologic, thrombocytopenia, anemia	Improvement
Fessel, 1980[109]	11	Neurologic, pulmonary, thrombocytopenia, cutaneous	Improvement: 64%
Isenberg et al., 1982[28]	20	Arthritis, pleurisy, vasculitis, fever, lymphadenopathy	Improvement: fever, arthritis, pleurisy, vasculitis, lymphadenopathy Occasional response: thrombocytopenia
Goldberg and Lidsky, 1984[110]	2	Subacute cutaneous lupus	Rapid improvement
Ballou et al., 1985[23]	11	Fever, arthritis, rash, thrombocytopenia, pneumonitis	Rapid improvement: 73%

Methotrexate

Methotrexate has been used in patients with corticosteroid-resistant lupus. Ten patients with fever, arthritis, and cutaneous lupus treated with weekly intravenous or daily oral methotrexate improved rapidly.[40] Of 10 patients with multiple nonrenal lupus manifestations treated with 7.5 mg weekly, seven showed benefit.[41]

Plasmapheresis

Most case series and open trials of plasmapheresis have been for renal lupus.[42] One open trial of plasmapheresis alone in four SLE patients (one with central nervous system lupus, two with arthritis, and one with thrombocytopenia) resulted in poor clinical outcome in all patients.[43] A second open trial of 14 SLE patients treated with plasmapheresis and concurrent conventional therapy resulted in improvement in 8, with joint and cutaneous symptoms responding best.[44] Concurrent immunosuppressive therapy may prevent or ameliorate the increased antibody production after removal of serum antibody and circulating immune complexes. A combination of lymphapheresis and plasmapheresis was beneficial in an open trial in 16 of 19 SLE patients receiving concurrent immunosuppression.[45]

Plasmapheresis has also been used to remove maternal anti-Ro (SS-A)[46] and in patients with antiphospholipid antibody syndrome resistant to conventional therapies.[47]

Intravenous Gamma Globulin

Intravenous gamma globulin may be helpful in some but not all SLE patients with severe thrombocytopenia.[48–51] It has been used (with other therapies) for pregnancy loss in antiphospholipid antibody syndrome.[52,53] Intravenous gamma globulin has been used for multiple nonrenal manifestations of lupus, including cutaneous vasculitis,[50,54] pancytopenia,[55] arthritis,[48,56] neurologic lupus,[56] and pericarditis.[57]

CONTROLLED CLINICAL TRIALS

Nonsteroidal Antiinflammatory Drugs

A 10-day randomized double-blind trial of ibuprofen versus aspirin demonstrated improvement in number of swollen joints, joint pain, and global assessment of arthritis only in the aspirin group.[58] However, ibuprofen has been shown to be efficacious for lupus arthritis in an open trial[11] with a longer treatment period.

Antimalarials

In two retrospective studies, before and after withdrawal of atabrine, patients were more likely to relapse after withdrawal of medication.[59,60] In a study of 5 patients taking amodiaquine, with a placebo crossover design, the placebo group relapsed within 1 to 3 months.[8] In a large retrospective study matching years on and off antimalarial drugs (predominantly chloroquine, although hydroxychloroquine, quinacrine, and triquin were also used), antimalarials reduced flares and were corticosteroid sparing. In addition, chloroquine reduced fever, fatigue, weight loss, and cutaneous lupus (Table 7–4).[61,62] In the Canadian Hydroxy-

TABLE 7–4
Antimalarial Drugs: Controlled Trials

STUDY	TREATMENT GROUP (N)	COMPARISON GROUPS (N)	STUDY DESIGN	OUTCOME
Rothfield, 1988[62]	Antimalarial (43)	Postwithdrawal (43)	Retrospective withdrawal study	Antimalarial use reduced corticosteroid dose and disease flares
Canadian Hydroxychloroquine Study Group, 1991[63]	Hydroxychloroquine (25)	Placebo (22)	Six-month randomized double-blind placebo-controlled withdrawal study	Antimalarial use reduced disease flares and increased time to flare
Ruzicka, 1992[111]	Hydroxychloroquine	Acitretin	8-week randomized double-blind	46% improved in acitretin group 50% improved in antimalarial group

TABLE 7–5
Intravenous Methylprednisolone: Controlled Trials

STUDY	TREATMENT GROUP (N)	COMPARISON GROUPS (N)	STUDY DESIGN	OUTCOME
Edwards et al., 1987[64]	1000 mg IV-MP for 3 days (11), other medications as needed	100 mg IV-MP for 3 days (10), other medications as needed	Randomized double-blind	45% 100 mg IV-MP vs. 60% 100 mg IV-MP responded
Mackworth-Young et al., 1988[65]	1000 mg IV-MP for 3 days (12), oral prednisolone 40–60 mg	Placebo (13), oral prednisolone 40–60 mg	Randomized double-blind	Greater improvement in IV-MP group (83%) at 14 days, but no difference at 28 days

chloroquine Study, which was a randomized, double-blind placebo-controlled withdrawal study, the relative risk of disease flare was 2.5 times higher in the placebo group and the time to a flare was shorter ($p = 0.02$). However, no significant differences in prednisone dose were found.[63]

Intravenous Methylprednisolone

One randomized double-blind trial of 1000 mg versus 100 mg doses of intravenous methylprednisolone found no difference in response (Table 7–5).[64] A second randomized double-blind trial of 1000 mg of intravenous methylprednisolone versus placebo in patients who were also treated with high doses of oral prednisolone found greater improvement in the methylprednisolone group at 14 days but not at 28 days.[65] Cutaneous and arthritis manifestations improved faster in the treatment group but did not reach a statistical difference.

Azathioprine

Because most controlled trials of azathioprine have included only patients with lupus nephritis, information on extrarenal manifestations is usually lacking. Three controlled trials that included data on nonrenal lupus reached conflicting conclusions (Table 7–6) with two studies finding that azathioprine reduced flares and corticosteroid requirements[66,67] and one finding no difference.[68]

Cyclophosphamide

The National Institutes of Health prospective controlled trials have clearly shown the benefit of cyclophosphamide in the treatment of lupus nephritis but lack data on nonrenal manifestations of lupus. One controlled trial of cyclophosphamide versus prednisone alone included four patients with nonrenal lupus (two in each group). In this trial, there were no responders in the group treated with cyclophosphamide alone.[69]

TABLE 7–6
Azathioprine: Controlled Trials

STUDY	TREATMENT GROUP (N)	COMPARISON GROUPS (N)	STUDY DESIGN	OUTCOME
Sztejnbok et al., 1971[66]	Prednisone and azathioprine (16)	Prednisone (19)	Nonblinded	Azathioprine use decreased morbidity, mortality, prednisone dose, and flares
Sharon et al., 1973[67]	Prednisone and azathioprine (7)	Prednisone (9)	Randomized withdrawal	Azathioprine reduced flares
Hahn et al., 1975[68]	Prednisone and azathioprine (11)	Prednisone (13)	Randomized trial	No reduction in mortality, flares, or prednisone dose in the azathioprine group

AUTHOR'S APPROACH TO MANAGEMENT

Routine screening of the patient with SLE should be performed at least every 3 months and should include an interval history, a directed physical examination, and laboratory monitoring including complete blood cell count, creatinine and cholesterol determinations, urinalysis, and, in patients in whom they have proven clinically useful, serum C3, C4, and anti-dsDNA. Monitoring of and lifestyle guidance in coronary artery disease risk factors, including smoking, obesity, hyperlipidemia, and hypertension, are an integral part of the quarterly visits. Hypertension should be aggressively managed by both nonpharmacologic and pharmacologic means. Hypertension is one of the major predictive variables for both renal failure and mortality in SLE.[7,70,71] Except for the avoidance of β-blocking agents in patients with Raynaud's phenomenon, antihypertensive agents of all classes can be used.

All SLE patients undergoing corticosteroid or immunosuppressive treatment should receive the pneumococcal pneumonia vaccine and yearly influenza vaccination. Patients should be counseled that infections, including bronchitis and urinary tract infections, should be brought to the physician's attention promptly. If possible, sulfa antibiotics should be avoided because of their propensity to cause allergy or disease flares in SLE.[72]

Because of the increased risk of cancer (even without exposure to alkylating agents), screening for malignant change should be instituted whenever or wherever appropriate. In the adult female SLE patient, this would include yearly pelvic examination and mammography (beginning in the age range of 35 to 40). Sunscreens should be used routinely, not just in photosensitive patients, to reduce cutaneous cancers.

Ongoing dental care is important to avoid a potential source of systemic infection and to avoid unnecessary caries due to secondary Sjögren's syndrome. Yearly ophthalmologic consultation is essential, not just to monitor antimalarial therapy but to screen for and treat glaucoma and posterior subcapsular cataracts secondary to corticosteroid therapy.

For purposes of the discussion to follow, 3 dosage forms of oral daily corticosteroids will be used, in prednisone equivalents: mild, 5 to 10 mg/day; moderate, 15 to 30 mg/day; and high, 40 to 60 mg/day.

Cutaneous Lupus

Malar rash, photosensitive rash elsewhere, and discoid lupus are approached in a similar manner. The patient is cautioned against ultraviolet (UV) light exposure, but not to the point of excessive paranoia. However, some patients have extreme sun sensitivity. Reducing their UV light exposure represents a major challenge to all caregivers and patient support systems. Sunscreens should be used not just to help cutaneous lupus, but to prevent skin cancer and to retard aging. Topical corticosteroid lotions and creams may have limited benefit (although fluorinated compounds should not be used on the face because of cutaneous atrophy), but their use should not delay the institution of systemic therapy.

Antimalarial agents remain the mainstay of treatment. Because of difficulty in obtaining quinacrine and concern about retinopathy with chloroquine, the agent of choice is hydroxychloroquine, with an average adult dose of 400 mg daily. Response usually begins within 1 month, and the full effect of treatment can be assessed at 3 months.

In many patients, antimalarial therapy is sufficient for cutaneous lupus. In the rare patient with allergic rash, severe gastrointestinal intolerance, or one of the unusual nervous system side effects (such as nightmares) of antimalarial therapy, it may be necessary to try alternative therapies. Retinoids, including isotretinoin or etretinate (in a patient practicing effective birth control), or dapsone (in a patient who is not G6PD-deficient) may be helpful. Dapsone may be the agent of choice for a rare form of cutaneous lupus, bullous lupus. In some cases, atabrine has been used with some success.

For very severe discoid lesions, intralesional corticosteroid injection may be necessary. Waiting weeks (or months) for control of disease by antimalarial therapy might allow irreversible scarring to occur. Similarly, low doses of corticosteroids (prednisone in doses of 5 to 20 mg/day) may be necessary for initial control of moderate cutaneous lupus, with rapid taper being the goal. Severe cutaneous vasculitis or severe discoid lupus (especially on areas such as the soles of the feet) may require intravenous pulse methylprednisolone (1000 mg/day for 3 days) to achieve initial control.

In the rare patient who requires a high maintenance dose of corticosteroid for severe vasculitic or other forms of cutaneous lupus, either azathioprine (100 to 150 mg/day) or methotrexate (initially 7.5 mg orally once a week) may play a corticosteroid-sparing role.

Raynaud's phenomenon is often seasonal, and not very severe in SLE patients. Patients with more severe symptoms benefit from the calcium channel blockers nifedipine and diltiazem. Purchase of battery-operated warming gloves and socks is a worthwhile investment.

Musculoskeletal Lupus

Nonsteroidal antiinflammatory agents are used in the initial management of polyarthralgias or polyarthritis. Many patients will require the addition of antimalarial therapy for adequate control.

Although corticosteroids in moderate to high doses are very effective for lupus arthritis, the long-term side effects do not justify their use for arthritis. If steroids are to be used at all, the lowest dose (usually 5 to 10 mg/day prednisone) should be employed, keeping the dosage just above the threshold for symptoms. A severe, incapacitating polyarthritis or myositis flare may require intravenous pulse methylprednisolone therapy (1000 mg/day for 3 days). Patients who require unacceptably high daily corticosteroid doses may do well with the addition of azathioprine or methotrexate (initially 7.5 mg orally once a week) as a corticosteroid-sparing agent. Lupus patients with features that overlap with rheumatoid arthritis ("rhupus") are good candidates for methotrexate therapy.

Cardiopulmonary Lupus (Including Serositis)

The initial management of severe serositis, either pericarditis or pleurisy with pleural effusion, may require intravenous pulse methylprednisolone therapy (1000 mg/day for 3 days) followed by oral prednisone at moderate or high dosage depending on the clinical severity. Milder forms of serositis can be managed with NSAIDs supplemented by low-dose prednisone as necessary. In a patient already taking a maintenance dose of an NSAID and low-dose prednisone, a mild exacerbation may be managed by temporarily increasing the prednisone dose to moderate levels, followed by a slow reduction back to the maintenance dose.

Interstitial lung disease can occur in an acute or chronic form in SLE. In a patient already on immunosuppressive therapy, the initial differential diagnosis requires a work-up for bacterial or opportunistic infection. Often a lung biopsy will be required to ascertain that the condition is due to SLE and to assess the degree of active inflammation. In many patients, high-dose corticosteroid therapy is required in the initial phases. The addition of azathioprine or alkylating agents is frequently necessary in patients with the chronic form. Serial monitoring of chest roentgenogram, pulmonary function tests (including single-breath diffusion capacity and helium lung volumes), and arterial blood gases is used to evaluate response.

Pulmonary hypertension in a mild, stable form may be detected by noninvasive cardiac echo Doppler in as many as 10% of SLE patients.[73] In the rare patient who progresses to severe pulmonary hypertension, the differential diagnosis includes recurrent pulmonary emboli or the presence of a hypercoagulable state. Management of idiopathic pulmonary hypertension with pulmonary artery pressures greater than 50 mm will usually require an initial right-heart catheterization to monitor response to therapy, including calcium-channel blockers and prostacyclin (if available as an investigational agent). Long-term anticoagulation is the rule. For follow-up, noninvasive monitoring with echo Doppler correlates well with catheterization.[73]

Libman-Sacks endocarditis is extremely rare in the poststeroid era. In many patients, antiphospholipid antibodies are found. If accompanied by embolic events, anticoagulation is necessary. Small lesions can be monitored by serial transesophageal echocardiograms, and treatment with corticosteroids and anticoagulation can be instituted if they enlarge.

Myocarditis or congestive heart failure is a very rare cardiac presentation or manifestation. Treatment with high-dose corticosteroids, usually initially pulse methylprednisolone (1000 mg/day for 3 days), is necessary. Coronary arteritis is also rare. Most cases of angina pectoris or myocardial infarction are due to premature atherosclerosis.

Hematologic Lupus

SLE patients with severe cytopenias require periodic laboratory monitoring to detect life-threatening declines in their blood counts.

Anemia in SLE can be due to bleeding in the gut, hemolysis, chronic disease, iron deficiency, or immunosuppressive therapy. When the cause is unclear, a bone marrow biopsy may be helpful. Hemolytic anemia can be managed with corticosteroids. If unacceptably high doses of daily prednisone are required, the addition of azathioprine as a steroid-sparing agent can be tried. In a few patients, Danocrine may be a useful adjunct. A severe hemolytic anemia may require intravenous pulse methylprednisolone, 1000 mg/day for 3 days, followed by a maintenance dose of prednisone.

Mild stable thrombocytopenia can be tolerated. Severe thrombocytopenia (platelet counts below 35,000) is treated with corticosteroids. For life-threatening thrombocytopenia, intravenous pulse methylprednisolone, 1000 mg/day for 3 days, is given initially. "Refractory" thrombocytopenia may require intravenous gamma globulin (after it is first ascertained whether there is IgA deficiency, a contraindication to its use). Danocrine may be tried, although it is variably successful. The patient with severe, persistent thrombocytopenia for more than 6 months, in whom alternative therapies have failed and who has developed complications from high-dose corticosteroids, is a candidate for splenectomy. Although it is not curative (and care must be taken to remove all accessory spleens), many patients require lower doses of medication for control of cytopenias after splenectomy. In rare cases, thrombocytopenia is a manifestation of TTP, and should be managed accordingly (with plasma exchange).

Constitutional Features

An occasional patient with SLE will have weight loss. Often this responds to a very small maintenance dose of prednisone in the range of 5 to 10 mg/day. Generalized lymphadenopathy is also rare in the adult SLE patient but usually responds rapidly to low-dose prednisone. Lymphadenopathy that is local or that does not respond to low-dose corticosteroid therapy should instigate a search for infection or malignancy.

Fever in a lupus patient is always a diagnostic and sometimes a therapeutic challenge. In an untreated patient, after a routine search for infection, fever can be attributed to SLE with some security. Nonsteroidal antiinflammatory agents can be used, but usually a low dose of corticosteroids is necessary to suppress fever. Patients should be counseled that mild elevations of temperature can be tolerated.

Fever in a lupus patient treated with corticosteroids or with immunosuppressive agents should be assumed to be due to infection until proven otherwise. Persistent high temperatures should be evaluated in the hospital setting. After appropriate bacterial (and often opportunistic organisms must be considered) cultures, an empiric course of antibiotic treatment may be necessary. If infection is ruled out, an increase in corticosteroid dose should control fever secondary to an underlying SLE flare. Sometimes an adjustment of the steroid dose timing along with a dose increase (from once a day to twice a day, or even from twice a day to four times a day) may be necessary to control the fever in a patient whose symptoms and signs appear recalcitrant to treatment. If fever occurs in the setting of activation of lupus in other organs, control of lupus activity elsewhere usually leads to resolution of fever, as well.

Cystitis

Acute interstitial cystitis may be a manifestation of SLE. Management consists of ruling out infection, imaging studies to confirm the presence of a thickened bladder wall, and mild to moderate doses of corticosteroids.

Gastrointestinal Lupus

A rare patient may require corticosteroid therapy for abdominal serositis or protein-losing enteropathy. The more serious, but still rare, manifestation of abdominal vasculitis requires therapy with high-dose corticosteroids (often initially intravenous methylprednisolone, 1000 mg daily for 3 days, followed by high dose intravenous methylprednisolone, 40 to 80 mg daily until stable, followed by cautious dose reduction).

Pregnancy

Pre-pregnancy counseling is important, but all too often the patient announces an unplanned pregnancy. It is optimum to have control of disease activity for at least six months before embarking on pregnancy, but successful pregnancies are the rule even if lupus is active at conception. However, there are certain stringent contraindications to pregnancy. First, women receiving cyclophosphamide (orally or intravenously) should not become pregnant because of the substantial risk of congenital defects. Methotrexate must be stopped before a woman becomes pregnant because it is an abortifacient and a teratogen. Second, women receiving warfarin should not become pregnant. Women who require anticoagulation should receive extensive counseling about the increased risk of thrombosis to themselves during pregnancy; if they still remained adamant about pregnancy, they should be switched to therapeutic doses of subcutaneous heparin while trying to conceive.

Before pregnancy the risks of pregnancy to both the fetus and to the woman should be assessed and reviewed with the patient (and, optimally, with the obstetrician). The risk of lupus flare in our Lupus Pregnancy Center is 60%, although most flares are mild or moderate. The risk of preterm birth is 45%, and the risk of pregnancy loss is 15%.[74] Women with anti-Ro (SS-A), especially if accompanied by anti-La (SS-B), will need to have fetal four-chamber echocardiograms performed during pregnancy to detect congenital heart block (or myocarditis) at an early and, presumably, treatable stage. Women with a history of pregnancy loss (two consecutive first-trimester spontaneous abortions or any late loss without known cause) should be tested for both anticardiolipin antibody and lupus anticoagulant. Women with severe renal insufficiency or with nephrotic syndrome are at increased risk of renal and pregnancy complications but may be able to have a successful pregnancy. Women with a history of preeclamptic toxemia or toxemia are candidates for daily low-dose aspirin (80 mg) therapy.[75] Maternal diastolic hypertension (90 mm Hg or higher) is a risk factor for preterm birth.[74] Alpha-methyldopa and hydralazine are the antihypertensive agents most widely used in pregnancy.

Management of medications during lupus pregnancy involves weighing of risk-benefit ratios and should be done on an individual basis, with the following guidelines. If azathioprine is necessary to control disease activity in crucial organs, it can be continued. NSAIDs should be avoided during the second and third trimesters because of potential adverse effects on labor and on the fetus.[76] Use of a NSAID for a very short period, however, might be permissible to treat a severe serositis or arthritis flare. Hydroxychloroquine use in pregnancy is a complex issue.[77] The theoretical concern is the potential for deposition in the fetal eye and ear. It is, of course, widely used in Africa and did not appear to cause any adverse effects during lupus pregnancies in one series.[78] It is illogical to stop it once pregnancy is recognized, because it is stored in tissues and, in any case, the fetus was already exposed during the first trimester. If hydroxychloroquine has been shown to be necessary to control disease activity, a good case can be made in the individual patient for continuing its use during pregnancy. Documentation of discussion of these issues with the patient and obstetrician is important.

Women with two or more first-trimester losses or one or more mid-trimester or late intrauterine losses, without known cause, should be evaluated for antiphospholipid antibodies. Women with pregnancy loss due to antiphospholipid antibody syndrome have a choice of regimens. In a clinical trial that did not include lupus patients, prednisone, 40 mg/day, with low-dose aspirin had efficacy equal that of subcutaneous heparin, 10,000 units twice a day, with low-dose aspirin. However, maternal morbidity was higher in the prednisone-treated group.[79] It is not necessary to use 40 mg of prednisone; 20 mg or less appears to be efficacious and less likely to cause maternal morbidity. If a woman with lupus and recurrent pregnancy loss already requires in the range of 20 mg of prednisone to control her SLE, low-dose aspirin can be added while she is trying to conceive. If a woman requires only low doses of prednisone, aspirin can be added while she is trying to conceive, and when she becomes pregnant the prednisone can be increased to 20 mg or alternatively, subcutaneous heparin can be added.

Monthly visits of all pregnant women with SLE to monitor and treat disease activity are important. Lupus flares that are mild or moderate may be managed with appropriate doses of oral prednisone. NSAIDs are usually avoided in the late second or third trimester. Severe lupus flares may require intravenous pulse methylprednisolone therapy or the addition of azathioprine. Cyclophosphamide, including intravenous pulse cyclophosphamide, must be avoided in the first trimester. Its use later in pregnancy can be justified only for life-threatening disease. Termination of pregnancy is not necessary to treat lupus flares and may, in fact, aggravate lupus activity. Referral to an obstetrician who specializes in high-risk cases is optimum, not just because of the increased frequency of fetal loss but, more important, because of the increased frequency of preterm birth (40%), which is due largely to preterm premature rupture of membranes and preeclamptic toxemia.

Antiphospholipid Antibody Syndrome

As many as 50% of patients with SLE will manifest the ability to make antiphospholipid antibodies (lupus anticoagulant or anticardiolipin antibody), often intermittently, when observed sequentially over time. Prophylactic therapy for SLE patients who produce antiphospholipid antibodies, but who have not had venous or arterial thrombosis (or vasculopathy), is not currently recommended.

Patients with venous thrombosis (usually deep venous thrombosis of the lower extremities) and either the lupus anticoagulant or anticardiolipin antibody can be treated initially with heparin or with thrombolytic therapy, as appropriate. Long-term anticoagulation with warfarin is strongly recommended because of the high recurrence rate.[80,81]

Initial management of patients with arterial thrombosis or vasculopathy is dictated by the site and the severity of the thrombotic event. Ischemic strokes may be treated initially with heparin, provided that there is no hemorrhagic complication. Myocardial infarction due to thrombosis may be treated initially with heparin, thrombolytic therapy, or angioplasty, as appropriate. Peripheral arterial emboli or thrombi may require emergency embolectomy/thrombectomy, thrombolytic therapy, angioplasty, or heparin. Long-term anticoagulation with warfarin appears to be preferable to antiplatelet therapy.[80]

In most cases, full anticoagulation, achieving an international normalized ratio (INR) of 3 to 4, is recommended.[80] Close monitoring of prothrombin time is necessary to reduce bleeding complications. Patients are switched to intravenous heparin before elective surgical procedures.

DRUG SIDE EFFECTS AND RECOMMENDED MONITORING SCHEDULES

Nonsteroidal Antiinflammatory Agents

For an in-depth discussion of NSAIDs, see Kelley et al., Chapter 43 (reference 112). Of 99 SLE pa-

tients exposed to an NSAID (including aspirin), 49.5% reported epigastric distress at some time; 7.1%, peptic ulcer disease; 9.1%, stomatitis; 4.0%, worsening renal insufficiency; 5.1%, bronchospasm; and 5.1%, urticaria/angioedema. Tinnitus was reported in 21.2%, vertigo in 7.1%, and an increase in ecchymoses in 34.3%.[82] Patients with mild epigastric distress can be managed initially with the introduction of an H_2-blocker. Patients with past peptic ulcer disease secondary to or aggravated by NSAIDs are candidates for misoprostol therapy. Low-dose prednisone is indicated in the high-risk patient who cannot tolerate NSAIDs.

Antimalarial Drugs (Hydroxychloroquine)

Reported side effects of antimalarial drugs include ocular toxicity (corneal deposits or retinopathy), cutaneous eruptions, gastrointestinal intolerance, and rare nervous system complaints, including myopathy. Of 104 SLE patients exposed to one or more antimalarial drugs, 22.1% had nausea, 15.4% had abdominal cramps, 12.5% had anorexia, and 9.6% had diarrhea. Only 5% (five patients) had any evidence of retinopathy; all were reversible. One of these five patients had renal insufficiency.

The risk of retinopathy from hydroxychloroquine is so low—only one patient in one series,[83] no patients among 73 in a second series,[84] and 3% to 4% in a third series[85]—that ophthalmologic monitoring every 6 months should be more than sufficient. In fact, it can be argued that ophthalmologic monitoring is not cost-effective for hydroxychloroquine alone and that it is more important to monitor for ocular effects of lupus itself or of corticosteroid therapy. This subject is reviewed in-depth in Kelley et al., Chapter 44 (reference 112).

Corticosteroids

Major side effects attributed to corticosteroid therapy include avascular necrosis of bone, osteoporosis (with or without fractures), steroid myopathy, diabetes mellitus, and increased frequency of infections. Corticosteroid therapy also increases the level of several cardiovascular risk factors, including cholesterol, hypertension, and obesity; this is one explanation of the association of corticosteroid use with premature atherosclerotic disease.[86] Of 170 SLE patients receiving corticosteroids, 21% developed avascular necrosis, 8% had recognized osteoporosis, 8% had steroid myopathy, and 7% had vertebral compression fractures; 7% had diabetes mellitus. Cutaneous fungal infections occurred in 18%, oral candida in 29%, and herpes zoster in 7%.[82]

Minor side effects of corticosteroid use include the cushingoid habitus, dermatologic toxicity, and neurologic symptoms. In the same group of 170 patients, 26% had a buffalo hump, 62% had moon facies, and 49% had truncal obesity. Dermatologic side effects included spontaneous ecchymoses (44%), impaired wound healing (32%), increased sweating (30%), new onset acne (28%), and striae (22%). Other minor side effects included insomnia (31%), and steroid mood change or psychosis (18%). Corticosteroids are discussed in Kelley et al., Chapter 48 (reference 112).

If detected at an early stage before collapse of the femoral head, core decompression of bone may prevent or delay the need for total joint replacement for avascular necrosis of the hip (the most frequently involved joint). Shoulder and knee avascular necrosis are less likely to require total joint replacement. Some avascular necrosis may be asymptomatic, and some regresses spontaneously.

All patients taking corticosteroids should receive supplemental calcium to achieve an intake of 1200 mg daily and vitamin D (as part of a daily multiple-vitamin regimen). Although not currently available, deflazacort may engender less osteoporosis. For the postmenopausal patient, estrogen replacement (with progesterone, if the uterus is intact) is recommended. Estrogen replacement may also decrease the risk of coronary artery disease. Estrogen replacement after menopause is not associated with lupus flares.[87] Etidronate may also be used for 2 weeks every 3 months. In the premenopausal patient, calcitonin and, possibly, biphosphonates may be useful.

In the patient who is hypercholesterolemic and who either already has atherosclerotic disease or has other major risk factors for atherosclerotic disease, referral to a registered dietitian for instruction in the Step II American Heart Association diet is recommended. For the patient with atherosclerotic disease who fails to achieve dietary control of hyperlipidemia, pharmacologic management can be instituted. We have found that lupus patients have a higher frequency of elevated creatine phosphokinase (CPK) level, usually asymptomatic, with both lovastatin and gemfibrozil than the general population; initial monthly monitoring of CPK level is recommended.

Intravenous Pulse Methylprednisolone

Pulse methylprednisolone therapy may lead to fluid overload, hypertension, and hyperglycemia. Rarely, it has been associated with cardiac arrhythmias, seizures, or steroid psychosis. Attention to fluid and electrolyte balance before and during therapy is important.[88]

Immunosuppressive Drugs

Major side effects of cytotoxic drugs include premature ovarian failure, hemorrhagic cystitis and bladder fibrosis, malignancy, bone marrow suppression, and infection. SLE patients taking oral or intravenous cyclophosphamide should be monitored monthly with interval history, directed physical examination, complete blood cell count, chemistry panel, and urinalysis. Pneumovax 23 and yearly influenza vaccination are recommended. Intravenous cyclophosphamide appears to be as efficacious as oral cyclophosphamide and at the present time is the preferred cytotoxic drug for severe SLE manifestations. It can be given with mesna to avoid the risk of hemorrhagic cystitis that occurs with oral cyclophosphamide use. Maintenance therapy with intravenous cyclophosphamide (dosage, timing, duration) remains unclear and needs further study.

Premature ovarian failure is more common in women over 30 years of age and after longer courses of cyclophosphamide (either oral or intravenous). If possible, to preserve fertility in younger patients, intravenous cyclophosphamide should be timed to coincide with the menses. Practically speaking, this may be difficult to achieve in the patient with irregular menses or because of the patient's work schedule.

Both cutaneous and gynecologic cancers can occur in cytotoxically treated patients. Cervical carcinoma is increased in black patients with lupus, patients without renal disease, and azathioprine-treated patients.[89] Use of sunscreens and yearly gynecologic examinations (including mammograms in women over 40 years of age) are important. Leukemias and lymphomas, which occurred in SLE patients treated with oral cyclophosphamide, appear to be rarer in patients exposed to intravenous cyclophosphamide. The mechanism of action and the immunoregulatory effect of the drugs are discussed in Kelley et al., Chapter 49 (reference 112).

CLINICAL PHARMACOLOGY AND DRUG INTERACTIONS

Nonsteroidal Antiinflammatory Drugs

Pharmacology. NSAIDs can be divided into those with short elimination half-times (ibuprofen, indomethacin, tolmetin, ketoprofen), intermediate half-times of 12 to 18 hours (naproxen, sulindac, diflunisal), and long half-times (piroxicam, nabumetone). Biotransformation includes hepatic metabolism to inactive metabolites, which are excreted renally. Indomethacin and sulindac have an enterohepatic circulation with fecal excretion.

Mechanism of Action. Although NSAIDs reversibly inactivate platelet cyclooxygenase, their in vivo action is also mediated through neutrophil function.[90]

Drug Interactions. Potential renal effects of NSAIDs, including sodium retention, hyperkalemia,[91] reduction in glomerular filtration rate, interstitial nephritis, and papillary necrosis, among others, can occur in SLE patients. A rare SLE patient may have fever and aseptic meningitis while taking ibuprofen, sulindac, or tolmetin. NSAID use may inhibit renal excretion of chlorpropamide, methotrexate, and lithium, and it may potentiate sulfonylurea hypoglycemics and warfarin because of protein-binding changes. Use of NSAIDs (other than nonacetylated salicylates) is considered high-risk therapy in anticoagulated patients because of the increased chance of bleeding. NSAIDs, in addition to aspirin, can also cause a drug hepatitis.

Antimalarials

Pharmacology. Chloroquine and hydroxychloroquine are water-soluble 4-aminoquinolones. They are rapidly absorbed in 2 to 4 hours, reaching a peak in 8 to 12 hours, with 50% transported by binding to serum proteins. Biotransformation of hydroxychloroquine results in two first-stage metabolites (chloroquine has one) that lead to a primary amine with a short half-life. The second stage of elimination has a half-life of 18 days. The clinical half-life is 50 to 52 hours.[92,93] The plasma concentration rises rapidly during the first week and then more slowly until equilibrium is reached by the fourth week. Fifty to sixty percent is excreted in the urine, with 8% to 10% of chloroquine and 15% to 24% of hydroxychloroquine excreted in the feces.[94] Hydroxychloroquine is also excreted in the bile.[95] Plasma concentrations are related to the daily dosage. Tissue levels are highest in melanin-containing tissues (choroid, ciliary body, inner ear), with most distributed in adrenals, spleen, lung, liver, and kidneys.[95] The concentration of antimalarial drug in the white blood cells is 100 to 200 times that in the plasma. It is concentrated in the epidermis of the skin, with an epidermis-to-corium ratio of between 5 and 15 times.[96] Chloroquine may persist in the retina for months to years.[97]

Mechanism of Action. Antimalarial drugs raise the pH within lysosomes, thereby interrupting the generation and presentation of antigenic peptides.[98] Other potential effects include a reduction of light absorption, inhibition of antigen-antibody complexes, antiinflammatory actions, and nucleoprotein binding (reviewed in reference 99).

Corticosteroids

Pharmacology. Corticosteroids bind to transcortin (corticosteroid-binding globulin) and to albumin, with only the unbound corticosteroid having biologic activity. Corticosteroids are inactivated by several pathways, including 11-dehydrogenation, which is accelerated by hyperthyroidism. Dihydro and tetrahydro corticosteroid derivatives are conjugated in the liver and excreted. Drugs, such as phenobarbital, that activate hepatic microsomal enzymes increase corticosteroid inactivation. Corticosteroids are classified into short-acting (hydrocortisone, prednisone, prednisolone, methylprednisolone), intermediate-acting (triamcinolone), and long-acting (betamethasone, dexamethasone) according to duration of ACTH suppression. Doses of prednisone greater than 15 mg/day cause adrenal suppression within 1 week. Doses of 5 mg or less of prednisone are not adrenally suppressive.[100]

Pharmacologic Effects. Corticosteroids bind to cytoplasmic receptors and then bind to DNA regions in target cells. Changes in the rate of DNA transcription, reflected in protein synthesis, then explain the effects of corticosteroids. Antiinflammatory effects include inhibition of leukocyte recruitment at inflammatory sites, decreased bactericidal activity, and reduced phagocytic activity.[101,102] Glucocorticoids also decrease the release of arachidonic acid, inhibiting prostaglandin synthesis. Immunosuppressive actions of corticosteroids include lymphopenia, with a reduction in the T inducer/helper subset. Corticosteroids inhibit antibody production and production of interleukin and other cytokines. They also affect cell-mediated immunity by decreasing proliferation in response to mitogens, inhibiting IL-2 production, and suppressing cutaneous delayed hypersensitivity. Some of these effects are dose- and time-dependent.

Drug Interactions. Corticosteroids can aggravate diabetes mellitus, congestive heart failure, and glaucoma. Corticosteroid-induced hypokalemia can predispose to digoxin toxicity and cardiac arrhythmias. Drugs that affect hepatic microsomal enzymes, such as phenobarbital, accelerate corticosteroid metabolism. Corticosteroids can reduce serum salicylate levels.

INVESTIGATIONAL DRUGS AND FUTURE DIRECTIONS

The major focus of clinical trials in lupus will continue to be the management of renal and neurologic lupus. It is hoped that data on the response of nonrenal, nonneurologic manifestations of lupus will result from these trials. The current trend to minimize corticosteroid doses and to emphasize combination therapies for nonrenal, nonneurologic lupus will continue.

Newer biologic therapies, including monoclonal antibodies, cytokine, lymphokine, and adhesion molecule agents, will eventually have a role in the treatment of SLE. Inasmuch as some of these agents are already being used successfully in the treatment of rheumatoid arthritis, a logical extension will be to use them for lupus arthritis. Current dosing regimens of available drugs, such as loading doses of antimalarial drugs, may be changed as a result of clinical trials already under way in rheumatoid arthritis.

The treatment of cutaneous lupus may benefit from studies of combinations of antimalarials, dapsone, and retinoids. Some investigational agents, such as thalidomide, may have limited applications. Severe cytopenias due to lupus may eventually be treated by growth factors. The eventual hope is that immunologic advances will lead to the development of peptide or other vaccines to prevent the disease and its characteristic flares.

REFERENCES

1. Pickering G, Bywaters EGL, Damielli JF, et al. Treatment of systemic lupus erythematosus with steroids: report to the Medical Research Council by the Collagen Diseases and Hypersensitivity Panel. Br Med J 1961;5257:915.
2. Posnick J. Systemic lupus erythematosus: the effect of corticotropin and adrenocorticoid therapy on survival rate. CA Med 1963;98:308.
3. Jessar RA, Lamont-Havers W, Ragan C. Natural history of lupus erythematosus disseminatus. Ann Intern Med 1953;38:717.
4. Harvey AM, Shulman LE, Tumulty PA, et al. Systemic lupus erythematosus: review of the literature and clinical analysis of 138 cases. Medicine 1954;33:291.
5. Ropes MW. Observations on the natural course of disseminated lupus erythematosus. Medicine 1964;43:387.
6. Wallace DJ, Dubois EL. Dubois' lupus erythematosus. 3rd ed. Philadelphia: Lea & Febiger, 1987.
7. Reveille JS, Bartolucci A, Alarcón GS. Prognosis in systemic lupus erythematosus: negative impact of increasing age at onset, black race, and thrombocytopenia, as well as causes of death. Arthritis Rheum 1990;33:37.
8. Dubois EL. Systemic lupus erythematosus: recent advances in its diagnosis and treatment. Ann Intern Med 1956;45:163.
9. Petri M, Conroy M, Caffentzis E, et al. The evolution of systemic lupus erythematosus (SLE) [Abstract]. Arthritis Rheum 1993;36 (9, suppl):S274.
10. Petri M, Genovese M, Engle E, et al. Definition, incidence and clinical description of flare in systemic lupus erythematosus: a prospective cohort study. Arthritis Rheum 1991;34:937.
11. Dubois EL. Ibuprofen for systemic lupus erythematosus [Letter]. N Engl J Med 1975;293:779.
12. Dubois EL. Management of systemic lupus erythematosus. Mod Treatment 1966;3:1245.
13. Marmont AM, Damasio E. The place of indomethacin in the treatment of SLE. In: Atti del Simposio Internazionale su Recenti Acquisizioni nella Terapia Antireumatica nonsteroidea. Turin: Minerva Medica, 1965:219.

14. Goldman L, Cole DP, Preston RH. Chloroquine diphosphate in treatment of discoid lupus erythematosus. JAMA 1953;152:1428.

15. Mullins JF, Watts FL, Wilson CJ. Plaquenil in the treatment of lupus erythematosus. JAMA 1956;161:879.

16. Ziff M, Esserman P, McEwen C. Observations on the course and treatment of systemic lupus erythematosus. Arthritis Rheum 1958;1:332.

17. Lewis HM, Frumess GM. Plaquenil in the treatment of discoid lupus erythematosus. Arch Dermatol 1956;73:576.

18. Jansen GT, Dillaha CJ, Honeycutt WM. Discoid lupus erythematosus: is systemic treatment necessary? Arch Dermatol 1965;92:283.

19. Callen JP. Chronic cutaneous lupus erythematosus. Arch Dermatol 1982;118:412.

20. Rowell NR. Treatment of chronic discoid lupus erythematosus with intralesional triamcinolone. Br J Dermatol 1962;74:354.

21. Dubois EL. Prednisone and prednisolone in the treatment of systemic lupus erythematosus. JAMA 1956;161:427.

22. Ropes MW. Systemic lupus erythematosus. Cambridge, Massachusetts: Harvard University Press, 1976.

23. Ballou SP, Kahn MA, Kushner I: Intravenous pulse methylprednisolone followed by alternate day corticosteroid therapy in lupus erythematosus: a prospective evaluation. J Rheumatol 1985;12:944.

24. Walton J, Watson BS, Ney RL. Alternate-day vs shorter-interval steroid administration. Arch Intern Med 1970;126:601.

25. Davies UM, Ansell BM. Central nervous system manifestations in juvenile systemic lupus erythematosus: a problem of management. J Rheumatol 1988;15:1720.

26. Lurie DP, Kahaleh MB. Pulse corticosteroid therapy for refractory thrombocytopenia in systemic lupus erythematosus. J Rheumatol 1982;9:311.

27. Oto A, Sozen T, Boyacioglu S. Pulsed methylprednisolone [Letter]. Ann Rheum Dis 1981;40:630.

28. Isenberg DA, Morrow WJW, Snaith ML. Methylprednisolone pulse therapy in the treatment of systemic lupus erythematosus. Ann Rheum Dis 1982;41:347.

29. Levitt JI. Deterioration of renal function after discontinuation of long-term prednisone-azathioprine therapy in primary renal disease. N Engl J Med 1970;282:1125.

30. Drinkard JP, Stanley TM, Dornfeld L, et al. Azathioprine and prednisone in the treatment of adults with lupus nephritis. Medicine 1970;49:411.

31. Cade R, Spooner G, Schlein E, et al. Comparison of azathioprine, prednisone, and heparin alone or combined in treating lupus nephritis. Nephron 1973;10:37.

32. Donadio JV Jr, Holley KE, Wagoner RD, et al. Treatment of lupus nephritis with prednisone and combined prednisone and azathioprine. Ann Intern Med 1972;77:829.

33. Carette S, Klippel JH, Decker JL, et al. Controlled studies on oral immunosuppressive drugs in lupus nephritis: a long-term follow-up. Ann Intern Med 1983;99:1.

34. Tsokos GC, Caughman SW, Klippel JH. Successful treatment of generalized discoid skin lesions with azathioprine. Arch Dermatol 1985;121:1323.

35. Shehade S. Successful treatment of generalized discoid skin lesions with azathioprine [letter]. Arch Dermatol 1986;122:376.

36. Boumpas DT, Barez S, Klippel JH, et al. Intermittent cyclophosphamide for the treatment of autoimmune thrombocytopenia in systemic lupus erythematosus. Ann Intern Med 1990;112:674.

37. Schulz EJ, Menter MA. Treatment of discoid and subacute lupus erythematosus with cyclophosphamide. Br J Dermatol 1971;86 (suppl 7):60.

38. Fricchione GL, Kaufman LD, Gruber BL, et al. Electroconvulsive therapy and cyclophosphamide in combination for severe neuropsychiatric lupus with catatonia. Am J Med 1990;88:442.

39. Kono DH, Klashman DJ, Gilbert RC. Successful IV pulse cyclophosphamide in refractory PM in 3 patients with SLE [Letter]. J Rheumatol 1990;17:982.

40. Miescher PA, Riethmüller D. Diagnosis and treatment of systemic lupus erythematosus. Semin Hematol 1965;2:1.

41. Rothenberg RJ, Graziano GM, Grandone JT, et al. The use of methotrexate in steroid-resistant systemic lupus erythematosus. Arthritis Rheum 1988;31:612.

42. Wallace DJ, Goldfinger D, Nichols S, et al. A controlled study on the use of plasmapheresis in steroid/immunosuppressive resistant systemic lupus erythematosus with nephrotic syndrome. In: Uda T, Shiokawa Y, Inoue N, eds. Proceedings of the First International Congress of the World Apheresis Association. Cleveland: ISAO Press, 1987:91.

43. Schlansky R, Dettoratius RJ, Pincus T, et al. Plasmapheresis in systemic lupus erythematosus: a cautionary note. Arthritis Rheum 1981;24:49.

44. Verrier-Jones J, Cumming RH, Bacon PA, et al. Evidence for a therapeutic effect of plasmapheresis in patients with SLE. Q J Med 1979;48:535.

45. Spiva DA, Cecere FA. The use of combination plasmapheresis/leukocytapheresis in the treatment of refractory systemic lupus erythematosus. Plasma Ther Trans Tech 1983;4:151.

46. Buyon JP, Swersky SH, Fox HE, et al. Intrauterine therapy for presumptive fetal myocarditis with acquired heart block due to systemic lupus erythematosus: experience in a mother with a predominance of SS-B (La) antibodies. Arthritis Rheum 1987;30:44.

47. Fullcher D, Stewart G, Exner T, et al. Plasma exchange and the anticardiolipin syndrome in pregnancy. Lancet 1989;2:171.

48. Kater L, Derksen\RHWM, Houwert DA, et al. Effect of plasmapheresis in active systemic lupus erythematosus. Neth J Med 1981;24:209.

49. Howard RF, Maier WP, Gordon DS, et al. Clinical and immunological investigation of intravenous human immunoglobulin (IVIG) therapy in SLE-associated thrombocytopenia [Abstract]. Arthritis Rheum 1989;32:S75.

50. Gaedicke G, Teller WM, Kohne E, et al. IgG therapy in systemic lupus erythematosus—two case reports. Blut 1984;48:387.

51. Maier WP, Gordon DS, Howard RF, et al. Intravenous immunoglobulin therapy in systemic lupus erythematosus-associated thrombocytopenia. Arthritis Rheum 1990;33:1233.

52. Katz VL, Thorp JM Jr, Watson WJ, et al. Human immunoglobulin therapy for preeclampsia associated with lupus anticoagulant and anticardiolipin antibody. Obstet Gynecol 1990;76:986.

53. Carreras LO, Pérez GN, Vega HR, et al. Lupus anticoagulant and recurrent fetal loss: successful treatment with gammaglobulin. Lancet 1988;II:393.

54. Ballow M, Parke A. The uses of intravenous immune globulin in collagen vascular disorders. J Allergy Clin Immunol 1989;84:608.

55. Akashi K, Nagasawa K, Mayumi T, et al. Successful treatment of refractory systemic lupus erythematosus with intravenous immunoglobulins. J Rheumatol 1990;17:375.

56. Lin RY, Racis SP. In vivo reduction of circulating C1q binding immune complexes by intravenous gammaglobulin administration. Int Arch Allergy Appl Immunol 1986;79:286.

57. Petersen HH, Nielsen H, Hansen M, et al. High-dose immunoglobulin therapy in pericarditis caused by SLE [Letter]. Scand J Rheumatol 1990;19:91.

58. Karsh J, Kimberly RA, Stahl NI, et al. Comparative effects of aspirin and ibuprofen in the management of systemic lupus erythematosus. Arthritis Rheum 1980;23:1401.

59. Christiansen JV, Nielsen JP. Treatment of lupus erythematosus with mepacrine: results and relapses during a long observation. Br J Dermatol 1956;68:73.

60. Buchanan R Jr, King H, Hamilton CM. Quinacrine in discoid lupus erythematosus. South Med J 1954;47:678.

61. Rudnicki RD, Gresham GE, Rothfield NF. The efficacy of antimalarials in systemic lupus erythematosus. J Rheumatol 1975;2:323.

62. Rothfield N. Efficacy of antimalarials in systemic lupus erythematosus. Am J Med 1988; 85(suppl 4A):53.

63. The Canadian Hydroxychloroquine Study Group. A randomized study of the effect of withdrawing hydroxychloroquine sulfate in systemic lupus erythematosus. N Engl J Med 1991;324:150.

64. Edwards JCW, Snaith ML, Isenberg DA. A double blind controlled trial of methylprednisolone infusions in systemic lupus erythematosus using individualized outcome assessment. Ann Rheum Dis 1987;46:773.

65. Mackworth-Young CG, David J, Morgan SH, et al. A double blind, placebo controlled trial of intravenous methylprednisolone in systemic lupus erythematosus. Ann Rheum Dis 1988; 47:496.

66. Sztejnbok M, Stewart A, Diamond H, et al. Azathioprine in the treatment of systemic lupus erythematosus: a controlled study. Arthritis Rheum 1971;14:639.

67. Sharon E, Kaplan D, Diamond HS. Exacerbation of systemic lupus erythematosus after withdrawal of azathioprine therapy. N Engl J Med 1973;288:122.

68. Hahn BH, Kantor OS, Osterland CK. Azathioprine plus prednisone compared with prednisone alone in the treatment of systemic lupus erythematosus. Ann Intern Med 1975;83:597.

69. Fries JF, Sharp GC, McDevitt HO, et al. Cyclophosphamide therapy in systemic lupus erythematosus and polymyositis. Arthritis Rheum 1973;16:154.

70. Studenski S, Allen NB, Caldwell DS, et al. Survival in systemic lupus erythematosus: a multivariate analysis of demographic factors. Arthritis Rheum 1987;30:1326.

71. Ginzler EM, Diamond HS, Weiner M, et al. A multicenter study of outcome in systemic lupus erythematosus. I. Entry variables as predictors of prognosis. Arthritis Rheum 1982;25:601.

72. Petri M, Allbritton J. Antibiotic allergy in SLE: a case-control study. J Rheumatol 1992;19: 265.

73. Simonson JS, Schiller NB, Petri M, et al. Pulmonary hypertension in systemic lupus erythematosus. J Rheumatol 1989;16:918.

74. Petri M, Howard D, Repke J, et al. The Hopkins Lupus Pregnancy Center: 1987–1991 update. Am J Reprod Immunol 1992;28:188.

75. Sibai BM, Caritis SN, Thom E, et al. Prevention of preeclampsia with low-dose aspirin in healthy, nulliparous pregnant women: the National Institute of Child Health and Human Development Network of Maternal-Fetal Medicine Units. N Engl J Med 1993;329:1213.

76. Norton ME, Merrill J, Cooper BAB, et al. Neonatal complications after the administration of indomethacin for preterm labor. N Engl J Med 1993;329:1602.

77. Levy M, Buskila D, Gladman DD, et al. Pregnancy outcome following first trimester exposure to chloroquine. Am J Perinatol 1991;8: 174.

78. Parke AL. Antimalarial drugs, systemic lupus erythematosus and pregnancy. J Rheumatol 1988;15:607.

79. Cowchock FS, Reece EA, Balaban D, Branch DN, Plouffe L. Repeated fetal losses associated with antiphospholipid antibodies: a collaborative randomized trial comparing prednisone

with low-dose heparin treatment. Am J Obstet Gynecol 1992;166:1318.

80. Rosove MH, Brewer PMC. Antiphospholipid thrombosis: clinical course after the first thrombotic event in 70 patients. Ann Intern Med 1992;117:303.

81. Derksen RHWM, de Groot PG, Kater L, et al. Patients with antiphospholipid antibodies and venous thrombosis should receive long term anticoagulant treatment. Ann Rheum Dis 1993;52:689.

82. Petri M, Howard D, Goldman DW. Side-effects of medications prescribed for systemic lupus erythematosus [Abstract]. Arthritis Rheum 1992; 35:S358.

83. Easterbrook M. Useful and diagnostic tests in the detection of early chloroquine retinopathy [Abstract]. Arthritis Rheum 1989;32:R8.

84. Morsman CD, Livesey SJ, Richards IM, et al. Screening for hydroxychloroquine retinal toxicity: is it necessary? Eye 1990;4:572.

85. Bernstein HN. Ophthalmologic considerations and testing in patients receiving long-term antimalarial therapy. Am J Med 1983;75(Suppl 1A):25.

86. Petri M, Lakatta C, Magder L, et al. Effect of prednisone and hydroxychloroquine on coronary artery disease risk factors in systemic lupus erythematosus: a longitudinal data analysis. Am J Med 1993;96:254.

87. Arden NK, Lloyd M, Spector TD, et al. The safety of estrogen replacement therapy (ERT) in systemic lupus erythematosus [Abstract]. Arthritis Rheum 1993;36(9 suppl):S64.

88. Wollheim FA. Acute and long-term complications of corticosteroid pulse therapy. Scand J Rheumatol 1983;54(suppl):27.

89. Ginzler E, Feldman D, Giovaniello G, et al. The association of cervical neoplasia (CN) and SLE [Abstract]. Arthritis Rheum 1989;32(4, suppl):S30.

90. Abramson SB, Weissmann G. The mechanisms of action of nonsteroidal antiinflammatory drugs. Arthritis Rheum 1989;32:1.

91. Kimberly RF, Bowden RE, Keiser HR, et al. Reduction of renal function by newer nonsteroidal antiinflammatory drugs. Am J Med 1978;64:804.

92. MacKenzie A. Dose refinements in long-term therapy of rheumatoid arthritis with antimalarials. Am J Med 1983;75(1A):40.

93. Carr RE, Gouras P, Gunkel RD. Chloroquine retinopathy: early detection by retinal threshold test. Arch Ophthalmol 1966;75:171.

94. Legros K, Rosner I, Berger C. Influence du niveau d'eclairement ambiant sur les modifications oculaires induites par l'hydroxychloroquine chez le rat. Arch Ophthalmol 1973;33: 417.

95. McChesney EW. Animal toxicity and pharmacokinetics of hydroxychloroquine sulfate. Am J Med 1983;75(1A):11.

96. Shaffer B, Cahn MM, Levy EJ. Absorption of antimalarial drugs in human skin: spectroscopic and chemical analysis in epidermis and corium. J Invest Dermatol 1958;30:341.

97. Tuffanelli DL, Abraham RK, Dubois EL. Pigmentation associated with antimalarial therapy: its possible relation to ocular lesions. Arch Dermatol 1963;88:419.

98. Fox RI, Kang H-I. Mechanism of action of antimalarial drugs: inhibition of antigen processing and presentation. Lupus 1993;2(suppl 1): S9.

99. Dubois EL. Antimalarials in the management of discoid and systemic lupus erythematosus. Semin Arthritis Rheum 1978;8:33.

100. Danowski TS, Bonessi JV, Sabeh G, et al. Probabilities of pituitary adrenal responsiveness after steroid therapy. Ann Intern Med 1964: 61:11.

101. Rinehart JJ, Sagone AL, Balcerzak SP, et al. Effects of corticosteroid therapy on human monocyte function. N Engl J Med 1975;292: 236.

102. Jones CJP, Morris KJ, Jayson MIV. Prednisolone inhibits phagocytosis by polymorphonuclear leukocytes via steroid receptor-mediated events. Ann Rheum Dis 1983;42:56.

103. Rogers J, Finn OA. Synthetic antimalarial drugs in chronic discoid lupus erythematosus and light eruptions. Arch Dermatol Syphilol 1954;70:61.

104. Pillsbury DM, Jacobson C. Treatment of chronic discoid lupus erythematosus with chloroquine (aralen). JAMA 1954;154:1330.

105. Cornbleet T. Discoid lupus erythematosus treatment with plaquenil. Arch Dermatol 1956;73:572.

106. Ponticelli C, Tarantino A, Pioltelli P, et al. High-dose methylprednisolone pulses in active lupus nephritis [Letter]. Lancet 1977;I:1063.

107. Dosa S, Cairns SA, Lawler W, et al. The treatment of lupus nephritis by methylprednisolone pulse therapy. Postgrad Med J 1978;54:628.

108. Eyanson S, Passo MH, Aldo-Benson MA, et al. Methylprednisolone pulse therapy for nonrenal lupus erythematosus. Ann Rheum Dis 1980;39:377.

109. Fessel JW. Megadose corticosteroid therapy in systemic lupus erythematosus. J Rheumatol 1980;7:486.

110. Goldberg JW, Lidsky MD. Pulse methylprednisolone therapy for persistent subacute cutaneous lupus [Letter]. Arthritis Rheum 1984;27: 837.

111. Ruzicka T, Sommerburg C, Goerz G, Kind P, Mensing H. Treatment of cutaneous lupus erythematosus with acitretin and hydroxychloroquine. Br J Dermatol 1992;127:513.

112. Kelley WN, Harris ED, Ruddy S, Sledge CB, eds. Textbook of rheumatology. 4th ed. Philadelphia: WB Saunders, 1993.

RENAL DISEASE IN SYSTEMIC LUPUS ERYTHEMATOSUS

Ellen M. Ginzler

The diagnosis, routine follow-up, and treatment of nephritis in patients with systemic lupus erythematosus (SLE) is based on knowledge of the renal histologic changes, serologic and clinical correlations with renal disease, and the natural history of the disease, as well as the expected response to therapeutic interventions. Our understanding of these various factors is derived from anecdotal reports in individual patients, from both small and large retrospective and prospective cohort studies, and from uncontrolled as well as randomized therapeutic trials. Statistical techniques have also been applied to use data from small studies or to correct for multiple factors that might have an influence on outcome. The following discussion will review what is generally accepted regarding the clinical features and prognosis of lupus nephritis, as well as what remains controversial, in order to provide an approach to the management of patients with this disease. In so doing, specific issues will be considered:

- What are the clinical correlations and the natural history of the various histologic forms of lupus nephritis?
- What is the role of renal biopsy in predicting outcome or in making therapeutic decisions?
- How should patients with SLE be followed in order to predict an exacerbation of nephritis at any early stage?
- Should serologic or other immunologic abnormalities alone be treated?
- What therapeutic modalities have demonstrated efficacy in controlled trials versus anecdotal reports?

- How should outcome be monitored? And what are the criteria for therapeutic success?
- What ancillary measures other than treatment of the acute exacerbation of nephritis should be considered in order to preserve renal function and prevent other, especially cardiovascular, features of morbidity?
- When progression to end-stage renal disease occurs, what is the expected course with chronic dialysis and/or renal transplantation?

For an in-depth discussion of the overall management of SLE patients, please see Kelley et al., Chapter 62 (reference 104).

HISTOLOGIC CLASSIFICATION OF LUPUS NEPHRITIS

The histologic classification of lupus nephritis is based on glomerular pathology, as described initially by Baldwin et al. in 1970[1] and in a subsequent modification by the World Health Organization (WHO), which includes immunofluorescent and electron microscopic findings.[2] Class I, an unusual finding in patients with SLE, represents a renal biopsy specimen that is normal on light microscopy and demonstrates no immune complex deposition on either immunofluorescence or electron microscopy. Normal light microscopy coincident with immune deposits, usually limited to the mesangium, is designated WHO Class IIA. Mesangial immune deposits accompanied by histologic change, including either increased mesangial matrix or areas of increased mesangial cellularity in some or all glomeruli sampled, is designated Class IIB, or mesangial lupus nephritis (Fig. 8–1A).

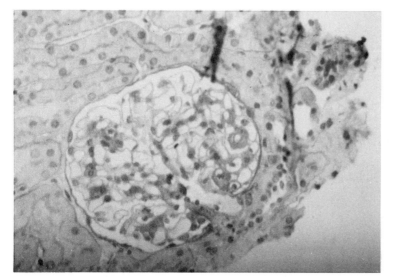

A

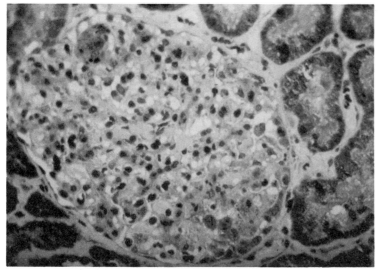

B

C

FIGURE 8–1

A, High-power light microscopic appearance of WHO Class IIB (mesangial) lupus nephritis showing mesangial thickening and mild mesangial hypercellularity with normal, patent capillary loops. **B,** High-power light microscopic appearance of Class III (focal proliferative) lupus nephritis showing segmental proliferation and basement membrane thickening of capillary tufts with other lobules of the glomerulus remaining normal. **C,** High-power light microscopic appearance of Class IV (diffuse proliferative) lupus nephritis showing generalized basement membrane thickening, endothelial cell proliferation, and infiltration with inflammatory cells.

Focal proliferative lupus nephritis, generally corresponding to WHO Class III, may include mesangial disease as well as more severe histologic abnormalities, including capillary endothelial cell proliferation, necrosis, and polymorphonuclear leukocyte infiltration (Fig. 8–1B). These changes are limited to some lobules of the glomerulus, while other glomeruli may be entirely unaffected. Immune complex deposition frequently extends beyond the mesangium to the subendothelial surface of the capillary basement membrane of some or all glomeruli.

Diffuse proliferative lupus nephritis, as originally described by Baldwin et al., includes disease within all lobules of the glomerulus, and essentially all glomeruli are affected (Fig. 8–1C). The membranoproliferative variant may show a predominance of capillary basement membrane thickening. However, proliferative changes, polymorphonuclear leukocyte infiltration, and subendothelial immune deposits are also characteristic. Epithelial crescents and totally sclerotic glomeruli are also well described but less frequent features of Class IV lupus nephritis.

Although it was originally believed that the various proliferative forms of lupus nephritis were distinct entities, it is now well accepted that progression from the milder to the more severe histologic forms occurs with time.[3–5] The nature of a continuum of severity of glomerular disease is also reflected in the WHO definition of Class IV nephritis, in which more than 50%, but not all, of the glomeruli have light microscopic changes as described above. In fact, the three glomeruli shown in Figure 8–1 were all found in the same biopsy specimen from a young woman in whom lupus nephritis had been clinically apparent for less than 1 year. Several years later, during an exacerbation of her renal disease, a repeat renal biopsy showed diffuse proliferative changes in 100% of the glomeruli in the biopsy specimen.

Membranous lupus nephritis, designated WHO Class V, is characterized by diffusely thickened glomerular capillary walls (Fig. 8–2). This histologic pattern, in which endothelial cell proliferation and polymorphonuclear leukocyte infiltration are absent, may represent a different pathophysiologic process from that which results in the proliferative forms of lupus nephritis. Furthermore, immune complexes are identified by immunofluorescence and electron microscopy only in the mesangium and the subepithelial, but not subendothelial, surface of the glomerular basement membrane in true membranous lupus nephritis. With treatment and healing of the proliferative forms of nephritis, the histologic appearance may resemble a membranous lesion, but some cellular proliferation and immune complex deposition generally remain.

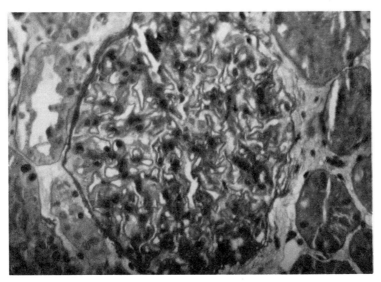

FIGURE 8–2
High-power light microscopic appearance of Class V (membranous) lupus nephritis showing diffuse basement membrane thickening without cellular proliferation or necrosis.

Nonglomerular pathology may also be present in lupus renal disease, generally as tubular fatty change or tubular atrophy in areas adjacent to glomerular abnormalities. Interstitial infiltration with mononuclear cells is generally a mild scattered phenomenon, but dense generalized infiltration may occasionally be the predominant histologic abnormality.

CLINICAL CORRELATIONS AND NATURAL HISTORY OF THE HISTOLOGIC LESIONS OF LUPUS NEPHRITIS

The severity of serologic (hypocomplementemia and anti-dsDNA antibodies) and clinical (active urinary sediment, proteinuria, azotemia, and hypertension) abnormalities in patients with active lupus nephritis generally parallels the severity of histologic change.[6] A random renal biopsy in an SLE patient with no clinical or serologic abnormalities might show Class IIA or IIB lesions: however, this histologic appearance would also be compatible with a few leukocytes or red blood cells in the urinary sediment as well as minimal proteinuria (200 to 500 mg/24 hours). Hypocomplementemia, an active urinary sediment containing cellular casts, and proteinuria of 1 to 2 g/24 hours typically accompany Class III lesions during active disease; a modest increase in serum creatinine to the range of 1.2 to 1.5 is not incompatible. Active Class IV lupus nephritis is characterized by the presence of antibodies to double-stranded DNA and hypocomplementemia, as measured by C3, C4, and CH50, in addition to the frequent findings of red blood cell casts and protein casts in the urine and nephrotic-range proteinuria. The development of azotemia is to be expected in more than 50% of patients with this lesion. Even with treatment and reversal of serologic abnormalities, some degree of persistent proteinuria and azotemia may be observed. Hypertension may be present initially, or it may be the consequence of treatment.

Differing clinically from the proliferative lesions, the hallmark of membranous lupus nephritis is severe proteinuria, which may reach the range of 10 to 15 g/24 hours. Moderate hypocomplementemia is present in up to 50% of patients, but antibodies to ds-DNA are rare, as is significant azotemia, especially early in the disease course. Hypertension is common, and the development of renal vein thrombosis, probably secondary to a general hypercoagulable state, is well described. Massive proteinuria, often accompanied by defects in renal tubular function such as renal tubular acidosis, may also be a marker for severe interstitial nephritis, even in the absence of significant glomerular damage.[7]

In considering the individual patient with lupus nephritis, however, it must be remembered that mean values for subsets of patients are just that; the variation from patient to patient in serologic parameters and degree of proteinuria or azotemia may be large, and a particular combination of clinical and serologic abnormalities may be compatible with more than one type of lesion. Similarly, it must be remembered that not all derangements in renal function can be attributed to active nephritis. Cardiovascular disease may result in hemodynamic changes which diminish glomerular filtration rate. The use of NSAIDs for nonrenal disease manifestations may result in a rising serum creatinine level secondary to an ischemic nephropathy induced by inhibition of prostaglandins or to an active interstitial nephritis without evidence of immune complex deposition.[8]

Just as the severity of clinical disease manifestations is generally directly related to the severity of the histologic lesions, the overall prognosis for preservation of renal function and patient survival is inversely related to the pathologic findings. The natural history of lupus nephritis, that is, a measure of survival and/or a determination of renal function in untreated patients, is difficult to establish. The series reported by Estes and Christian[9] in 1971 does, however, reflect an era before the general use of high-dose corticosteroids and immunosuppressive drugs and a time when dialysis was not generally available. From the first appearance of overt renal disease, 5-year survival was only about 50%, with less than 30% 5-year survival in patients with renal biopsy evidence of diffuse proliferative or membranous nephritis.[9] Other early series observed patients with mesangial and focal lesions on biopsy to have survival rates similar to that of patients without clinical renal disease. Diffuse proliferative nephritis, on the other hand, was associated with survival rates as poor as 47% at 2 years and 29% at 5 years after biopsy.[5] Contrast this with the recent report by Moroni et al.[10] documenting a major improvement in outcome. Of 34 patients with lupus nephritis first seen between 1964 and

1980, six died within 1 to 62 months and three progressed to end-stage renal disease. Among the remaining 25, 18 had diffuse proliferative nephritis on initial renal biopsy; 13 of the 18 had normal renal function, and 15 had <1 g proteinuria/per 24 hours at last observation 11 to 27 years later. Furthermore, the incidence of disease exacerbations fell significantly after the tenth year of follow-up.

There is controversy concerning the natural history of the membranous form of lupus nephritis, especially in the absence of adherence to the strict criteria for its designation, as outlined above. Maintenance of normal renal function and overall survival is generally good in pure membranous disease, even among patients with persistent nephrotic syndrome.[11] In the recent series reported by Pasquali et al.,[12] two of 26 patients with pure Class V disease died of cerebrovascular accidents, two progressed to end-stage renal disease more than 10 years after biopsy, and three others developed renal insufficiency 3.5 to 10.9 years after biopsy. Survival rates to death or end-stage renal disease were 96% at 5 years and 92% at 10 years.[12]

IMMUNOLOGIC PREDICTORS OF DISEASE ACTIVITY

If one accepts the premise that treatment can alter the natural history of lupus renal disease, it becomes increasingly important to identify disease activity at an early stage, before irreversible pathologic changes associated with permanent functional impairment ensue. The notion that immunochemical measures were predictive of disease activity was first proposed by Schur and Sandson[13] in 1968. They found elevated anti-DNA titers in 57% of patients in association with active nephritis. Among 32 patients tested serially, 22 had a 50% or greater fall in serum CH_{50} level; 19 of the 22 subsequently had an exacerbation of nephritis. Other investigators have subsequently noted similar correlations between hypocomplementemia and increased evidence of DNA binding with active renal disease; however, a number of discrepancies between serologic and clinical activity have also been noted. Lightfoot and Hughes[14] followed 16 patients with serial serum samples; in 21 of 28 instances in which anti-DNA antibodies became elevated, the titers remained abnormal until a clinical flare occurred after 60 to 450 days; however,

only 10 instances included an exacerbation of renal disease.[14] In three instances anti-DNA titer reverted to normal spontaneously, and in four it remained abnormal without a clinical flare at the end of the study. Among the same patients, low levels of CH_{50} resolved spontaneously in 16 of 35 instances, most of which occurred in patients with prior renal disease. Gladman et al.[15] also identified 14 patients with persistently low C3 and CH_{50} levels who remained untreated and free of clinical renal manifestations for a mean of 4.25 years.

Since these early studies, many other investigators have attempted with varying degrees of success to correlate specific complement components and both anti-DNA antibodies and circulating immune complexes by various immunochemical techniques with clinical manifestations of active nephritis.[16–20] Several recent long-term prospective studies have been reported. In one, which stressed the predictive value of anti-dsDNA antibodies, measurement by the Farr assay was generally superior to ELISA or *Crithidia luciliae* methods.[21] All renal flares were accompanied by increases in anti-DNA titer, which were frequently characterized by a biphasic pattern, with a gradual increase in antibody level during the first phase followed by a rapid increase a few months to weeks before clinical disease exacerbation. Interestingly, 23% of the renal flares in this series were not accompanied by a fall in C3 or C4 levels.

In 1991 the Lupus Nephritis Collaborative Study Group reported their observations on 12 patients with severe nephritis studied serially over 12 to 77 months through 25 renal and 16 nonrenal relapses.[22] C3 and C4 were measured by both nephelometry and radial immunodiffusion. During remission C3 tended to be normal by both methods, whereas C4 showed no such tendency. Decreases in C3 by both methods predicted relapse with 95% sensitivity and 85% specificity, compared with 56% sensitivity and 54% specificity for C4. This appears to be due to the much broader range of normal of C4, which is characterized by a high prevalence of at least one null allele in normal subjects (up to 40%) as well as in SLE patients (up to 80%).

Discordance between levels of complement components and clinical evidence of active nephritis may be related not only to congenital and acquired complement deficiencies but also to increases in complement components as acute phase reactants. Buyon et al.[23] have suggested that levels of complement split products better reflect disease activity and impending flares than do traditional complement components. They serially measured Ba, Bb, SC5b-9, and C4d in 86 patients, subset initially by clinical status as inactive, moderately active, or severely active (including acute renal disease with rising serum creatinine, cellular sediment, or increasing proteinuria). The mean values of all complement split products were highest in the group with the most severe disease, with an elevated C4d level having the highest degree of sensitivity for an exacerbation within the next 3.5 months, occurring in 86% of such patients, compared with increased Ba or SC5b-9 levels in 73% of the patients with a subsequent flare. Bb, on the other hand, was the most specific for active disease; 81% of patients who did not flare had normal levels, versus 60% for Ba, 67% for SC5b-9, and 69% for C4d. In comparison, fewer than 50% of the patients with low C3, C4, or CH_{50} levels had a subsequent disease flare.

Can a consensus be reached from the disparate results of these numerous studies that will permit a logical approach to management of the individual patient with SLE and either no previous renal disease or established prior clinical nephritis? It appears that no single measure is a reliable predictor of impending or even currently active nephritis. A specific parameter may, however, be consistently associated with disease activity in a given patient, so that a pattern emerges over time. In the newly diagnosed SLE patient, frequent monitoring may increase the likelihood of identifying that pattern of serologic abnormalities. Furthermore, the absolute value of each parameter may be less important than the appearance of changes in level or titer. Practically, technical and financial considerations make C3 and anti-dsDNA the most useful predictors of active nephritis in most patients. Should monitoring of complement split products become more cost-effective, they may replace conventional complement components as the parameters of choice to monitor.

Investigators continue to seek new immunochemical measures that will serve as better predictors of disease activity and distinguish between activity in different organ systems. For example, activated T-lymphocytes produce the cytokine interleukin-2 and are induced to secrete interleukin-2 receptors on their cell surface, which can then be measured as a soluble form in the serum (sIL-2R). sIL-2R has been shown to be elevated in a number of autoimmune conditions, with increased levels in SLE and even higher mean levels during active disease.[24–26] A recent study found that sIL-2R levels were highest among SLE patients with active nephritis and that 9 of 10 patients undergoing a renal flare had a significant increase in sIL-2R, whereas only 6 of 10 had either increased anti-DNA antibodies or decreased CH_{50}, suggesting that sIL-2R may be a more reliable marker than conventional measures.[27]

Similar attempts have been made to identify products of immune activation in the urine of patients with SLE, which would provide a simple and less invasive means of frequent monitoring. Anti-RNA polymerase I antibodies and neopterin have been measured, but neither marker has been shown to distinguish between renal and nonrenal involvement.[28–29]

Whatever immunochemical markers are chosen to monitor disease activity, changes in these levels should signal the clinician that a therapeutic decision is in order. Treating serologic abnormalities in the absence of clinical disease features might prevent serious manifestations, irreversible organ damage or both; on the other hand, it might subject the patient to potentially toxic therapy despite the possibility of spontaneous remission of immunologic activity. My own approach, especially in patients whose disease is newly diagnosed or who had no prior evidence of clinical renal disease, is to increase the frequency of monitoring of clinical parameters such as urinalysis, degree of proteinuria, serum creatinine, and blood pressure, as well as nonrenal features of activity, but not to treat abnormal serologic conditions alone. In patients with well-established disease and a clear pattern of serologic abnormalities preceding clinical manifestations, early treatment may abort subsequent disease activity.

THE ROLE OF RENAL BIOPSY IN MANAGEMENT OF PATIENTS WITH LUPUS NEPHRITIS

Despite the fact that much of our understanding of the natural history of lupus nephritis is based on renal biopsy studies, some investigators have suggested that renal biopsy is an invasive and expensive procedure in which the information regarding glomerular class yields no marginal predictive value regarding outcome beyond that provided by clinical data.[30] Investigators at the National Institutes of Health have proposed, however, that more specific features of glomerular and tubulointerstitial disease reflecting histologic activity and chronicity are both predictive of outcome and beneficial in identifying subsets of patients with lupus nephritis who are most likely to respond to aggressive therapy.[31,32] In a large retrospective study examining demographic and clinical variables as well as renal biopsy activity and chronicity indexes, Nossent et al.[33] found that only a chronicity index greater than 3 predicted renal survival. Although neither Esdaile et al.[34] nor Schwartz et al.[35] were able to show a marginal contribution to the prediction of renal failure when chronicity index scores were added to clinical information, Esdaile et al. have commented that it is necessary to classify patients on the basis of renal severity in order to demonstrate the relationship of disease activity to outcome.[36] The ongoing controversy may be explained by a recent analysis by the Lupus Nephritis Collaborative Study Group, which failed to demonstrate reproducibility of the activity and chronicity indexes by different pathologists, concluding that these measures are too subjective to be used as prognosticators or therapeutic guides.[37]

Considering the foregoing caveats, it remains important to establish guidelines regarding the decision to perform renal biopsy. When immunochemical and clinical parameters clearly indicate active disease and the pattern of abnormalities is consistent with a particular histologic type, it is reasonable to initiate therapy without a biopsy. When the pattern of abnormal results is inconsistent or the possibility of non-lupus-related abnormalities such as diabetes mellitus or NSAID-induced nephropathy is a consideration, renal biopsy is appropriate before a course of therapy is initiated. When clinical features such as advanced azotemia or hypertension suggest the possibility of irreversible disease, review of the pathologic changes may provide the clinician with a rational approach to treatment. Statistical considerations aside, it may not be necessary to compute the actual value of the activity or chronicity index to become more comfortable with the probability of therapeutic response in the individual patient.

CORTICOSTEROID THERAPY FOR LUPUS NEPHRITIS

For more than three decades, the use of corticosteroids has been accepted as appropriate initial therapy for active lupus nephritis. Pollak et al.[38] showed that prednisone in a dose of 15 to 20 mg/day did not alter survival in patients with nephritis, but when high-dose oral prednisone (60 to 100 mg/day) was given for 6 months in an uncontrolled trial, greater survival and reduction in azotemia were observed. Other anecdotal reports supporting this finding followed.[1,39-40] In fact, these early observations have rendered the conducting of randomized placebo-controlled clinical trials of corticosteroids as essentially unethical. Recognizing the significant short- and long-term morbidity attributed to high-dose oral steroids, including cushingoid features, hyperglycemia or frank diabetes, myopathy, hypertension, an increase in pyogenic and opportunistic infections, and avascular necrosis, investigators have sought to devise steroid regimens that minimize toxicity. Ackerman.[41] reported improvement in renal function in five of seven patients with lupus nephritis treated with 100 to 120 mg of prednisone every other day. Cushingoid changes were avoided, and stabilization of renal function was maintained with subsequent tapering of the steroid dose. In my experience, an alternate-day steroid regimen is rarely successful in suppressing constitutional symptoms, azotemia, or proteinuria associated with active disease but may minimize toxicity as a maintenance regimen in steroid-dependent patients whose disease flares with tapering of medication.

A regimen of intravenous pulse methylprednisolone (1 g/day for 3 consecutive days) for severe lupus nephritis was first advocated in 1976 by Cathcart et al.,[42] who hypothesized that this extremely high dose of steroids would rapidly reverse the pathologic findings of inflammation and clinical deterioration in renal function, allowing for subsequent treatment with steroids in a dose necessary only to control extrarenal disease manifestations. Indeed, in five of seven patients so treated renal function returned to baseline within 1 month, and all patients demonstrated reversal of immunologic abnormalities. Subsequent larger uncontrolled series with longer follow-up have confirmed an initial response to pulse methylprednisolone therapy in about 50% of instances, with responders being characterized by more recent deterioration in renal function and more profound abnormalities of immunochemical measures.[43,44] Even among patients with an initial response, however, improvement was neither complete nor sustained in most.[44] A quasirandomized unblinded study of pulse methylprednisolone compared with high-dose prednisone in pediatric patients with diffuse nephritis concluded that long-term effects on renal function were similar in both groups, although there was more rapid improvement in glomerular filtration rate (GFR) with pulse therapy.[45] One small double-blind controlled study examined the efficacy of 1 year of monthly pulse methylprednisolone compared with placebo.[46] The five patients in the treatment group showed a significant improvement in serum creatinine levels, whereas the four patients in the placebo group did not. After an additional 2 years of follow-up, renal function remained stable in the treatment group but deteriorated further in the placebo group.

There is no doubt that pulse methylprednisolone therapy is useful for initial treatment of acute lupus nephritis, especially in the presence of recent deterioration in renal function. It is unlikely, however, that this regimen can be successfully followed immediately by treatment with zero- or low-dose prednisone. It is generally necessary to continue conventional high-dose steroids for at least several weeks, as well as to consider addition of another immunosuppressive agent as a maintenance regimen. Furthermore, it is essential that attention be paid to preexisting hypertension and edema, as a single course of pulse methylprednisolone may result in marked salt and fluid retention.

IMMUNOSUPPRESSIVE AGENTS IN THE TREATMENT OF LUPUS NEPHRITIS

Immunosuppressive agents other than corticosteroids have for many years been added to the therapeutic regimen of patients with lupus nephritis in order to reverse acute clinical and immunologic abnormalities and to maintain remission. In considering the efficacy of these agents, it is important to keep in mind that these two goals are different and that various drugs may be appropriate for one or both goals. In several early uncontrolled studies, azathioprine, a purine analog, appeared to be associated with improvement in azotemia and proteinuria in 50% to 100% of patients with severe lupus nephritis.[47–50] Among the series of 47 azathioprine-treated patients with diffuse proliferative and membranous nephritis reported by Barnett et al.,[50] survival was 82% at 5 years and 74% at 10 years. In a prospective randomized trial that included 35 patients, Sztejnbok et al.[51] observed decreased mortality and morbidity, lower steroid requirements, and better maintenance of renal function after 1 to 4 years among azathioprine-treated patients.[51] These findings were confirmed at the same institution in a larger, uncontrolled retrospective comparison study.[52] Survival was not improved in the azathioprine group during the first 6 months of therapy; however a subsequent survival benefit and steroid sparing were observed. Other studies failed to show a survival benefit with azathioprine; this included two controlled trials of 2 and 3 years' duration in 24 and 16 patients, respectively.[53,54]

As with azathioprine, early experience with the nitrogen mustard derivative cyclophosphamide in patients with SLE began in the 1960s and 1970s. Feng et al.[55] treated 42 patients, 31 of whom had evidence of nephritis, with oral cyclophosphamide for periods of 6 months to 7 years.[55] Responses ranged from sustained clinical remission in 16 patients to death in five, along with the common toxicity of amenorrhea and infection. Donadio et al.[56] reported the results of a controlled trial of oral cyclophosphamide plus prednisone compared with prednisone alone, in which no difference in outcome was seen between the two groups at the end of 6 months, with improvement in 84% of the patients.[56] During a 4-year follow-up, recurrent nephritis occurred more often in the group treated with prednisone only; however, survival and the prevalence of stable or improved renal function were similar in both groups.[57] In a series of reports from the National Institutes of Health with increasingly longer duration of follow-up, in which patients with diffuse proliferative or membranous nephritis were randomized to receive prednisone alone or low-dose prednisone in combination with oral cyclophosphamide or azathioprine, no substantial benefit with either immunosuppressive agent was noted with regard to patient survival or renal function.[58–60]

In addition to the obvious problems with drawing conclusions from anecdotal series, most of the controlled trials of immunosuppressive therapy for lupus nephritis conducted in the 1970s and early 1980s suffered from methodologic difficulties, including small numbers of patients, noncomparable groups, and short follow-up. Potential trends in the direction of a positive association with a treatment regimen

were likely to be missed. Felson and Anderson[61] performed a meta-analysis of all published randomized trials comparing prednisone alone with prednisone plus azathioprine or cyclophosphamide (Table 8–1). They found that patients who received an immunosuppressive drug had significantly less renal deterioration or progression to end-stage renal disease and were significantly less likely to die of renal disease. Overall mortality and deaths from nonrenal causes were not different in the two groups.

To avoid hemorrhagic cystitis in patients receiving cyclophosphamide, the National Insti-

TABLE 8–1

Results of Pooled Analysis Comparing Immunosuppressive Therapy Plus Steroids With Steroids Alone in the Treatment of Lupus Nephritis*

| | NO OF PATIENTS | | OUTCOME RATE (λ) | | |
	STEROIDS ALONE	COMBINED THERAPY	STEROIDS ALONE	COMBINED THERAPY	P VALUE
All Studies	113	137			
Renal deterioration	37	27	0.0096	0.0048	0.006
ESRD	24	16	0.0058	0.0028	0.023
Nephritis-related death	19	12	0.0049	0.0022	0.024
All deaths	32	29	0.0083	0.0052	0.066
Studies Using CYCLO	60	59			
Renal deterioration	18	11	0.0070	0.0043	0.190
ESRD	10	7	0.0035	0.0027	0.561
Nephritis-related death	5	4	0.0019	0.0015	0.739
All deaths	11	12	0.0043	0.0047	0.835
Studies Using AZA	68	62			
Renal deterioration	27	15	0.0115	0.0061	0.047
ESRD	18	9	0.0068	0.0036	0.102
Nephritis-related death	15	8	0.0062	0.0033	0.135
All deaths	26	16	0.0111	0.0068	0.095
Patients With DPGN	72	91			
Renal deterioration	28	19	0.0097	0.0045	0.008
ESRD	19	10	0.0060	0.0023	0.012
Nephritis-related death	14	7	0.0048	0.0016	0.017
All deaths	21	21	0.0073	0.0050	0.207
Patients Without DPGN on Biopsy	9	14			
Renal deterioration	3	3	0.0079	0.0040	0.416
ESRD	1	2	0.0026	0.0026	0.986
Nephritis-related death	1	1	0.0026	0.0013	0.642
All deaths	2	2	0.0052	0.0027	0.506

*ESRD denotes end-stage renal disease; CYCLO, cyclophosphamide; AZA, azathioprine; and DPGN, diffuse proliferative glomerulonephritis.

From Felson DT, Anderson J. Evidence for the superiority of immunosuppressive drugs and prednisone over prednisone alone in lupus nephritis: results of a pooled analysis. N Engl J Med 1984;311:1528. Reprinted by permission of the *New England Journal of Medicine*.

tutes of Health added to the randomized trial of lupus nephritis a group of patients receiving intravenous cyclophosphamide, given monthly in incremental doses (0.5 to 1.0 g/m³ body surface area) for three successive doses, followed by a maintenance dose every 3 months.[59] Toxicity in the early phases of the study was minimal; however, this regimen had no clear therapeutic advantage over prednisone alone or in combination with oral immunosuppressive agents. Improved preservation of renal function associated with intravenous cyclophosphamide plus low-dose prednisone, in comparison with high-dose prednisone alone, became apparent only after 5 years of follow-up.[62] The most recent report from this randomized study, in which the duration of follow-up extended beyond 15

years for some patients, indicated better preservation of renal function for all patient groups receiving cyclophosphamide, with the most significant benefit in the intravenous cyclophosphamide group (Fig. 8–3).[63] Although the original intention of the investigators was to continue the study protocol indefinitely, study drugs were terminated if clinical remission was sustained for at least 18 months. In all treatment groups, progression to renal failure was significantly more frequent among patients with a high chronicity score on renal biopsy.

More prolonged monthly therapy with intravenous cyclophosphamide has been used by various investigators, including an uncontrolled series of 16 pediatric patients who were treated with 6 monthly pulses followed by maintenance

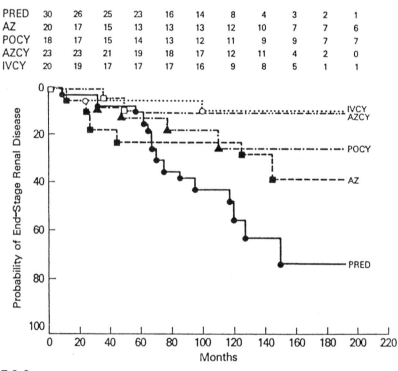

FIGURE 8–3

Probability of progression to end-stage renal disease in the study population by treatment group (prednisone only [PRED]; azathioprine [AZ]; oral cyclophosphamide [POCY]; oral azathioprine plus oral cyclophosphamide [AZCY]; and intravenous cyclophosphamide [IVCY]). Survival curves are shown, with end-stage renal disease as the outcome. The number of patients at risk in each group is shown for each 20-month time point. The curves for the AZCY, IVCY, and POCY groups were significantly different from that of the control (PRED) group ($P = 0.0011$, $P = 0.0025$, and $P = 0.032$, respectively). The AZ group did not differ significantly from the PRED group ($P = 0.09$). The Mantel statistic from which the P values (versus PRED) were obtained were AZ 2.872, POCY 4.619, AZCY 10.571, and IVCY 9.169. The 95% confidence intervals at the 120-month (10-year) point were as follows: PRED 0.67–0.23, AZ 0.93–0.49, POCY 0.97–0.53, AZCY 1.00–0.78, and IVCY 1.00–0.74. (From Steinberg AD, Steinberg SC. Long-term preservation of renal function in patients with lupus nephritis receiving treatment that includes cyclophosphamide versus those treated with prednisone only. Arthritis Rheum 1991;34:945.)

pulses every 3 months.[64] All were placed on this regimen because of steroid-unresponsive or steroid-dependent manifestations of nephritis, including renal insufficiency or nephrotic syndrome. All but one of the eight children with initial azotemia had substantial improvement in creatinine clearance within 6 months.

The toxic effects of intravenous cyclophosphamide are numerous and vary widely in frequency. Nausea during administration and occasionally lasting several days thereafter may limit patients' willingness to continue therapy. Pretreatment with antiemetics is essential. Another less common gastrointestinal side effect is diarrhea. Hyponatremia with seizures secondary to vigorous hydration has been reported[64] as an acute side effect. Both short- and long-term therapy may be associated with bone marrow suppression and an increased risk of infection and activation of herpes zoster. As the cumulative dose of cyclophosphamide increases with time, the development of subtle or obvious alopecia is noted. Similarly, the risk of secondary amenorrhea is increased, related not only to the number of doses of cyclophosphamide received but also to the age of the patient at initiation of therapy.[65] Hemorrhagic cystitis may occur, even with hydration, and bladder cancer has been reported.[66] The increased risk of lymphoproliferative malignancies that has been documented with prolonged oral cyclophosphamide therapy has so far not been reported with the intravenous regimen.

GOALS IN THE MONITORING OF THERAPEUTIC EFFICACY

If one accepts the conclusions of the studies described above that initial treatment of active nephritis with corticosteroids is indicated, supplemented in some patients with an immunosuppressive agent, it is still necessary to outline a plan for decision making with regard to the appropriate regimen and for monitoring of the immunologic and clinical response. As stated previously, my approach is not to treat immunochemical abnormalities in the absence of clinical manifestations unless a pattern of exacerbations after changes in serologic findings has already been established in a given patient. I also believe that therapy must be tailored to the individual, taking into account the patient's lifestyle and personal wishes. Treatment for

proteinuria or active urinary sediment, in the absence of the nephrotic syndrome, azotemia, or serious nonrenal manifestations, can usually be managed with prednisone in moderate doses (40 to 60 mg/day) and renal biopsy is not essential. Serologic and clinical parameters should be monitored weekly to biweekly, with upward adjustments in steroid dose if significant worsening of clinical markers ensues. If azotemia or the nephrotic syndrome is present, I prefer to have a renal biopsy before deciding on a supplemental immunosuppressive regimen for acute therapy; however I am comfortable with institution of intravenous pulse methylprednisolone for deteriorating renal function, even should a biopsy be contraindicated or the patient refuse it. In the absence of biopsy documentation of Class IV nephritis with histologic evidence of active lesions, I am likely to err on the side of aggressive treatment (i.e., institution of intravenous cyclophosphamide).

One should expect renal function and proteinuria to improve within 1 to 2 weeks after the institution of therapy, whereas improvement in hypocomplementemia (especially C3) and anti-DNA titers may lag behind by several weeks.[67] Tapering of prednisone may begin when a therapeutic response is sustained and clinical parameters have stabilized for at least 2 weeks, unless significant toxicity (hyperglycemia, intractable edema or hypertension, steroid psychosis) requires more urgent reduction in dose. It is important to be aware that a partial response may occur, with either improvement in immunochemical parameters but failure to reverse azotemia or proteinuria or improvement in clinical markers with persistent serologic abnormalities. The goal of normalization of serum complement levels is laudatory but not always possible. Laitman et al.[68] recently reported the results of an ongoing study of 39 patients with lupus nephritis in whom an attempt was made to maintain normal CH_{50} levels with prednisone and the addition of azathioprine in nonresponders. Twenty-five patients achieved normal CH_{50} levels within 6 months, and immunosuppressive therapy was then tapered but continuously readjusted to the lowest dose that preserved normal CH_{50} and maintained clinical remission. Seventeen patients had continuous control of CH_{50}, eight of the 25 responders became persistently hypocomplementemic, and 14 failed to achieve normal CH_{50} within the first 6 months; these 14 were subsequently treated on the basis of clinical considerations only. No differences were observed in clinical or histologic features during the first 6 months in complement-controlled versus complement-uncontrolled patients. After a mean 10-year follow-up, however, patients in the normal CH_{50} group had significantly better renal function, less diastolic hypertension, and better overall survival than either group of complement-uncontrolled patients.

I favor institution of intravenous cyclophosphamide for patients with documented Class IV nephritis and active lesions, as well as for patients with azotemia and/or membranous nephropathy with steroid-resistant nephrotic syndrome. In general, my approach is to continue monthly intravenous administration of cyclophosphamide for 6 months, followed by maintenance doses every 3 months. I follow serologic parameters and renal function at least monthly, especially just after beginning the maintenance schedule. Should there be a deterioration in either laboratory or clinical status, I decrease the interval between doses to 6 to 8 weeks, until a stable status is maintained. Unless significant toxicity develops, I usually continue maintenance intravenous cyclophosphamide during at least 1 year of sustained remission, and 2 years if the patient has developed azotemia during a prior exacerbation.

Cyclophosphamide is excreted almost completely by the kidneys as an active metabolite, so that impaired renal function results in a prolonged half-life and a potential for increased bone marrow suppression. In mild renal insufficiency (GFR < 50 ml/min), no reduction in dose is generally necessary, whereas reductions to 75% of the usual dose for moderate renal insufficiency (GFR 50 to 10 ml/min) and 50% for severe renal insufficiency (GFR < 10 ml/min) are recommended.[69]

I find azathioprine to be especially useful as a steroid-sparing agent in patients whose disease, although nonazotemic and nonnephrotic, flares with tapering or in whom exacerbations are frequent. It is also appropriate to treat patients with azathioprine when they are no longer willing to tolerate the side effects of cyclophosphamide or to use it initially in young patients who wish to preserve ovarian function.

When conventional therapy fails and life-threatening disease manifestations are present, the use of new, experimental therapies is warranted but only if the patient understands the potential for toxicity and the possible lack of efficacy. With the ready availability of chronic dialysis, withdrawal of steroids, immunosuppressive agents, or both may also be appropriate, allowing for progression to end-stage renal disease. This option may preserve patient survival at the expense of renal function.

UNPROVEN, ANECDOTAL, AND EXPERIMENTAL THERAPIES

There are several reasons to consider therapies other than those outlined above, the most obvious of which is that a substantial proportion of patients fail to respond completely and progression to end-stage renal disease continues to occur. In addition, therapeutic manipulations based on pathophysiologic mechanisms other than glomerular immune complex deposition have been proposed. Plasmapheresis, designed to remove antigen-antibody complexes from the circulation, was advocated in the late 1970s in patients with severe nephritis, especially when unresponsive to steroids. Verrier Jones[70] treated eight patients in whom he demonstrated a fall in circulating immune complexes and anti-DNA titers. In five patients, cessation of plasmapheresis was followed by a rapid rebound in immune complexes and antibody to pretreatment levels. Subsequently, in anecdotal reports, several investigators have suggested synchronization of plasmapheresis with pulse cyclophosphamide in order to take advantage of the plasmapheresis-induced proliferation of pathogenetic clones, with subsequent clonal deletion by large doses of cytotoxic drugs during a period of increased B-cell vulnerability.[71,72] Even before the results of a large-scale controlled trial in 86 patients by the Lupus Nephritis Collaborative Study Group were reported, the initial enthusiasm for this therapeutic modality was dampened because of its invasive nature and considerable cost. It has now been shown that treatment with plasmapheresis plus a standard regimen of prednisone and cyclophosphamide does not result in more significant clinical improvement of severe lupus nephritis than the standard regimen alone.[73]

High-dose intravenous immunoglobulins have been used to treat SLE patients with drug-resistant, life-threatening disease manifestations, especially profound thrombocytopenia. Lin et al.[74] reported the use of this aggressive therapeutic modality in nine patients who had lupus nephritis with azotemia and nephrotic syndrome unresponsive to methylprednisolone pulse therapy and cyclophosphamide. All were treated with 400 mg/kg body weight human gamma globulin for 5 consecutive days.[74] Creatinine clearance, proteinuria, and anti-DNA titers improved in all nine patients, and in all seven who had a second renal biopsy 2 months after the course of treatment there was a dramatic decrease in intensity of immune complex deposition. Two subsequent anecdotal reports describe an additional three patients with severe unresponsive lupus nephritis whose condition improved with intravenous immunoglobulin; one of these patients had a prolonged remission in association with monthly therapy over 20 months.[75,76]

Cyclosporin A, a fungal polypeptide with immunosuppressive activity, has become the most common agent used to suppress rejection of renal transplants. It has also been used with varying efficacy in the treatment of patients with active lupus. Isenberg et al.[77] treated five patients at a dose of 10 mg/kg/day; no patient was able to tolerate more than 7 weeks of therapy because of side effects, including nephrotoxity and angioedema. Feutron et al.,[78] on the other hand, had better success in 13 pediatric patients with steroid-resistant disease treated for a mean period of 12 months with an average of 5 mg/kg/day.[78] Eight patients were able to taper their steroid dose on the basis of clinical symptoms, although serologic measures did not improve. Nephrotoxicity was reversible with lowering of the dose; however, elevated blood pressure required control with antihypertensive medications in eight patients. In the largest uncontrolled study reported to date, Favre et al.[79] treated 26 patients with unresponsive lupus nephritis by continuing steroids and replacing the immunosuppressive drug with cyclosporin in an average dose of 5 mg/kg/day.[79] Results were generally favorable, with improvement in global disease activity and decrease in proteinuria in all patients. Nephrotic-range proteinuria, originally present in 19 patients, was reduced below 1 g/24 hours at 9 months in all 19. Serum creatinine levels increased somewhat during the first 6 months of therapy and then returned to baseline or better. Despite this promising anecdotal experience, clinicians appear reluctant to enter patients in a randomized double-blind trial of cyclosporin, given its potential nephrotoxicity.

Achieving immunosuppression via total lymphoid irradiation had been suggested as an alternative to cytotoxic therapy. The largest series, which was not randomized, was reported by Strober et al.,[80] who treated 15 SLE patients who had diffuse nephritis that was unresponsive to steroids and azathioprine, as well as a high chronicity index on renal biopsy, with a total dose of 2000 rad over a 4- to 6-week period. There was significant improvement in serum creatinine level, urinary protein excretion, and anti-DNA antibody titer, with a significant reduction in the mean prednisone requirement. With posttreatment follow-up as long as 6 years, 13 of the 15 patients remained alive with stable renal function. One died of a nonrenal cause at 13 months, and one progressed to renal failure at 24 months. Infection was the most common complication in this series; its potential catastrophic nature was stressed in another anecdotal report on two patients who received total lymphoid irradiation without clinical benefit.[81]

Immunosuppressive therapy has been directed at reversing the abnormal immunologic events that lead to inflammation and secondary tissue injury and dysfunction. Treatment designed to prevent the inflammatory process with the use of dietary supplementation with fish oil, which contains naturally occurring marine lipids rich in the n-3 fatty acids eicosapentaenoic acid and docosahexaenoic acid, has been suggested. These substances substitute for arachidonic acid in the cyclooxygenase and lipoxygenase pathways and have been shown to retard the development of nephritis in murine models of SLE. Results from preliminary trials in human beings have been inconsistent.[82,83] Clark et al.[84] recently completed a 1-year double-blind crossover study of dietary fish oil supplementation in 21 patients with stable lupus nephritis.[84] They found no improvement in renal function or reduction in disease activity, as reflected by C3, C4, and anti-dsDNA antibody levels. Serum very low density lipoprotein cholesterol was markedly decreased. It may not be unexpected that preexisting renal disease does not reverse or that immunochemical measures of disease activity are unaffected. As fish oil suppresses the inflammatory response elicited by immune complex deposition, it may merely prevent tissue damage without changing the underlying immunologic dysfunction. Its usefulness, therefore, might be in preventing further damage, rather than reversing existing abnormalities. It is likely that a much larger series of patients, treated for a significantly longer period of time, would be required to show a benefit of this generally inexpensive and nontoxic intervention.

Conventional immunosuppressive therapy has general effects on the immune system. One anecdotal report employing the concept of specific immunotherapy documented the use of anti-CD4 monoclonal antibody in a man with steroid and immunosuppressive refractory SLE, including azotemia and nephrosis.[85] Clinical improvement lasted for 1 month. The number of CD4 cells fell by 50% within 1 day and remained decreased for a month. In vitro studies showed that production of anti-DNA antibodies by the patient's cultured peripheral blood mononuclear cells was significantly inhibited after treatment.

A number of other potential therapeutic modalities have been based upon nonimmunologic pathophysiologic mechanisms. In 1973 Kincaid-Smith[86] suggested that obliteration of glomerular capillaries in lupus nephritis might result not only from immunoglobulin deposition but also from fibrin, which has been identified by immunofluorescence in renal biopsy specimens. Several uncontrolled series subsequently reported clinical improvement in manifestations of nephritis in patients treated with intravenous heparin.[87,88] Reversal of glomerular thrombosis with the defibrinating agent ancrod, the venom of the Malayan pit viper, has recently been described in a series of 22 SLE patients, most with deteriorating renal function. Long-term follow-up (mean 58 months) noted three nonrenal deaths, progression to end-stage renal disease in 11 patients a mean of 27 months after therapy, and stabilization of renal function in eight patients.[89] With increasing attention to the antiphospholipid syndrome and its associated thrombotic manifestations, interest may be renewed in the use of anticoagulation as a treatment for SLE patients, such as those described in a recent report with the insidious development of renal insufficiency in the presence of anticardiolipin antibodies or the lupus circulating anticoagulant.[90]

The clinical manifestations of renal disease in SLE may be mediated in part by hemodynamic mechanisms, as suggested by recent beneficial results of treatment with thromboxane antagonists in a small randomized double-blind crossover study[91] and by the improvement observed in eight patients treated with intravenous prostaglandin E1 therapy.[92]

THE RELATIONSHIP OF HYPERTENSION TO OUTCOME

In addition to modalities designed to treat active manifestations of lupus renal disease, it is now well accepted that other conservative measures may protect renal function, decrease patient morbidity, and prolong survival. Attention to the maintenance of normal blood pressure is probably the most important of these measures. Budman and Steinberg[93] demonstrated the independence of hypertension and active nephritis with their observations in 36 patients that hypertension was not correlated with the degree of proteinuria, hematuria, serum complement, urinary casts, or biopsy findings of necrosis or interstitial inflammation. Studies in several large lupus cohorts have documented that hypertension early in the course of disease is an important predictor of mortality. Reveille et al.[94] found that both systolic and diastolic hypertension present within 6 months of SLE diagnosis were associated with decreased survival. Seleznick and Fries[95] similarly identified systolic hypertension as the only significant risk factor for mortality, when statistical corrections were made for the multiple variables they studied. Ward and Studenski[96] recently showed the association between diastolic hypertension at the onset of nephritis with the development of end-stage renal disease. Among the 41 of 160 patients who progressed to renal failure, the median times were >273 months, 146 months, and only 7 months among patients with normal blood pressure, mild hypertension, and severe hypertension, respectively.[96] Ginzler et al.[97] recently reported a long-term retrospective study in a cohort of 685 patients, which was designed to examine the continuous effect of hypertension at any time in the course of the disease on subsequent renal deterioration, end-stage renal disease, and mortality. They found that, independent of measures of active nephritis, hypertension is a potent risk factor for adverse renal outcomes, as well as for death from any cause.[97]

MANAGEMENT OF END-STAGE RENAL DISEASE

Some patients may have renal failure as a consequence of unresponsive active nephritis, even with the many therapeutic modalities currently available. Others, however, may slowly progress to end-stage renal disease in the absence of immunochemical measures of disease activity, presumably secondary to irreversible renal damage leading to a combination of progressive glomerulosclerosis, vascular disease, interstitial fibrosis, and/or tubular atrophy.[98] It is important to recognize this subset of patients, so that they are not put at increased risk of toxic manifestations of immunosuppressive therapy, such as infection, in a futile attempt to reverse azotemia. The most critical period with regard to morbidity and mortality appears to be the first several months on dialysis, especially for patients who have progressed to renal failure during an acute episode of SLE and who continue to have disease manifestations. As remission is achieved, maintenance dialysis may continue to be complicated by an increased incidence of infection, compared with that in patients with other causes of renal failure.[99] Furthermore, although it is true that the frequency and severity of extrarenal disease manifestations decrease with end-stage renal disease, SLE exacerbations do occur and should be treated accordingly. Occasionally, in fact, patients receiving long-term maintenance dialysis will develop new organ system manifestations that were not present before the onset of renal failure.

An initial reluctance to perform renal transplantation in patients with SLE appears to have been overcome. Numerous centers have reported their experience with both live donor and cadaver transplants,[100-103] with general agreement that the risk of recurrent disease in the transplanted kidney is low. In the series of 16 transplants in 14 patients reported by Goss et al.[100] overall survival was 95% after a mean follow-up of 44 months, and the mean serum creatinine level was 1.4 mg/dl. Goss et al. found that graft survival was similar in patients undergoing short- or long-term dialysis before transplant and suggested that the development of recurrent nephritis in the transplanted kidney may be related to the presence of antinuclear antibodies and anti-DNA antibodies both before and after transplant (Table 8–2). It is important, therefore, to continue frequent monitoring of the serologic as well as the clinical status of pa-

TABLE 8–2
Predictors of Renal Allograft Survival in Patients With Systemic Lupus Erythematosus

	GRAFT SURVIVAL	GRAFT FAILURE
Transplants, *n*	10	6
Mean duration of dialysis pretransplant, *mo*	27.9	47.8
Mean duration of graft survival, *mo*	43.6	9.2
Mean serum creatinine at last follow-up or at graft failure, *mg/dl*	1.4	Data not given
Pretreatment serologies		
Patients positive for ANAs, *n*	2	2
Patients positive for anti-DNA, *n*	2	1
Patients with hypocomplementemia, *n*	1	0
Posttreatment serologies		
Patients positive for ANAs, *n*	4	2
Patients positive for anti-DNA, *n*	1	1
Patients with hypocomplementemia, *n*	1	0

ANAs—antinuclear antibodies.
From Ginzler EM, Antoniadis I. Clinical manifestations of systemic lupus erythematosus, measures of disease activity and long-term complications. Cur Opinion Rheumatol 1992;4:672.
Based on data from Goss JA, Cole BR, Jendrisak MD, et al. Renal transplantation for systemic lupus erythematosus and recurrent lupus nephritis: a single center experience and a review of the literature. Transplantation 1991;52:805.

tients who have received renal transplants. Although it may be difficult at times to distinguish between mild transplant rejection and recurrent nephritis, treatment with increased doses of immunosuppression (steroids and/or other immunosuppressive drugs) should have a beneficial effect on either and may prevent loss of the transplanted kidney.

REFERENCES

1. Baldwin DS, Lowenstein J, Rothfield NF, et al. The clinical course of the proliferative and membranous forms of lupus nephritis. Ann Intern Med 1970;73:929.
2. McCluskey RT. Lupus nephritis. In: Sommers SC, ed. Kidney pathology decennial 1966–1975. New York: Appleton-Century-Crofts, 1975:437.
3. Ginzler EM, Nicastri AD, Chen C-K, et al. Progression of mesangial and focal to diffuse lupus nephritis. N Engl J Med 1975;291:693.
4. Zimmerman SW, Jenkins PG, Shelp WD, et al. Progression from minimal or focal to diffuse proliferative lupus nephritis. Lab Invest 1975;32:665.
5. Baldwin DS, Gluck MC, Lowenstein J, et al. Lupus nephritis: clinical course as related to morphologic forms and their transitions. Am J Med 1977;62:12.
6. Appel GB, Silva FG, Pirani CL, et al. Renal involvement in systemic lupus erythematosus (SLE): a study of 56 patients emphasizing histologic classification. Medicine 1978;57:371.
7. Brentjens JR, Sepulveda M, Baliah T, et al. Interstitial immune complex nephritis in patients with systemic lupus erythematosus. Kidney Int 1975;7:342.
8. Ling BN, Bourke E, Campbell WG Jr, et al. Naproxen-induced nephropathy in systemic lupus erythematosus. Nephron 1990;54:249.
9. Estes D, Christian CL. The natural history of systemic lupus erythematosus by prospective analysis. Medicine 1971;50:85.
10. Moroni G, Banfi G, Ponticelli C. Clinical status of patients after 10 years of lupus nephritis. Q J Med 1992;84:681.
11. Donadio JV Jr, Burgess JH, Holley KE. Membranous lupus nephropathy: a clinicopathologic study. Medicine 1977;56:527.
12. Pasquali S, Banfi G, Zucchelli A, et al. Lupus membranous nephropathy: long-term outcome. Clin Nephrol 1993;39:173.
13. Schur P, Sandson J. Immunologic factors and clinical activity in SLE. N Engl J Med 1968;278:533.
14. Lightfoot RW, Hughes GRV. Significance of persisting serologic abnormalities in SLE. Arthritis Rheum 1976;19:837.
15. Gladman DD, Urowitz MB, Keystone EC. Serologically active clinically quiescent systemic lupus erythematosus: a discordance between clinical and serologic features. Am J Med 1979;66:210.
16. Bardana EJ Jr, Harbeck FJ, Hoffman AA, et al. The prognostic and therapeutic implications of DNA:anti-DNA immune complexes in systemic lupus erythematosus (SLE). Am J Med 1975;59:515.
17. Harkiss GD, Hazleman BL, Brown DL. A longitudinal study of circulating immune complexes, DNA antibodies and complement in patients with systemic lupus erythematosus: an analysis of their relationship to disease activity. J J Lab Clin Med 1979;2:275.
18. Abrass CK, Nies KM, Louie JS, et al. Correlation and predictive accuracy of circulating immune complexes with disease activity in patients with systemic lupus erythematosus. Arthritis Rheum 1980;23:273.
19. Swaak AJG, Groenwold J, Aarden LA, et al. Prognostic value of anti-dsDNA in SLE. Ann Rheum Dis 1982;41:388.
20. Valentijn RM, van Overhagen H, Hazevoet HM, et al. The value of complement and immune complex determinations in monitoring disease activity in patients with systemic lupus erythematosus. Arthritis Rheum 1985;28:904.
21. ter Borg EJ, Horst G, Hummel EJ, et al. Measurement of increases in anti-double stranded DNA antibody levels as a predictor of disease exacerbations in systemic lupus erythematosus: a long-term prospective study. Arthritis Rheum 1990;33:634.
22. Ricker DM, Hebert LA, Rohde R, et al. Serum C3 levels are diagnostically more sensitive and specific for systemic lupus erythematosus activity than are serum C4 levels. Am J Kidney Dis 1991;18:678.
23. Buyon JP, Tamerius J., Belmont HM, et al. Assessment of disease activity and impending flare in patients with systemic lupus erythematosus: comparison of the use of complement split products and conventional measurements of complement. Arthritis Rheum 1992;35:1028.
24. Campen DH, Horwitz DA, Quismorio FP, et al. Serum levels of interleukin-2 receptor and activity of rheumatic diseases characterized by immune system activation. Arthritis Rheum 1988;31:1358.
25. Ward MM, Dooley MA, Christenson VD, et al. The relationship between soluble interleukin 2 receptor levels and antidouble stranded DNA antibody levels in patients with systemic lupus erythematosus. J Rheumatol 1991;18:235.
26. Wong KL, Wong RPO. Serum soluble interleukin 2 receptor in systemic lupus erythematosus: effects of disease activity and infection. Ann Rheum Dis 1991;50:706.
27. Laut J, Senitzer D, Petrucci R, et al. Soluble interleukin-2 receptor levels in lupus nephritis. Clin Nephrol 1992;35:179.
28. Picking WL, Smith C, Petrucci R, et al. Anti-RNA polymerase I antibodies in the urine of

patients with systemic lupus erythematosus. J Rheumatol 1990;17:1308.

29. Lim KL, Jones AC, Brown NS, et al. Urine neopterin as a parameter of disease activity in patients with systemic lupus erythematosus: comparisons with serum sIL-2R and antibodies to dsDNA, erythrocyte sedimentation rate, and plasma C3, C4, and C3 degradation products. Ann Rheum Dis 1993;52:429.

30. Fries JF, Porta J, Liang MH. Marginal benefit of renal biopsy in systemic lupus erythematosus. Arch Intern Med 1978;138:1386.

31. Austin HA III, Muenz LR, Joyce KM, et al. Prognostic factors in lupus nephritis: contribution of renal histologic data. Am J Med 1983;75:382.

32. Austin HA III, Muenz LR, Joyce KM, et al. Diffuse proliferative lupus nephritis: identification of specific pathologic features effecting renal outcome. Kidney Int 1984;25:689.

33. Nossent HC, Henzen-Logmans SC, Vroom TM, et al. Contribution of renal biopsy data in predicting outcome in lupus nephritis: analysis of 116 patients. Arthritis Rheum 1990;33:970.

34. Esdaile JM, Levinton C. Federgreen W, et al. The clinical and renal biopsy predictors of long-term outcome in lupus nephritis: a study of 87 patients and review of the literature. Q J Med 1989;72:779.

35. Schwartz MM, Bernstein J, Hill GS, et al. Predictive value or renal pathology in diffuse proliferative lupus glomerulonephritis. Lupus Collaborative Study Group. Kidney Int 1989;35:891.

36. Goulet J-R, Mackenzie T, Levinton C, et al. The long-term prognosis of lupus nephritis: the impact of disease activity. J Rheumatol 1993;20:59.

37. Schwartz MM, Lan S-P, Bernstein J, et al. Irreproducibility of the activity and chronicity indices limits their utility in the management of lupus nephritis. Am J Kidney Dis 1993;21:374.

38. Pollak VE, Pirani CL, Schwartz FD. The natural history of the renal manifestations of systemic lupus erythematosus. J Lab Clin Med 1964;63:537.

39. Mackay IR, Chan D, Robson G. Prednisolone treatment of lupus nephritis: effect of high doses on course of disease, renal function, histological lesions, and immunological reactions. Aust Ann Med 1970;2:123.

40. Boelaert J, Morel-Maroger L, Mery J-P. Renal insufficiency in lupus nephritis. Adv Nephrol 1974;4:249.

41. Ackerman GL. Alternate-day steroid therapy in lupus nephritis. Ann Intern Med 1970;72:511.

42. Cathcart ES, Idelson BA, Scheinberg MA, et al. Beneficial effects of methylprednisolone "pulse" therapy in diffuse proliferative lupus nephritis. Lancet 1976;1:163.

43. Kimberly RP, Lockshin MD, Sherman RL, et al. High-dose intravenous methylprednisolone pulse therapy in systemic lupus erythematosus. Am J Med 1981;70:817.

44. Isenberg DA, Morrow WJW, Snaith ML. Methyl prednisolone pulse therapy in the treatment of systemic lupus erythematosus. Ann Rheum Dis 1982;41:347.

45. Barron KS, Person DA, Brewer EJ Jr, et al. Pulse methylprednisolone therapy in diffuse proliferative nephritis. J Pediatr 1982;101:137.

46. Liebling MR, McLaughlin K, Boonsue S, et al. Monthly pulses of methylprednisolone in SLE nephritis. J Rheumatol 1982;9:543.

47. Hayslett JP, Kashgarian M, Cook CD, et al. The effect of azathioprine on lupus glomerulonephritis. Medicine 1972;51:393.

48. Drinkard JP, Stanley TM, Dornfeld L, et al. Azathioprine and prednisone in the treatment of adults with lupus nephritis. Medicine 1970;49:411.

49. Shelp WD, Bloodworth JMB Jr, Rieselbach RE. Effect of azathioprine on renal histology and function in lupus nephritis. Arch Intern Med 1971;128:566.

50. Barnett EV, Dornfeld L, Lee DBN, et al. Long-term survival of lupus nephritis patients treated with azathioprine and prednisone. J Rheumatol 1978;5:275.

51. Sztejnbok M, Stewart A, Diamond H, et al. Azathioprine in the treatment of systemic lupus erythematosus: a controlled study. Arthritis Rheum 1971;14:639.

52. Ginzler E, Sharon E, Diamond H, et al. Long-term maintenance therapy with azathioprine in systemic lupus erythematosus. Arthritis Rheum 1975;18:25.

53. Hahn B, Kantor O, Osterland K. Azathioprine plus prednisone compared with prednisone alone in the treatment of SLE. Ann Intern Med 1975;83:592.

54. Donadio JV, Holley KE, Wagoner RD, et al. Further observations in the treatment of lupus nephritis with prednisone and combined prednisone and azathioprine. Arthritis Rheum 1974;17:573.

55. Feng PH, Jayaratnam FJ, Tock EPC, et al. Cyclophosphamide in treatment of systemic lupus erythematosus: 7 years' experience. Br Med J 1973;2:450.

56. Donadio JV, Holley KE, Ferguson RH, et al. Progressive lupus glomerulonephritis: treatment with prednisone and combined prednisone and cyclophosphamide. Mayo Clin Proc 1976;51:484.

57. Donadio JV, Holley KE, Ferguson RH, et al. Treatment of diffuse proliferative lupus nephritis with prednisone and combined prednisone and cyclophosphamide. N Engl J Med 1978;299:1151.

58. Decker JL, Klippel JH, Plotz PH, et al. Cyclophosphamide or azathioprine in lupus glomerulonephritis: a controlled trial: results at 28 months. Ann Intern Med 1975;83:606.

59. Dinant HJ, Decker JL, Klippel JH, et al. Alternative modes of cyclophosphamide and aza-

thioprine therapy in lupus nephritis. Ann Intern Med 1982;96:728.

60. Carette S, Klippel JH, Decker JL, et al. Controlled studies of oral immunosuppressive drugs in lupus nephritis. Ann Intern Med 1983; 99:1.

61. Felson DT, Anderson J. Evidence for the superiority of immunosuppressive drugs and prednisone over prednisone alone in lupus nephritis: results of a pooled analysis. N Engl J Med 1984;311:1528.

62. Austin HA III, Klippel JH, Balow JE, et al. Therapy of lupus nephritis: controlled trial of prednisone and cytotoxic drugs. N Engl J Med 1986;314:614.

63. Steinberg AD, Steinberg SC. Long-term preservation of renal function in patients with lupus nephritis receiving treatment that includes cyclophosphamide versus those treated with prednisone only. Arthritis Rheum 1991;34:945.

64. Lehman TJA, Sherry DD, Wagner-Weiner L, et al. Intermittent intravenous cyclophosphamide therapy for lupus nephritis. J Pediatr 1989; 114:1055.

65. Boumpas DT, Austin HA III, Vaughan EM, et al. Risk for sustained amenorrhea in patients with systemic lupus erythematosus receiving intermittent pulse cyclophosphamide therapy. Ann Intern Med 1993;119:366.

66. Ortiz A, Gonzalez-Parra E, Alvarez-Costa G, et al. Bladder cancer after cyclophosphamide therapy for lupus nephritis. Nephron 1992;60:378.

67. Lloyd W, Schur PH. Immune complexes, complement, and anti-DNA in exacerbations of systemic lupus erythematosus (SLE). Medicine 1981;60:208.

68. Laitman RS, Glicklich D, Sablay LB, et al. Effect of long-term normalization of serum complement levels on the course of lupus nephritis. Am J Med 1989;87:132.

69. Seyffart G. Drug dosage in renal insufficiency. Dordrecht, The Netherlands: Kluwer Academic Publishers, 1991:167.

70. Verrier Jones J, Robinson MF, Parciany RK, et al. Therapeutic plasmapheresis in systemic lupus erythematosus: effect on immune complexes and antibodies to DNA. Arthritis Rheum 1981;24:1113.

71. Schroeder JO, Euler HH, Loffler H. Synchronization of plasmapheresis and pulse cyclophosphamide in severe systemic lupus erythematosus. Ann Intern Med 1987;107:344.

72. Dau PC, Callahan J, Parker R, et al. Immunologic effects of plasmapheresis synchronized with pulse cyclophosphamide in systemic lupus erythematosus. J Rheumatol 1991;18:270.

73. Lewis EJ, Hunsicker LG, Lan S-P, et al. A controlled trial of plasmapheresis therapy in severe lupus nephritis. N Engl J Med 1992;326:1373.

74. Lin C-Y, Hsu H-C, Chiang H. Improvement of histological and immunological change in steroid and immunosuppressive drug-resistant lupus nephritis by high-dose intravenous gamma globulin. Nephron 1989;53:303.

75. Akashi K, Nagasawa K, Mayumi, et al. Successful treatment of refractory systemic lupus erythematosus with intravenous immunoglobulins. J Rheumatol 1990;17:375.

76. Winder A, Molad Y, Ostfeld I, et al. Treatment of systemic lupus erythematosus by prolonged administration of high dose intravenous immunoglobulin: report of 2 cases. J Rheumatol 1993;20:495.

77. Isenberg DA, Snaith ML, Morrow WJW, et al. Cyclosporin A for the treatment of systemic lupus erythematosus. Int J Immunopharmacol 1981;3:163.

78. Feutren G, Querin S, Noel LH, et al. Effects of cyclosporin in severe systemic lupus erythematosus. J Pediatr 1987;111:1063.

79. Favre H, Miescher PA, Huang YP, et al. Cyclosporin in the treatment of lupus nephritis. Am J Nephrol 1989;9(suppl 1):57.

80. Strober S, Farinas C, Field EH, et al. Lupus nephritis after total lymphoid irradiation: persistent improvement and reduction of steroid therapy. Ann Intern Med 1987;107:689.

81. Ben-Chetrit E, Gross DJ, Braverman A, et al. Total lymphoid irradiation in refractory systemic lupus erythematosus. Ann Intern Med 1986;105:58.

82. Westberg G, Tarkowski A. Effect of MaxEPA in patients with SLE. Scand J Rheumatol 1990;19:137.

83. Walton AJE, Snaith ML, Locniskar M, et al. Dietary fish oil and the severity of symptoms in patients with systemic lupus erythematosus. Ann Rheum Dis 1991;50:463.

84. Clark WF, Parbtani A, Naylor CD, et al. Fish oil in lupus nephritis: clinical findings and methodological implications. Kidney Int 1993; 44:75.

85. Hiepe F, Volk H-D, Apostoloff E, et al. Treatment of severe systemic lupus erythematosus with anti-CD4 monoclonal antibody (Letter). Lancet 1991;338:1529.

86. Kincaid-Smith P. The role of coagulation in the obliteration of glomerular capillaries. In: Kincaid-Smith P, Mathew TH, Lovell Becker D, eds. Glomerulonephritis. New York: Wiley, 1973:871.

87. Suc JM, Conte J, Mignon-Conte M. Treatment of glomerulonephritis with indomethacin and heparin. In: Kincaid-Smith P, Mathew TH, Lovell Becker D, eds. Glomerulonephritis. New York: Wiley 1973;927.

88. Cade R. Spooner F, Schlein E, et al. Comparison of azathioprine, prednisone, and heparin alone or combined in treating lupus nephritis. Nephron 1973;10:37.

89. Hariharan S, Pollak VE, Kant KS, et al. Diffuse lupus nephritis: long-term observations in patients treated with ancrod. Clin Nephrol 1990; 34:61.

90. Leaker B, McGregor A, Griffiths M, et al. Insidious loss of renal function in patients with anticardiolipin antibodies and absence of overt nephritis. Br J Rheumatol 1991;30:422.

91. Pierucci A, Simonetti BM, Pecci G, et al. Improvement of renal function with selective thromboxane antagonism in lupus nephritis. N Engl J Med 1989;320:421.
92. Lin C-Y. Improvement in steroid and immunosuppressive drug resistant lupus nephritis by intravenous prostaglandin E1 therapy. Nephron 1990;55:258.
93. Budman DR, Steinberg AD. Hypertension and renal disease in systemic lupus erythematosus. Arch Intern Med 1976;136:1003.
94. Reveille JD, Bartolucci A, Alarcon GS. Prognosis in systemic lupus erythematosus: negative impact of increasing age at onset, black race, and thrombocytopenia, as well as causes of death. Arthritis Rheum 1990;33:37.
95. Seleznick MJ, Fries JF. Variables associated with decreased survival in systemic lupus erythematosus. Semin Arthritis Rheum 1991;21:73.
96. Ward MM, Studenski S. Clinical prognostic factors in lupus nephritis: the importance of hypertension and smoking. Arch Intern Med 1992;152:2082.
97. Ginzler EM, Felson DT, Anthony JM, et al. Hypertension increased the risk of renal deterioration in systemic lupus erythematosus. J Rheumatol 1993;20:1694.
98. Fries JF, Powers R, Kempson RL. Late-stage lupus nephropathy. J Rheumatol 1974;1:166.
99. Cheigh JS, Stenzel KH. End-stage renal disease in systemic lupus erythematosus. Am J Kidney Dis 1993;21:2.
100. Goss JA, Cole BR, Jendrisak MD, et al. Renal transplantation for systemic lupus erythematosus and recurrent lupus nephritis: a single-center experience and a review of the literature. Transplantation 1991;52:805.
101. Sumrani N, Miles AM, Delaney V, et al. Renal transportation in cyclosporine-treated patients with end-stage lupus nephropathy. Transplant Proc 1992;24:1785.
102. Contreras-Rodriguez JL, Bordes-Aznar J, Alberu J, et al. Kidney transplantation in systemic lupus erythematosus: experience from a reference center in Mexico. Transplant Proc 1992;24:1798.
103. Bitker MO, Barrou S, Ourhama S, et al. Renal transportation in patients with systemic lupus erythematosus. Transplant Proc 1993;25:2172.
104. Kelley WN, Harris ED, Ruddy S, Sledge CB, eds. Textbook of rheumatology, 4th ed. Philadelphia: WB Saunders, 1993.

THE NEUROPSYCHIATRIC MANIFESTATIONS OF SYSTEMIC LUPUS ERYTHEMATOSUS

Harry G. Bluestein

"Lupus can do everything . . ." is the opening of a favorite aphorism regarding systemic lupus erythematosus (SLE). It reflects the wide range of clinical manifestations of the disease. Virtually every organ system can be affected by SLE immune-mediated mechanisms. As the immunopathogenic mechanisms underlying lupus began to be studied and understood in the 1950s and 1960s, primarily through animal models of lupus nephritis, it seemed logical to extrapolate the findings of an immune complex–mediated vasculitis to other organs. Subsequent pathologic studies have confirmed the primacy of small-vessel vasculitis in the immunopathogenesis of most tissue damage in SLE but not in the nervous system.

In many ways nervous system involvement can be viewed as a microcosm of systemic LE. The aphorism opening this chapter, although coined to describe the multisystem nature of lupus, also accurately reflects its neuropsychiatric manifestations. Lupus activity in the nervous system has produced virtually every clinical manifestation that a pathologic process in the nervous system can produce. From the ends of the nervous system at the neuromuscular junction, through the peripheral and cranial nerves and the spinal cord to the central nervous system with gross disturbances in motor function, to abnormalities in the regulation of motor function by the cerebellum and basal ganglia, to defects in the highest cerebral functions of reasoning, memory, and reality testing, there is no part of the nervous system that lupus has not affected.

PATHOGENESIS

Historically, the immunopathogenesis of neuropsychiatric lupus was assumed to be the same as for other organ systems. Clinicians commonly used quasipathologic terms such as *CNS vasculitis* and *lupus cerebritis* as names for nervous system involvement in lupus. However, beginning in the late 1960s, pathologic studies revealed that true vasculitis and other signs of tissue inflammation are relatively uncommon and that those pathologic features cannot account for most of the neuropsychiatric effects of SLE.[1–3] Since then, evidence has accumulated implicating several different immunopathogenic mechanisms. Autoantibodies reacting with neuronal membrane molecules have been associated with the more common central nervous system (CNS) abnormalities (reviewed in reference 4). There is a high correlation of the presence of those antibodies within the nervous system, as measured in cerebrospinal fluid, with active neuropsychiatric disease due to lupus.[5] Noninflammatory vasculopathy and associated nervous tissue infarcts are also associated with neurologic dysfunction, primarily with those manifestations that have a more focal presentation. Those focal manifestations correlate well with anticardiolipin and other antiphospholipid autoantibodies and are thought to represent thrombotic events (reviewed in reference 6). Thus neuropsychiatric lupus cannot be viewed as a monolithic entity. Rather, it is a collection of a variety of clinical manifestations of one or a combination of pathologic events, which could include neuron-reactive autoantibodies, the sequelae of the antiphospholipid syndrome, or immune complex–mediated vasculitis.

NATURAL HISTORY

The natural history of the neuropsychiatric manifestations of lupus is not well defined. Studies of factors that affect prognosis in SLE generally have implicated nervous system disease as a major cause of morbidity and mortality, second only to renal disease among the many clinical manifestations of lupus.[7–11] An analysis of the prognosis of individual neuropsychiatric manifestations[9] revealed a generally good outcome for diffuse CNS involvement without significant organic mental dysfunction. A high proportion of patients with seizures or nonorganic psychoses had little or no residual neuropsychiatric dysfunction. In contrast, the outcome was poorer in those patients with organic brain syndrome in terms of both survival and the development of chronic cerebral dysfunction. Morbidity in the form of residual neurologic deficit was also common among patients with focal neurologic disorders.

The impact of neurologic disease on mortality in SLE appears to be diminishing in recent times. In the first half of this century, nervous system disease was reportedly responsible for 25% of the deaths in SLE patients.[7,8,12] In more recent times that figure has dropped to approximately 10%.[7,8,10,11] The change coincided with the availability of aggressive immunotherapeutic modalities as well as improvement in overall SLE survival. Thus there is reason to believe that the natural history of lupus neuropsychiatric disorders can be improved by medical management.

DIFFERENTIAL DIAGNOSIS

This chapter opened with the reminder that "lupus can do everything . . . ." The aphorism concludes with "but not everything is lupus." The clinical manifestations of neuropsychiatric lupus, particularly the more common ones, are mimicked by a variety of other pathogenic processes to which lupus patients are particularly susceptible. Nervous system infection, changes in mentation secondary to metabolic abnormalities, encephalopathy, stroke, or intracranial hemor-

rhage from hypertension, and neuropsychiatric side effects of medications used to treat SLE must be considered and ruled out before treatment is directed at lupus-caused CNS disease. NSAID-induced meningitis in SLE patients should not be forgotten.

In a consideration of medication-induced CNS dysfunction in lupus, initial thoughts focus on corticosteroid therapy, and the possibility of "steroid psychosis" deserves special attention. Steroid psychosis is well recognized[13,14] and is frequently placed high on the list of differential diagnoses of lupus patients with a psychotic presentation. However, virtually all large clinical studies of neuropsychiatric lupus have emphasized that steroid psychosis is uncommon.[7,15–18] Corticosteroid therapy causes fewer than 10% of the psychotic events that occur in patients with lupus. Steroid psychosis should be considered when a significant change in corticosteroid dose preceded the onset of the psychiatric manifestations. There are clinical features that can help to distinguish between the steroid and lupus causes of psychoses. Steroid psychosis tends to be nonorganic in character; that is, it is not accompanied by the classic features of organic mental syndrome (diminished consciousness and cognitive impairment) or other signs of organic neurologic dysfunction. Almost all patients with lupus-caused psychosis have accompanying organic mental syndrome. Other signs of organicity accompanying psychosis that implicate lupus as the cause include concurrent focal neurologic signs or the presence of visual, tactile, or olfactory hallucinations. If any of these signs of organicity are present, or if the psychosis occurs in the setting of increased systemic activity of the SLE, the event is most likely lupus induced.

GENERAL CONSIDERATIONS IN THERAPY

A discussion of the therapy of neuropsychiatric manifestations of SLE is hampered by the absence of documentation of the effectiveness of any therapeutic modality by controlled studies. Current approaches to treatment have been based on retrospective analyses of the results obtained with empirically derived treatment protocols or on anecdotal reports of a small number of cases. The mainstay of therapy for the neuropsychiatric manifestations of SLE is corticosteroids. This evolved primarily from the writings of Dubois who, in the 1950s, recommended the aggressive use of corticosteroids, initiating therapy with the equivalent of 1 mg/kg/d of prednisone and doubling it each day until the patient responded.[19] Follow-up studies some years later documented decreased mortality from CNS disease after the initiation of that therapeutic program.[8] Dubois' work had a profound impact, which led to the use of some heroic steroid dosages that, in turn, led to increasing complications. The enthusiasm for high-dose steroids was tempered considerably by a study published in the mid 1970s that documented a high death rate from infection in patients treated with more than 100 mg of prednisone equivalent per day for more than 2 weeks.[20] As a result, steroid therapy now is generally given either as a daily dose of 1 to 1.5 mg/kg/d of prednisone equivalent, or it is initiated with a regimen of daily pulses of 1 g of methylprednisolone given intravenously for 2 or 3 days followed by a daily dose in the range of 0.6 to 1 mg/kg/d of prednisone equivalent.[21,22] The relative effectiveness and risk of toxicity of "pulse" versus fixed daily corticosteroid dosage remain controversial. In our experience, morbidity and mortality, especially from opportunistic infections, have been significantly higher among patients treated with pulse therapy, and we have not been impressed with a commensurately greater therapeutic effectiveness. Thus we rarely use that modality of treatment for neuropsychiatric disease.

During the 1980s, after a number of reports of successful treatment of lupus nephritis with plasmapheresis,[23-26] that therapeutic modality was applied to patients with steroid-resistant neuropsychiatric manifestations. Several studies, mostly anecdotal, described a good outcome.[27-29] No controlled studies of CNS disease have been done; with the appearance of some controlled studies of the effects of plasmapheresis on lupus nephritis, which showed no statistically significant therapeutic benefit,[30,31] enthusiasm for this mode of treatment has receded. In the 1980s we used plasmapheresis to treat four patients with life-threatening steroid-resistant neuropsychiatric lupus. Two patients died of infectious complications directly related to technical problems with the procedure; one patient with thrombotic thrombocytopenic purpura made a good recovery; and the fourth

patient showed no appreciable change. We do not use plasmapheresis as a standard mode of therapy for lupus neuropsychiatric disease and would consider using it only as a last resort measure in life-threatening situations.

In this decade, following the documented successful use of intermittent pulse intravenous cyclophosphamide therapy in the treatment of lupus nephritis, there have appeared several small uncontrolled retrospective studies or anecdotal case reports suggesting an important therapeutic role for that immunosuppressive regimen in treating steroid-resistant neuropsychiatric lupus.[32-36] We have a larger and more successful experience with that form of treatment than we do with plasmapheresis or "pulse" steroid therapy. Although it is not free of serious side effects, especially infection, it is the most effective modality we have seen for corticosteroid-resistant disease. The appropriate clinical settings for its use will be discussed below.

THERAPY OF DIFFUSE NEUROPSYCHIATRIC MANIFESTATIONS

Given the variety of different clinical features with different pathogenic bases, it is evident that a review of the management of lupus neuropsychiatric manifestations should be divided into discussions of the various clinical entities that fall under that rubric. Historically, the clinical manifestations of nervous system involvement in lupus had been grouped into neurologic or psychiatric categories. In reality, however, the majority of patients will have psychiatric and neurologic problems. Based on our current understanding of the pathogenesis of neuropsychiatric lupus, it is more useful to categorize the nervous system events into "diffuse" and "focal" groups (Table 9–1). The diffuse manifestations represent global dysfunction of the CNS. That category includes the two most prototypic features of lupus neuropsychiatric disease—(1) organic mental syndrome characterized by reduced mental function spanning the spectrum from encephalopathic diminished consciousness to obvious impairment of cognitive function expressed as defective short-term memory, diminished attention, or dyscalculia, and (2) seizure disorders, most typically of the grand mal type. The diffuse manifestations are the most common forms of neuropsychiatric lupus, each occurring in 15% to

TABLE 9–1

Nervous System Involvement in Systemic Lupus Erythematosus

MANIFESTATION	OCCURRENCE RATE (%)
Diffuse Cerebral Dysfunction	
Organic mental syndrome	20
Psychosis	15
Seizure disorder	15
Focal Neurologic Disease	
Cranial neuropathy	12
Peripheral neuropathy	10
Stroke	4
Chorea	3
Transverse myelitis	1

20% of SLE patients. There is a strong association between the diffuse neuropsychiatric manifestations and neuron-reactive autoantibodies in the cerebrospinal fluid. Focal neurologic manifestations, in order of frequency, include cranial and peripheral neuropathies, strokes, chorea and other movement disorders, and transverse myelitis. Several of the focal manifestations, especially stroke, chorea, and transverse myelitis, have been linked pathogenically with antiphospholipid autoantibodies and the hypercoagulable state. While this is a somewhat simplistic summary of the current state of understanding of the pathogenesis of neuropsychiatric lupus, it provides, to a limited extent, a useful framework for understanding the current approaches to therapy of the various manifestations of SLE.

Acute onset of the diffuse neuropsychiatric manifestations of lupus requires therapeutic intervention. For most of them, the approach to therapy is two-pronged: (1) control of the acute neuropsychiatric manifestation with neuroactive drugs and (2) suppression of the immunopathogenic mechanisms responsible for the nervous system dysfunction. Control of agitation or panic is an important early therapeutic goal of lupus patients with acute or chronic organic mental dysfunction and/or psychosis. Haloperidol (Haldol) is generally quite effective and is the most frequently used neuroleptic agent. For severely agitated psychotic patients, the addition of a sedating neuroleptic such as chlorpromazine (Thorazine) may be needed.

Acute cerebral dysfunction, with or without psychosis, should be treated with an immuno-

suppressive regimen. In very severe cases, such as those involving diminished states of consciousness, I recommend relatively high-dose parenteral therapy with approximately 2 mg/kg/d of methylprednisolone given intravenously in four divided doses. If there is a good therapeutic response, the dose is slowly tapered and the patient is switched to oral prednisone at 60 mg/d initially in divided doses, followed by a slow, steady taper. If there is no response within 7 days (less if the patient's condition is rapidly deteriorating), I initiate a course of pulse intravenous cyclophosphamide (0.75 to 1 g/m^2 body surface area) on a monthly basis and, at the same time, slowly taper the corticosteroid dose.

In less life-threatening situations, the patient may be treated with oral prednisone, which can be given in a dose that is significantly higher than the dose the patient had been taking before the onset of the neuropsychiatric problem. If the patient had been taking 25 mg of prednisone a day or less, the dosage should be raised to 60 mg daily in divided doses. If the patient had been taking higher amounts, the dose should be raised to 80 to 100 mg/d. Tapering of the prednisone should begin when there is a good clinical response or after 14 days of therapy, even in the setting of inadequate response. If the organic mental dysfunction does not respond to steroids, we initiate a course of pulse intravenous cyclophosphamide, using the regimen just described.

Patients with *chronic organic brain syndrome* who present because of increasing agitation or psychosis should be controlled with neuroleptic agents, but a careful reevaluation should precede initiation of aggressive therapy for lupus activity. If the psychiatric disturbance is not accompanied by clear-cut signs of worsening lupus activity or other new neurologic dysfunction, and if the chronic mental dysfunction is the result of a poor response to aggressive therapy for lupus in the past, it is unlikely that there will be a therapeutic response to high-dose corticosteroids or cyclophosphamide, and the risks of those therapies are not justified.

Seizure disorders in lupus are generally controllable with standard anticonvulsant therapies. Phenytoin (Dilantin) is commonly used despite the evidence that it and several other anticonvulsants may induce a lupuslike syndrome.[37–40] There is no evidence that those agents that precipitate drug-induced lupus (e.g., phenytoin, procainamide, or hydralazine) alter disease activity in patients with idiopathic SLE; they can be used therapeutically in the appropriate clinical setting.

Patients with a new seizure disorder of acute onset generally present in the setting of active lupus activity, and the seizures often accompany other neuropsychiatric manifestations of lupus. Seizures more frequently occur with organic mental syndromes than would be expected by chance. In such settings, aggressive therapy for organic mental syndromes (see acute cerebral dysfunction above) should be followed. Seizures occurring with active SLE but no other diffuse CNS disease should be treated with more moderate steroid doses of 1 mg/kg/d of prednisone equivalent. If a lupus patient has a single acute seizure with no recurrence after a year of therapy with anticonvulsants, there is a high degree of likelihood that the anticonvulsant can be discontinued without a return of seizure activity. If seizures do recur at any point, it is likely that chronic epilepsy has developed and the patient will need lifelong anticonvulsant treatment.

Lupus patients with a prior history of epileptic seizures need to be treated with an improved anticonvulsant regimen, but they may not need to be treated for active lupus. If the seizures are occurring together with other manifestations of lupus-induced CNS involvement or in the setting of a generalized flare-up of SLE, then more aggressive lupus therapy is appropriate. If the lupus disease overall is stable, however, optimization of the anticonvulsant regimen should be sufficient.

THERAPY OF FOCAL NEUROPSYCHIATRIC MANIFESTATIONS

Cranial and peripheral neuropathies are the most common of the focal neuropsychiatric features of lupus. Each occurs in about 10% of lupus patients at some time during the course of their disease. Among the cranial neuropathies, involvement of motor and sensory nerves related to the eye is most common.[2,41–45] The pathogenesis of that involvement is not defined. Ophthalmoplegias secondary to pathology in the nerves serving the extraocular muscles tend to be short lived, respond well to moderate increases in corticosteroids, and on some occasions disappear spontaneously without any change in therapy. Optic neuritis, on the other

hand, needs to be treated more aggressively. Parenteral methylprednisolone, either the "pulse" steroid regimen or the daily split-dose regimen described above, often restores vision during the first few attacks; however, in those patients with recurrent optic neuritis, resistance to corticosteroids often develops, necessitating immunosuppressive therapy. Cyclophosphamide, given as monthly intravenous boluses, is often effective. Trigeminal neuralgia is another cranial neuropathy associated with SLE. It typically affects sensory fibers, producing the characteristic tic douloureux chronic pain syndrome but generally spares motor function. Trigeminal neuralgia responds poorly to corticosteroids. Carbamazepine (Tegretol) and phenytoin (Dilantin) have been moderately successful in controlling the nerve pain.

Several types of peripheral neuropathies occur in SLE. Transitory mild to moderate polyneuropathy, predominantly affecting sensory fibers, is the most common, accounting for almost two thirds of the peripheral neuropathies seen in lupus patients.[46] This type of neuropathy, in which symptoms are generally annoying but not severe, usually does not improve significantly with more aggressive treatment of the SLE. Mononeuritis multiplex accounts for up to one third of the peripheral neuropathies that occur in SLE.[9,47,48] The pathologic condition underlying the mononeuritis is usually a necrotizing vasculitis of the vasonervorum. Vasculitis has also been implicated in a relatively rare but severe widespread polyneuropathy.[48–51] Both of those vasculitis-associated neuropathies should be treated with moderately high doses of corticosteroids. Cyclophosphamide should be used in steroid-resistant cases in the setting of biopsy-proven lupus vasculitis affecting nerves.

Stroke is a relatively common focal neurologic manifestation of SLE, affecting about 5% of lupus patients at some time during the course of their illness.[46,52] Stroke may result from a variety of pathologic processes, each of which is treated differently. Most commonly, it is an ischemic event caused by arterial thrombosis[53–55] or, less commonly, by thromboembolism from Libman-Sacks endocarditis.[56–58] Both of these types of stroke have been linked to antiphospholipid antibodies and are thought to represent the antiphospholipid syndrome occurring in lupus.[6,57–60] Cerebral infarctions tend to occur in isolation without other neuropsychiatric manifestations of lupus, usually in the setting of stable lupus activity, and they are typically recurrent. Patients with strokes due to arterial thrombosis should be treated with anticoagulation, heparin initially and then warfarin (Coumadin).[6,61] Unless complications of the therapy develop, anticoagulation should be continued indefinitely. There is evidence of a high incidence of recurrent strokes if the anticoagulation is discontinued.[62] There is also evidence that anticoagulation is more effective in preventing recurrent strokes if the International Normalization Ratio (INR) of treated/control prothrombin time is maintained in the 3 to 4 range[63] instead of the usual 2 to 3 range. There are more bleeding complications at the higher ratios, however, and I recommend a target ratio of 2.5. Lupus patients with transient ischemic attacks, often associated with antiphospholipid antibodies, should be treated with low-dose aspirin (80 to 300 mg/d) or another platelet antagonist. Treatment of lupus with high-dose corticosteroids or other immunosuppressive drugs will not reduce the recurrence of thrombotic events.[64]

Other focal neurologic manifestations of SLE associated with antiphospholipid antibodies include chorea[65-67] and spinal cord pathosis occurring as transverse myelitis.[68-70] *Chorea* is relatively uncommon in lupus but is the most frequently encountered movement disorder, affecting 2% or 3% of lupus patients at some time during the course of their illness. The choreiform movements tend to last for weeks but are usually self-limited. Chorea generally does not recur. Despite the strong association with antiphospholipid antibodies, therapy with platelet antagonists or anticoagulants has not been reported or recommended. Corticosteroids have been used, but since the condition usually resolves spontaneously within weeks there is no certainty of their necessity or effectiveness.

Transverse myelitis affects perhaps 1% of lupus patients at some time during the course of their illness. Although relatively uncommon, it is the cause of considerable morbidity, often resulting in lower-extremity paralysis and loss of sphincter control.[71-73] It occurs most commonly in the mid to low thoracic spine. A variety of pathologic mechanisms have been documented in different cases. Ischemic necrosis or the cord due to involvement of the anterior spinal artery is the common final pathway in most cases. Antiphospholipid-related arterial thrombosis is well documented and the most common cause; however, lupus arteritis has been described, as has compression of the anterior spinal artery by steroid-induced excessive fat accumulation. Corticosteroids have been the mainstay of therapy. Corticosteroids may stabilize or prevent worsening of the transverse myelitis, but there is little evidence that therapy reverses the neurologic deficit or alters prognosis.[71] With the recent interest in the use of intravenous cyclophosphamide to treat neuropsychiatric lupus, several published reports have described significant reversal of the neurologic deficits of transverse myelopathy with monthly pulse cyclophosphamide in conjunction with high-dose corticosteroids.[32,35,36] There are now 11 cases treated with that regimen described in the literature. Six patients reportedly recovered completely or improved significantly, two died without recovery (one of infection, the other of a pulmonary embolus), one did not change, and two recovered temporarily and then suffered a relapse. One of the relapses was followed by partial improvement when a second course of treatment was given. In some cases, the failure to respond to the cyclophosphamide regimen could be blamed on the time between onset of the myelopathy and the initiation of treatment. Therapy was begun within the first week of the event in those who responded but not until more than 1 month after the event in some of the unsuccessfully treated patients. The proportion of patients with a good outcome is significantly higher than expected from therapy with corticosteroids alone,[71,74] but the number of patients treated with the cyclophosphamide regimen in published reports is still quite small. More experience will be needed before it is known whether the therapeutic benefit will be sufficient to justify the increased toxicity of the cyclophosphamide therapy. Because of the occurrence of antiphospholipid antibodies and arterial thrombosis, it is surprising that there are no reports on the use of anticoagulation. In fact, one authority has recommended heparin therapy,[75] but there is no indication that anyone has found it efficacious. At present, given the poor prognosis of transverse myelitis, the cyclophosphamide plus corticosteroid regimen is recommended for patients with profound neurologic deficit from myelopathy due to lupus.

OTHER NERVOUS SYSTEM–RELATED CLINICAL MANIFESTATIONS

Intractable headaches of the vascular type, with or without visual auras, occur more frequently in SLE than in age- and sex-matched control populations. Some studies report a correlation between "lupus headache" and increased lupus activity affecting other organs,[76,77] whereas others report that lupus headaches follow a course that is independent of other clinical or laboratory manifestations of lupus.[78] Those cases in which there are concurrent changes on electroencephalograms or brain scans or in cerebrospinal fluid (CSF) have lent credence to the speculation that some lupus headaches are caused by lupus-induced vascular disease. However, analysis of the epidemiology and natural history of these migrainelike headaches in lupus reveals no significant differences between headaches occurring in lupus patients and in patients with idiopathic migraine. Despite the uncertainty regarding the importance of lupus immunopathology in their pathogenesis, on a practical level, management of lupus headaches should not be different from that of intractable headaches in patients without SLE. Lupus patients are treated with the same medical regimens used for patients with idiopathic migraine or chronic headache. Beyond determining whether the nonsteroidal antiinflammatory drug the patient may be taking is causing the headache, therapy for lupus itself should be adjusted independent of considerations of headache.

Pseudotumor cerebri, a form of benign intracranial hypertension without focal neurologic dysfunction, is an uncommon neurologic manifestation associated with SLE.[79–81] Headache and papilledema are the usual presenting manifestations. It is generally unaccompanied by other signs of active lupus, and its pathogenesis is not known. We have managed our few patients with pseudotumor cerebri with nothing but repeated drainage of CSF by spinal tap to reduce intracranial pressure. In those cases, the signs of pseudotumor disappeared within months without other therapeutic intervention. Despite its lack of association with other lupus disease activity or with antiphospholipid antibodies, treatment with corticosteroids, anticoagulation, or platelet antagonists has been suggested.[75] That has not been necessary in our limited experience.

CONCLUSION

The heterogeneous collection of clinical features and the neuropathologic processes that are included in the neuropsychiatric manifestations of SLE require a variety of therapeutic approaches. The therapies have evolved empirically, for the most part, although attempts have been made, after the fact, to provide a rationale for them based on scientific insights into the pathogenesis of the neurologic dysfunction. The apparent beneficial results only sometimes seem logical on scientific grounds. In fact, diagnosis and treatment of the neuropsychiatric manifestations of SLE remain largely an imperfect art. Better diagnostic tests and controlled therapeutic trials are sorely needed, particularly for those neuropsychiatric manifestations associated with high morbidity and mortality. The trend in recent years toward faddish shifts in therapies as early optimistic anecdotal reports of new treatments appear reflects a lack of confidence in current regimens, which can change only with convincing data documenting therapeutic efficacy. The frequency of the serious neuropsychiatric manifestations is such that cooperative national or international studies with standardized treatment protocols will be needed to provide the data on which to base rational therapeutic decisions.

REFERENCES

1. Johnson RT. Neurology and neuropathologic observations in lupus erythematosus. N Engl J Med 1962;266:895.
2. Johnson RT, Richardson EP. The neurological manifestations of systemic lupus erythematosus: a clinical-pathological study of 24 cases and review of the literature. Medicine 1968;47:337.
3. Ellis SG, Verity MA. Central nervous system involvement in systemic lupus erythematosus: a review of neuropathologic findings in 57 cases, 1955–1977. Semin Arthritis Rheum 1979;8:212.
4. Bluestein HG. Antibodies to neurons. In: Wallace DJ, Hahn BH, eds. Dubois' lupus erythematosus. 4th ed. Philadelphia: Lea & Febiger, 1993:260.
5. Bluestein HG, Williams GW, Steinberg AD. Cerebrospinal fluid antibodies to neuronal cells: association with neuropsychiatric manifestations of systemic lupus erythematosus. Am J Med 1981;70:240.
6. Asherson RA. Antiphospholipid antibodies and syndromes. In: Lahita RG, ed. Systemic lupus erythematosus. 2nd ed. New York: Churchill Livingstone, 1992:587.
7. Dubois EL, Tuffanelli DL. Clinical manifestations of systemic lupus erythematosus: computer analysis of 520 cases. JAMA 1964;190:104.

8. Dubois EL, Wierzchowiecki M, Cox MB, et al. Duration and death in systemic lupus erythematosus: an analysis of 249 cases. JAMA 1974; 227:1399.

9. Estes D, Christian CL. The natural history of systemic lupus erythematosus by prospective analysis. Medicine 1971;50:85.

10. Wallace DJ, Podell T, Weiner J, et al. Systemic lupus erythematosus—survival patterns: experience with 609 patients. JAMA 1981;245:934.

11. Rosner S, Ginzler EM, Diamond HS, et al. A multicenter study of outcome in systemic lupus erythematosus. II. Causes of death. Arthritis Rheum 1982;25:612.

12. Klemperer P, Pollack D, Baehr G. Pathology of disseminated lupus erythematosus. Arch Pathol 1941;32:569.

13. Hall RCW, Popkin MK, Stickney SK, et al. Presentation of the steroid psychoses. J Nerv Ment Dis 1979;167:229.

14. Lewis DA, Smith RE. Steroid-induced psychiatric syndromes: a report of 14 cases and a review of the literature. J Affective Disord 1983;5:319.

15. O'Connor JF. Psychoses' association with systemic lupus erythematosus. Ann Intern Med 1959;51:526.

16. Ropes MW. Systemic lupus erythematosus. Cambridge, Massachusetts: Harvard University Press, 1976.

17. Stern M, Robbins ES. Psychoses in systemic lupus erythematosus. Arch Gen Psychiatry 1960;3:205.

18. Fessel WJ, Solomon GF. Psychosis and systemic lupus erythematosus: review of the literature and case report. Calif Med 1960;92:266.

19. Dubois EL. Systemic lupus erythematosus: recent advances in its diagnosis and treatment. Ann Intern Med 1956;45:163.

20. Sergent JS, Lockshin MD, Klemper MS, et al. Central nervous system disease in systemic lupus erythematosus: therapy and prognosis. Am J Med 1975;58:644.

21. Kimberly RP, Lockshin MD, Sherman RI, et al. High-dose intravenous methylprednisolone pulse therapy in systemic lupus erythematosus. Am J Med 1981;70:817.

22. Price J, Klestov A, Beacham B, et al. A case of cerebral systemic lupus erythematosus treated with methylprednisolone pulse therapy. Aust NZ J Psychiatry 1985;19:184.

23. Jones JV, Cumming RH, Bacon PA, et al. Evidence for a therapeutic effect of plasmapheresis on patients with systemic lupus erythematosus? Q J Med 1979;48:555.

24. Leaker BR, Becker GJ, Dowling JP, et al. Rapid improvement in severe lupus glomerular lesions following intensive plasma exchange associated with immunosuppression. Clin Nephrol 1986; 25(5):236.

25. Lockwood CM, Pussell B, Wilson CB, et al. Plasma exchange in nephritis. Adv Nephrol 1979;8:383.

26. Sharon Z, Roberts JL, Fennel JS, et al. Plasmapheresis in lupus nephritis. Plasma Therapy 1982; 3:165.

27. Smith GM, Leyland MJ. Plasm exchange for cerebral lupus erythematosus. Lancet 1987;1:103.

28. Unterweger B, Klein G, Fleischhacker WW. Plasma exchange for cerebral lupus erythematosus [Letter]. Biol Psychiatry 1988;24:946.

29. Tanter Y, Rifle G, Chalopin JM, et al. Plasma exchange in central nervous system involvement of systemic lupus erythematosus. Plasma Ther Transfus Technol 1987;8:161.

30. Hebert L, Nielsen E, Pohl M, et al. Clinical course of severe lupus nephritis during the controlled trial of plasmapheresis therapy. Kidney Int 1987;31:201.

31. Lewis E, Lachin J. Primary outcomes in the controlled trial of plasmapheresis therapy in severe lupus nephritis. Kidney Int 1987;31:208.

32. Boumpas DT, Yamada H, Patrones NJ, et al. Pulse cyclophosphamide for severe neuropsychiatric lupus. Q J Med 1991;81:975.

33. LaRochelle G, Lacks S, Borenstein D. IV cyclophosphamide therapy of steroid resistant neuropsychiatric SLE (NPSLE) [Abstract]. Arthritis Rheum 1990;33(5):R21.

34. Von Feldt J, Ostrov BE. The use of cyclophosphamide in the treatment of CNS lupus [Abstract]. Arthritis Rheum 1990;33(5):R21.

35. Barile L, Lavalle C. Transverse myelitis in systemic lupus erythematosus—the effect of IV pulse methylprednisolone and cyclophosphamide. J Rheumatol 1992;19:370.

36. Klaiman MD, Miller SD. Transverse myelitis complicating systemic lupus erythematosus: treatment including hydroxychloroquine. Am J Phys Med Rehabil 1993;72:158.

37. Alarcon-Segovia D. Drug induced lupus syndromes. Mayo Clin Proc 1969;44:664.

38. Lee SL, Rivero I, Siegel M. Activation of systemic lupus erythematosus by drugs. Arch Intern Med 1966;117:620.

39. Dabbous IA, Idriss HM. Occurrence of systemic lupus erythematosus in association with ethosuccimide therapy (case report). J Pediatr 1970; 76:617.

40. AlBalla S, Fritzler MJ, Davis P. A case of drug-induced lupus due to carbamazepine. J Rheumatol 1987;14:599.

41. Hackett ER, Martinez RP, Larson PF, et al. Optic neuritis in SLE. Arch Neurol 1974;31:9.

42. Meyer MW, Wild JW. Unilateral internuclear ophthalmoplegia in SLE. Arch Neurol 1975;32: 486.

43. Evans OB, Lexow SS. Painful ophthalmoplegia in systemic lupus erythematosus. Ann Neurol 1978;4:584.

44. April RS, Van Sonnenberg E. A case of neuromyelitis optica (Devics syndrome) in SLE: clinicopathologic report and review of the literature. Neurology 1976;26:1066.

45. Jabs DA, Miller NR, Newman SA, et al. Optic neuropathy in systemic lupus erythematosus. Arch Ophthalmol 1986;104:564.

46. Feinglass EJ, Arnett FC, Dorsch CA, et al. Neuropsychiatric manifestations of systemic lupus erythematosus: diagnosis, clinical spectrum, and

relationship to other features of the disease. Medicine 1976;55(4):323.

47. Dubois E. Clinical picture of systemic lupus erythematosus. In: Dubois E, ed. Lupus erythematosus. Los Angeles: USC Press, 1974:305.

48. Clark EC, Bailey AA. Neurological and psychiatric signs associated with systemic lupus erythematosus. JAMA 1956;160:455.

49. McGehee HA, Shulman LE, Tumulty AP, et al. Systemic lupus erythematosus: review of the literature and clinical analysis of 138 cases. Medicine 1954;33(4):291.

50. Heptinstall RH, Sowry GSC. Peripheral neuritis in SLE. Br Med J 1952;1:525.

51. Bailey AA, Sayre GP, Clark EC. Neuritis associated with systemic lupus erythematosus: report of 5 cases with necropsy in 2. Arch Neurol Psychiatr 1956;75:251.

52. Kitagawa Y, Gotoh F, Koto A, et al. Stroke in systemic lupus erythematosus. Stroke 1990;21:1533.

53. Trevor RP, Sondhemier FK, Fessel WJ, et al. Angiographic demonstration of major cerebral vessel occlusion in systemic lupus erythematosus. Neuroradiology 1972;4:202.

54. Fields RA, Sibbitt WL, Toubbeh H, et al. Neuropsychiatric lupus erythematosus, cerebral infarctions, and anticardiolipin antibodies. Ann Rheum Dis 1990;49(2):114.

55. Dubois E. Clinical picture of systemic lupus erythematosus. In: Dubois E, ed. Lupus erythematosus. Los Angeles: USC Press, 1974:410.

56. Fox IS, Spence AM, Wheelis RF, et al. Cerebral embolism in Libman-Sacks endocarditis. Neurology 1980;30:487.

57. Asherson RA, Lubbe WF. Cerebral and valve lesions in SLE: association with antiphospholipid antibodies. J Rheumatol 1988;15:539.

58. Young SM, Fisher M, Sigsbee A, et al. Cardiogenic brain embolism and lupus anticoagulant. Ann Neurol 1989;26:390.

59. Asherson RA, Gibson DG, Evans DW, et al. Diagnostic and therapeutic problems in two patients with antiphospholipid antibodies, heart valve lesions and transient ischemic attacks. Ann Rheum 1988;47(11):947.

60. Trimble M, Bell DA, Brien W, et al. The antiphospholipid syndrome: prevalence among patients with stroke and transient ischemic attacks. Am J Med 1990;88(6):593.

61. Lockshin MD. Which patient with antiphospholipid antibody should be treated and how? Rheum Dis Clin North Am 1993;19:235.

62. Asherson RA, Chan JK, Harris EN, et al. Anticardiolipin antibody, recurrent thrombosis, and warfarin withdrawal. Ann Rheum Dis 1985;44:823.

63. Rosove MH, Brewer PM. Antiphospholipid thrombosis: clinical course after the first thrombotic event in 70 patients. Ann Intern Med 1992;117:303.

64. Asherson RA, Baguley E, Pal C, et al. The antiphospholipid syndrome: the five year follow-up. Ann Rheum Dis 1991;50:805.

65. Hadron PY, Bouchez B, Wattel A, et al. Chorea, systemic lupus erythematosus, circulating anticoagulant. J Rheumatol 1986;13:991.

66. Asherson RA, Derksen RH, Harris EN, et al. Chorea in systemic lupus erythematosus and "lupus-like" disease: association with antiphospholipid antibodies. Semin Arthritis Rheum 1987;16(4):253.

67. Khamashita MA, Gil A, Anciones B, et al. Chorea in systemic lupus erythematosus: association with antiphospholipid antibodies. Ann Rheum Dis 1988;47:681.

68. Lavalle C, Pizarro S, Drenkard C, et al. Transverse myelitis: manifestation of systemic lupus erythematosus strongly associated with antiphospholipid antibodies. J Rheumatol 1990;17:34.

69. Marabani M, Zoma A, Hadley D, et al. Transverse myelitis occurring during pregnancy in a patient with systemic lupus erythematosus. Ann Rheum Dis 1989;48:160.

70. Hardie RJ, Isenberg DA. Tetraplegia as a presenting feature of systemic lupus erythematosus complicated by pulmonary hypertension. Ann Rheum Dis 1985;44:491.

71. Kewalramani LS, Saleem S, Bertrand D. Myelopathy associated with systemic lupus erythematosus (erythema nodosum). Paraplegia 1978;16:282.

72. Warren RW, Kredich DW. Transverse myelitis and acute central nervous system manifestations of systemic lupus erythematosus. Arthritis Rheum 1984;27:1058.

73. Al-Husaini A, Jamal GA. Myelopathy as the main presenting feature of systemic lupus erythematosus. Eur Neurol 1985;24:94.

74. Propper DJ, Bucknall RC. Acute transverse myelopathy complicating systemic lupus erythematosus. Ann Rheum Dis 1989;48:512.

75. Wallace DJ, Metzger AL. Systemic lupus erythematosus and the nervous system. In: Wallace DJ, Hahn BH, eds. Dubois' lupus erythematosus. 4th ed. Philadelphia: Lea & Febiger, 1993:370.

76. Abel T, Gladman DD, Urowitz MB. Neuropsychiatric lupus. J Rheumatol 1980;7:325.

77. Brandt KD, Lessel S. Migrainous phenomenon in systemic lupus erythematosus. Arthritis Rheum 1978;21:7.

78. Isenberg DA, Meyrick-Thomas D, Snaith ML, et al. A study of migraine in systemic lupus erythematosus. Ann Rheum Dis 1982;41:30.

79. Bettman JW Jr, Daroff RB, Sanders MD, et al. Papilledema and asymptomatic intracranial hypertension in systemic lupus erythematosus: a fluorescein angiographic study of resolving papilledema. Arch Ophthalmol 1968;80:189.

80. Silderberg DH, Laties AM. Increased intracranial pressure in disseminated lupus erythematosus. Arch Neurol 1973;29:88.

81. Del Guidice GC, Scher CA, Athreya BH, et al. Pseudotumor cerebri and childhood systemic lupus erythematosus. J Rheumatol 1986;13:748.

10

VASCULITIS

E. William St. Clair

The major vasculitic syndromes encompass a broad spectrum of clinical disorders (see Table 10–1 for a partial listing of the recognized syndromes).[1,2] These diagnostic categories have many overlapping clinical, laboratory, and histopathologic features, a fact that has created much nosologic confusion and impeded the development of a standard nomenclature. The American College of Rheumatology, however, has recently proposed classification criteria that may help establish some uniformity in disease definition.[3] The severity of disease manifestations and prognosis varies considerably across disease categories and even within the same category. Vasculitis can trigger a mild skin disease of short duration or a devastating illness that languishes menacingly during a waxing and waning course. To add to the confusion, patients may evolve over time from one diagnostic category to another. Such diversity not only poses diagnostic challenges but also shapes management by requiring clinical end points to define the period of therapy.

This chapter addresses the treatment of polyarteritis nodosa, Churg-Strauss syndrome, Wegener's granulomatosis, isolated central nervous system (CNS) vasculitis, essential mixed cryoglobulinemia, Henoch-Schönlein purpura, hypersensitivity vasculitis, and Cogan's syndrome. (For more detail on pathogenesis, see Conn et al., Vasculitis and Related Disorders, in Kelley et al., reference 12). Treatment of other vasculitic syndromes, including temporal arteritis, Takayasu's arteritis, Kawasaki's disease, and vasculitis associated with connective tissue disease, is considered elsewhere in this volume.

TABLE 10–1
Classification of the Vasculitic Syndromes

Polyarteritis nodosa group
  Classic polyarteritis nodosa
  Churg-Strauss syndrome
  Polyangiitis overlap syndrome
Wegener's granulomatosis
Hypersensitivity vasculitis
  Essential mixed cryoglobulinemia
  Henoch-Schönlein purpura
  Serum sickness
  Vasculitis associated with malignancies
  Vasculitis associated with other primary disorders
Isolated central nervous system vasculitis
Kawasaki's disease
Giant cell arteritides
  Temporal arteritis
  Takayasu's arteritis
Miscellaneous vasculitides (Cogan's syndrome, Behçet's syndrome)

POLYARTERITIS NODOSA AND CHURG-STRAUSS SYNDROME

The pathologic hallmark of polyarteritis nodosa (PAN) is a small and medium-sized necrotizing arteritis involving multiple organ systems. Its clinical features include fever, weight loss, cutaneous ulcers, livedo reticularis, muscle pain and weakness, arthralgias and arthritis, neuropathy, abdominal pain, ischemic bowel, testicular pain or tenderness, hypertension, and renal failure. While PAN classically spares the lung, a polyangiitis overlap syndrome has been described with PAN-like features and pulmonary involvement.[4]

Microscopic polyarteritis is a pathologic lesion characterized by focal segmental necrotizing glomerulonephritis without interlobar or intralobar artery involvement; it often accompanies histopathologic evidence of a small and medium-sized vessel vasculitis in other organ systems.[5] In most schemes, microscopic polyarteritis is classified with the PAN group of systemic necrotizing vasculitides. Hepatitis B[6-8] and hepatitis C[9,10] infection may play a role in the pathogenesis of systemic PAN and distinguish other subsets of this disease. Not to be confused with microscopic polyarteritis, cutaneous PAN is a clinical variant of necrotizing vasculitis that primarily targets the skin and subcutaneous tissue and does not usually progress to systemic involvement.[11]

The foremost manifestations of Churg-Strauss syndrome (CSS), also called allergic angiitis and granulomatosis, are asthma, pulmonary vasculitis, and peak eosinophil counts exceeding $1.5 \times 10^9/L$.[12-15] The heart, nervous system, gastrointestinal and urinary tracts, and joints are the other principal targets of this systemic necrotizing vasculitis. Only a minority of patients exhibit severe renal disease. CSS must be differentiated from other clinical disorders associated with marked eosinophilia, such as eosinophilic leukemia, hypereosinophilic syndrome, Loeffler's syndrome, chronic eosinophilic pneumonia, eosinophilic gastroenteritis, parasitic infections, and bronchopulmonary aspergillosis.

Laboratory studies in patients with PAN and CSS reflect chronic inflammation (e.g., acute phase reactants) and injury to various organ systems. They are nonspecific, however, for diagnostic purposes. Finding the typical arteriographic abnormalities[16] or the histopathologic changes of necrotizing vasculitis in the wall of the artery[17] is critical for diagnosis.

Natural History of Disease

Our understanding of the natural history of PAN and CSS derives from clinical observations made before the introduction of glucocorticoids. These clinical and histopathologic descriptions did not take into account the major subdivisions of systemic vasculitis. Instead, PAN as well as CSS and other vasculitic syndromes fell into the broader category of "periarteritis nodosa." Researchers at the Mayo Clinic found that patients with periarteritis nodosa who were seen between 1946 and 1962 and left untreated had 1- and 5-year survival rates of 35% and 13%, respectively.[18] A worse outcome was predicted by initial presentation with renal and gastrointestinal disease, with most early deaths being caused by active vasculitis. These observations were reproduced by studies from other major medical centers[19,20] and a community hospital.[21]

In a similar retrospective analysis, patients with CSS fared no better without therapy than the periarteritis nodosa group as a whole, exhibiting a 1-year survival of 4%.[22] Allergic rhinitis and asthma, the prodrome to CSS, preceded the onset of vasculitis by as long as 7 years.[22] Deaths in CSS have most often resulted from pulmonary compromise, cardiac failure, renal failure, or cerebral hemorrhage.[13,22]

Uncontrolled Treatment Studies

Glucocorticoids are now widely accepted as efficacious therapy for systemic necrotizing vasculitis, a conclusion supported by retrospective studies. In patients with PAN, glucocorticoid therapy has been associated with survival rates of 60% to 71% at 1 year and 48% to 55% at 5 years.[18-21,23] An important milestone in the management of PAN and CSS was the advent of cytotoxic therapy.[19,24-26] In 1979 Fauci et al.[26] reported that treatment with 2 mg/kg/d of oral cyclophosphamide produced a high rate of remissions in 17 patients with PAN whose disease had been refractory to previous glucocorticoid therapy. Although three of the patients in this study died, the other 14 patients achieved a complete or partial remission and within a few months tolerated a reduction in glucocorticoid doses to a less toxic, alternate-day regimen. Since the patients in this study had disease of more than 2 years duration upon initiation of cytotoxic therapy, it is difficult to separate the individual effects of natural history of disease, previous glucocorticoid therapy, and cytotoxic agents on clinical outcomes. In agreement with these results, researchers from the University of California at Los Angeles found that treatment of PAN with both glucocorticoids and cytotoxic agents yielded a 5-year survival rate of 80%, contrasting with a 5-year survival rate of 53% for a comparable group treated only with glucocorticoids.[19] The experience at the Mayo Clinic, however, did not show improved outcomes with cytotoxic therapy.[23] In most of these open treatment studies, much of the mortality occurs in the first 2 years of disease. Thus, nonrandom allocation into different treatment groups of patients in various stages of disease may bias the survival analysis, making it impossible to draw any definite conclusions about the therapeutic effects of cytotoxic agents in this setting.

Glucocorticoids and cytotoxic agents also have been widely employed in the treatment of CSS. At one medical center, patients with CSS who received 40 to 60 mg of prednisone or its equivalent demonstrated 1- and 5-year survival rates of 90% and 62%, respectively.[27] Most deaths in this group resulted from myocardial infarction and cardiac failure. Another study found that 15 of 16 CSS patients who were treated with glucocorticoids alone were alive after a mean follow-up of 38 months.[15] Instances of clinical disease unresponsive to glucocorticoids could often be brought under control with azathioprine[27,28] or cyclophosphamide.[27]

Prospective Clinical Trials

The Cooperative Study Group for Polyarteritis Nodosa has been the pacesetter in conducting prospective treatment trials in systemic vasculitis. In one trial, they found that initial treatment of PAN and CSS with prednisone plus plasma exchange (PE) or prednisone alone produced nearly identical remission rates and similar 7-year survival rates of 83% and 79%, respectively.[29] Most of the 16 patients in whom the assigned treatment was stopped because of lack of efficacy were then treated with oral cyclophosphamide for disease control. These results argue against using PE for the routine treatment of systemic vasculitis. They are also informative because they provide a contemporary prognostic view of PAN and CSS after initial therapy with glucocorticoids alone. The 7-year survival rate of 80% in this trial surpasses the 50% long-term survival rates of glucocorticoid-treated patients from retrospective studies. Earlier diagnosis, differences in case mix, and vital lessons learned in exploiting the therapeutic benefits of glucocorticoids in systemic vasculitis may explain the superior outcomes from the prospective trial. Overall, these studies suggest that cytotoxic therapy may not be required for all patients with PAN.

In another clinical trial, 71 patients with PAN or CSS were randomized to receive initial treatment with either prednisone plus PE or prednisone, PE, and oral cyclophosphamide.[30] Both treatment groups achieved similar remission and survival rates, although the group receiving oral cyclophosphamide suffered fewer relapses during follow-up. Only two patients in the prednisone plus PE group deteriorated during the first 6 months of treatment. Age over 55 years and an elevated serum creatinine level at presentation predicted a worse outcome. Although initiation of therapy with oral cyclophosphamide did not enhance overall survival in PAN and CSS, this approach was still favored by the trial's investigators because it prolonged the disease-free period.

Some studies suggest that hepatitis B viral (HBV) infection worsens outcomes in PAN.[31] Although glucocorticoids are clearly indicated for the treatment of PAN, they may potentially complicate the course of HBV infection by impairing the immune response to this virus. It is known, for example, that glucocorticoid therapy reduces survival in HBV-associated chronic liver disease.[32] Also, sudden cessation of immunosuppressive therapy may reconstitute cell-mediated immunity in HBV-infected patients and provoke a fulminant hepatitis.[33] The outcome of HBV infection can be monitored with circulating markers of viral replication. Disappearance of hepatitis B surface antigen (HB_sAg) correlates with elimination of HBV infection. HBe-antigen (HB_eAg) seroconversion is a favorable prognostic sign and parallels a large drop in liver HBV-DNA.[34] Although some information may be gained by serologic monitoring of HBV infection, its treatment implications in regard to PAN are unclear.

Antiviral therapy might be expected to improve the treatment of patients with PAN and HBV infection. The Cooperative Study Group for Polyarteritis Nodosa has studied the outcome of 33 patients with PAN and HBV infection in an open trial of glucocorticoids, PE, and vidarabine A therapy.[35] Twenty-four of the patients recovered completely from their vasculitis, a result not dissimilar from that of glucocorticoid-treated PAN patients without HBV infection. During the trial, circulating HB_eAg and HB_sAg cleared in 12 and 5 of the patients, respectively. Since most studies fail to confirm the treatment efficacy of vidarabine A in chronic hepatitis B,[34] this antiviral drug probably had little effect on the outcomes in this trial.

Chronic hepatitis B, however, may respond favorably to interferon-α therapy.[36] The immunomodulatory effects of interferon-α are complex and may theoretically hasten the progression of vasculitis. In fact, treatment with interferon-α can provoke various autoimmune phenomena, including vasculitis.[36] Until further study, interferon-α therapy should be reserved for HBV-related liver disease.

Long-Term Experience

Relapses can punctuate the course of PAN for many years after onset. In one study, at least one relapse was recorded in 23 of 83 (28%) patients with PAN who survived longer than 3 months and were treated with prednisone and cyclophosphamide therapy.[37] Despite aggressive therapy, about 10% to 20% of patients with PAN and CSS die 5 to 10 years after onset of their illness because of active disease or a disease- or treatment-related complication.[18,19,21,23,26,29,30] Most early deaths result from a perforated viscus, massive gastrointestinal hemorrhage, myocardial infarction, cerebrovascular accident, or renal failure due to active disease. A minority die of infections during immunosuppressive therapy. Concomitant HBV infection in PAN may increase the risk of chronic liver failure.[7,8,31]

Management

Patients with active PAN or CSS are treated with high doses of glucocorticoids. Some judgment can be exercised in deciding whether to initially combine these drugs with a cytotoxic agent. In my view, serious visceral organ system disease, such as mononeuritis multiplex, CNS deficits, congestive heart failure, renal involve-

ment, or evidence of mesenteric ischemia, justifies the addition of oral cyclophosphamide to the initial treatment regimen. Patients with PAN who lack serious visceral organ involvement can be managed initially with glucocorticoids alone and, failing immediate improvement, subsequently treated with oral cyclophosphamide.

Certain factors may modify this treatment approach. For example, a concurrent diabetic state may support the initial use of cytotoxic therapy to allow more rapid reduction in the glucocorticoid dose and better control of hyperglycemia. Conversely, other considerations, such as diagnostic uncertainty, compliance issues, or a patient's concern about drug side effects, may militate against use of a cytotoxic agent.

The glucocorticoids most commonly prescribed are prednisone or methylprednisolone (orally or intravenously) in starting doses of 1 to 2 mg/kg/d. A protocol for initiating glucocorticoid therapy without concomitant cytotoxic agents in systemic vasculitis is shown in Table 10–2. Treatment is begun in rapidly progressing disease with divided daily doses of glucocorticoids, which are more immunosuppressive and potentially toxic than equivalent doses of the same preparation given once a day. A 70 kg person, for example, would be treated initially with prednisone or methylprednisolone in doses of 15 to 30 mg four times daily. Glucocorticoids are then converted from divided daily doses to a single morning dose in accordance with the time required to control disease activity, usually 7 to 10 days. If possible, the period of divided dose therapy should not exceed 7 to 10 days to minimize

---

TABLE 10–2

A Protocol for Initiating Glucocorticoid Therapy Without Concomitant Cytotoxic Agents in Systemic Necrotizing Vasculitis

GLUCOCORTICOID PREPARATION	ROUTE	DOSE AND FREQUENCY	TIME FROM ONSET OF THERAPY
Methylprednisolone	IV	20 mg q6h	Day 1
Methylprednisolone	IV	40 mg q12h	Day 5
Prednisone	Oral	60 mg/d	Day 10
Prednisone	Oral	60 mg/d	Week 4
Prednisone	Oral	40 mg/d	Week 8
Prednisone	Oral	20 mg/d	Week 12
Prednisone	Oral	40 mg alt w/ 30 mg/d	Week 17
Prednisone	Oral	40 mg alt w/ 20 mg/d	Week 18
Prednisone	Oral	40 mg alt w/ 10 mg/d	Week 19
Prednisone	Oral	40 mg qod	Week 20

alt w/ = alternating with.

glucocorticoid-related complications. With clinical improvement, the prednisone dose can be tapered over the first 2 weeks of therapy to a single morning dose of 60 to 80 mg and over the next 3 to 4 months to 20 mg/d. The daily prednisone dose may then be converted to an alternate-day schedule, an approach I favor, or reduced further in small decrements (e.g., 2.5 mg) until reaching the lowest dose that effectively controls the disease. Concomitant cytotoxic therapy usually allows more rapid reduction in prednisone dose, starting about 4 weeks after initiation of therapy, and an earlier conversion of the daily prednisone regimen to an alternate-day schedule (e.g., at 3 to 4 months).

The initial dose of cyclophosphamide for treatment of systemic vasculitis is 1 to 2 mg/kg/d (usually given orally); this dose is later adjusted, depending on the peripheral leukocyte count (see below). More fulminant vasculitis may warrant initiation of cyclophosphamide at a dose of 4 mg/kg/d for 3 days, followed by a dosage reduction within 7 days to 2 mg/kg/day. Azathioprine (2 mg/kg/d) is far less effective than cyclophosphamide in inducing remission but may serve as an alternative in this situation.[26]

The treatment of disease unresponsive to cyclophosphamide therapy may take two directions. First, the daily dose of cyclophosphamide can be increased by 25 mg increments until the peripheral leukocyte and neutrophil counts approach 3000/mm³ and 1500/mm³, respectively (see below). Sometimes higher doses of cyclophosphamide are tolerated when the prednisone dose is increased, preferably keeping the alternate-day schedule. A second option is experimental therapy, which may involve a trial of intravenous pulse methylprednisolone, intermittent high-dose cyclophosphamide, or cyclosporin A (see below).

The tolerance of the myeloid compartment to cyclophosphamide usually wanes with prolonged treatment because of diminishing bone marrow reserves. The cyclophosphamide dose is reduced only if the peripheral leukocyte count drops below 3000/mm³. Azathioprine may sustain remission if unacceptable side effects result from oral cyclophosphamide therapy.[37,38] The patient should receive oral cyclophosphamide for 12 months after a complete remission followed by a gradual withdrawal of the drug over 2 to 3 months in 25 to 50 mg decrements.

Cutaneous PAN generally requires less immunosuppression because of its lack of systemic manifestations and favorable long-term prognosis. Local measures and high-potency topical or intralesional glucocorticoids may be tried as the first approach. Salicylates, dipyridamole, sulfapyridine, pentoxifylline, and dapsone are only variably effective in the treatment of cutaneous PAN,[11,39] but they may be useful in individual cases. Severe, rapidly progressive skin disease can respond to prednisone in doses of up to 1 mg/kg/d.

Some patients with chronic skin lesions may not improve with glucocorticoids or may suffer excessive complications from the prolonged use of these drugs. In this situation, low-dose weekly oral methotrexate (7.5 to 20 mg/wk) may promote healing of skin lesions and act as a steroid-sparing agent.[40] Although oral cyclophosphamide is effective in the treatment of systemic vasculitis, it less consistently induces remissions of cutaneous PAN. Moreover, combining oral cyclophosphamide with daily doses of glucocorticoids can predispose the patient to bacterial infections of nonhealing skin lesions. Thus cytotoxic agents are used with caution in cutaneous PAN. Since the major clinical manifestations of cutaneous PAN are painful skin ulcers, local therapy aimed at protecting the wound, decreasing superficial infection, and promoting healing are often the most productive avenues of therapy.

Clinical Pharmacology and Drug Interactions

Glucocorticoids can produce a myriad of biologic effects. (For more detail, see Axelrod, Glucocorticoids, in Kelley et al., reference 42.) After moving across the cell membrane, they complex with high-affinity receptors and enter the nucleus, where they change the transcription of specific genes. The products of these genes regulate diverse intracellular and extracellular events associated with cellular activation and inflammation. Glucocorticoids interfere with endothelial cell function, inhibit recruitment of circulating leukocytes to sites of tissue inflammation, and block proinflammatory mediator production.[41] Pharmacologic doses of glucocorticoids suppress the hypothalamic-pituitary-adrenal axis, reducing endogenous cortisol production.

Glucocorticoid preparations differ in relative potency, sodium-retaining properties, and biologic half-life. Those most commonly used to treat vasculitis are the short-acting preparations—prednisone and methylprednisolone. Because of their longer biologic half-life, the longer-acting preparations such as dexamethasone exhibit a much greater "steroid effect" than equivalent doses of shorter-acting agents. A single daily dose of dexamethasone, for example, suppresses cortisol production for more than 48 hours and thus is not suitable for long-term daily administration.

Because glucocorticoids are inactivated in the liver, drugs that induce hepatic microsomal enzyme activity, such as phenytoin, barbiturates, and rifampin, may accelerate the elimination of glucocorticoids.[42] Glucocorticoids may also speed the metabolism of salicylates in the liver, lowering the serum salicylate levels.[42] Pharmacologic doses of glucocorticoids can change the need for antihypertensive medications or the insulin requirements of patients with diabetes mellitus.

Cyclophosphamide is a potent immunosuppressive drug. (For more detail, see Fauci and Young, Immunoregulatory Agents, in Kelley et al., reference 43.) It inhibits cellular activity by alkylating DNA, which cross-links the DNA coil and introduces coding errors during DNA synthesis and transcription.[43] Thus rapidly dividing cells are its principal target. In doses applicable to vasculitis therapy, cyclophosphamide inhibits lymphocyte proliferation more strongly than neutrophil proliferation, resulting in a greater degree of lymphopenia than neutropenia. Cyclophosphamide also downregulates both B cell and T cell function.[43]

Hepatic microsomal enzymes are involved in the activation of cyclophosphamide. Drugs that induce these enzymes may alter the conversion of cyclophosphamide from its inactive to its active form. More importantly, the elimination and detoxification of cyclophosphamide may be prolonged in patients with liver or renal dysfunction.

Drug Side Effects and Recommended Monitoring

Glucocorticoid complications are more pronounced with longer-acting preparations, more frequent administration, and prolonged use. Physicians should be alert for the occurrence of these toxicities. The initiation of high-dose glucocorticoids may produce sudden and dramatic hyperglycemia in susceptible persons. Patients should be warned about polyuria and polydipsia. An intervening serious illness or a surgical procedure may warrant temporary administration of "stress doses" of glucocorticoids because of HPA suppression.[44] Unless contraindicated, 400 IU of vitamin D and 1000 to 1500 mg of elemental calcium can be given daily to retard the development of glucocorticoid-induced osteoporosis. (See Chapter 22 for a more detailed discussion of this issue.)

Cyclophosphamide therapy is associated with substantial toxicity. The most common side effects are dose-related and include gastrointestinal intolerance, hair loss, and myelosuppression.[45] Its myelosuppressive actions can be a major factor in the development of serious infections. Patients receiving cyclophosphamide have frequent infections from common bacterial pathogens, opportunistic organisms, and herpes zoster; these infections occur most often in patients who are receiving concurrent daily doses of prednisone.[46,47] Keeping the prednisone dose on an alternate-day schedule appreciably lowers the risk of infection.

The cyclophosphamide dose must be adjusted on an individual basis to avoid excessive myelosuppression. With renal impairment (e.g., serum creatinine >2 mg/dl), the initial dose can be reduced by 25% to 50%, although the level of renal function does not reliably correlate with the maximum tolerated dose. The cyclophosphamide dose is held constant for the first 10 days to 2 weeks of therapy, with subsequent dosage adjustments to keep the total leukocyte count above 3000/mm^3 and the neutrophil count above 1500/mm^3. The peripheral leukocyte count begins to drop 8 to 14 days after starting cyclophosphamide or increasing its dose. Thus measured counts in peripheral blood do not reflect suppression of the marrow from the current dose but, rather, from the dose taken 1 to 2 weeks earlier. Waiting until the leukocyte counts drop below safe limits almost invariably results in prolonged myelosuppression. Such unwanted toxicity can be avoided by monitoring the rate of decline in the peripheral leukocyte count, anticipating its nadir, and making the appropriate dosage adjustment before the full myelosuppressive effects of the current dose are realized. Recovery from myelosuppression takes 18 to 25 days.

Glucocorticoids influence the numbers of circulating neutrophils by stimulating their release from the bone marrow and inhibiting their adhesion to vascular endothelium. Treatment with high doses of glucocorticoids often increases the peripheral leukocyte count to 10,000 to 20,000/mm^3. About 2 weeks into the treatment of systemic vasculitis, the usual practice of consolidating the glucocorticoid dose to once a day, combined with the delayed myelosuppressive effects of cyclophosphamide, can result in a rapid fall in the leukocyte count that must be closely monitored to ensure an appropriate level of immunosuppression. Cyclophosphamide overdosage can be averted by checking the peripheral leukocyte count at least twice weekly for the first 3 weeks of therapy (or possibly longer until the counts level off in a safe range) and making prompt dosage adjustments. Subsequently, the peripheral leukocyte counts can be monitored on a weekly basis and every 2 weeks after 2 months of constant dosing.

The teratogenicity of cyclophosphamide mandates that effective birth control practices be maintained during the treatment period. Cyclophosphamide interferes with the development of oocytes and spermatocytes and can promote gonadal fibrosis and clinical sterility. These gonadal effects frequently produce oligomenorrhea and amenorrhea in women and decreased libido, impotence, and azoospermia in men. The risk of permanent sterility appears to be dose-related and higher in women over 30 years of age.[48] Concomitant use of oral contraceptives by women during cyclophosphamide therapy may reduce the incidence of sterility.[49] Before initiation of treatment with cyclophosphamide, male patients should be advised about banking sperm to aid future conception.

Acrolein, a toxic metabolite of cyclophosphamide, can irritate the bladder and promote hemorrhagic cystitis, bladder fibrosis, and transitional and squamous cell carcinoma.[45,50] Two preventive measures may lessen the frequency of bladder complications. One widely accepted approach is maintenance of a liberal fluid intake of several liters daily. Mesna, or 2-mercaptoethanesulfonate, has also been advocated for prophylaxis[51] and is available for intravenous use. The parenteral solution can be taken orally because it is 29% to 81% bioavailable by this route and stable for up to 24 hours in a variety of beverages.[52]

The urine should be examined every month during cyclophosphamide therapy to monitor for signs of bladder toxicity. Unexplained hematuria, unless it clears rapidly, demands an immediate diagnostic evaluation, including urology consultation and cystoscopy. The occurrence of severe cystitis usually requires discontinuation of oral cyclophosphamide. On the other hand, mild cystitis that resolves quickly can be managed by reemphasizing the need for good hydration and resuming the cyclophosphamide at a 25 to 50 mg lower dose. Hematuria also can signal a neoplastic change in the bladder mucosa. To screen for bladder cancer, a urine cytologic examination is performed yearly in patients whose total cyclophosphamide dose exceeds 10 g. Neoplastic changes have been detected in the bladder mucosa up to 11 years after the completion of cyclophosphamide therapy.[51] Thus, after cyclophosphamide therapy, patients must have annual surveillance for potential bladder neoplasms. An overall scheme for monitoring oral cyclophosphamide therapy is outlined in Table 10–3.

A major concern of long-term cyclophosphamide therapy is delayed appearance of malignant disease, mostly leukemias and lymphomas.[53] Since the risk of these secondary malignant conditions is greater with higher total doses of cyclophosphamide, the need for this drug should be reexamined in those patients who have received it for more than 2 years.

Investigational Drugs and Future Directions

Intravenous pulse glucocorticoid therapy (e.g., 0.5 to 1 g of methylprednisolone daily for 3 days) has shown efficacy in the treatment of PAN and CSS[54,55] and may be useful as a therapeutic alternative in refractory disease. In addition, potentially less toxic cyclophosphamide regimens have been tried in patients with systemic vasculitis. Intermittent high-dose cyclophosphamide therapy (500 to 750 mg/m^2 given intravenously every month for 6 months) is as effective as daily oral cyclophosphamide in treating lupus nephritis[56] and may also produce therapeutic benefits in PAN and CSS.[57-59] High-dose cyclophosphamide therapy can be administered as a single intravenous bolus, as routinely done in the management of lupus nephritis, or as multiple oral doses over a 3-day period.[37] A cautionary note concerning alternative cyclophospha-

TABLE 10–3

**Recommended Monitoring of Patients Receiving Oral Cyclophosphamide (CYC)
for the Treatment of Systemic Necrotizing Vasculitis**

TIME PERIOD*	MONITORING TESTS	COMMENTS
Weeks 1–3	CBC twice a week	Carefully note the rate of decline in peripheral leukocyte count; adjust CYC dose to keep leukocyte count >3000/mm³ and neutrophil count >1500/mm³
Weeks 3–8	CBC every week	As above
	Urinalysis every month	Hematuria may indicate cystitis
Week 9 until end of therapy	CBC every 2 weeks	As above
	Urinalysis every month	As above
	Urine cytology every year	Screen for bladder cancer
After therapy	Urine cytology every year	Maintain bladder cancer surveillance indefinitely

*Time period refers to the period after initiation of CYC therapy. CBC = Complete blood cell count.

mide regimens has been sounded by recent studies which indicate that intermittent high-dose cyclophosphamide does not sustain remissions in Wegener's granulomatosis (WG) as long as daily oral cyclophosphamide.[60] Especially deserving of further study, however, are treatment regimens in which an initial induction course of daily oral cyclophosphamide is followed by a longer period of intermittent high-dose cyclophosphamide as maintenance therapy.[37]

Cyclosporin A is a powerful immunoregulatory agent that can effectively suppress active systemic vasculitis, although it may be frequently toxic at the doses necessary to control disease.[61] Treatment with cyclosporin A has been initiated at doses of 5 mg/kg/d and, depending on the clinical response and tolerability, gradually reduced to doses of 1 to 3 mg/kg/d for long-term maintenance.

A greater understanding of disease mechanisms has afforded new horizons for treatment. Alluring targets for novel therapies currently under investigation include potential pathogenic T cell populations, proinflammatory cytokines such as interleukin-1 and tumor necrosis factor, and an array of cell-adhesion molecules that mediate immune cell interactions and movement of leukocytes into inflamed tissue.[1] This approach has seen only limited application in systemic vasculitis. In one study, treatment with a combination of two monoclonal antibodies transiently reduced the number of circulating T cells and improved clinical disease manifestations in four patients with refractory systemic vasculitis.[62,63] Such in-

novative therapies will undoubtedly be the focus of more research in the future.

WEGENER'S GRANULOMATOSIS

Wegener's granulomatosis is a necrotizing vasculitis with a predilection for the upper and lower respiratory tracts and kidneys.[13] Otitis media, mucosal ulceration, nasal perforation and deformity, and sinusitis dominate the upper airway involvement. The most common symptoms of lower airway disease are cough and hemoptysis. Chest radiographs of patients with symptoms as well as those who have no symptoms may show bilateral nodular infiltrates and cavities. In addition to respiratory and renal disease, other features of WG include ocular inflammation, retroorbital masses, arthritis, mononeuritis multiplex, cerebral arteritis, and vasculitic skin lesions. Many investigators emphasize the variable prognosis for patients with WG and its relationship to sites of clinical involvement. Concomitant respiratory and renal disease has been termed "generalized WG," which, without aggressive immunosuppressive therapy, portends a grave prognosis. A less ominous course is taken by patients with "limited WG," a subgroup with respiratory disease and no clinical evidence of kidney involvement.[64,65]

The erythrocyte sedimentation rate (ESR) is a useful laboratory test in WG because elevated values correlate with clinical disease activity. Antineutrophil cytoplasmic antibodies (C-ANCA) also have diagnostic significance in this disease because they occur in sera from 88% to 96% of patients with active, generalized WG.[66-68] The frequency of a positive C-ANCA test drops to 67% in patients with locally active disease[68] and to 41% to 43% in patients with inactive disease.[66] False-positives are noted in fewer than 5% of cases.[66,67] Temporal changes in the C-ANCA titer may correlate with clinical disease activity and predict a relapse.[68,69] However, the evidence to date does not justify the use of this serological marker as the sole basis for initiating or increasing immunosuppressive therapy.[70]

Depending on the biopsy site, areas of disease involvement in WG may exhibit histologic evidence of necrotizing granulomatous vasculitis, necrotizing granuloma without vasculitis, or acute and chronic inflammation. The diagnosis is most often confirmed by the pathologic findings from an open-lung biopsy, which are also valuable in excluding possible infection and other conditions that may resemble WG such as lymphomatoid granulomatosis or lymphoma. Other biopsy sites may be equally informative, although biopsy specimens from upper airways notoriously yield nondiagnostic material. Despite the apparent predictive value of a positive C-ANCA test, this result has not been shown to reliably substitute in clinical practice for a tissue diagnosis.

Natural History of Disease

The initial clinical and histopathologic descriptions of patients with WG portray a rapidly fatal course without therapy. Such patients survive a mean of 5 months and die of uremia, respiratory failure, or disseminated vasculitis.[71] Some with limited WG survive longer and succumb later to respiratory complications or progression to renal failure.

Treatment Studies and Long-Term Experience

Although treatment with glucocorticoids extends the mean survival of WG patients to 12 months,[72] vastly improved outcomes followed the adoption of oral cyclophosphamide as standard therapy.[73] Researchers from the National Institutes of Health (NIH) have summarized their experience in treating 158 patients with WG who had been followed for 1229 patient-years.[66,74,75] Nearly all of the patients in

this group had received initial treatment with 1 mg/kg/d of prednisone and 2 mg/kg/d of oral cyclophosphamide, with subsequent reduction of the prednisone dose to an alternate-day schedule and maintenance of daily oral cyclophosphamide for 12 months after a complete remission. With this therapy, 91% of the patients showed clinical improvement, and 75% attained a complete remission.[66] About half of the group had at least one relapse, and nearly the same number sustained a remission that lasted more then 5 years.[66]

Disease- and treatment-related morbidity were common in this patient population and included chronic sinus dysfunction (47%), chronic renal insufficiency (42%), hearing loss (35%), nasal deformities (28%), pulmonary insufficiency (17%), tracheal stenosis (13%), and visual loss (8%). Complications attributed to cyclophosphamide were cystitis (43%), hair loss (17%), bladder cancer (2.8%), and myelodysplasia (2%).[66] Overall, the rate of bladder cancer was 33 times higher than in the general population. Two patients developed non-Hodgkin's lymphoma, an 11-fold increase in overall risk. Glucocorticoid therapy was associated with transient cushingoid features in most patients, cataracts (21%), fractures (11%), diabetes mellitus (8%), and avascular necrosis (3%).[66] Slightly more than half of the women of childbearing age could not become pregnant or had ovarian failure after more than 1 year of cyclophosphamide therapy.[66] Nearly half of the patients required at least one hospitalization for treatment of a serious infection, usually bacterial.[66] Eight fungal, six *Pneumocystis carinii*, and two mycobacterial infections, as well as 34 episodes of herpes zoster, occurred during follow-up.[66]

Twenty percent of the patients in this study died.[66] Death was due to active WG or a disease- or treatment-related complication in 13% of the patients, with deaths resulting from renal disease (3%), pulmonary disease (3%), a combination of pulmonary and renal disease (1%), infection (3%), and cancer (2.5%).

Prospective Clinical Trials

The toxic nature of oral cyclophosphamide therapy has motivated researchers to investigate alternative, less hazardous therapies for WG. In an open, prospective trial, NIH workers found intermittent high-dose cyclophosphamide therapy to be less effective than daily oral cyclophosphamide in sustaining complete remissions of WG,[60] a conclusion supported by one other study.[76] More promising results have been obtained using methotrexate in WG patients without immediately life-threatening disease. In one study, oral MTX at 20 mg/wk, combined with standard glucocorticoid therapy, produced marked improvement in 22 of 29 WG patients with this clinical profile.[77] Most improved patients remained in complete remission after a mean follow-up of 14.5 months.

Management

The initial treatment of active WG consists of 1 mg/kg/d of prednisone (or its equivalent) and 2 mg/kg/d of oral cyclophosphamide, as described above for PAN. Initial treatment with prednisone alone may be cautiously undertaken in selected patients with limited WG who lack pulmonary and other serious organ system involvement.

Apart from the general principles of glucocorticoid and cyclophosphamide therapy described above, several issues pertain specifically to the management of WG. Chronic sinus inflammation, a predominant feature of WG, impairs mucosal immunity and increases susceptibility to infection, usually from *Staphylococcus aureus*. Frequent irrigation to relieve nasal crusting and blocked airways, surgical procedures to drain impacted sinuses, and antibiotics are often necessary for management of chronic nasal and sinus disease. Worsening nasal or sinus disease may result from infection, active WG, or both and, if unresponsive to local measures and antibiotic therapy, may require tissue biopsy for diagnosis.

Certain ocular manifestations in WG, such as conjunctivitis, episcleritis, and anterior uveitis, can be successfully treated with topical glucocorticoid preparations.[78] In contrast, active scleritis and optic nerve vasculitis threaten vision and call for greater concern. These more serious eye conditions demand immediate ophthalmologic evaluation to assess the need for systemic immunosuppressive therapy. A retro-orbital mass, another worrisome ocular manifestation, can also jeopardize vision and warrant emergency orbital decompression.

Investigational Drugs and Future Directions

Investigators are striving to find an alternative to oral cyclophosphamide because of its potentially serious complications. The results achieved with low-dose weekly oral MTX, as described above, are preliminary and await confirmation.[77] This approach, however, may ultimately prove useful in treating WG patients with non-life-threatening disease or intolerance to oral cyclophosphamide.

Considerable interest has focused on the role of trimethoprim-sulfamethoxazole (T/S) in the treatment of WG.[79-84] Since infection has long been suspected to trigger WG, any beneficial effects from T/S could stem from this drug's antimicrobial properties. In reviewing published cases, it is difficult to dissect the specific effects of T/S therapy in WG because of some uncertain diagnoses, concurrent use of other immunosuppressive agents, and the potential impact of T/S on coexisting sinus infection. Insufficient evidence exists at this writing to conclude that T/S can replace glucocorticoids or oral cyclophosphamide in the treatment of WG.

Several other therapies have been tried successfully in WG; these include intravenous pulse methylprednisolone,[85,86] cyclosporin A,[61,87] intravenous gamma globulin,[88] and etoposide.[89] These experimental agents may be considered for treatment of patients with cyclophosphamide-resistant disease. With improved awareness of WG and its clinical spectrum, future management may entail a more staged approach using therapeutic agents with less toxicity to control mild disease.

ISOLATED CNS VASCULITIS

Isolated CNS vasculitis is a rare disorder involving the arteries of the brain and, less frequently, the spinal cord.[90] Some investigators also refer to this condition as granulomatous angiitis of the nervous system or primary angiitis of the CNS. Its diverse clinical features include headache, psychiatric manifestations, confusion, seizures, and a countless array of cerebrovascular syndromes. Multifocal CNS disease most strongly suggests this diagnosis.

Magnetic resonance imaging (MRI) typically highlights the widespread nature of this disease in showing numerous areas of increased signal intensity scattered throughout the cerebral hemispheres, cerebellum, brain stem, and spinal cord. Cerebral arteriography may reveal narrowing or dilatation of small arteries or appear normal if the involved arteries are too small to be imaged by this procedure. These abnormal MRI and arteriographic findings, while suggestive of the diagnosis, can be mimicked by infection, tumor, and other pathologic processes. For this reason, the "gold standard" for diagnosing isolated CNS vasculitis is histopathologic evidence of vessel inflammation in the brain or spinal cord. Leptomeningeal and/or parenchymal brain biopsy is often performed to evaluate patients with suspected isolated CNS vasculitis, but the diagnostic utility of this procedure is compromised by the frequent occurrence of false-negative results, which have been reported in up to 25% of patients with this disorder.[91]

Natural History of Disease

Isolated CNS vasculitis, if left untreated, leads to a devastating and nearly always fatal outcome.[90,92,93] In the first reported cases, the diagnosis was usually not made until late in the course of the disease or after death. Without therapy, the disease pursues a rapid downhill course, terminating with the development of severe CNS deficits, intractable seizures, and coma.

Uncontrolled Treatment Studies

Because of the rarity of isolated CNS vasculitis, analysis of treatment efficacy has been based on isolated case reports and small case series. These uncontrolled observations suggest that glucocorticoid therapy markedly decreases the mortality and morbidity associated with isolated CNS vasculitis, although nearly half of the patients treated solely with these agents suffer permanent neurologic deficits.[90,92,93] Further improvement in survival and neurologic recovery has been seen when glucocorticoids are combined with daily oral cyclophosphamide.[90–95] Active disease previously uncontrolled with glucocorticoids has responded to the addition of daily oral cyclophosphamide. Calabrese et al.,[91] however, have described a group of patients (mostly women) with isolated CNS vasculitis whose disease follows a relatively benign course and may not require cytotoxic therapy.

Long-Term Experience

Among survivors of isolated CNS vasculitis, more than one third are left with some neurologic impairment.[93] The permanent deficits tend to be severe and include hemiparesis, cortical blindness, quadriplegia, and incontinence.[93,94] Earlier recognition and treatment of patients with isolated CNS vasculitis have probably improved patient outcomes in recent years.

Management

The pharmacologic management of isolated CNS vasculitis is similar to that of systemic vasculitis. Undoubtedly, timely therapy and the potential reversibility of neurologic lesions are major factors in determining outcome. Patients with severe multifocal disease (the majority of cases) are generally treated with glucocorticoids and oral cyclophosphamide in the same manner as patients with PAN (see above). A trial of glucocorticoids alone may be considered in selected patients with mild neurologic dysfunction or who have contraindications to the use of oral cyclophosphamide .

The treatment response should be evaluated by serial neurologic examinations and cerebrospinal fluid analyses (if indicated), as well as by monitoring CNS abnormalities using MRI brain scanning and cerebral arteriography. For example, an MRI brain scan and a cerebral arteriogram (if positive) are often repeated 8 to 12 weeks after the start of therapy to help assess the treatment response and adjust immunosuppressive therapy. Disease progression in the face of glucocorticoid therapy justifies the addition of daily oral cyclophosphamide. With clinical improvement, the prednisone can be tapered to an alternate-day schedule and the oral cyclophosphamide maintained for an additional 12 months after complete remission. Treatment failure calls for careful reappraisal of the original diagnosis and, if appropriate, CNS biopsy.

ESSENTIAL MIXED CRYOGLOBULINEMIA (CRYOGLOBULINEMIA WITH VASCULITIS)

Essential mixed cryoglobulinemia (EMC) is characterized by recurrent purpura, arthralgias/arthritis, hepatomegaly, splenomegaly, nervous system deficits, and glomerulonephritis.[96] By definition, type II or type III serum cryoglobulins must also be present for diagnosis. Recurrent episodes of abdominal pain, pulmonary hemorrhage, and myocardial infarction are among its less common clinical features and reflect the potentially widespread nature of this illness. Recent studies show a striking association between EMC and hepatitis C virus (HCV) infection, suggesting a role for this virus in pathogenesis.[97,98] Although a high prevalence of HBV infection has been reported in patients with EMC,[99] other studies have failed to confirm this association.[100]

Histopathologic examination of skin lesions in EMC reveals perivascular inflammation with varying degrees of leukocytoclasis. The glomerular lesion displays focal or diffuse proliferative changes and intraglomerular thrombi. IgG, IgM, and C3, the most prevalent immunoreactants, produce intense granular staining of peripheral capillary loops and massive staining of intraluminal thrombi.[101] Electron microscopy can reveal electron-dense subendothelial deposits with a peculiar fibrillar or crystalloid structure. These morphologic patterns are also found in the serum cryoprecipitate. Other involved organ systems show histopathologic evidence of a small-vessel vasculitis.

Natural History of Disease and Long-Term Experience

The natural history of EMC can not be determined accurately because most patients with this condition have received immunosuppressive therapy. EMC most likely resembles PAN in its overall prognosis. The episodes of purpura last 3 to 10 days and recur sporadically over a period of years.[101,102] Confluent purpura on the lower legs may evolve into deep ulcers that are susceptible to infection with progression to osteomyelitis.[101,102]

Renal disease develops in a majority of patients and may emerge with the first episode of purpura or, more frequently, several years after the onset of skin and joint disease.[100–103] In one study of 44 patients with EMC, renal involvement was heralded by acute renal failure (two cases), hematuria and proteinuria accompanied by a slow rise in serum creatinine level (six patients), nephrotic syndrome with proteinuria ≥3 g/24 h (eight patients), or hematuria or proteinuria <3 g/24 h with a normal serum creatinine level (28 patients).[103] Hypertension frequently occurs in patients with renal involvement. After initial presentation, the renal lesion pursues a variable course.[100–103] A partial or complete remission of renal disease occurs in nearly one third of the patients. The remainder progress in

an indolent fashion or suffer acute, reversible exacerbations. Whereas earlier workers claimed that progression to chronic renal failure was common in EMC, recent evidence provides a more optimistic outlook and suggests that chronic renal failure develops in only about 10% of the cases.[100]

Most deaths in EMC result from cardiovascular disease, cerebral hemorrhage, or infection.[101,103] Many cardiovascular deaths occur in patients with severe hypertension, although autopsy in two cases found evidence of coronary arteritis.[101] Hypertension and cerebral arteritis are factors in cerebrovascular deaths.[101,103] Infections of chronic, deep skin ulcers can predispose to death from sepsis.[101,103]

Uncontrolled Treatment Studies

The symptoms of cutaneous vasculitis have been successfully managed with salicylates and nonsteroidal antiinflammatory drugs (NSAIDs).[101] Severe visceral organ system manifestations of disease may respond to treatment with glucocorticoids, cytotoxic agents, or PE, or a combination of these measures. For example, renal disease has improved with high doses of glucocorticoids and cyclophosphamide, chlorambucil, or azathioprine, although it can progress despite treatment with the full gamut of immunosuppressive modalities.[100,101,103,104] Intravenous pulse methylprednisolone therapy also may control active nephritis in this setting and induce remissions of extrarenal disease.[101]

PE has theoretic value in EMC because it rapidly removes circulating immune complexes and hence eliminates potentially pathogenic serum cryoglobulins.[105] Although PE reduces the cryocrit (quantitative measure of serum cryoglobulins), studies have not always found a consistent relationship between a high cryocrit and disease activity.[105,106] Disease manifestations can rebound when PE is stopped without concurrent immunosuppressive drug therapy.[106] Cryofiltration has been proposed as a safe and effective alternative to PE because it removes only the cryoprecipitable material from the circulation.[107,108]

Prospective Trials

Interferon-α is effective for the treatment of HCV-associated hepatitis.[109] Prompted by this observation, interferon-α therapy was examined by Ferri et al.[110] in a prospective crossover trial of patients with EMC because of the association between this vasculitic syndrome and HCV infection. Patients were eligible for this trial only if they had liver or neurologic involvement and no clinical evidence of renal disease. HCV infection was documented in 25 of 26 patients with EMC who entered this trial. Interferon-α therapy was associated with statistically significant reductions in the purpura score, liver enzyme values, and cryocrit.[110] On withdrawal of interferon-α, patients often developed a rebound in disease manifestations. Two patients dropped out of the study, one because of a progressive peripheral neuropathy and the other because of the new onset of glomerulonephritis. These results are preliminary and do not support the general use of interferon-α for the treatment of EMC; however, this intervention may be considered in the treatment of patients with HCV-related liver disease independent of vasculitic manifestations.

Management

Uncontrolled observations and the experience of treating other vasculitides form the basis of management of EMC. Episodes of purpura and joint symptoms in EMC are dealt with conservatively using salicylates or NSAIDs. Leg ulcers should be aggressively treated with local measures, such as support stockings and Unna's boots, before systemic therapy is considered. Progressive, severe skin disease may occasionally require treatment with glucocorticoids or cytotoxic agents.

The severity of nephritis in EMC largely determines the use of immunosuppressive therapy. Kidney biopsy can evaluate the morphologic activity and chronicity of the renal lesion and aid treatment decisions. Initial treatment of nephritis consists of 1 mg/kg/d of prednisone and 1 to 2 mg/kg/d of oral cyclophosphamide, as described for PAN. PE may be useful as a supplementary treatment measure, but the data supporting its value are lacking. In more severe cases, intravenous pulse methylprednisolone (e.g., 1 g/d for 3 days) may offer further treatment benefits. The duration of immunosuppressive therapy hinges on the therapeutic response, resembling the approach taken in PAN and WG. Treatment of extrarenal manifestations is analogous to that of

renal disease, with the decision to use glucocorticoids, cytotoxic agents, or both guided by the site of involvement and disease activity.

HENOCH-SCHÖNLEIN PURPURA (ANAPHYLACTOID PURPURA)

Henoch-Schönlein purpura (HSP) is a multisystem disease that primarily affects the skin, joints, gastrointestinal tract, and kidneys.[111] This illness most commonly strikes children, although it occurs in adults. The key clinical feature is a purpuric rash that involves the lower extremities and buttocks. The majority of patients experience joint pain and swelling. Abdominal pain commonly occurs in HSP and may be complicated by gastrointestinal hemorrhage or, rarely, intussusception. Approximately 40% of the patients develop some degree of renal involvement, ranging from microscopic hematuria to acute nephritis and nephrotic syndrome.

In addition to the urinary findings, laboratory studies may reveal mild leukocytosis and an elevated ESR. A characteristic clinical picture with a normal platelet count is usually sufficient for a clinical diagnosis. Biopsy of the purpuric skin lesions reveals a leukocytoclastic vasculitis and prominent IgA deposition in the vessel walls, confirming its vasculitic nature.

Natural History of Disease

The acute illness usually lasts about 4 weeks, but more than one third of the cases persist longer.[112,113] Recurrent episodes of HSP occur in 12% to 40% of children and are reminiscent of the initial clinical presentation, although milder.[112,113] Age greater than 5 years at presentation has been associated with increased renal disease.[114]

Kidney involvement accounts solely for the long-term morbidity and mortality in HSP. Most studies of unselected HSP cases suggest that progression to chronic renal failure occurs in fewer than 5%.[115,116] Kobayashi et al.[115] retrospectively classified 203 Japanese children with HSP according to their renal findings at presentation. They found no abnormalities in 80 (39%), minimal hematuria or proteinuria in 83 (41%), and heavy proteinuria or hematuria in 40 (20%). Many children in the latter group suffered multiple recurrences of nephritis for more than 1 year. Only four cases (2%) showed progressive deterioration in renal function. Adults with HSP have been reported with both a higher[117,118] and a similar[119] frequency of renal disease as children with HSP.

The extent of hematuria, proteinuria, and renal dysfunction at presentation correlates with greater morphologic severity of glomerular disease,[113,114,120] which in turn is associated with worse long-term renal outcomes.[113,114,121] Despite these clinicopathologic correlations, extended follow-up has revealed unexpected deterioration in several HSP patients with only mild renal manifestations at the initial assessment.[121] Furthermore, the predictive value of an initial biopsy is poor because many patients with severe glomerular changes will completely recover from their illness.[121] For these reasons, a renal biopsy is not recommended in the routine initial evaluation of HSP patients.

Treatment Studies

The evidence to date does not show that immunosuppressive therapy alters the natural history of HSP. Glucocorticoids play only a limited role in the treatment of HSP. In the acute illness, they can promptly relieve severe abdominal pain and arrest gastrointestinal hemorrhage.[112] Glucocorticoids and cytotoxic agents have been prescribed during the acute illness to prevent serious renal disease, but they do not appear to change long-term outcomes.[112,113,122]

In a recent prospective trial, 168 children with HSP lacking renal abnormalities at presentation were assigned to receive either no treatment or 1 mg/kg/d of prednisone for 2 weeks.[123] None of the patients in the prednisone-treated group developed clinical signs of nephropathy; microscopic hematuria, proteinuria, or both appeared within 2 to 6 weeks after recovery from the acute illness in 10 of the untreated patients. These abnormalities resolved within 1 year in eight of these children, whereas in the other two children the urinary findings persisted without decline in renal function. Although this study suggests that prednisone therapy may reduce the incidence of early HSP renal disease, it does not address the critical question of whether glucocorticoids prevent progression to chronic renal failure. Given the low incidence of chronic renal failure in HSP and the long natural history of the renal lesion,

an interventional trial would require a large number of patients and many years of follow-up to detect a therapeutic effect. An international group is currently conducting a prospective trial involving large numbers of children with HSP to determine whether early cyclophosphamide therapy can protect against the development of renal disease.[124]

Management

Most children and adults with HSP can be managed conservatively as outpatients during their acute illness. Antibiotics may be necessary to treat an infection that has been appropriately documented by Gram stain or culture. Salicylates and other NSAIDs are the cornerstone of therapy and can alleviate symptoms from purpura and joint manifestations. Patients with severe abdominal pain or other gastrointestinal complications require hospitalization. Severe abdominal pain, melena, or hematemesis usually responds promptly to 1 mg/kg/d of prednisone, which should not be continued longer than 2 weeks. Persistence of abdominal pain beyond 24 hours or a tender abdominal mass may be a sign of intussusception. Such findings call for further diagnostic evaluation and surgical consultation. Hypertension in patients with renal involvement can be treated with standard antihypertensive medications.

HYPERSENSITIVITY VASCULITIS

Hypersensitivity vasculitis defines a heterogenous group of vasculitic disorders in which the predominant pathologic lesion is inflammation of arterioles, capillaries, and venules. Although virtually any organ system or vessel size can be attacked in this condition, skin manifestations and biopsy evidence of leukocytoclastic vasculitis dominate the clinical and histopathologic picture. The cutaneous disease can variously appear as purpura, urticaria-like lesions, bullous lesions, ulcers, erythematous plaques, or nodules.[125,126] Less frequently, hypersensitivity vasculitis may produce vessel inflammation outside the skin, leading to joint, kidney, liver, lung, heart, or nervous system involvement.[125–127]

As the name implies, hypersensitivity vasculitis is thought to represent an immune response to an antigenic stimulus resulting from exposure to an environmental toxin, foreign protein, drug, tumor antigen, infectious agent, or self-antigen. Historically, several clinical syndromes have been included under the general heading of hypersensitivity vasculitis: serum sickness, HSP, EMC, vasculitis associated with malignancies, and vasculitis associated with other primary disorders.[127] These subgroups are distinctive enough to be considered separately from a diagnostic and prognostic standpoint. Hypersensitivity vasculitis is a diagnosis usually reserved for patients with a small-vessel vasculitis that lack these unique additional clinical features.

Natural History of Disease

Serum sickness occurs after exposure to a foreign antigen (e.g., heterologous horse serum) and typically produces a 2- to 4-week self-limited bout of fever, urticaria, arthralgias, and lymphadenopathy. The clinical course of patients with hypersensitivity vasculitis, however, is more unpredictable. In one study of 82 patients with this condition, the clinical course was characterized as acute (56%), chronic (28%), or relapsing (16%), with recurring episodes of skin disease separated by intervals of months to years.[125] The subgroup of patients with drug-related hypersensitivity vasculitis also have a highly variable course. The interval between disease onset and resolution in one large study ranged from 1 day to 10 months; 12 of 100 patients had symptoms that lasted more than 1 month.[126]

Uncontrolled Treatment Studies

Identification and then discontinuation of a potentially inciting drug is effective therapy for most cases of hypersensitivity vasculitis. Skin involvement can respond to treatment with topical glucocorticoids, antihistamines, and NSAIDs.[125] In patients with chronic or relapsing disease, Callen[128] has reported success with oral colchicine in a dose of 0.6 mg twice daily. Other agents, including hydroxychloroquine, dapsone, and azathioprine, have also been occasionally effective in treating this condition. Although systemic glucocorticoids can suppress the development of skin lesions, their withdrawal is invariably followed by new eruptions.

Management

The first step in treating hypersensitivity vasculitis is removal of the offending antigen. Since this process is often self-limited, it is treated conservatively with local measures, including topical glucocorticoids, protective dressings, Unna's boots, and antihistamines and NSAIDs. Treatment with colchicine, hydroxychloroquine, dapsone, or azathioprine may be considered in patients with chronic or relapsing disease. Evidence does not support the prolonged use of glucocorticoids or cytotoxic agents for treating hypersensitivity vasculitis. However, in rare cases, such as severe bullous or ulcerative disease, this approach may be undertaken with caution. The occasional patient with serious or life-threatening systemic involvement may require treatment with 40 to 60 mg/d of prednisone followed by a 2- to 3-month taper to the lowest dose that effectively controls the disease.

COGAN'S SYNDROME

Cogan's syndrome (CS) is a rare disorder characterized by recurrent episodes of bilateral ocular inflammation and vestibuloauditory dysfunction. The hallmark of the ocular involvement is interstitial keratitis, a patchy mononuclear cell infiltrate in the cornea that causes eye discomfort, redness and photophobia.[129] Other types of ocular inflammation, including conjunctivitis, iritis, episcleritis/scleritis, posterior uveitis, vitritis, choroiditis, and retinal vasculitis, may accompany interstitial keratitis.[129] Vestibuloauditory disease, the other major feature of CS, provokes sudden and debilitating attacks resembling Meniere's disease that consist of nausea, vomiting, decreased hearing, and severe vertigo. About half of the CS cases are characterized by simultaneous onset of ocular and vestibuloauditory symptoms; whereas in the remainder the disease unfolds as isolated ocular and vestibuloauditory events occurring within months of each other.[130]

Systemic inflammatory disease arises commonly in CS and may produce constitutional symptoms, CNS manifestations, cutaneous lesions, and systemic necrotizing vasculitis.[129-131] Widespread vasculitis develops in about 10% of CS patients and can affect either large vessels (resembling Takayasu's disease) or medium vessels (PAN-like).[130] Aortic insufficiency with aortitis has been reported in up to 10% of patients with CS.[131]

Natural History of Disease

The ocular outcomes in CS are excellent unless the course is complicated by posterior segment inflammation (e.g., scleritis, vitritis, posterior uveitis). Interstitial keratitis, conjunctivitis, and iritis target the anterior segment of the eye and only rarely cause visual loss. In some of the original cases described by Cogan, however, recurrent bouts of interstitial keratitis resulted in decreased visual acuity from corneal scarring and vascularization.[132,133] In contrast, ocular inflammation of the posterior segment, if left unchecked, can rapidly destroy ocular tissue and cause permanent visual loss. Blindness has been reported in about 5% of CS patients and results from ocular inflammation beyond the anterior segment.[129,131]

Hearing loss, sometimes asymmetrical, is the major cause of morbidity in CS. Deafness was noted in 21 of 78[130] ears in one recent series and 78 of 156[131] ears in another previous review. Vestibular symptoms usually resolve, although mild oscillopsia may persist in the minority of cases. Cochlear hydrops can develop as a consequence of prolonged disease and produce hearing fluctuations from hormonal changes (e.g., menstrual cycle in women), ingestion of salty foods, allergic conditions, or an upper respiratory illness. Such hearing fluctuations are clinically indistinguishable from those of inflammatory origin.

Treatment Studies

Prompt treatment of interstitial keratitis with topical glucocorticoids usually prevents corneal scarring and vascularization.[130,134] The rare occurrence of severe visual loss from corneal scarring has been surgically treated with corneal transplantation. Posterior segment ocular disease has responded variably to treatment with systemic glucocorticoids, cyclophosphamide, and cyclosporin A.[61,129,135,136]

Acute hearing loss may be at least partially restored by systemic prednisone therapy 1 to 2 mg/kg/d.[135] Some evidence suggests that prompt therapy with systemic glucocorticoids can reduce chronic hearing loss.[137] Acute hearing loss resistant to glucocorticoid therapy has been managed successfully with oral cyclophosphamide, methotrexate, and azathioprine therapy;[135] however, the true efficacy of these agents is uncertain, given the variable nature of the

disease. Patients with permanent deafness from CS have benefited from cochlear implants.

Aortic insufficiency due to aortitis has improved after treatment with glucocorticoids and cytotoxic agents.[129] Other patients have required aortic valve replacement.[128,131,138] Large- and medium-vessel vasculitis in CS can be controlled with prednisone, oral cyclophosphamide, and cyclosporin A.[61,129,130] Occlusive vascular disease from coronary[129] and mesenteric[139] arteritis has necessitated surgical bypass to correct end-organ ischemia.

Management

Interstitial keratitis and iritis are satisfactorily managed with mydriatics and topical glucocorticoid therapy. Ocular signs and symptoms generally improve within 3 to 7 days after the start of therapy. A poor treatment response may signal the presence of another disease process such as chlamydial infection, which can mimic the ocular manifestations of CS.[140] Episcleritis and scleritis also usually resolve with topical glucocorticoid therapy. In contrast, nodular scleritis, posterior uveitis, and retinal artery disease often demand systemic therapy consisting initially of 1 to 2 mg/kg/d of prednisone for 1 month, followed by a gradual dosage taper over the next 2 to 3 months (see Table 10–2). Serious ocular inflammation that progresses despite glucocorticoid therapy can be treated with oral cyclophosphamide or cyclosporin A.[136] Since such cytotoxic therapy is potentially hazardous, end points must be set to define the period of therapy.

Audiograms are obtained routinely to quantify hearing loss and follow the response to therapy. Patients with acute hearing loss are initially given a 2-week trial of prednisone at a dose of 1 mg/kg/d. This dose of prednisone is usually maintained for an additional 2 weeks with a favorable treatment response and tapered within 6 to 8 weeks to an alternate-day regimen as long as auditory acuity is preserved. Some patients require continuous low doses of prednisone on a daily or alternate-day schedule to prevent further deterioration in hearing, whereas others can stop prednisone for variable periods and maintain their hearing. Patients whose auditory acuity does not improve with glucocorticoids may be treated with oral cyclophosphamide (1 to 2 mg/kg/d), metho-

TABLE 10–4
Guidelines for Initial Therapy of the Major Vasculitic Syndromes

DISEASE CATEGORY	INITIAL THERAPY	INITIAL REMISSION RATE WITH STANDARD THERAPY
PAN and CSS	Prednisone 1 mg/kg/d (mild disease)	More than 80%
	Prednisone 1 mg/kg/d + oral cyclophosphamide 1–2 mg/kg/d (serious disease)	
Isolated CNS vasculitis	Same as above	50–75%
Wegener's granulomatosis	Prednisone 1 mg/kg/d + oral cyclophosphamide 1–2 mg/kg/d	75%
Essential mixed cryoglobulinemia	Prednisone 1 mg/kg/d + oral cyclophosphamide 1–2 mg/kg/d (serious organ system disease)	Variable
Henoch-Schönlein purpura	Antihistamines, NSAIDs	More than 80%
Hypersensitivity vasculitis	Antihistamines, NSAIDs	More than 75%
	Colchicine (chronic cases)	
Cogan's syndrome	Topical steroids (ocular)	Hearing stabilized in 50%
	Prednisone 1 mg/kg/d (acute hearing loss)	

NSAIDs = Nonsteroidal antiinflammatory drugs (avoid in patients with renal insufficiency).

trexate (7.5 to 20 mg/wk), or azathioprine (2 mg/kg/d). Since the benefits of these agents are uncertain, therapeutic response criteria are mandatory to define the period of treatment.

The heart should be periodically examined for signs of aortic insufficiency. Cardiac symptoms, signs of heart failure, or clinical evidence of a valvular abnormality may merit further diagnostic evaluation with two-dimensional echocardiography or cardiac catheterization. The treatment of systemic inflammatory vascular disease in CS parallels that described for PAN.

CONCLUDING REMARKS

The management of the major vasculitic syndromes is summarized in Table 10–4. These recommendations serve as treatment guides, recognizing that the standard approach can entail modification in individual cases. Beyond current therapy, future progress in the management of vasculitis likely will come from new insights into disease pathogenesis. Advances of this kind may suggest novel therapies, which will need to be tested in prospective clinical trials. These studies are difficult to perform because of the relatively low incidence of most vasculitic syndromes. Hence, one institution usually cannot enroll enough patients in any single disease category to meet the sample size requirements of a definitive clinical study. Accomplishing this task will require the cooperative efforts of researchers at multiple institutions.

ACKNOWLEDGMENTS

The author thanks David Pisetsky, Rex McCallum, Nancy Allen, and Barton Haynes for reviewing this chapter and providing needed advice and criticism. Appreciation is also extended to my other valued colleagues, John Rice and David Caldwell, who have taught me much about vasculitis and its treatment.

REFERENCES

1. Haynes BF. Vasculitis: pathogenic mechanisms of vessel damage. In: Gallin JI, Goldstein IM, Snyderman R, eds. Inflammation: basic principles and clinical correlates. 2nd ed. New York: Raven Press 1992.
2. Fauci AS, Haynes BF, Katz P. The spectrum of vasculitis: clinical, pathologic, immunologic, and therapeutic considerations. Ann Intern Med 1978;89:660.
3. Hunder GG, Arends WP, Bloch DA, et al. The American College of Rheumatology 1990 criteria for the classification of vasculitis. Arthritis Rheum 1990;33:1065.
4. Leavitt RY, Fauci AS. Polyangiitis overlap syndrome: classification and prospective clinical experience. Am J Med 1986;81:79.
5. Savage COS, Winearls CG, Evans DJ, et al. Microscopic polyarteritis: presentation, pathology, and prognosis. Q J Med 1985;56:467.
6. Gocke DJ, Hsu K, Morgan C, et al. Association between polyarteritis and Australia antigen. Lancet 1970;2:1149.
7. Sergent JS, Lockshin MD, Christian CL, et al. Vasculitis with hepatitis B antigenemia: long-term observations in nine patients. Medicine 1976;55:1.

8. McMahon BJ, Heyward WL, Templin DW, et al. Hepatitis B–associated polyarteritis nodosa in Alaskan Eskimos: clinical and epidemiologic features and long-term follow-up. Hepatology 1989;9:97.

9. Quint L, Deny P, Guillevin L, et al. Hepatitis C virus in patients with polyarteritis nodosa: prevalence in 38 patients. Clin Exp Rheumatol 1991;9:253.

10. Carson CW, Conn DL, Czaja AJ, et al. Frequency and significance of antibodies to hepatitis C virus in polyarteritis nodosa. J Rheumatol 1993;20:304.

11. Diaz-Perez JL, Winkelmann RK. Cutaneous periarteritis nodosa: a study of 33 cases. In: Wolff K, Winkelmann R, eds. Major problems in dermatology. Philadelphia: WB Saunders 1980:273.

12. Conn DL, Hunder GG, O'Duffy JD. Vasculitis and related disorders. In: Kelley WN, Harris ED, Ruddy S, Sledge CB, eds. Textbook of rheumatology. 4th ed. Philadelphia: WB Saunders, 1993:1077.

13. Churg J, Strauss L. Allergic granulomatosis, allergic angiitis, and periarteritis nodosa. Am J Pathol 1951;27:277.

14. Lanham JG, Elkon KB, Pusey CD, et al. Systemic vasculitis with asthma and eosinophilia: a clinical approach to the Churg-Strauss syndrome. Medicine 1984;63:65.

15. Lanham JG, Churg J. Churg-Strauss syndrome. In: Churg A, Churg J, eds. Systemic vasculitis. New York: Igaku-Shoin, 1991:101.

16. Ewald EA, Griffin D, McCune WJ. Correlation of angiographic abnormalities with disease manifestations and disease severity in polyarteritis nodosa. J Rheumatol 1987;14:952.

17. Lie JT. Diagnostic histopathology of major systemic and pulmonary vasculitic syndromes. Rheum Dis Clin North Am 1990;16:269.

18. Frohnert PP, Sheps SG. Long-term follow-up study of periarteritis nodosa. Am J Med 1967; 43:8.

19. Lieb ES, Restivo C, Paulus HE. Immunosuppressive and corticosteroid therapy of polyarteritis nodosa. Am J Med 1979;67:941.

20. Report to the Medical Research Council by the Collagen Diseases and Hypersensitivity Panel. Treatment of polyarteritis nodosa with cortisone: results after three years. Br Med J 1960; 1:1399.

21. Scott DGI, Bacon PA, Elliott PJ, et al. Systemic vasculitis in a district general hospital 1972–1980: clinical and laboratory features, classification and prognosis of 80 cases. Q J Med 1982;51:292.

22. Rose GA, Spencer H. Polyarteritis nodosa. Q J Med 1957;26:43.

23. Cohen RD, Conn DL, Ilstrup DM. Clinical features, prognosis, and response to treatment in polyarteritis nodosa. Mayo Clin Proc 1980;55:146.

24. Fauci AS, Doppman JL, Wolff SM. Cyclophosphamide-induced remissions in advanced polyarteritis nodosa. Am J Med 1978;64:890.

25. Turna S, Chaimovitz C, Szylman P, et al. Periarteritis nodosa in the kidney: recovery following immunosuppressive therapy. JAMA 1976; 235:280.

26. Fauci AS, Katz P, Haynes BF, et al. Cyclophosphamide therapy of severe systemic necrotizing vasculitis. N Engl J Med 1979;301:235.

27. Chumbley LC, Harrison EG, DeRemee RA. Allergic granulomatosis and angiitis (Churg-Strauss syndrome): report and analysis of 30 cases. Mayo Clin Proc 1977;52:477.

28. Cooper BJ, Bacal E, Patterson R. Allergic angiitis and granulomatosis. Arch Intern Med 1978;138:367.

29. Guillevin L, Fain O, Lhote F, et al. Lack of superiority of steroids plus plasma exchange to steroids alone in the treatment of polyarteritis nodosa and Churg-Strauss syndrome. Arthritis Rheum 1992;35:208.

30. Guillevin L, Jarrousse B, Lok C, et al. Long-term follow-up after treatment of polyarteritis nodosa and Churg-Strauss angiitis with comparison of steroids, plasma exchange and cyclophosphamide to steroids and plasma exchange: a prospective randomized trial of 71 patients. J Rheumatol 1991;18:567.

31. Guillevin L, Le Thi Huong D, Gayraud M. Systemic vasculitis of the polyarteritis nodosa group and infections with hepatitis B virus: a study in 98 patients. Eur J Intern Med 1989;1:97.

32. Perillo RP. Antiviral therapy of chronic hepatitis B: past, present, and future. J Hepatol 1993; 17(suppl 3):S56.

33. Lam KC, Lai CL, Ng RP, et al. Deleterious effect of prednisolone in HBsAg-positive chronic active hepatitis. N Engl J Med 1981;304:380.

34. Johnson RJ, Couser WG. Hepatitis B infection and renal disease: clinical, immunopathogenetic, and therapeutic considerations. Kidney Int 1990;37:663.

35. Guillevin L, Lhote F, Jarrousse B, et al. Treatment of polyarteritis nodosa and Churg-Strauss syndrome: a meta-analysis of 3 prospective controlled trials including 182 patients over 12 years. Ann Med Intern 1992;143:405.

36. Perillo RP. Interferon in the management of chronic hepatitis B. Dig Dis Sci 1993;38:577.

37. Gordon M, Luqmani RA, Adu D, et al. Relapses in patients with a systemic vasculitis. Q J Med 1993;86:779.

38. Haynes BF, Allen NB, Fauci AS. Diagnostic and therapeutic approach to the patient with vasculitis. Med Clin North Am 1986;70:355.

39. Cupps TR, Fauci AS. The vasculitides. Philadelphia: WB Saunders, 1981:42.

40. Jorizzo JL, White WL, Wise CM, et al. Low-dose weekly methotrexate for unusual neutrophilic vascular reactions: cutaneous polyarteritis nodosa and Behcet's disease. J Am Acad Dermatol 1991;24:973.

41. Haynes BF. Glucocorticosteroid therapy. In: Wyngaarden JB, Smith LH Jr, Bennett JC, eds. Cecil's textbook of medicine. Philadelphia: WB Saunders, 1992:104.

42. Axelrod L. Glucocorticoids. In: Kelley WN, Harris ED, Ruddy S, Sledge CB, eds. Textbook of rheumatology. 4th ed. Philadelphia: WB Saunders, 1993:779.

43. Fauci AS, Young KR Jr. Immunoregulatory agents. In: Kelley WN, Harris ED, Ruddy S, Sledge CB, eds. Textbook of rheumatology. 4th ed. Philadelphia: WB Saunders, 1993:797.

44. Orth DN, Kovacs WJ, Debold CR. The adrenal cortex. In: Wilson JD, Foster DW, eds. Williams' textbook of endocrinology. Philadelphia: WB Saunders, 1992:532.

45. Fraiser LH, Kanekal S, Kehrer JP. Cyclophosphamide toxicity. Characterizing and avoiding the problem. Drugs 1991;42:781.

46. Bradley JD, Brandt KD, Katz BP. Infectious complications of cyclophosphamide treatment for vasculitis. Arthritis Rheum 1989;32:45.

47. Sen RP, Walsh TE, Fisher W, et al. Pulmonary complication of combination therapy with cyclophosphamide and prednisone. Chest 1991; 99:143.

48. Boumpas DT, Austin HA, Vaughn EM, et al. Risk for sustained amenorrhea in patients with systemic lupus erythematosus receiving intermittent pulse cyclophosphamide therapy. Ann Intern Med 1993;119:366.

49. Chapman RM, Sutcliffe SB. Protection of ovarian function by oral contraceptives in women receiving chemotherapy for Hodgkin's disease. Blood 1981;58:849.

50. Stein JP, Skinner EC, Boyd SD, et al. Squamous cell carcinoma of the bladder associated with cyclophosphamide therapy for Wegener's granulomatosis. J Urol 1993;149:588.

51. Shepherd JD, Pringle LE, Barnett MJ, et al. Mesna versus hyperhydration for the prevention of cyclophosphamide-induced hemorrhagic cystitis in bone marrow transplantation. J Clin Oncol 1991;9:2016.

52. Goren MP, Lyman BA, Li JT. The stability of mesna in beverages and syrup for oral administration. Cancer Chemother Pharmacol 1991; 28:298.

53. Escalante A, Kaufman RL, Beardmore TD. Acute myelocytic leukemia after the use of cyclophosphamide in the treatment of polyarteritis nodosa. J Rheumatol 1989;16:1147.

54. Guillevin L, Rosser J, Cacoub P, et al. Methylprednisolone in the treatment of Wegener's granulomatosis, polyarteritis nodosa and Churg-Strauss angiitis. APMIS (suppl) 1990;19:98.

55. MacFayden R, Tron V, Keshmiri M, et al. Allergic angiitis of Churg and Strauss syndrome: response to pulse methylprednisolone. Chest 1987;91:629.

56. Austin HA, Klippel JH, Balow JE. Therapy of lupus nephritis: controlled trial of prednisone and cytotoxic drugs. N Engl J Med 1986;314:614.

57. Fort JG, Abruzzo JL. Reversal of progressive necrotizing vasculitis with intravenous pulse cyclophosphamide and methylprednisolone. Arthritis Rheum 1988;31:1194.

58. De Vita S, Neri R, Bombardieri S. Cyclophosphamide pulses in the treatment of rheumatic diseases: an update. Clin Exp Rheumatol 1991;9:179.

59. Chow C, Li EKM, Lai FM. Allergic granulomatosis and angiitis (Churg-Strauss syndrome): response to pulse intravenous cyclophosphamide. Ann Rheum Dis 1989;48:605.

60. Hoffman GS, Leavitt RY, Fleisher TA, et al. Treatment of Wegener's granulomatosis with intermittent high-dose intravenous cyclophosphamide. Am J Med 1990;89:403.

61. Allen NB, Caldwell DS, Rice JR, et al. Cyclosporin A therapy for Wegener's granulomatosis. In: Gross WL, ed. ANCA-associated vasculitides: immunological and clinical aspects. New York: Plenum Press, 1993:473.

62. Mathieson PW, Cobbold SP, Hale G, et al. Monoclonal antibody therapy in systemic vasculitis. N Engl J Med 1990;323:250.

63. Lockwood CM, Thiru S, Isaacs JD, et al. Long-term remission of intractable systemic vasculitis with monoclonal antibody therapy. Lancet 1993;341:1620.

64. Carrington CB, Liebow AA. Limited forms of angiitis and granulomatosis of Wegener's type. Am J Med 1966;41:497.

65. Cassan SM, Coles DT, Harrison EG. The concept of limited forms of Wegener's granulomatosis. Am J Med 1970;49:366.

66. Hoffman GS, Kerr GS, Leavitt RY, et al. Wegener granulomatosis: an analysis of 158 patients. Ann Intern Med 1992;116:488.

67. Nölle B, Specks U, Lüdemann J, et al. Anticytoplasmic autoantibodies: their immunodiagnostic value in Wegener granulomatosis. Ann Intern Med 1989;111:28.

68. Cohen Trevaert JW, van der Woude FJ, Fauci AS, et al. Association between active Wegener's granulomatosis and anticytoplasmic antibodies. Arch Intern Med 1989;149:2461.

69. Specks U, Wheatley CL, McDonald TJ, et al. Anticytoplasmic autoantibodies in the diagnosis and follow-up of Wegener's granulomatosis. Mayo Clin Proc 1989;64:28.

70. Kerr GS, Fleisher TA, Hallahan CW, et al. Limited prognostic value of changes in antineutrophil cytoplasmic antibody titer in patients with Wegener's granulomatosis. Arthritis Rheum 1993;36:365.

71. Walton EW. Giant-cell granuloma of the respiratory tract (Wegener's granulomatosis). Br Med J 1958;2:265.

72. Fred HL, Lynch EC, Greenberg SD, et al. A patient with Wegener's granulomatosis exhibiting unusual clinical and morphologic features. Am J Med 1964;37:311.

73. Hollander D, Manning RT. The use of alkylating agents in the treatment of Wegener's granulomatosis. Ann Intern Med 1967;67:393.

74. Fauci AS, Wolff SM. Wegener's granulomatosis: studies in eighteen patients and a review of the literature. Medicine 1973;52:535.

75. Fauci AS, Haynes BF, Katz P, et al. Wegener's granulomatosis: prospective clinical and thera-

peutic experience with 85 patients for 21 years. Ann Intern Med 1983;98:76.

76. Drosos AA, Sakkas LI, Goussia A, et al. Pulse cyclophosphamide therapy in Wegener's granulomatosis: a pilot study. J Intern Med 1992; 232:279.

77. Hoffman GS, Leavitt RY, Kerr GS, et al. The treatment of Wegener's granulomatosis with glucocorticoids and methotrexate. Arthritis Rheum 1992;35:1322.

78. Haynes BF, Fishman ML, Fauci AS, et al. The ocular manifestations of Wegener's granulomatosis: fifteen years experience and review of the literature. Am J Med 1977;63:131.

79. DeRemee RA, McDonald TJ, Weiland LH. Wegener's granulomatosis: observations on treatment with antimicrobial agents. Mayo Clin Proc 1985;60:27.

80. West BC, Todd JR, King JW. Wegener granulomatosis and trimethoprim-sulfamethoxazole. Ann Intern Med 1987;106:840.

81. Leavitt RY, Hoffman GS, Fauci AS. Response: the role of trimethoprim/sulfamethoxazole in the treatment of Wegener's granulomatosis. Arthritis Rheum 1988;31:1073.

82. Israel HL. Sulfamethoxazole-trimethoprim therapy for Wegener's granulomatosis. Arch Intern Med 1988;148:2293.

83. DeRemee RA. The treatment of Wegener's granulomatosis with trimethoprim/sulfamethoxazole: illusion or vision? Arthritis Rheum 1988;31:1068.

84. Valeriano-Marcet J, Spiera H. Treatment of Wegener's granulomatosis with sulfamethoxazole-trimethoprim. Arch Intern Med 1991;151: 1649.

85. Alloway JA, Cupps TR. High dose methylprednisolone for retroorbital Wegener's granulomatosis. J Rheumatol 1993;20:752.

86. Chapman PT, O'Donnell JL. Respiratory failure in Wegener's granulomatosis: response to pulse intravenous methylprednisolone and cyclophosphamide. J Rheumatol 1993;20:504.

87. Harley N, Ihle B. Wegener's granulomatosis— use of cyclosporin A: a case report. Aust NZ J Med 1990;20:71.

88. Tuso P, Moudgil A, Hay J, et al. Treatment of antineutrophil cytoplasmic autoantibody-positive systemic vasculitis and glomerulonephritis with pooled intravenous gammaglobulin. Am J Kidney Dis 1992;20:504.

89. D'Cruz D, Payne H, Timothy A, et al. Response of cyclophosphamide-resistant Wegener's granulomatosis to etoposide. Lancet 1992; 340:425.

90. Sigal LH. Cerebral vasculitis. In: McCarty DJ, Koopman WJ, eds. Arthritis and allied conditions. 12th ed. Philadelphia: Lea & Febiger, 1993:1131.

91. Calabrese LH, Gragg LA, Furlan AJ. Benign angiopathy: a distinct subset of angiographically defined primary angiitis of the central nervous system. J Rheumatol 1993;20:2046.

92. Sigal LH. The neurologic presentation of vasculitic and rheumatologic syndromes. Medicine 1987;66:157.

93. Calabrese LH, Mallek JA. Primary angiitis of the central nervous system: report of 8 new cases, review of the literature, and proposal for diagnostic criteria. Medicine 1987;67:20.

94. Cupps TR, Moore PM, Fauci AS. Isolated angiitis of the central nervous system: prospective diagnostic and therapeutic experience. Am J Med 1983;74:97.

95. Moore PM. Diagnosis and management of isolated angiitis of the central nervous system. Neurology 1989;39:167.

96. Meltzer M, Franklin EC, Elias K, et al. Cryoglobulinemia: a clinical and laboratory study. II. Cryoglobulins and rheumatoid factor activity. Am J Med 1966;40:837.

97. Agnello V, Chung RT, Kaplan LM. A role for hepatitis C virus infection in type II cryoglobulinemia. N Engl J Med 1992;327:1490.

98. Misiani R, Bellavita P, Fenili D, et al. Hepatitis C virus infection in patients with essential mixed cryoglobulinemia. Ann Intern Med 1992;117:573.

99. Gorevic PD, Kassar HJ, Levo Y, et al. Mixed cryoglobulinemia: clinical aspects and long-term follow-up of 40 patients. Am J Med 1980; 69:287.

100. Popp JW Jr, Dienstag JL, Wands JR, et al. Essential mixed cryoglobulinemia without evidence for hepatitis B infection. Ann Intern Med 1980;92:379.

101. D'Amico G, Colasanti G, Ferrario F, et al. Renal involvement in essential mixed cryoglobulinemia. Kidney Int 1989;35:1004.

102. Frankel AH, Singer DRJ, Winearls CG, et al. Type II essential mixed cryoglobulinemia: presentation, treatment and outcome in 13 patients. Q J Med 1992;82:101.

103. Tarantino A, De Vecchi A, Montagnino G, et al. Renal disease in essential mixed cryoglobulinemia: long-term follow-up of 44 patients. Q J Med 1981;197:1.

104. Germain MJ, Anderson RW, Keane WF. Renal disease in cryoglobulinemia type II: response to therapy. Am J Nephrol 1982;2:221.

105. Geltner D, Kohn RW, Gorevic P, et al. The effect of combination therapy (steroids, immunosuppressives, and plasmapheresis) on 5 mixed cryoglobulinemia patients with renal, neurologic, and vascular involvement. Arthritis Rheum 1981;24:1121.

106. Ferri C, Moriconi L, Gremignai G, et al. Treatment of the renal involvement in mixed cryoglobulinemia with prolonged plasma exchange. Nephron 1986;43:246.

107. McLeod BC, Sassetti RJ. Plasmapheresis with return of cryoglobulin-depleted autologous plasma (cryoglobulinpheresis) in cryoglobulinemia. Blood 1980;55:866.

108. Sawada K, Segal AM, Malchesky PS, et al. Rapid improvement in a patient with leukocyto-

clastic vasculitis with secondary mixed cryoglobulinemia treated with cryofiltration. J Rheumatol 1991;18:91.

109. Hoofnagle JH, Muller KD, Jones B, et al. Treatment of chronic non-A non-B hepatitis with recombinant human alpha-interferon. N Engl J Med 1986;315:1575.

110. Ferri C, Marzo E, Longombardo G, et al. Interferon-α in mixed cryoglobulinemia patients: a randomized, crossover-controlled trial. Blood 1993;81:1132.

111. Cassidy JT. Systemic lupus erythematosus, juvenile dermatomyositis, scleroderma, and vasculitis. In: Kelley WN, Harris ED, Ruddy S, Sledge CB, eds. Textbook of rheumatology. 4th ed. Philadelphia: WB Saunders 1993:1243.

112. Allen DM, Diamond LK, Howell DA. Anaphylactoid purpura in children (Schönlein-Henoch syndrome). Am J Dis Child 1960;99:833.

113. Meadow SR, Glasgow EF, White RH, et al. Schönlein-Henoch nephritis. Q J Med 1972; 41:241.

114. Meadow SR. The prognosis of Henoch Schönlein nephritis. Clin Nephrol 1978;9:87.

115. Koskimies O, Mir S, Rapola J, et al. Henoch-Schönlein nephritis: long-term prognosis of unselected patients. Arch Dis Child 1981;56:482.

116. Kobayashi O, Wada H, Okawa K, et al. Schönlein-Henoch's syndrome in children. Contrib Nephrol 1977;4:48.

117. Faull RJ, Woodroffe AJ, Aarons I, et al. Adult Henoch-Schönlein nephritis. Aust NZ J Med 1987;17:396.

118. Fogazzi GB, Pasquali S, Moriggi M, et al. Long-term outcome of Schönlein-Henoch nephritis in the adult. Clin Nephrol 1989;31:60.

119 Cream JJ, Gumpel JM, Peachey RDG. Schönlein-Henoch purpura in the adult: a study of 77 adults with anaphylactoid or Schönlein-Henoch purpura. Q J Med 1970;39:461.

120. Niaudet P, Levy M, Broyer M, et al. Clinicopathologic correlations in severe forms of Henoch-Schönlein purpura nephritis based on repeat biopsies. Contrib Nephrol 1984;40: 250.

121. Goldstein AR, White RHR, Akuse R, et al. Long-term follow-up of childhood Henoch-Schönlein nephritis. Lancet 1992;339:280.

122. Saulsbury FT. Corticosteroid therapy does not prevent nephritis in Henoch-Schönlein purpura. Pediatr Nephrol 1993;7:69.

123. Mollica F, Li Volti S, Garozzo R, et al. Effectiveness of early prednisone treatment in preventing the development of nephropathy in anaphylactoid purpura. Eur J Pediatr 1992; 151:140.

124. White RHR. Henoch-Schönlein purpura. In: Churg A, Churg J, eds. Systemic vasculitides. New York: Igaku-Shoin, 1990:203.

125. Ekenstam E, Callen JP. Cutaneous leukocytoclastic vasculitis: clinical and laboratory features of 82 patients seen in private practice. Arch Dermatol 1984;120:484.

126. Haber MM, Marboe CC, Fenoglio JJ Jr. Vasculitis in drug and serum sickness. In: Churg A, Churg J, eds. Systemic vasculitides. New York: Igaku-Shoin, 1990:305.

127. Cupps TR, Fauci AS. The vasculitides. Philadelphia: WB Saunders 1981:50.

128. Callen JP. Colchicine is effective in controlling chronic cutaneous leukocytoclastic vasculitis. J Am Acad Dermatol 1985;13:193.

129. Haynes BF, Kaiser-Kupfer MI, Mason P, et al. Cogan's syndrome: studies in thirteen patients, long-term follow-up, and a review of the literature. Medicine 1980;59:426.

130. McCallum RM, Haynes BF. Cogan's syndrome. In: Pepose JS, Holland GN, Wilhelmus KR, eds. Ocular infection and immunity. St. Louis: Mosby–Year Book (in press).

131. Vollersten RS, McDonald TJ, Younge BR, et al. Cogan's syndrome: 18 cases and a review of the literature. Mayo Clin Proc 1986;61:344.

132. Cogan DG. Nonsyphilitic interstitial keratitis and vestibuloauditory symptoms: report of four additional cases. Arch Ophthal 1949;42:42.

133. Cogan DG. Syndrome of nonsyphilitic interstitial keratitis and vestibuloauditory symptoms. Arch Ophthal 1945;33:144.

134. Cobo LM, Haynes BF. Early corneal findings in Cogan's syndrome. Opthalmology 1984;91:903.

135. McCallum RM. Cogan's syndrome. In: Franunfelder FT, Hampton R, eds. Current ocular therapy. 4th ed. Philadelphia: WB Saunders 1993 (in press).

136. Allen NB, Cox CC, Cobo M, et al. Use of immunosuppressive agents in the treatment of severe ocular and vascular manifestations of Cogan's syndrome. Am J Med 1990;88:296.

137. McCallum RM. Cogan's syndrome: clinical features and outcomes. Arthritis Rheum 1992; 35(suppl):S51.

138. Bielory L, Conti J, Frohman L. Cogan's syndrome. J Allergy Clin Immunol 1990;85:808.

139. LaRaja RD. Cogan syndrome associated with mesenteric vascular insufficiency. Arch Surg 1976;111:1028.

140. Darougar S, John AC, Viswalingam M, et al. Isolation of *Chlamydia pssittaci* from a patient with interstitial keratitis and uveitis associated with otological and cardiovascular lesions. Br J Ophthalmol 1978;62:709.

CHAPTER 1

POLYMYALGIA RHEUMATICA, TEMPORAL (GIANT CELL) ARTERITIS, AND TAKAYASU'S ARTERITIS

Gregory C. Gardner

Polymyalgia rheumatica and temporal arteritis began to emerge separately as clinical syndromes in the 1930s. Their recognition has probably been aided by the increasing life expectancy in the industrialized nations, since most of the cases occur in the sixth and seventh decades. The relationship between polymyalgia rheumatica and giant cell arteritis was recognized in the late 1950s, but for the purpose of this discussion we will consider the treatment of the two separately. Takayasu's arteritis is histologically similar to giant cell arteritis, but it has a dissimilar epidemiology and vascular distribution. This chapter will address treatment of these three diseases, with emphasis on more recent developments in the field. (For a general discussion of the epidemiology, etiopathogenesis, and differential diagnosis of giant cell arteritis and polymyalgia rheumatica, see Hunder in Kelley et al., reference 38.)

POLYMYALGIA RHEUMATICA

Natural History of Polymyalgia Rheumatica

In 1888 Bruce reported on a disease he named "senile rheumatic gout" in five patients 60 to 70 years of age.[1] They had widespread muscular and joint stiffness and, although the symptoms were quite disabling, complete recovery occurred in 1 to 2 years in all of the patients. Since that time, the syndrome we now know as polymyalgia rheumatica has been given a variety of names, including secondary fibrositis, periar-throsis humeroscapularis, peri-extraarticular rheumatism, anarthritic rheumatoid arthritis, pseudopolyarthrite rhizomelique, and polymyalgia arteritica.[2] Barber[3] first used "polymyalgia rheumatica" as a term to denote the syndrome in 1957, and this designation was adopted but not without some debate.

A 1960 paper by Ian Gordon[4] is useful for its description of the precorticosteroid course of the disease. In that report, Gordon describes 21 patients with polymyalgia rheumatica and in some detail records the course of eight patients who had never received corticosteroids. He divided the course of the illness into two stages based on his experience with these patients. Stage 1 is characterized by severe pain and stiffness of the proximal musculature. In six of the patients, the disease reached its maximum intensity within a few weeks of the onset of symptoms; for the other two the maximum intensity was at approximately 4 to 5 months after symptoms first appeared. Stiffness to the point of being incapacitating occurred in two patients but lasted less than 4 months. This first stage lasted an average of 18 months, with a range of 9 to 30 months. Gordon's stage 2 is characterized by mild morning stiffness or stiffness after prolonged sitting, although the patient generally believed that the disease was essentially cured. The sedimentation rate continued to be mildly elevated in this stage but was much reduced from the initial level. This stage lasted an average of 15 months, with a range of 7 to 25 months. The disease then remitted completely, and there were no recurrences in any of these eight patients during the observation period of up to 5 years. All patients were treated during the more severe periods of the disease with bed rest, exercises, salicylates, and in some cases phenylbutazone, but these effected only mild relief. The shortest disease duration was 24 months and the longest was 50 months, with the average being 33 months.

As first suggested by Gordon, recurrence of disease (once the patient is free of medication and symptoms) is relatively uncommon. Infrequent recurrence was reported in other early studies[2] and more recently recurrence was seen in only 4 of 93 patients followed during a 10-year period at the Mayo Clinic[5] and 19 of 114 patients followed for 12 years at St. Peter's Hospital in Surrey, England.[6] In the latter study, 90% of the recurrences were within 1 year of discontinuation of corticosteroids and almost 50% were within the first 6 months.

One of the more important aspects of the natural history of polymyalgia rheumatica is the possible development of giant cell arteritis. A review of the literature regarding the incidence of a positive temporal artery biopsy in clinically pure polymyalgia rheumatica by Healey and Wilske[7] revealed numbers ranging from 6% to 41%. The important question is how often a patient with clinically pure polymyalgia rheumatica develops clinical giant cell arteritis. Chuang et al.[5] found over a 10-year period that 9 of 90 patients with clinically pure polymyalgia rheumatica went on to develop manifestations of giant cell arteritis between 1 month and $2^1/_2$ years after first presenting with polymyalgia rheumatica.[5] Spiera and Davison[8] reported that only 4 of 400 patients seen in their clinic developed giant cell arteritis after first presenting with only polymyalgia rheumatica. Delecoeuillerie et al.[9] reported a 7% incidence of giant cell arteritis developing in 132 patients with clinically pure polymyalgia rheumatica. Of interest, the presence or absence of a positive temporal artery biopsy in this group was not predictive of who would go on to develop giant cell arteritis, as none of the nine patients with clinically pure polymyalgia rheumatica with a positive temporal artery biopsy developed clinical giant cell arteritis during the 10-year follow-up period. This last concept is further strengthened by Behn et al.,[6] who found that only 2 of 11 patients with clinically pure polymyalgia rheumatica and positive temporal

artery biopsies developed clinical giant cell arteritis in spite of what appears to have been corticosteroid levels typically used to treat polymyalgia rheumatica. A dissenting voice comes from Jones and Hazleman[10] who reported that 42% of their patients with polymyalgia rheumatica seen over a 5-year period developed giant cell arteritis, although they pointed out that their hospital-based study may have been biased toward more severe disease.

In general, the recent literature suggests that temporal artery biopsy is unnecessary in patients with clinically pure polymyalgia rheumatica. A small minority of patients with clincially pure polymyalgia rheumatica develop giant cell arteritis, and several reports have commented on the rarity of blindness or other significant consequences in the patients who do. This is probably due to the fact that these patients are under medical observation and are usually warned about the symptoms of giant cell arteritis.

Treatment of Polymyalgia Rheumatica

The efficacy of low-dose corticosteroids in the treatment of polymyalgia rheumatica has long been recognized. There have been few controlled trials regarding the treatment of polymyalgia rheumatica, but an abundance of long-term treatment experience has been reported in the literature. Nonsteroidal antiinflammatory drugs (NSAIDs) will be considered first, followed by corticosteroids and, finally, other immunosuppressive medications.

Nonsteroidal Antiinflammatory Drugs

Salicylates were the first medications used to treat polymyalgia rheumatica, with some reports citing partial to complete relief of musculoskeletal symptoms[3,10,11] and others finding minimal benefit.[4] Other nonsteroidal agents have been used with similar results. One of the more complete reports on the utility of nonsteroidal medications was offered by Chuang et al.[5] Of their 93 patients, 39 were treated with aspirin (30 patients) or other nonsteroidal agents. Of the remaining 54, 37 patients were initially tried on aspirin or nonsteroidal agents, but, because of inefficacy, corticosteroids were used. Patients treated without corticosteroids appeared to have had a milder disease, requiring a median of only 8 months of treatment compared with a median of 17 months for those treated with corticosteroids. The patients who received aspirin and nonsteroidal medications had a more gradual resolution of symptoms than those who took corticosteroids, but at 3 months the clinical improvement was judged to be the same and the sedimentation rates were not significantly different. Relapse (increased symptoms while the patient was still on medication) was unusual for the noncorticosteroid-treated patients but very common for those given corticosteroids; it typically occurred with lowering of the corticosteroid dose, a point to be discussed below.

In selected patients with polymyalgia rheumatica, salicylates and other nonsteroidal medications appear to be effective, although clearly corticosteroids are the preferred mode of therapy. The routine use of salicylates or other nonsteroidal medications as first-line agents in the treatment of polymyalgia rheumatica is a decision the physician and the patient will have to weigh on the basis of severity of disease, patient risk factors for side effects of corticosteroids or nonsteroidal agents, patient preferences, and medication costs. Patience is required for those of us who are used to the rapid relief afforded by corticosteroids; a more gradual improvement occurs with the nonsteroidal agents. In addition to initial treatment, salicylates or other nonsteroidal agents may find a niche in the treatment of polymyalgia rheumatica in combination with corticosteroids to control symptoms and help reduce the cumulative dose of steroidal medications, especially once the more severe "stage 1" symptoms have abated.

Corticosteroids

In the past, there have been several schools of thought with regard to the treatment of polymyalgia rheumatica. Some have maintained that polymyalgia rheumatica is a form of vasculitis and that all patients should be treated with high-dose corticosteroids. Others have believed that treatment of polymyalgia rheumatica should be influenced by the temporal artery biopsy. The other school of thought presents temporal arteritis and polymyalgia rheumatica as a spectrum of disease, with clinically pure polymyalgia as a benign disease needing only low-dose corticosteroid treatment. The latter has emerged as the predominant thinking in the recent literature, for reasons presented previously, with the main controversies in the treat-

ment of polymyalgia rheumatica presently centering around the lowest dose of corticosteroids one can use to control symptoms initially and the length of treatment.

In the study from the Mayo Clinic by Chuang et al.,[5] the median initial dose of corticosteroids for polymyalgia was 20 mg, with a wide dosing range (5 to 100 mg). Behn et al.[6] found that most of their patients could be adequately controlled with just 10 mg of prednisone per day and that few needed upward adjustment when compared with those patients started on between 5 and 9 mg of prednisone. Delecoeuillerie et al.[9] treated 75% of their 132 patients with polymyalgia rheumatica with 7 to 12 mg of prednisone while the remaining 25% received 15 to 30 mg. Patients treated with higher doses were thought to have more corticosteroid side effects without any apparent additional benefit; therefore the authors recommended initial dosing at or below 15 mg of prednisone. Lundberg and Hedfors[13] gave their 40 patients with polymyalgia rheumatica a mean dose of 18 mg of prednisolone and thought that a reasonable initial dosing regimen consisted of 10 mg twice a day. They suggested a twice-daily schedule based on the insufficient relief in their patients over a full 24-hour period. Spiera and Davison[14] treated 54 of 56 patients with 10 mg of prednisone, with only two patients requiring 15 mg.

In one of the only controlled trials of corticosteroid dosing in polymyalgia rheumatica by Kyle and Hazleman,[15] all 19 patients who received 20 mg of prednisolone achieved initial control of symptoms during the first month, whereas 14 of 20 treated with 10 mg had complete symptomatic relief.[15] The remaining six patients in this latter group were controlled when the prednisolone dose was raised to either 15 or 20 mg.

Suggested Approach (Table 11–1)

In general, a range of 10 to 15 mg of prednisone taken as a single morning dose appears to be a reasonable initial treatment for the majority of patients with polymyalgia rheumatica. It is generally recommended that they call within a few days to determine their respose to therapy. If one starts at 10 mg, the dose can be increased to 12.5 or 15 mg if there is an incomplete response; on rare occasions, the dose can be increased to a

TABLE 11-1
Treatment of Polymyalgia Rheumatica

Initial therapy: 10–15 mg of prednisone as a single dose

Partial response: Increase dose to 12.5–20 mg as single dose or give part as an evening dose, especially if there are persistent AM symptoms

Taper: 1 month at control dose, then decrease by 1 mg every 2–4 weeks

Length of therapy: Mean length of therapy is 2 years

Corticosteroid-sparing medication:
Methotrexate, hydroxychloroquine, dapsone, azathioprine, monthly injectable methylprednisolone, NSAIDs

maximum of 20 mg/d. If the patient does well symptomatically during the day but has continued early morning stiffness only, a small portion of the total dose given in the evening (i.e., 2.5 mg or even 5.0 mg) may be more useful than an increased total dose. This nighttime dose is the first to be tapered.

Most authors generally maintain the initial dose for 1 month and then begin a slow taper. The speed of corticosteroid taper has received only limited attention in the literature. Chuang et al.[5] reviewed the frequency of relapse and the speed of corticosteroid taper. Patients whose doses were tapered at a median of 5 mg/mo experienced two to four relapses, whereas those tapered at a median of 2.9 mg/mo did not have any relapses. Kyle and Hazleman[15] also reported relapse in 7 of 20 patients during the second month of treatment when tapering from 10 to 5 mg of prednisolone in decrements of 2.5 mg every 2 weeks. Small reductions (i.e., 1 mg) in corticosteroid dose may result in fewer relapses than less frequent but larger dose reductions; reductions of the prednisone dose by 1 mg until symptoms return is recommended. If symptoms return, the patient resumes the previous dose and after 2 to 4 weeks a slow taper is resumed. Many patients are willing to cope with minor stiffness as a trade-off for less corticosteroid while other patients want complete resolution of symptoms despite the potential toxicity of corticosteroids. Patients may plateau at a given dose, with resistance to further tapering. These patients may need prolonged therapy at this level. Patients should be given written instructions on dose tapering, and dose modifications can frequently be handled with a telephone consultation.

Tapering corticosteroids in actual practice is an art and depends on a variety of factors that make each patient or situation somewhat different. Some of these issues include dose, rapidity, and completeness of initial response, tolerability of prednisone, actual and potential side effects, ability of the patient to follow complicated tapering instructions, and convenience/costs of monitoring schedules. In general, doses should be tapered by 1 mg every 2 to 4 weeks in an effort to reduce the dose gradually to avoid steroid withdrawal symptoms and yet keep above a threshold when polymyalgia rheumatica symptoms might occur.

Length of Therapy

Treatment periods have ranged from 1 month[5] to more than 10 years. Ayoub et al.[16] found that of their 75 patients, 21% were off corticosteroids by 1 year, 53% by 2 years, 73% by 3 years, and 84% by 4 years. Four patients were still taking corticosteroids at 7 years. Studies in the United States have in general indicated a shorter period of treatment than those from Europe.[17] It is usually safe to tell the patient to count on approximately 2 years of therapy, but the treatment period could be longer. It is difficult to predict early in the course of therapy which patients with polymyalgia rheumatica will require more prolonged treatment, although, as noted previously, patients who respond to nonsteroidal agents alone may have a much shorter course.[5] Treatment is only suppressive, and in the less symptomatic phase of the disease a nonsteroidal agent may help in the corticosteroid taper.[17]

Alternative Corticosteroid Regimen

An alternative to traditional corticosteroid regimens uses intermittent corticosteroid injections to reduce the amount of corticosteroids.[18] Dasgupta et al. administered 120 mg of methylprednisolone to 16 patients by intramuscular injections every 3 weeks for 12 weeks and then tapered the doses monthly. All patients responded to initial therapy; at 1 year, 13 patients were receiving 40 to 60 mg of medication by injection each month. Three patients required a return to more traditional dosing after an initial response. At 12 weeks, there was no evidence of hypothalamic-pituitary-adrenal axis suppression.

Side effects in the remaining 13 patients after 12 months of therapy included only minor bruising in three patients.

Corticosteroid-Sparing Medications

Factors that influence corticosteroid side effects include high initial doses, cumulative dose, maintenance dose, and length of treatment.[17] In patients who are at risk of corticosteroid side effects, even at the low doses used in polymyalgia rheumatica, or who are not able to taper the dose, other options would be useful. Unfortunately, there has been only limited experience with other second-line antirheumatic therapy. The French literature includes two reports published in the 1960s discussing the utility of hydroxychloroquine (400 to 600 mg/d) in polymyalgia rheumatica.[19,20] Dapsone has also been used with variable results.[21,22] Its usefulness is generally limited by hematologic toxicity. Azathioprine was reported to have a modest corticosteroid-sparing effect in 31 patients with either polymyalgia rheumatica, temporal arteritis, or both in a double-blind placebo-controlled trial.[23] At 52 weeks of treatment, the placebo group was receiving a mean dose of 4.2 ± 0.58 mg of prednisolone compared with 1.9 ± 0.84 mg for the azathioprine group. Whether a 2 mg difference at the end of 1 year is clinically important, given their potential side effects, drug cost, and monitoring costs of azathioprine, is debatable.

There has been one report on the use of methotrexate in polymyalgia rheumatica.[24] Another study compared the utility of azathioprine and methotrexate in patients with polymyalgia and/or temporal arteritis.[25] Forty-two patients were randomized to azathioprine plus prednisolone or methotrexate plus prednisolone. Patients were treated for 9 months and then switched to the other treatment schedule. At the end of 18 months, 85% of the patients preferred methotrexate. Methotrexate was reported to have a stronger disease-modifying and steroid-sparing effect. Based on the general acceptance of methotrexate in rheumatoid arteritis under similar circumstances, this agent would seem to be the most reasonable alternative for steroid-resistant polymyalgia rheumatica.

Other Treatment Considerations

Prevention and treatment of corticosteroid-induced osteoporosis is essential.[26] Patients are encouraged to use supplemental calcium and vitamin D. A regular weight-bearing exercise program to maintain weight and to prevent corticosteroid-induced myopathy and corticosteroid-associated bone loss is recommended. (For additional details see Chapter 22 by Leboff and Wade.) Deflazacort has been studied as a potential bone-sparing corticosteroid in patients with inflammatory conditions, including polymyalgia rheumatica.[27] Patients with polymyalgia rheumatica often have shoulder capsulitis, rotator cuff weakness, or both. Once the stiffness of the polymyalgia rheumatica is controlled with corticosteroids, patients may need physical therapy to improve shoulder rage of motion and restrengthen the rotator cuff muscles.

TEMPORAL (GIANT CELL) ARTERITIS

Natural History of Temporal Arteritis

Temporal arteritis may have been first described in the tenth century, but credit for its description is given to Hutchinson,[28] who described an 80-year-old patient with red streaks on his head and scalp pain while wearing his hat. Hutchinson named this illness "arteritis of the aged." Some 40 years later, in the 1930s and 1940s, visual complications of the disease and the presence of widespread arteritis in some patients were recognized. Horton et al.[29] described the histologic findings in the temporal artery and described the giant cells and granulomatous nature of the vasculitis. Some authors prefer the term *giant cell arteritis* to *temporal arteritis* to avoid the notion of a limited vascular distribution, but giant cells are not unique to this form of vasculitis, and thus the best terminology for "temporal arteritis" is still a matter of debate. In this chapter, both terms are interchangeable and will be used for convenience.

Kilbourne and Wolff[30] summarized the initial 21 cases of temporal arteritis in the English-language literature in a review paper published in 1946, before the introduction of corticosteroids. Temporal arteritis was considered a disease of older Caucasians. All 21 patients had nonspecific systemic complaints and headache. One third experienced partial or complete permanent visual loss. The duration of the disease ranged from 1 to 20 months, with rare patients having recurrences. Elevation of the sedimentation rate was not recognized as an important diagnostic clue.

One year later, Andersen[31] reviewed 57 cases in the English-language and non-English-language literature, noting the marked elevation of the sedimentation rate in most patients, and put the risk of significant visual symptoms at 40%. Thirteen of the 57 developed permanent blindness. The course of the disease was generally less than 30 months; in 12 of the patients the disease was less than 1 year in duration. Seven of the 57 patients were believed to have died as a result of their disease, with causes including four cerebral vascular accidents, two coronary occlusions, and one hemorrhage.

One of the transitional studies (patients treated with and without corticosteroids) is useful for its contrast of the natural history of temporal arteritis. Russell[32] reported on 35 cases seen between 1947 and 1958 and divided the disease into three stages: headache, ocular complications, and systemic complications. Patients ranged in age from 59 to 85 years of age, with an average of 73 years. Most patients had vague symptoms preceding the onset of headache. All 35 patients complained of head pain, and in only two was it a minor symptom. Sixteen patients had permanent visual impairment, with complete bilateral blindness occurring in five patients. Russell documented the efficacy of corticosteroids in the prevention of blindness as compared with salicylates. None of the 10 patients treated with corticosteroids before the appearance of visual symptoms experienced visual failure, whereas 5 of 13 patients treated with salicylates before visual symptoms had significant visual loss. Russell also recognized the inability of corticosteroids to salvage vision, once fixed abnormalities had occurred. He also reported on the systemic sequelae in several patients. Two developed a generalized arteritis, 2 developed a significant peripheral neuropathy, and 3 had coexisting proximal muscle pain and weakness. The association with "polymyalgia rheumatica" was still speculative at this time, but a rapid response to corticosteroids was noted. Reference was made to Bagratuni,[33] who reported on a condition called "anarthritic rheumatoid arthritis," which describes what we today classify as polymyalgia rheumatica. Corticosteroid doses between 30 and 50 mg of prednisone were recommended for the first few weeks and then tapered to a maintenance dose of 10 to 20 mg. Therapy for those without visual symptoms was recommended for 6 months, while those with symptoms were treated for 18 months.

The association between temporal arteritis and polymyalgia rheumatica was strengthened by reports in the late 1950s and the 1960s. Data from the Mayo Clinic estimated that 50% of the patients with temporal arteritis developed polymyalgia rheumatica.[34] Polymyalgia may first appear as the corticosteroids are tapered.[35] There are several reports that suggest that the coexistence of temporal arteritis and polymyalgia rheumatica lengthens the mean duration of therapy by 8 months.[6,9,13]

Treatment of Temporal Arteritis

Visual prognosis is the most important issue when the treatment of temporal arteritis is discussed. High-dose corticosteroids have been the standard treatment for 3 decades, but recently the need for such aggressive and intensive therapy has been questioned. It was recognized that corticosteroids protected patients from developing visual loss and that most patients developed visual sequelae before the institution of corticosteroids.

Improved Visual Prognosis in Temporal Arteritis

Aiello et al.[36] reported the visual prognosis over a 5-year period in 245 patients with temporal arteritis. Thirty-four permanently lost some vision as a result of temporal arteritis (14%); 32 of the 34 patients had visual impairment before corticosteroids were started. Of the two patients who developed permanent visual sequelae after the diagnosis of temporal arteritis was made, only one was receiving corticosteroids. The other patient had not been taking any corticosteroids for 1 year and the visual loss occurred during a recurrence of her temporal arteritis. The risk of permanent visual damage once corticosteroids were started was 1% (0.5% if only patients taking corticosteroids are considered). Three patients with visual loss before corticosteroids were started had further loss soon after treatment was initiated, whereas five patients experienced an improvement in their vision. These data suggest that, once corticosteroids are initiated, vision-threatening disease rarely occurs if a deficit was not already present. The 30% to 60% incidence of significant visual loss in the precorticosteroid era has given way to an incidence in the range of 10% to 20%.[36,37] Figures from Scandinavia describe a less than 10% incidence of visual loss over the last decade.[37]

Corticosteroids

Recent Data Concerning Lower-Dose Corticosteroid Therapy.

The standard protocols for treating temporal arteritis have used doses of 45 to 60 mg of prednisone or prednisolone, generally in divided doses, for 1 month. After 1 month, doses were reduced by 10% of the total dose per week until a maintenance level of 5 to 7.5 mg/d was achieved.[38,39] Higher doses have been suggested for those who do not respond in the first 3 to 4 days.

Hunder et al.[40] reported that 45 mg of prednisone given as a single daily dose suppressed the inflammation in the majority of patients with temporal arteritis but was not as effective as 45 mg split into three daily doses. The amount and severity of corticosteroid side effects were no different between the split- and single-dose groups. Alternate-day therapy for temporal arteritis did not suppress the inflammation.

It has been suggested that doses lower than 45 mg/d could be effective in temporal arteritis without significantly increasing the risk of visual injury. Paulley and Hughes[41] reported that 20 mg of prednisolone (10 mg twice a day) was adequate for most patients with temporal arteritis, although some patients needed up to 90 mg/d to control symptoms and signs of inflammation.

Behn et al.[6] prospectively evaluated the corticosteroid regimens of 68 patients with temporal arteritis. Dosing ranged from 5 to 60 mg/d. Three patients initially given 5 to 9 mg required an increase in the prednisolone dose, 7 of 18 patients initially started on 10 mg needed an increase, and only 1 of 33 patients given 20 mg needed to have their dose elevated. All 14 patients started on more than 20 mg did not need to have their dose increased, and these included patients with visual symptoms. None of the patients had permanent visual loss after corticosteroid therapy was started. In an update to this study, the authors retrospectively evaluated 96 patients with temporal arteritis. A review of the initial dosing regimens included 35 patients started on less than 20 mg of prednisolone, 42 patients on 20 mg, and 19 patients started on more than 20 mg of prednisolone per day for temporal arteritis.[42] One half of the patients in the first group needed dose adjustments, while only two patients in the second group and one in the third group required any increase in their prednisolone dose. Only one patient had visual changes, and that person was in the third group. The authors concluded that 20 mg of prednisolone was sufficient to treat most patients with temporal arteritis and more than 20 mg had no additional benefit.

Delecoeuillerie et al.[9] retrospectively reviewed the course of 78 patients with temporal arteritis and analyzed disease progression and corticosteroid side effects by initial corticosteroid dose. Subgroup I consisted of 25 patients started on 10 to 20 mg of prednisolone, subgroup II consisted of 28 patients initially started on 21 to 59 mg of prednisolone, and subgroup III consisted of 25 patients started on 60 to 90 mg, and this latter subgroup included all 12 patients who had visual symptoms at presentation. One patient each in the first two subgroups had disease progression (the patient in subgroup I stopped corticosteroids against medical advice), whereas four of the patients in subgroup III had disease progression. In subgroup I, 7% had significant corticosteroid-related side effects compared with 33% and 60% for subgroups II and III respectively. This included two deaths in subgroup II and one in subgroup III that were directly related to the corticosteroids. Of importance, duration of treatment, percentage of patients who experienced remission during the study period, and relapses did not differ among the three subgroups. However, the interpretation of this study should be circumspect and cautious since the patients did not appear to be randomly assigned to different dosages.

Lundberg and Hedfors[13] concluded from their study of 46 patients with temporal arteritis that 10 mg of prednisolone twice daily was sufficient to suppress the inflammation in temporal arteritis without undue risk of visual complications and avoided the excess corticosteroid side effect of higher doses.

These data certainly suggest that patients with temporal arteritis who do not have vision-threatening or generalized arteritis can be treated with lower doses of corticosteroids than previously recommended. Patients treated with lower dose regimens do not seem to have a more prolonged disease or more frequent relapses or run a risk of visual impairment in excess of those treated in a more conservative (higher dose) manner.

Suggested Approach (Table 11–2)

Treatment of Patients Without Visual Involvement. Even though the argument from the published literature in favor of lower-dose corticosteroids in many patients with temporal arteritis is compelling, confirmatory studies are needed. Currently, patients who have symptoms and signs of temporal arteritis without visual symptoms or evidence of large-artery involvement (see below) are started on a dose of 30 to 40 mg of prednisone. A temporal artery biopsy should be performed within the next several days and no longer than 1 week after steroid initiation to avoid the effect that corticosteroids may have on the biopsy results. The biopsy specimen should be 4 to 5 cm in length; multiple cuts should be done for histologic sampling because of the tendency of the inflammation to skip segments of the artery. The biopsy should be performed on all patients with suspected temporal arteritis, as histologic confirmation is useful, particularly since patients may be committed to long-term immunosuppressive therapy. Generally a unilateral biopsy of sufficient size is positive in 85% of patients with the disease. In the setting of a negative biopsy a contralateral biopsy increases the yield to approximately 95%. A pathologist with experience in interpreting the histology is essential; the absence of giant cells does not exclude the diagnosis of temporal arteritis.

After 1 month of prednisone in doses of 30 to 40 mg/d, the prednisone dose is tapered. Multiple strategies have been used, but one approach involves a slow weekly reduction by about 10% of the total daily dose per week. For a reappearance of symptoms, the patient is directed to return to the previous level at which symptoms were controlled, and after 2 weeks the taper is attempted again at the same or a slower rate. As with polymyalgia rheumatica, small weekly decrements may be better tolerated than less frequent, larger decreases in the corticosteroid dose. It should be pointed out that some patients' symptoms may not be adequately controlled even with the initial dose of 30 to 40 mg/d, and in these cases the dose can be increased to 60 or 80 mg. An alternative but essentially similar tapering approach is to use a graduated, stepwise decrement of dosing. For example, once the patient is controlled on 40 mg for 1 month, the dose can be lowered to 30, 25, 20, 17.5, 15, and 12.5 mg every 2 to 4 weeks. Below 12.5 mg the dose should be dropped by 1 mg decrements. The speed of tapering is also influenced by a variety of factors described above in the section on polymyalgia rheumatica. For "flares" of disease once tapering has begun, in this alternative scheme it is usually not necessary to go beyond a return to 40 mg of prednisone.

The erythrocyte sedimentation rate can be used as a general indicator of disease activity. It should be checked during the first several visits to assure the patient and the physician that the inflammation is responding to therapy. Some physicians and patients are quite keyed into the sedimentation rate and respond to minor asymptomatic changes in the sedimentation rate with increases in the corticosteroid dose that may be unnecessary. The symptom-free patient who now develops an increase in the sedimentation rate should be followed closely for a possible flare of the disease. Generally the prednisone dose is not increased in this setting if the patient is truly free of symptoms. The patient who has responded clinically to prednisone but has a persistently elevated sedimentation rate should be investigated for a nontemporal arteritis cause of the elevated sedimentation rate.

TABLE 11–2
Treatment of Temporal Arteritis

Initial therapy: 30–40 mg of prednisone in divided doses for patients without significant visual symptoms or evidence of large-artery involvement
  60–80 mg for patients with visual symptoms or evidence of large-artery involvement
    Megadose corticosteroids for patients with an acute visual deficit on presentation
Taper: 1 month at the control dose and then taper by 10% of the daily dose each week. Maintenance dose, 5–7.5 mg.
Length of therapy: Mean length of therapy is probably 2 years
Corticosteroid-sparing medication: Methotrexate, dapsone, azathioprine, cyclophosphamide

The patient should be educated on the symptoms that portend serious problems, even though these are rare once corticosteroids have been started. Patients are instructed to call immediately regarding any symptoms of concern.

Treatment of Patients With Visual Involvement. For patients with visual symptoms but no visual loss at the time of presentation, 60 to 80 mg of prednisone, in divided doses, is generally used. All patients with visual symptoms should see an ophthalmologist for a baseline visual examination and should be evaluated for an alternative cause of the visual symptoms. There are also several reports documenting the efficacy of "megadose" corticosteroid therapy in restoring vision in patients with acute visual loss.[36,43–47] Successful megadose therapy has been provided by high-dose oral therapy,[45] intravenous ACTH,[46] and intravenous methylprednisolone.[36,43,44] The latter has been given in doses ranging from 500 mg/d for 2 days up to 1000 mg every 12 hours for 5 days without any significant short-term side effects. Beneficial effects of this megadose therapy above and beyond those of simple high-dose oral therapy may include prevention of cellular membrane breakdown via inhibition of lipid peroxidation and hydrolysis by superoxide radicals released during tissue injury and also reduction of certain vasoactive by-products of arachidonic acid metabolism, thus promoting blood flow to the ischemic tissue.[43] Although such therapy is warranted in situations of acute visual loss, it has not been universally successful.[48]

Treatment of Other Manifestations. Among patients with temporal arteritis, 10% to 15% may have large-artery involvement.[38] Arteries most often involved include the carotid, subclavian, axillary, and brachial. Patients may present with claudications, Raynaud's phenomenon, or both. If large-artery involvement is suspected, angiography is recommended to confirm the diagnosis, and thereafter noninvasive Doppler studies can be used to follow the course of the vasculitis while the patient is under treatment. Therapy should be the same as for temporal arteritis with visual symptoms inasmuch as significant sequelae such as aortic rupture can occur and such complications may be avoided if high-dose corticosteroid treatment is instituted as soon as possible. All patients with temporal arteritis should be evaluated for large-artery involvement by measuring blood pressures in both arms and carefully auscultating arteries for bruits.

Length of Therapy

The length of therapy for temporal arteritis is similar to that for polymyalgia in that the majority of patients can be taken off corticosteroids after 2 to 3 years. Lundberg and Hedfors[13] found that all 21 patients with only temporal arteritis were off corticosteroids by 24 months, whereas 60% of the 25 patients with a combination of temporal arteritis and polymyalgia were off treatment by 24 months. Eighty percent of the latter group were off corticosteroids by 30 months, and 90% had stopped treatment by 36 months. Some patients may need therapy for a prolonged period. Andersson et al.[49] reported that 25% of their 90 patients followed prospectively were still taking corticosteroids at 9 years, although most of these were taking less than 5 mg of prednisolone. Except for the presence of polymyalgia rheumatica, no other feature of temporal arteritis has been associated with the need for more prolonged therapy. At least two reports have suggested that the presence of jaw claudications is more common in those patients with visual sequelae and other complications and may be a reason to consider higher initial corticosteroid dosing.[9,36]

Recurrent disease (disease that occurs when the patient is off corticosteroids) should be treated as if it were the initial disease presentation, and decisions about corticosteroid dosing should be made as suggested above. Recurrences usually occur during the first year off corticosteroids.

Corticosteroid-Sparing Medications

There has not been a great deal of information regarding corticosteroid-sparing agents in the treatment of temporal arteritis. As with polymyalgia rheumatica, dapsone has been used with mixed results.[21,22] Azathioprine has also been used.[23] Cyclophosphamide has been reported to be of benefit in two case series,[50,51] but in one series all the patients were also treated with 6-mercaptopurine.[50] Methotrexate compared favorably with azathioprine for the treatment of temporal arteritis.[24] Three patients with polymyalgia rheumatica associated with temporal arteritis who could not be tapered from their corticosteroids were treated with 7.5 to 12.5 mg of oral methotrexate each week with good results.[25] Methotrexate was also thought to be helpful in reducing the cumulative dose of corticosteroids needed for the treatment of temporal arteritis when compared with historical controls.[52,53] Methotrexate is now the agent of choice of many rheumatologists for patients who are having difficulty tapering the corticosteroids within the above proscribed time frame. The starting dose is 7.5 mg orally per week, and after 1 month of therapy with methotrexate further reduction in the corticosteroids is attempted. If not successful, the dose of methotrexate is increased in 2.5 mg increments to a maximum of 20 mg every 2 to 4 weeks as necessary. If there is no response to 20 mg given orally, intramuscular methotrexate can be tried in doses of up to 25 mg/wk.

Other Treatment Considerations

Attention should be directed toward prevention of corticosteroid-induced bone loss. Patients need to be warned about the effects of the corticosteroids on their appetite and sleep. Serum glucose levels and blood pressure should be monitored when corticosteroid doses are high. These important issues are discussed by Leboff and Wade in Chapter 22.

TAKAYASU'S ARTERITIS

Natural History of Takayasu's Arteritis

"Takayasu's arteritis" was actually described first by Savory[54] in 1856 but was later named after Takayasu,[55] who described peculiar vascular changes in the retina of a young Japanese woman. Most of the early cases were reported from Japan, but the disease has been described worldwide.

The course of Takayasu's arteritis is typically intermittent, with exacerbations of the disease that eventually lead to the development of progressive vascular ischemia.[56] A minority of patients may have unremitting disease activity or disease activity followed by a spontaneous remission. It is a common cause of renovascular hypertension among young people in Asia.[57] Unfortunately, Takayasu's arteritis is not generally as benign and self-limited a disease as polymyalgia rheumatica or even temporal arteritis. Significant morbidity and mor-

tality have been associated with this disease, although more recent treatment regimens may have changed the outlook for the patients affected with this illness.

In 1953, Ask-Upmark[58] described the outcome in 28 patients with "pulseless disease" reported in the American and European literature to augment the then described 58 cases from Japan. Twenty-seven of the 28 patients were females, ranging in age from 15 to 58 years with an average age of 30. The emphasis of the disease on the thoracic portion of the aorta and the brachiocephalic arteries was noted; the sedimentation rate was observed to be a useful laboratory parameter. Six of the 28 patients died of either cerebral ischemia or renovascular hypertension. Ask-Upmark was the first to report the use of corticosteroids for the treatment of Takayasu's arteritis and believed that a short course of 50 mg of cortisone was of no benefit.

Ishikawa[59] followed the course of 54 Japanese patients seen over an 18-year period and reported on their outcome. He classified these patients on the basis of certain complications, which included retinopathy, secondary hypertension, aortic regurgitation, and aortic or arterial aneurysm. Group I patients were without any of the above complications; group II patients had one complication and were subgrouped into IIa or IIb, depending on the severity of the complication; and, finally, group III patients had two or more complications. The overall 5-year survival rate was 83%, but in those patients classified as IIb or III the survival rate was only 66% at 5 years. Causes of death were usually related to congestive heart failure or cerebrovascular accidents, and almost all of the patients who died had secondary hypertension. Ishikawa emphasized the importance of early recognition of the disease, inasmuch as patients in group III had a 14-year hiatus between onset of symptoms and the diagnosis, compared with an average of only 6.7 years for group I patients. The 17% mortality at 5 years is similar to that found in other long-term studies of Takayasu's arteritis reported at the time of or before the Ishikawa article but is not much different from the survival reported by Ask-Upmark in the precorticosteroid era!

A more optimistic outcome for patients with Takayasu's arteritis was reported by Hall et al.,[60] with a 5-year survival of 94%. This improvement was attributed to earlier diagnosis (median time from onset of symptoms to diagnosis was 18 months), liberal use of corticosteroids, and aggressive control of hypertension.

Treatment of Takayasu's Arteritis

The treatment issues for Takayasu's arteritis include control of systemic symptoms and the prevention and/or control of vascular insufficiency. The data from the Mayo Clinic suggests that outcome can be improved if the disease can be recognized early and suppression of the granulomatous vascular inflammation achieved prior to the development of fibrous intimal hyperplasia.[60] Treatment modalities have included corticosteroids, cyclophosphamide, methotrexate, surgery to bypass occluded arterial segments, and more recently angioplasty.

Corticosteroid Therapy for Takayasu's Arteritis

The earliest uses of corticosteroids in Takayasu's arteritis were for short-term treatment of the acute phase of the disease.[58,61,62] Fraga et al.[63] used a regimen of 30 mg of prednisone for 9 weeks, tapered to a maintenance dose of 5 to 10 mg. None of the 12 patients so treated had any progression of their disease during an average follow-up of 2 years. Seven previously absent pulses returned, and 15 arteries with decreased pulsation did not worsen. Fraga et al. also reported the utility of the sedimentation rate for monitoring disease activity.

Hall et al.[60] also found that long-term corticosteroid therapy in which suppression of the sedimentation rate was achieved was useful in controlling symptoms. In 8 of 16 patients in whom pulses were absent, the pulses returned. Hall et al. commented that 30 mg of prednisone was not sufficient in some patients and up to 100 mg/d was used. Other immunosuppressants were generally not needed, although 3 of 32 patients were reported to be receiving additional immunosuppressants. Twelve of their patients also underwent a variety of surgical procedures.

Shellhammer et al.,[64] from the National Institutes of Health, used corticosteroids to treat 16 patients with active inflammatory Takayasu's arteritis. Eight patients responded on a regimen of prednisone, 1 mg/kg for 1 month followed when possible by a gradual taper to an every-other-day schedule. If the taper could not be done or if there

was evidence of disease progression, the patient was considered for therapy with oral cyclophosphamide. All seven patients treated with cyclophosphamide were able to have their corticosteroid doses reduced to alternate days (six patients) or to discontinue corticosteroids completely (one patient). Four of six patients who were given cyclophosphamide for progressive disease obtained control of the arteritis with the combined protocol. Overall, five of the seven patients were thought to benefit from the addition of cyclophosphamide. There were no major treatment complications for those treated with cyclophosphamide over an average period of 27 months per patient. There were no deaths due to Takayasu's arteritis over an average follow-up of 56 months. Seven patients required surgical therapy.

Overall, medical therapy for Takayasu's arteritis consisting of corticosteroids with or without a cytotoxic agent seems able to control the systemic symptoms as well as the identifiable inflammatory arteritis. The medications are usually given in doses to keep the sedimentation rate within the normal range. Even so, many patients continue to have problems with vascular insufficiency, despite often aggressive therapy, and require surgical procedures to improve blood flow. This may relate to the length of time the disease has been present relative to the institution of therapy. In addition, these reports generally lack information on long-term side effects of therapy for this chronic illness.

Recently, methotrexate has emerged as a potentially useful agent for the treatment of Takayasu's arteritis. Hoffman et al.,[65] from the National Institutes of Health, used methotrexate in a relatively treatment-resistant group of patients with Takayasu's arteritis and found that 81% achieved disease remission while taking methotrexate (average, 17 mg/wk), with 50% of the responders sustaining corticosteroid-free remissions for an average of 18 months.[65] Other case reports have added to the positive results of methotrexate in this disease.[66,67]

Suggested Approach (Table 11–3)

Diagnosis in the earliest phases of the disease is important and probably contributes to an improved outcome. Diagnosis requires angiographic demonstration of typical vascular changes and should be done before modification by therapy whenever possible. This will

TABLE 11-3
Treatment of Takayasu's Arteritis

Initial therapy: 40–60 mg of prednisone in divided doses
Taper: After 1 month at the initial control dose, begin a reduction by 10% of the daily dose per week to maintenance dose of 5–7.5 mg/d. Introduce methotrexate if unable to taper to acceptable level. Follow ESR, Doppler studies.
Length of therapy: Variable
Corticosteroid-sparing medication: Methotrexate, cyclophosphamide
Surgical therapy: Angioplasty, bypass surgery for ischemic symptoms not responsive to medical therapy

confirm the diagnosis and guide prednisone dosing on the basis of location of vascular involvement. Prednisone in a dose of 40 to 60 mg in divided doses is a reasonable range for the initial control of the inflammatory vascular disease and systemic symptoms in most patients. The higher dosing range is most appropriate for patients with vascular involvement of the head and neck and the renal arteries. The sedimentation rate is a useful parameter to titrate the corticosteroid dosing, as most studies note a direct correlation between disease activity and sedimentation rate level. After 1 month, a gradual reduction of the dose can be started, similar to that for temporal arteritis. If the disease symptoms and the sedimentation rate cannot be controlled with prednisone, low-dose methotrexate can be added. Methotrexate should be dosed according to the recommendations given for methotrexate treatment in temporal arteritis. Since many of the patients are women of childbearing age, it is imperative that birth control issues be adequately addressed. Cyclophosphamide should be reserved for severe disease that is unresponsive to the above and to date has been administered only orally for this disease. Besides the sedimentation rate, the course of the disease can be followed by noninvasive duplex ultrasonograpy.[68] Since the disease can be intermittent, patients may be able to be withdrawn from medications between exacerbations.

Surgical Therapy of Takayasu's Arteritis

Bypass surgery has been used to treat the vascular insufficiency associated with this disease. The disease is often so slowly progressive that some patients are able to develop collateral circulation. The site of disease activity and the size of the vessels involved make many of the fixed lesions amenable to surgical bypass. More recently, percutaneous transluminal angioplasty has been used successfully to treat these lesions.[60,66,69] Some of the reports have commented that vascular grafts or postangioplasty lesions have a greater chance of reoccluding if the active inflammatory disease is not controlled.[60,66] Other surgical procedures performed include aortic valve replacement, carotid endarterectomy, and aneurysm repair.

Other Treatment Recommendations

Measures to prevent osteoporosis are as important with this disease as with the other two previously discussed diseases. Hypertension, when present, should be addressed to prevent some of the significant sequelae caused by this disease complication. Finally, if cyclophosphamide is used, fertility issues need to be discussed with the patient. Treating a patient with Takayasu's arteritis who is pregnant limits the treatment options to prednisone only. Patients with more severe disease complicated by hypertension or heart disease will need a team effort and a recognition that prednisone treatment may exacerbate hemodynamic abnormalities.

REFERENCES

1. Bruce W. Senile rheumatic gout. Br Med J 1888; 2:811.
2. Hunder GG, Disney TF, Ward LE. Polymyalgia rheumatica. Mayo Clin Proc 1969;44:849.
3. Barber HS. Myalgic syndrome with constitutional effects: polymyalgia rheumatica. Ann Rheum Dis 1957;16:230.
4. Gordon I. Polymyalgia rheumatica. Q J Med 1960;29:273.
5. Chuang TY, Hunder GG, Ilstrup DM, Kurland T. Polymyalgia rheumatica: a 10 year epidemiologic and clinical study. Ann Int Med 1982;97: 672.
6. Behn AR, Perera T, Myles AB. Polymyalgia rheumatica and corticosteroids: how much for how long? Ann Rheum Dis 1983;42:374.
7. Healey LA, Wilske KR. The systemic manifestations of temporal arteritis. New York: Grune & Stratton, 1978.
8. Spiera H, Davison S. Treatment of polymyalgia rheumatica. Arthritis Rheum 1982;25:120.
9. Delecoeuillerie G, Joly P, Cohen De Lara A, Paolaggi JB. Polymyalgia rheumatica and temporal arteritis: a retrospective analysis of prog-

nostic features and corticosteroid regimens. Ann Rheum Dis 1988;47:733.

10. Jones JG, Hazleman BL. Prognosis and management of polymyalgia rheumatica. Ann Rheum Dis 1981;40:1.

11. Davidson S, Speira H, Plotz CM. Polymyalgia rheumatica. Arthritis Rheum 1966;9:18.

12. Bagratuni L. Prognosis in anarthritic rheumatoid syndrome. Br Med J 1963;1:513.

13. Lundberg I, Hedfors E. Restricted dose and duration of corticosteroid treatment in patients with polymyalgia rheumatica and temporal arteritis. J Rheumatol 1990;17:1340.

14. Speira H, Davidson S. Long-term follow-up of polymyalgia rheumatica. Mt Sinai J Med 1978; 45:225.

15. Kyle V, Hazleman BL. Treatment of polymyalgia rheumatica and giant cell arteritis. I. Steroid regimens in the first two months. Ann Rheum Dis 1989;48:658.

16. Ayoub WT, Franklin CM, Torretti D. Polymyalgia rheumatica: duration of therapy and long-term outcome. Am J Med 1985;79:309.

17. Kyle V, Hazleman BL. Stopping steroids in polymyalgia rheumatica and giant cell arteritis. Br Med J 1990;300:344.

18. Dasgupta B, Gray J, Fernandez L, Olliff C. The treatment of polymyalgia rheumatica with injections of depot methylprednisone. Ann Rheum Dis 1991;50:942.

19. Weissenbach R, Nobilliot A, Freneaux R, Coste F. Pseudo-polyarthrite rhizomelique. Sem Hop Paris 1963;39:2073.

20. de Seze S, Lequesne M, Veber A. Le rheumatisme inflammatorie des ceintures ou pseudopolyarthrite rhizomelique avec 45 observations. Sem Hop Paris 1965;41:711.

21. Doury P, Pattin S, Eulry F, Thabaut A. The use of dapsone in the treatment of giant cell arthritis and polymyalgia rheumatica. Arthritis Rheum 1983;26:698.

22. Fowler B, Dideriksen K, Stentoft J, Jensen MK. Dapsone in temporal arteritis and polymyalgia rheumatica. J Rheumatol 1988;15:879.

23. De Silva M, Hazleman BL. Azathioprine in giant cell arteritis/polymyalgia rheumatica: a double-blind study. Ann Rheum Dis 1986;45:136.

24. Settas L, Dimitriadis G, Sfetsios T, Disa E, Souliou E, Tourkantonis A. Methotrexate versus azathioprine in polymyalgia rheumatica-giant cell arteritis: a double blind, cross over trial. Arthritis Rheum 1991;34(suppl):S72.

25. Krall PA, Mazanec DJ, and Wilke W. Methotrexate for corticosteroid-resistant polymyalgia rheumatica and giant cell arteritis. Cleve Clin J Med 1989;56:253.

26. Adachi JD, Bensen WG, Hodsman AB. Corticosteroid-induced osteoporosis. Semin Arthritis Rheum 1993;22:375.

27. Gray RES, Doherty SM, Golloway J, Coulton L, De Broe M, Kanis JA. A double-blind study of deflazacort and prednisone in patients with chronic inflammatory disorders. Arthritis Rheum 1991; 34:287.

28. Hutchinson J. Diseases of the arteries: on a peculiar form of thrombotic arteritis of the aged which is sometimes productive of gangrene. Arch Surg (London) 1989;1:323.

29. Horton BT, Magath TB, Brown GE. An undescribed form of arteritis of the temporal vessels. Proc Staff Meet Mayo Clin 1932;7:700.

30. Kilbourne ED, Wolff HG. Cranial arteritis: a critical evaluation of the syndrome of "temporal arteritis" with a report of a case. Ann Intern Med 1946;24:1.

31. Andersen T. Arteritis temporalis (Horton): a survey of a case with glaucoma. Acta Med Scand 1947;128:151.

32. Russell RWR. Giant cell arteritis: a review of 35 cases. Q J Med 1959;112:471.

33. Bagratuni L. Anarthritis rheumatoid disease. Lancet 1956;2:694.

34. Huston KA, Hunder GG. Giant cell (cranial) arteritis: a clinical review. Am Heart J 1980; 100:99.

35. Huston KA, Hunder GG, Lie JT, Kennedy RH, Elveback LR. Temporal arteritis: a 25 year epidemiologic, clinical, and pathologic study. Ann Intern Med 1978;88:162.

36. Aiello PD, Trautmann JC, McPhee TJ, Kunselman AS, Hunder GG. Visual prognosis in giant cell arteritis. Ophthalmology 1993;100:550.

37. Fledelius HC, Nissen KR. Giant cell arteritis and visual loss: a 3 year retrospective hospital investigation in a Danish county. Acta Ophthalmol 1992;70:801.

38. Hunder GG. Giant cell arteritis and polymyalgia rheumatica. In: Kelley WM, Harris ED, Ruddy S, Sledge CB, eds. Textbook of rheumatology. 4th ed. Philadelphia: WB Saunders, 1993.

39. Wilske KR. Polymyalgia rheumatica and giant cell (temporal) arteritis. In: Roth SH, Calabro JJ, Paulus HE, Wilken RF, eds. Rheumatic therapeutics. New York: McGraw-Hill, 1985.

40. Hunder GG, Sheps SG, Allen GL, Joyce JW. Daily and alternate-day corticosteroid regimens in treatment of giant cell arteritis: comparison in a prospective study. Ann Intern Med 1975;82: 613.

41. Paulley JW, Hughes JP. Giant cell arteritis, or arteritis of the aged. Br Med J 1960;2:1562.

42. Myles AB, Perrera T, Ridley MG. Prevention of blindness in giant cell arteritis by corticosteroid treatment. Br J Rheumatol 1992;31:103.

43. Matzkin DC, Slamovits TL, Sach R, Burde RM. Visual recovery in two patients after intravenous methylprednisolone treatment of central retinal artery occlusion secondary to giant cell arteritis. Ophthalmology 1992;99:68.

44. Diamond JP. Treatable blindness in temporal arteritis. Br J Ophthalmol 1991;75:432.

45. Lipton RB, Solomon S, Wertenbaker C. Gradual loss and recovery of vision in temporal arteritis. Arch Intern Med 1985;145:2252.

46. Parsons-Smith G. Sudden blindness in cranial arteritis. Br J Ophthalmol 1959;43:204.

47. Rosenfeld SI, Kosmorsky GS, Klingele TG, Burde RM, Cohn EM. Treatment of temporal

arteritis with ocular involvement. Am J Med 1986;80:143.

48. Slavin ML, Margolis AJ. Progressive anterior ischemic optic neuropathy due to giant cell arteritis despite high-dose intravenous corticosteroids. Arch Ophthalmol 1988;106:1167.

49. Andersson R, Malmvall B, Bengtsson B. Long-term corticosteroid treatment in giant cell arteritis. Acta Med Scand 1986;220:465.

50. De Vita S, Tavoni A, Jeracitano G, Gemignani G, Dolcher MP, Bombardieri S. Treatment of giant cell arteritis with cyclophosphamide pulses. J Intern Med 1992;232:373.

51. Ustinger PD. Treatment of steroid non-responsive giant cell arteritis with Cytoxan. Arthritis Rheum 1982;25(suppl):S31.

52. Hernandez C, Fernandez B, Ramos P, Estrada V, Perez-Venegas J, Banares A. Giant cell arteritis: MTX as a steroid-sparing agent. Arthritis Rheum 1991;34(suppl):S73.

53. Jover JA, Morado C, Collado P, et al. Methotrexate treatment in giant cell arteritis: long term follow-up [Abstract]. Arthritis Rheum 1993;36:S141.

54. Savory WS. Case of a young woman in whom the main arteries of both upper extremities and of the left side of the neck were throughout completely obliterated. Med Chir Trans Lond 1856; 39:205.

55. Takayasu M. Case with unusual changes of the central vessels in the retina. Acta Soc Ophthalmol Jap 1908;12:554 (in Japanese).

56. Conn DL, Hunder GG. Vasculitis and related disorders. In: Kelley WM, Harris ED, Ruddy S, Sledge CB, eds. Textbook of rheumatology. 4th ed. Philadelphia: WB Saunders, 1993.

57. Malhotra KK, Sharma RK, Prabhaker S, et al. Aortoarteritis as a major cause of renovascular hypertension in the young. Indian J Med Res 1983;77:487.

58. Ask-Upmark E. On the pulseless disease outside Japan. Acta Med Scand 1954;149:164.

59. Ishikawa K. Natural history and classification of occlusive thromboaortopathy (Takayasu's disease). Circulation 1978;57:27.

60. Hall S, Barr W, Lie JT, Stanson AW, Kazmier FJ, Hunder GG. Takayasu's arteritis: a study of 32 North American patients. Medicine 1985; 64:89.

61. Nakao K, Ikeda M, Kimata S, et al. Takayasu's arteritis: clinical report of eighty-four cases and immunological studies of seven cases. Circulation 1967;35:1141.

62. Gibbons TB, King RL. Obliterative brachiocephalic arteritis (pulseless disease). Circulation 1957;15:845.

63. Fraga A, Mintz G, Valle L, Flores-Izquierdo G. Takayasu's arteritis: frequency of systemic manifestations and favorable response to maintenance steroid therapy with adrenocorticosteroids. Arthritis Rheum 1972;15:617.

64. Shelhammer JH, Volkman DJ, Parrillo JE, Lawley TJ, Johnston MR, Fauci AS. Takayasu's arteritis and its therapy. Ann Intern Med 1985; 103:121.

65. Hoffman GS, Leavitt RY, Kerr GS, Rottem M, Sneller MC, Fauci AS. Treatment of Takayasu's arteritis with methotrexate. Arthritis Rheum 1993;36(suppl):S96.

66. Liang GC, Nemickas R, Madayag M. Multiple percutaneous transluminal angioplasties and low dose pulse methotrexate for Takayasu's arteritis. J Rheumatol 1989;16:1370.

67. Mevorach D, Leibowitz G, Brezis M, Raz E. Induction of remission in a patient with Takayasu's arteritis by low dose pulses of methotrexate. Ann Rheum Dis 1992;51:904.

68. Reed A, Fincher RE, Nichols FT. Takayasu's arteritis in a middle-aged caucasian woman: clinical course correlated with duplex ultrasound and angiography. Am J Med Sci 1989;298:324.

69. Hodgins GW, Dutton JW. Transluminal dilitation of Takayasu's arteritis. Can J Surg 1984; 27:355.

12

SCLERODERMA

Fredrick M. Wigley

Alan K. Matsumoto

Scleroderma is a chronic disfiguring disease that can change every aspect of a person's life. The skin manifestations of scleroderma not only alter the patient's appearance but frequently cause major hand and limb disability. Patients must also cope with fatigue, cold intolerance, pain, decreased exercise tolerance, and a general inability to fully perform their usual role in life. As a consequence, emotional problems such as fear, anxiety, misconceptions, and depression are common among patients with scleroderma.[1]

Scleroderma can be equally frustrating for the physician. Because scleroderma is an uncommon rheumatic disease, physicians have less experience with the problems that afflict these patients. In addition, although several features of the disease are seemingly monotonous, the course of scleroderma is highly variable and the overall outcome cannot be completely predicted. Visceral involvement is relatively silent until an irreversible stage develops. At the same time, no treatment has been proven uniformly successful in either prevention or reversal of the disease process.

Effective management of the patient with scleroderma begins with a solid patient-doctor relationship. The patient must feel comfortable and have confidence that his or her care is well directed. The physician must be sensitive to the patient's needs, both physical and emotional. This usually requires frequent and regular contact. Careful education is important so that the patient and the family understand the rationale and limitations of the treatment. The patient must understand that while the course of scleroderma is a chronic one, it is also quite variable in expression and not uniformly "progressive."

Designing a management program frequently involves other subspecialists and health professionals. Consultation with an experienced expert in the management of scleroderma is helpful especially in patients with early disease when decisions about treatment options are especially critical. Experimental treatments are best done in conjunction with an academic center that is conducting controlled clinical trials.

A comprehensive evaluation and baseline studies (Table 12–1) give an important frame of reference for future management, and early detection of organ involvement provides an opportunity to prevent irreversible damage. Every patient with a diagnosis of scleroderma should have a baseline chest radiograph, electrocardiogram, and pulmonary function testing in addition to a complete physical examination. Several scleroderma-specific measurements are helpful in assessing status over time. These include the

---

TABLE 12–1

Baseline Evaluation of the Scleroderma Patient

- Complete history and physical examination with special attention to cardiopulmonary and gastrointestinal complaints
- Measurement of total body skin score, size of maximal oral aperture, patient global assessment
- Routine laboratory work including complete blood cell count, chemistries, urinalysis; in addition, thyroid function testing, creatinine kinase, and aldolase
- Chest x-ray, electrocardiogram, complete pulmonary function testing with diffusing capacity, and echocardiogram with Doppler studies

---

degree of skin thickening by documentation of a total body skin score, size of maximal oral aperture, and a patient global evaluation of current status. In addition to a complete blood cell count, measurement of electrolytes, urinalysis, and general chemistry determinations, the laboratory assessment should include measurement of muscle enzymes (creatine kinase, aldolase) and thyroid function testing. Active myositis and hypothyroidism are common and may not be clinically obvious. Specific autoantibodies can be helpful in defining disease subsets and predicting outcome. (For more detail see Seibold, Chapter 66, in Kelley et al., reference 112.) Other special testing is dictated by the clinical situation.

NATURAL HISTORY OF SCLERODERMA

The natural history of scleroderma is different for patients with limited skin disease than for patients with diffuse skin changes. Patients with limited scleroderma have an indolent course with little change in visceral involvement over the lifetime of the patient. Skin changes are indeed limited, and therefore aggressive treatment directed at the skin is inappropriate. In patients with limited scleroderma, it is prudent to evaluate them periodically to allow early detection of significant visceral involvement. No drug has been shown to alter the disease course in patients with limited disease; however, there are drugs that might improve organ function, prevent further visceral damage, or help alleviate the complications of tissue injury.

In patients with diffuse skin disease, the natural course of disease is generally aggressive in the early years with rapidly changing skin involvement and concurrent or subsequent significant visceral disease; particularly the gastrointestinal tract, lung, heart, and kidney. (For more detail, see Seibold, Chapter 66, in Kelley et al., reference 112.) After approximately a 1- to 3-year period, the patient may "stabilize" with a very indolent course and a gradual deterioration of a damaged organ. Some patients seem to wax and wane, and some improve. Improvement of the skin changes is quite common during this period of stabilization. In the active or early stage of diffuse disease, it is appropriate to consider treatment with "disease-modifying" drugs. Patients who have ad-vanced, thickened skin may or may not be treatable; patients who have begun a spontaneous regression should not be treated. All patients should be sequentially evaluated for visceral involvement and then considered for organ-specific treatment.

RATIONALE FOR TREATMENT APPROACH

Our current understanding of scleroderma would suggest that there is a complex interplay of at least four different biologic processes that are prominent in the disease: inflammation, an autoimmune process, fibrosis, and a chronic noninflammatory small-vessel vasculopathy. (For more detail, see Seibold, Chapter 66, in Kelley et al., reference 112.) Each of these processes is a potential target for therapeutic intervention. Current therapy has primarily focused on preventing or reversing fibrosis or controlling the immune system. Numerous drugs have been tried in the treatment of scleroderma, mostly in small numbers of patients or in open and uncontrolled trials. There is no drug that is generally accepted as helpful or that has been proven useful in a rigorous controlled trial. Therefore the risks and benefits of almost all of the drugs that have been used as disease modifying agents in scleroderma remain unknown.

For several reasons, research into the drug treatment of scleroderma has been less than ideal.[2] First, the pathogenesis of scleroderma is yet unsolved; therefore, the rationale for currently used medications is often theoretical rather than proven. Most academic research centers do not follow a large enough number of patients for a definitive clinical trial. There are also different subsets of scleroderma, each with its own unique clinical course and probably unique response to treatment. In addition, the course of the disease is highly variable, with periods of waxing and waning activity. Fibrosis and tissue atrophy are the final stages of scleroderma and may not respond to treatment. Many trials have been too short in duration or have chosen an inappropriate outcome variable to determine the usefulness of the agent being tested. Therefore clinical trials in scleroderma need to select a large enough uniform population of patients who have the potential for recovery.

DRUGS USED AS "DISEASE-MODIFYING AGENTS" IN SCLERODERMA

Excellent recent reviews of the drugs used in the treatment of scleroderma have been published.[3,4] This section will highlight agents that are currently used in the treatment of scleroderma, recognizing that no drug has been proven to change the natural course of scleroderma.

D-Penicillamine (DPA).

(For more detail see Jaffe, Chapter 46, in Kelley et al., reference 112.)

D-Penicillamine was first thought to be useful in scleroderma because of its ability to alter maturation of collagen by decreasing intermolecular cross-linking of collagen, increasing soluble collagen, and inhibiting collagen biosynthesis, thus thinning the skin. Although DPA is currently widely used in the treatment of scleroderma, there has been no randomized placebo-controlled trial to prove its efficacy or to define the appropriate dose and duration of therapy.

Patients need to understand that although DPA has been used with some reported success, it has not been absolutely proven to be efficacious. Most of the data supporting the use of DPA suggest that it primarily improves the skin with some suggestion of improved lung function and survival. However, if benefit is to be expected, it may not be noted for at least 6 months after the start of therapy, and therefore treatment should be directed toward early active disease. During this 6-month period, severe skin changes may occur, particularly facial changes and irreversible finger and hand contracture. Approximately two thirds of patients are reported to improve. Some investigators have suggested that this long interval before improvement is secondary to the long time necessary for skin remodeling to occur,[4] whereas others have countered that the natural course of untreated patients shows the same gradual improvement.

Steen et al.[5] reported one of the first large experiences with D-penicillamine in which only patients with diffuse disease were treated. Seventy-three patients who had received DPA for at least 6 months (mean 24 months, range 6 to 68 months) were compared with forty-five patients who were not treated with the drug. The DPA-treated patients had a greater decrease in skin thickness, less new visceral involvement (primarily renal disease), and a greater 5-year survival rate than the untreated group (DPA 88% versus no DPA 66%). Although no optimal dose was determined in this study, 40% of the responders improved after taking a maximum daily DPA dose of 750 mg. The untreated control group was not randomized; nor were they necessarily followed concurrently with the DPA-treated patients.

A second large survey of patients treated in an open uncontrolled experience was reported by Jimenez and Sigal.[6] This study is unique in that patients were included only if they had early (less than 18 months), rapidly progressive (an increase of greater than 30% in the extent of skin involvement in the preceding 6 months) disease. There was no comparison control group. Of the 60 patients who received 750 mg of DPA for at least 6 months, 58 demonstrated improvement in their skin (65% to 16% of total body surface). Little progression of renal or lung involvement was seen, and a survival rate of 88.3% was reported. In this study, the skin condition continued to worsen for the first 6 months of DPA administration before showing improvement.

The toxicity of DPA is significant in patients with scleroderma. Reviewed by Steen et al.,[7] 47% of 259 patients developed drug toxicity and 29% had to stop the use of DPA. Adverse reactions were seen most commonly during periods of rapid dose changes. Toxicity was similar to that seen in rheumatoid arthritis and include rash or pruritus (15%), proteinuria (9%), gastrointestinal symptoms (8%), dysgeusia (3%), oral ulcers (3%), leukopenia (2%), thrombocytopenia (4%), myasthenia gravis (2%), and pemphigus (2%).

There is currently under way a large multi-centered prospective parallel double-blinded trial in which patients with early diffuse scleroderma are being randomized to either low-dose (125 mg every other day) or high-dose (1000 mg every day) DPA. The results of this trial will be most helpful in giving us guidance about the role of DPA in the management of scleroderma.

Three types of patients are considered appropriate for treatment with DPA: The patient with early diffuse skin disease, the patient with early skin involvement that has included the hands and forearms, and patients with established diffuse skin changes who are clearly flaring with progressive skin changes. Patients should not be treated with DPA if they have skin changes limited to the fingers (CREST syndrome), if there are definite clinical signs of regression or stability, or if the skin changes are late and represent atrophic or inactive disease. Some may consider DPA for treatment of active scleroderma lung disease or other internal organ involvement, but the data as to whether DPA has any significant role for visceral disease are inconclusive.

D-Penicillamine should be started at 125 or 250 mg/d (Table 12–2). The daily dose can be increased at intervals of 6 weeks to 3 months by increments of 250 mg. The maximal dose is 1000 to 1500 mg daily. The dose should not be increased if the patient shows improvement or if potential toxicity is suspected. The maximal dose should be maintained for a minimum of 6 months after there is no further improvement and then tapered. Although specific data are not available to determine the maintenance dose or duration, it is recommended that a dose of 250 mg/d be continued unless toxicity occurs or a long remission is established.

DPA should be carefully monitored for toxicity (Table 12–2). Not all toxicity is related to dose; some occurs early in therapy (rash, proteinuria), and others late in the course of treatment (autoimmune disease). It is recommended that clinical and laboratory parameters be followed, first at 2-week intervals, and then monthly until a stable maximum dose is established. Once a stable dose is established, the patient should be seen and laboratory data should be obtained at intervals of 1 to 2 months. A complete blood cell count looking for leukopenia and thrombocytopenia and a urinalysis should be done at each safety visit. If protein or abnormal sediment is detected on urinalysis, then the drug should be stopped and a 24-hour urine collected to quantitate the total protein excretion. Mild proteinuria of less than 500 mg can be tolerated and the drug can be continued with careful serial assessment of renal function and proteinuria. Any worsening would dictate discontinuation of drug, with no rechallenge. Proteinuria usually occurs after 3 months of therapy and most commonly is secondary to an immune-complex mediated membranous nephropathy. Rarely, rapidly progressive glomerulonephritis may occur.[8] Long-term monitoring should be done to detect proteinuria, cytopenias, and the late onset of autoimmune diseases, including myasthenia gravis, pemphigus, myositis, and lupuslike reactions.

In summary, DPA is currently the drug of first choice in early disease when cutaneous disease is the dominant clinical problem. Although studies have suggested that DPA is helpful for internal organ involvement and may improve survival, the data are not solid enough for a final judgment.

Colchicine. Initial uncontrolled trials of colchicine reported disappointing results.[9,10] However, a randomized double-blind crossover trial of 1 mg/d of colchicine versus placebo for 3 months was conducted in 1979 and suggested some benefit.[11] Despite the lack of objective measurable changes, 9 of the 14 patients who completed the trial, believed they had improved while taking colchicine. These same investigators then entered patients into a long-term uncontrolled trial of colchicine.[12] Nineteen patients took an average dose of 10.1 mg colchicine per week for an average of 39 months. Generally, in patients treated less than 5 years into the course of their disease, there was improvement or stability in subjective measures of skin elasticity, measures of grip strength, fingertip-to-palm distance, mouth opening, dysphagia, and pulmonary function testing. A second placebo-controlled crossover trial of 28 patients treated with 2 mg/d versus placebo for 9 months failed to confirm that colchicine was beneficial to skin or visceral involvement.[13] All studies to date have major study design problems, and therefore the

---

TABLE 12–2

Guidelines for Use of D-Penicillamine in Systemic Sclerosis

- Use only in patients with early diffuse disease who demonstrate a definite change in skin in the preceding 2 months
- Start with 250 mg daily and increase slowly at 2- or 3-month intervals, moving to a maximal dose of 1000–1500 mg daily
- Maintain therapy for at least 1 year; if no benefit, discontinue treatment
- Monitor clinical status, complete blood cell count, platelet count, and urinalysis every month
- Early toxicities (few months): dermatitis, altered taste, pemphigus pruritus, fever
- Late toxicities (1–2 years): stomatitis, nausea, leukopenia, thrombocytopenia, proteinuria, autoimmune disease

role of colchicine in the treatment of scleroderma is unknown. We do not recommend the use of colchicine.

Potassium Para-aminobenzoate Acid (PABA).

In both normal and scleroderma dermal fibroblasts, PABA inhibits glycoaminoglycan production.[14] However, there has been no evidence that PABA inhibits collagen synthesis. Zarafonetis et al.[15] have reported their uncontrolled experience with PABA in 224 patients with scleroderma. Ninety percent of the patients treated with PABA showed a mild to moderate improvement while taking PABA, 8 to 12 g daily for 8 to 24 months, whereas only 19% of 96 patients who were not treated with PABA showed similar improvement. PABA-treated patients had less progression of lung involvement and increased survival when compared with the untreated group. The first large double-blinded placebo-controlled trial found no improvement in skin mobility or skin thickening in patients treated with PABA compared with those given placebo.[16] PABA cannot be recommended in the treatment of scleroderma.

Dimethyl Sulfoxide (DMSO).

DMSO has been reported to be an analgesic, a vasodilator, an antiinflammatory, and a cytoprotective agent. Although there are a number of uncontrolled studies suggesting some benefit of topical DMSO, the overall experience is controversial and, therefore, the use of DMSO cannot be recommended in the treatment of scleroderma. Scherbel[17] has reported some modest benefit in terms of grip strength and skin softening following 50% to 70% topical DMSO, whereas Binnick et al.[18] found no benefit in skin induration, ischemic ulcers, or range of motion in 20 patients treated for 3 to 15 months. The largest double-blind study found no benefit for healing of digital ulcers and no study has demonstrated any benefit for visceral involvement.[19] Some analgesic effect on painful digital ulcers may occur with topical DMSO; however, a number of severe skin reactions were reported with the use of the 70% solution.[19]

Immunosuppressive Agents.

Autoantibody production, inflammatory cellular infiltrates, and cytokine increases suggest that scleroderma is an autoimmune inflammatory disease dependent on T cell function and other cells of the immune system. Therefore a number of therapies have been designed to target components of the immune system. Unfortunately, most of these studies have been uncontrolled trials that mixed patients with both limited and diffuse disease and patients at various stages of disease. It is difficult to make a judgment about immunosuppressive therapy, but in general these agents have been disappointing.

The use of corticosteroids has not been completely studied. However, it is the general impression that corticosteroids do not influence the course of scleroderma. Corticosteroids should be used only in patients with a specific organ problem that may be responsive, such as inflammatory myositis, a polyarthritis that is unresponsive to a nonsteroidal antiinflammatory drug or rapid progressive pulmonary fibrosis (see section on specific organ therapy). Topical corticosteroids have been used on the skin in patients with localized morphea or during the early edematous pruritic stage of scleroderma when skin is rapidly worsening. Although not a proven risk, it has been suggested that oral corticosteroids may precipitate a normotensive renal crisis.

Chlorambucil is an alkylating agent with immunosuppressive properties. An unblinded trial of chlorambucil in 11 patients with scleroderma suggested some benefit,[20] whereas another trial in 21 patients reported no effect.[21] Furst et al.[22] conducted a 3-year parallel double-blind placebo-controlled trial of chlorambucil in 65 patients with scleroderma. Although the chlorambucil group had evidence of immunosuppression manifested by decreases in white blood cell count, lymphocyte counts, and platelet counts compared with the control group, the drug had no clinical advantage over placebo in terms of both skin score and internal organ involvement.

Azathioprine is an immunosuppressive agent that was studied in an open uncontrolled trial involving 21 patients with various forms and stages of scleroderma for an average of 14 months' follow-up.[23] A starting dose 150 mg/d was used and adjusted during the trial to a maximum of 250 mg/d. Eight patients were subjectively improved, seven were judged unchanged, two progressed, and one was lost to follow-up. Judgment on the role of azathioprine can hardly be made on the basis of this study, and azathioprine is not recommended.

5-Fluorouracil (5-FU) was found to soften fibrotic skin when applied topically and to improve the skin in a patient with scleroderma when 5-FU was used as part of a chemotherapeutic program for breast cancer.[24] Twelve patients with scleroderma, in an open labeled uncontrolled trial of 5-FU, demonstrated improvement in skin scores (mean total score from 36 to 22) and visceral involvement.[24] An additional international collaborative study randomized patients with scleroderma to either 5-FU or placebo.[25] The 5-FU was given in a dose of 12 mg/kg/d for 4 days, then 6 mg/kg for 2 days, followed by weekly doses of 12.5 mg/kg for a total of 6 months. Mild improvement in skin score was found in those receiving 5-FU compared with the placebo group, but there was no effect on internal organ involvement. It does not appear that 5-FU is very helpful in scleroderma, and it cannot be recommended.

Methotrexate (MTX) has been used in uncontrolled trials in the treatment of scleroderma. The rationale is the potential antiinflammatory and immunosuppressive effects of MTX and the success of this agent in the management of other autoimmune diseases. (For more detail see Weinblatt, Chapter 47, in Kelley et al., reference 112.) One unblinded study used a dosage of MTX of 15 mg/wk given intramuscularly for the first 6 months and then orally thereafter.[26] Seven of the eight patients had a 25% improvement in skin score but no significant visceral improvement.[26] A placebo-controlled double-blind trial was reported in abstract.[27] Patients with early or progressive disease were randomized to receive either placebo or MTX, 15 to 25 mg intramuscularly per week. There was no significant difference in skin score or in subjective measures of well-being between the treatment groups after 24 weeks.[27] The role of MTX in the treatment of scleroderma is unresolved, but MTX probably should be limited to the treatment of steroid-resistant active polymyositis until more research is done.

Cyclosporine was reported to be helpful in an open study of eight patients with scleroderma.[28] Skin score improved at 6 months, and four patients had improvement in baseline hypoxia. However, a reduction of renal function was reported in four patients in the trial. It has also been reported that a patient with scleroderma and renal transplant developed rapid renal failure during immunosuppressive therapy that included cyclosporine.[29] In a 48-week open safety study of cyclosporine in 10 scleroderma patients, Clements et al.[30] found that the skin score improved in all of the patients and significantly improved (greater than 35%) in 6 of the 10 patients, while cardiac and pulmonary organ involvement remained stable. This improvement in the skin was significant when compared with a historical control group. However, there was frequent dose-related and usually transient renal toxicity.[30] The use of FK506, a drug with properties similar to cyclosporine, is also currently being studied in patients with scleroderma.

Total lymphoid irradiation (TLI) has been used in immunosuppressive therapy for scleroderma.[31] The rationale for using TLI has been supported by its reported use in rheumatoid arthritis and systemic lupus erythematosus. Six scleroderma patients were randomized to either TLI or no therapy.[31] Despite good evidence of immunosuppression, there was no clinical benefit. Of note was the fact that severe pulmonary and gastrointestinal progression was reported in the TLI-treated patients.[31]

Antithymocyte globulin has been used because of the postulated central role of T cells in the pathogenesis of scleroderma. One patient with aplastic anemia and scleroderma-like syndrome was treated daily for 10 days with 15 mg/kg body weight.[32] The skin sclerosis improved and remained better after 5 months of follow-up. The same investigators treated two patients with scleroderma and reported a decrease in palpable skin induration and improvement in pulmonary function in both patients.[33] A randomized trial of intravenous saline solution versus antithymocyte globulin was reported in abstract.[34] Six months after treatment, skin score and lung function were not altered by treatment. Significant side effects, including fever and serum sickness, occurred during antithymocyte treatment.

Photopheresis has been used to treat T cell–dependent disorders, including cutaneous T cell lymphoma, pemphigus, and murine graft-versus-host disease.[35] Its use in scleroderma is based on the hypothesis that the inflammation and subsequent fibrosis in scleroderma are mediated by T cells. A multicentered single-blinded trial of photopheresis versus DPA in early diffuse scleroderma was reported in 1992.[36] The investigators reported photopheresis was marginally more beneficial than DPA at 6 months but was not different than DPA at 10 months. The reported benefit of photopheresis was limited to the skin without significant effects in other organ systems. Photopheresis is costly and is associated with study-related morbidities, including problems with repeated cannulations for access in this population. A number of study design flaws (including an unexplained differential drop-out rate in the two treatment arms) do not permit conclusions to be drawn from the report. The place of photopheresis in the treatment of scleroderma has not been defined as yet; more controlled investigations are needed and ongoing.[37]

Other Agents.   Several additional agents and therapeutic approaches have been reported in the treatment of scleroderma. However, the data, although of interest, is inconclusive and their use cannot be recommended. Some of these agents include factor XIII,[38,39] interferon-alpha,[40] interferon-gamma,[41] isotretinoin,[42] griseofulvin,[43] plasma exchange,[44,45] disodium edetate (EDTA),[46,47] N-acetlycysteine,[48] cyclofenil,[49] dextran infusion,[50] and kerotifen.[51]

FUTURE APPROACHES

The future is exciting for the development of new therapies for scleroderma. Investigations into the pathogenesis of scleroderma have suggested that specific cytokines are important mediators of fibrosis. Therapy that inhibits or down-regulates the production of specific cytokines may target a key factor that provokes the fibroblast and promotes the propagation of tissue fibrosis. Inhibitors of transforming growth factor-beta is one example of this type of approach.[52] Understanding the molecular mechanisms of gene regulation, cytokine production or collagen production by fibroblast may reveal methods to control the activation of the tissue fibroblast.

Rather than using global immunosuppressive drugs, targeting specific immune cells or targeting the ability of inflammatory and immune cells to traffic into target tissues may be an effective approach. Examples of this approach would include inhibitors of key adhesion molecules that are upregulated in the tissues and blood vessels of scleroderma patients, inhibition of specific autoreactive T cell clones, or regulation of antigen-processing cells.

A fundamental understanding of the chronic vasculopathy that is so widespread and prominent in scleroderma is a major key to developing effective new treatment. Controlling abnormal vascular reactivity and vascular occlusion is difficult without reversing the basic pathologic process and fibrosis of the blood vessel. Preventing tissue ischemia and reperfusion tissue injury is yet another major puzzle to unravel in scleroderma. Potential approaches include vasodilator therapy, prevention of coagulation, fibrinolysis therapy, interference with cell trafficking by blocking important adhesion molecules, and the use of antioxidants to reduce tissue damage.

THE AUTHORS' APPROACH

Most of the drugs that have been studied as disease-modifying agents in scleroderma have focused on the skin as the major important outcome variable. Certainly, the skin involvement is the most obvious problem to the scleroderma patient, particularly early in the disease. However, the systemic-visceral disease often dominates later treatment decisions as these issues emerge as clinically important and potential life-threatening problems. One should also recognize that the placebo arm of several studies has demonstrated that the skin (and visceral disease) can remain quite stable or improve after the initial insult of active disease.[53] The treatment approach must be comprehensive without focusing solely on the skin. It must also recognize both the shortcomings and the toxicity of our current available drugs. Aggressive use of experimental therapy in the stable patient or the patient with limited disease is not indicated.

DPA is considered the first drug to be tried in a patient with early disease (see above). However, in order to understand how to appropriately use DPA (or other drug therapy) in scleroderma, patients who are candidates for treatment should be considered for participation in a controlled clinical trial. If the patient is unable or unwilling to participate in a research trial, then it is reasonable to start DPA as the drug of first choice. If DPA fails or a significant toxicity develops, then the patient should be reevaluated for the tempo of the disease at that time. New therapy should be limited to patients with progressive disease. Therapy directed at specific organ dysfunction (see specific section) may improve the quality of the patient's life and be more important than potentially toxic and experimental drugs. Patients who have continued evidence of skin progression and who do not have treatment programs dictated by specific organ involvement (see specific section) should be considered for experimental treatment. Low-dose weekly methotrexate and cyclosporine are agents that we currently use in this situation.

ORGAN-SPECIFIC TREATMENT

Management of Scleroderma Lung (Fig. 12–1)

Lung involvement, usually associated with interstitial fibrosis, is a major factor in the morbidity and mortality of patients with scleroderma. Evidence correlating gallium scanning, bronchoalveolar lavage (BAL), and open lung biopsy has demonstrated that the pulmonary fibrosis is often preceded by an inflammatory alveolitis, which persists over time.[54] BAL is a safe and sensitive means to evaluate for the presence of an alveolitis.[55] In fact, a prospective study suggested that the presence of an alveolitis correlates with increased dyspnea and reductions in lung volume and diffusing capacity.[56] On initial evaluation and subsequent visits, patients with the diagnosis of systemic sclerosis should be asked specifically about cardiopulmonary complaints: cough, exertional dyspnea, pedal edema, chest pain, orthopnea. All patients regardless of symptoms should undergo a chest x-ray and complete pulmonary function testing (PFT). Attempts should be made to clinically distinguish the patients who have an "ac-

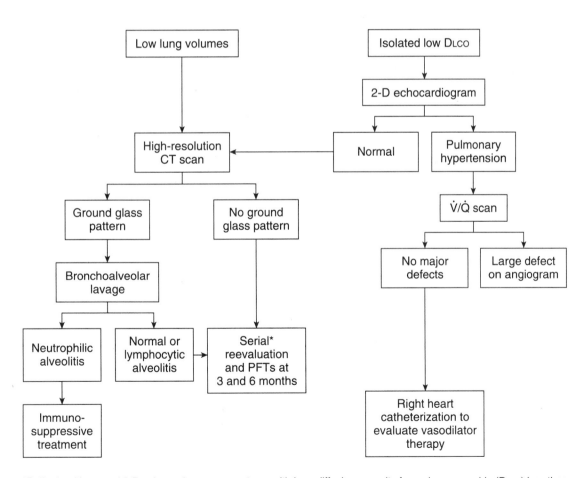

*Patients with normal 2-D echo and severe symptoms with lung diffusing capacity for carbon monoxide (D_{LCO}) less than 50% predicted who do not have evidence of alveolitis should be considered for right heart catheterization.

FIGURE 12–1
Pulmonary symptoms and/or documented decline in pulmonary function tests (PFTs).

tive" alveolitis from the patients who have stable, chronic, fibrotic lung changes. The patients with an active alveolitis are candidates for antiinflammatory treatment and, if left untreated, are at greater risk of declines in lung function.

Patients who have progressive pulmonary symptoms or have progressive declines of greater than 10% in lung function on serial PFTs at 3-month intervals, suggestive of an active process, should undergo a high-resolution computed tomography (CT) scan. If a "ground-glass" pattern indicative of an alveolitis is seen on the CT scan,[57] BAL is then used to confirm and characterize the alveolitis. Patients with progressive symptoms or deteriorating lung function, who also have a negative CT scan, may be followed with serial PFTs at 3-month intervals. If symptoms worsen or if lung function continues to decline despite a CT scan that does not demonstrate an alveolitis, patients should then undergo BAL.

Although there is no uniformly agreed-upon therapeutic approach to the interstitial fibrosis of the lung in scleroderma, patients with deteriorating lung function and objective evidence by BAL of an active, polymorphonuclear alveolitis should be considered for aggressive treatment. An alveolitis is considered to be present if the number of cells exceeds the normal control values established for each individual laboratory. Treatment of patients with a predominantly lymphocytic infiltrate is controversial; some suggest that this subset of patients may follow a benign course.[58] These patients, as well as those with normal BAL, can be followed by lung-function testing at 3- to 6-month intervals.

One treatment approach has been the use of antiinflammatory/immunosuppressive agents in the subset of patients with alveolitis. Corticosteroids have been used without clinical benefit[54] except in isolated case reports.[59,60] Corticosteroids did not suppress the alveolitis in four scleroderma patients treated with prednisone 1 mg/kg/d for 1 to 1.5 months, tapering by 5 mg every 10 days to a baseline of 0.25 mg/kg/d.[54] Similarly, corticosteroids alone have had little effect in suppressing the neutrophilic alveolitis seen in idiopathic pulmonary fibrosis (IPF).[61,62] The use of cyclophosphamide in addition to corticosteroids has been promising both in IPF[62] and scleroderma.[63] Recently, 14 scleroderma patients were treated with oral cyclophosphamide, 1 to 2 mg/kg/d, together with less than 10 mg/d

of prednisone. Twelve patients showed either a stable or improved forced vital capacity (FVC) and a stable diffusing capacity (DLCO) at 18 to 24 months of follow-up.[63] Although another study found no clinical benefit from chlorambucil, the investigators did not select for treatment patients who had an active alveolitis.[22]

It is recommended that the subset of patients with evidence on BAL of an active neutrophilic alveolitis be treated with a combination of prednisone and cyclophosphamide. Treatment is initiated with cyclophosphamide, 2 mg/kg/d orally, together with a tapering dose of prednisone starting at 0.5 mg/kg/d and tapering to less than 10 mg daily within the first 6 to 8 weeks. Therapy is reevaluated with a repeat BAL and PFTs at 6 months. If patients respond by an improvement in BAL and improvement or stabilization on PFTs, treatment is continued for 1 year. The patient is then followed by symptoms and lung-function testing every 3 months. Should patients have deterioration in PFTs and recurrent symptoms associated with active alveolitis, therapy is reinstituted for an additional year. Other immunosuppressive regimens can be tried, but there are little data to give guidance. Patients need to understand that immunosuppressive therapy is experimental (not proven) and is associated with significant potential risk.

Two studies limited by their retrospective designs show modest benefit of DPA in scleroderma lung.[64,65] However, the difference between treated and untreated groups was probably not clinically significant; nor was there any data on the subset of patients with active alveolitis and declining lung function.

Although pulmonary artery hypertension is a frequent complication of the interstitial parenchymal changes, it is usually indolent in nature and less worrisome than isolated pulmonary hypertension seen primarily in patients with limited scleroderma. Isolated pulmonary hypertension should be suspected in patients whose pulmonary complaints appear in the absence of evidence of interstitial fibrosis. It is especially difficult to detect mild to moderate pulmonary hypertension by physical findings. In one study, however, a DLCO less than 55% predicted and a ratio of FVC (% predicted)/DLCO (% predicted) of greater than 1.4 strongly correlated with the development of isolated pulmonary hypertension.[66] It is recommended that all patients with scleroderma with cardiopulmonary symptoms or pulmonary function abnormalities have an echocardiogram with Dopplers (2-D ECHO) to noninvasively determine whether there is evidence of pulmonary hypertension. If significant pulmonary hypertension is present, a ventilation perfusion scan should be done to rule out pulmonary embolism. If there is a high suspicion of emboli, then confirmation by pulmonary arteriography is recommended.

Treatment of primary pulmonary hypertension (PPH) and pulmonary hypertension secondary to scleroderma is controversial, with no universally accepted regimens. A consensus statement by the American College of Chest Physicians on pulmonary hypertension has recently been published.[67] Recommendations applicable to patients with pulmonary hypertension secondary to scleroderma include supplemental oxygen, diuretics in patients with significant right heart failure, anticoagulation, vasodilator therapy, and, if necessary, heart-lung transplantation.

Hypoxic pulmonary vasoconstriction occurs in both PPH and scleroderma,[68] and patients should undergo testing to look for resting and exercise-induced oxygen desaturation. In cases of significant desaturation, supplemental resting or ambulatory oxygen should be used. Anticoagulation, although not formally studied in the scleroderma population, has been demonstrated to significantly increase survival rates in PPH.[69] It is recommended that scleroderma patients with severe pulmonary hypertension and with no contraindication for anticoagulation be treated with warfarin.

Vasodilator therapy with calcium channel blockers, angiotensin-converting enzyme inhibitors, and recently intravenous prostacyclin analogs have been used for both scleroderma and PPH. In PPH, high doses of calcium channel blockers (mean daily dose nifedipine 172 mg, diltiazem 720 mg) improved pulmonary artery pressures and survival.[70] Both acute and chronic administration of nifedipine (10 to 30 mg every 8 hours) to patients with CREST syndrome produced a significant reduction of pulmonary artery pressures.[71] The angiotensin-converting enzyme inhibitor captopril has been disappointing in the treatment of PPH. However, captopril reverses the renovascular complications of scleroderma, and in a small study of eight CREST patients with mild to moderate pulmonary hypertension captopril, 12.5 to 50 mg, reduced pulmonary artery pressures.[72] Thus, captopril should not be totally excluded from future studies on pulmonary hypertension secondary to scleroderma. Experimental treatment with the intravenous prostacyclin (epoprostenol), chronically infused through a portable pump, has shown promise in improving the hemodynamic and symptomatic responses in PPH.[73] However, acute administration of a prostacyclin analogue, iloprost, failed to improve diffusing capacity in patients with scleroderma.[74] More studies with both long-term and short-term infusion with prostacyclin need to be done in both scleroderma and PPH.

Patients with evidence of pulmonary hypertension are considered eligible for a trial of vasodilator therapy. They should be hospitalized for monitoring and right heart catheterization; therapy is then instituted with short-acting preparations of nifedipine, with doses titrated to systemic blood pressure, pulmonary artery pressure, and cardiac output. Systemic hypotension, increased right heart failure, and negative inotropy are frequent complications. Patients who respond are maintained on nifedipine over a long term and are followed clinically. We do not recommend corticosteroids or immunosuppressive therapy for pulmonary hypertension in the absence of an active alveolitis.

Pleural reactions are a common finding but are usually clinically silent. When active pleuritis is present, other causes should be considered. A short course of a nonsteroidal antiinflammatory drug is usually effective. All scleroderma patients with lung involvement should be given both influenza and pneumococcal vaccines. They should be treated with antibiotics at the first signs of purulent bronchitis or pulmonary infection.

Long-term, aspiration may be clinically important, even in patients without severe myositis and pharyngeal muscle involvement. Patients with reflux symptoms should be treated aggressively (see "Management of the Gastrointestinal Tract"). Nocturnal wakenings due to choking or shortness of breath, recurrent pneumonias, recent onset of hoarseness, and unexplained bronchospasm are suggestive of chronic aspiration. The incidence of carcinoma of the lung has been reported to be increased in patients with scleroderma. However, the risk is not sufficient to recommend increased surveillance in the absence of clinical suspicion and other risk factors.

Management of the Gastrointestinal Tract

Involvement of the gastrointestinal tract in scleroderma is almost universal, but the severity of the clinical problem is highly variable and generally unpredictable. A vasculopathy or muscular atrophy with fibrosis causes neuromuscular dysfunction throughout the gastrointestinal tract and, as a consequence, a loss of normal coordinated motility. Unfortunately, no therapeutic intervention has been shown to prevent or alter the natural course of the gastrointestinal involvement.

Facial scleroderma can make chewing difficult, and a small oral aperture often precludes normal dental care. In addition, hand deformities, muscle weakness, and disease of the temporomandibular joint may all complicate care of the mouth and accelerate caries and loss of teeth. Adaptive devices such as an electric toothbrush are helpful, and more frequent dental visits for cleaning and surveillance are prudent. Dry mucous membranes (the sicca syndrome) are frequent in scleroderma and may dampen normal taste and appetite and complicate dental care (see Chapter 5, Sjögren's syndrome). Frequent small meals and avoidance of large difficult-to-chew foods are most helpful. Some patients will require liquid supplements to maintain adequate caloric intake.

Dysphagia is generally caused by esophageal dysmotility. Patients who have difficulty initiating a swallow or who have regurgitation of food into the upper airway may have a superimposed neuromuscular disease such as DPA-induced myasthenia gravis or polymyositis affecting the striated muscles of the oral pharynx.

A high prevalence of esophagitis is present in patients with scleroderma as a result of abnormal motility and decreased acid clearance from the esophagus.[75] This damage may be associated with ulceration, blood loss, and (rarely) a Barrett's esophagus (predisposing to carcinoma) or stricture. Therefore patients with a diagnosis of scleroderma should be evaluated aggressively for esophageal disease. Because there is no medication that reverses the disease process, treatment is directed at symptomatic disease or complications of abnormal motility. Patients may be

without symptoms and yet have significant esophageal disease. However, patients with normal motility studies rarely have esophagitis.[75] A barium swallow is useful to rule out esophageal stricture but is insensitive as a measurement of dysmotility. Ideally, every patient with a diagnosis of scleroderma should have a motility study by either cineesophagography or manometry. If these studies are abnormal, then endoscopy should be done, even if the patient does not have symptoms. In practice, patients may be treated empirically if symptoms of reflux or dysphagia are present. Those who fail a therapeutic trial or have signs of gastrointestinal blood loss should have motility studies or endoscopy. The presence of esophagitis warrants aggressive therapy and careful follow-up to document healing.

Esophagitis in scleroderma may be difficult to treat. Nondrug treatment should include not filling the stomach before bedtime, elevation of the head of the bed, eating small frequent meals, avoidance of tightly fitting clothing, and discontinuation of smoking. Calcium channel blockers, often used for Raynaud's phenomenon, may worsen reflux by decreasing lower esophageal sphincter tone and may have to be stopped. A histamine (H_2) receptor blocker can be used in patients with reflux or dysphagia. However, the esophagitis may be resistant to histamine receptor blockers, and therefore careful follow-up documenting resolved symptoms or endoscopic examination is recommended. Antacids are not recommended as sole therapy because they often cause diarrhea and are less effective than H_2 blockers.[76] Sulcrafate (1 g 4 times daily) may be added to the H_2 blocker, but most patients who have refractory reflux and esophagitis will likely benefit from the use of omeprazole (20 to 40 mg daily) alone. Omeprazole inhibits the activity of H^+/K^+-ATPase and dramatically inhibits gastric acid, thus healing refractory esophagitis.[77] Short-term therapy is safe, and studies of long-term use have not shown an increase in gastric tumors in human beings. Although it is recommended that patients rest from omeprazole periodically, many patients with scleroderma require continuous therapy. Although not yet well studied in scleroderma, the use of omeprazole is justified, given the improved quality of life and the presumed decrease in esophageal damage that omeprazole provides. In scleroderma, symptoms may not directly correlate with the degree of reflux or with resolution of the esophagitis. Therefore, the judgment as to when gastrointestinal studies are done must be based on the overall status of the patient and on laboratory parameters.

Studies suggest that promotility drugs may improve esophageal and gastric emptying if used early in scleroderma, before advanced fibrosis and muscle atrophy occur. Metoclopramide and cisapride have been reported to be helpful in scleroderma.[78–81] Cisapride is preferable to metoclopramide because it has less central nervous system toxicity. The effect of cisapride on lower esophageal sphincter (LES) pressure in scleroderma is controversial.[80,81] Horowitz et al.[79] reported significant improvement in gastric emptying after 10 mg by mouth four times daily but no definite effect on esophageal emptying.[79] Cisapride can be tried by starting at 10 mg 30 to 60 minutes before meals and at bedtime. Cisapride may also improve intestinal transit and small-bowel motility in patients with pseudoobstruction. Although objective documentation of improved motility would be ideal, improvement of symptoms is generally reasonable as a measure of drug effectiveness. Patients who continue to have reflux, dysphagia, or weight loss should be restudied to assess whether esophagitis or stricture is present and to determine whether the motility problem is reversible. Another prokinetic drug is erythromycin, a motilin receptor agonist. Intravenous erythromycin (150 mg) has been shown in scleroderma patients to lower esophageal pressure and improve gastric (fundi) waves, suggesting that it may be helpful in reflux disease or gastroparesis.[82] It is recommended that a small dose of erythromycin (25 mg 1 hour before meals) be tried if cisapride is not helpful.

Feeding tubes bypassing esophageal strictures or severe gastroparesis can be tried. However, generally patients also have significant small-bowel aperistalsis, and tube feeding is usually not successful. Surgical repair has been reported successful in the treatment of esophageal strictures.[83] However, many patients can be managed with periodic endoscope-guided dilatation.

Small-bowel involvement causes abnormal peristalsis that manifests itself clinically as intermittent distention and pain, alternating diarrhea and constipation, pseudoobstruction, and rarely malnutrition from malabsorption secondary to bacterial overgrowth. Most pa-

tients tolerate mild symptoms and, in the absence of weight loss, need no specific therapy except a sensible diet and appropriate natural fiber intake. Calcium channel blockers may aggravate small-bowel motility problems and should be avoided in the problematic patient. Likewise, narcotics and barium studies may lead to impaction and a bowel crises. If weight loss or signs of malnutrition are present during a reasonable caloric intake, then an evaluation for malabsorption should be done. A comprehensive work-up may include fecal fat collection, a breath test to determine whether there is bacterial overgrowth, cultures of duodenal contents, and motility studies. However, a trial of cyclic intermittent antibiotics (1 to 2 weeks of each month) such as ampicillin, tetracycline, trimethoprim-sulfamethoxazole, or metronidazole is reasonable in the patient with suspected or proven malabsorption. Clinical parameters can be followed; these include caloric intake, number of bowel movements, and weight. Proper replacement of calcium, iron, fat-soluble vitamins, vitamin B_{12} replacement, and supplemental protein or medium-chain triglycerides may be necessary.

Cisapride may improve small-bowel motility and should be tried in patients who have symptoms. Octreotide, a synthetic octapeptide analog of somatostatin, has been reported in several cases to help patients with scleroderma-related intestinal pseudoobstruction.[84] Octreotide is given at 50 μg daily in subcutaneous injections. Clinical improvement is monitored. Side effects include depression of normal feeding responses (therefore it should be given at nighttime) and hypoglycemia. The experience thus far has been limited to a few cases.[84] Our personal experience has been disappointing and without any long-term or consistent success.

Leuprolide acetate, gonadotropin-releasing hormone administered once daily at a dose of 0.5 mg subcutaneously, was reported to improve bowel function in five subjects with severe nonscleroderma bowel disfunction.[85] This agent has not been tested in scleroderma, but we have had modest success in one patient with chronic pseudoobstruction secondary to scleroderma. It is evident that any prokinetic drug must be used early in disease before irreversible end-stage muscle atrophy or fibrosis.

Severe malabsorption or pseudoobstruction that is unresponsive to medical management would be treated with total parenteral nutrition (TPN).[86] These patients can be cycled onto feeding for 12 hours at night so that they are free for other activities during the day. Although long-term TPN may be necessary, some patients will have significant improvement in bowel function after relatively short-term TPN. TPN should be continued until the patient has reached normal weight and nutritional status and can demonstrate adequate oral intake.

Acute episodes of pseudoobstruction are best treated with bowel rest and decompression. Surgical resection of atonic sections of bowel have been reported successful in individual cases, but generally surgical resection is not helpful because of the widespread nature of the bowel disease. The rare complication of pneumatosis cystoides intestinalis is best treated conservatively with bowel decompression, oxygen therapy (70% to 100% inhaled oxygen), and antibiotics (metronidazole).[87,88]

Colonic involvement is also common but usually asymptomatic.[89,90] However, wide-mouthed diverticula may rupture, causing a bowel crisis and peritonitis. Scleroderma involving the colon or anorectal area may cause distention, constipation, diarrhea, or incontinence. Most patients can be managed with administration of a synthetic fiber such as Metamucil to increase the stool bulk and yet maintain a soft stool. Low doses of diphenoxylate hydrochloride with atropine sulfate (Lomotil) or loperamide hydrochloride (Imodium) may be used to control diarrhea. Caution should be taken with these agents or narcotics that can precipitate atonic bowel or pseudoobstruction. Surgical correction of rectal prolapse has been reported to improve incontinence, but the surgery may be difficult because of local tissue fibrosis.

Management of Kidney Involvement

Since the first description of the use of captopril to treat renal crisis in 1979,[91,92] angiotensin-converting enzyme (ACE) inhibitors have revolutionized management of scleroderma kidney. The use of captopril or the long-acting ACE inhibitor enalapril rapidly controls blood pressure and stabilizes renal function.[93,94] Efficacy of the newer ACE inhibitors—lisinopril, ramipril, fosinopril, and benazepril—have not been reported. Therapy with ACE inhibitors should be instituted in all patients who have any hypertension (>140/90), particularly in the presence of renal insufficiency. It is the general impression that early treatment of mild or modest hypertension with ACE inhibitors has dramatically reduced the incidence of renal crisis. Hypertension in the absence of a renal crisis should be treated with small doses of either captopril (12.5 mg three times a day) or enalapril (2.5 mg daily). Patients with evidence of scleroderma renal crisis should be hospitalized and treated aggressively with the short-acting agent, captopril (Table 12–3). Patients with hypertension who cannot take an ACE inhibitor should be treated with a calcium channel blocker alone or in combination with other antihypertensive medications.

Patients who are intravascularly volume depleted are particularly susceptible to ACE inhibitor–induced hypotension. Therefore patients taking diuretics and other vasodilators should be monitored carefully for hypotension. Blood pressure, renal function, and potassium level should be monitored carefully during therapy in all patients.

Helfrich et al.[95] reviewed the records of 131 patients encountered over 33 years who presented with acute renal failure thought to be due to scleroderma. Of these patients, 11% had normal recorded blood pressure, atypical for scleroderma renal crisis. The normotensive group had more microangiopathic hemolytic anemia, thrombocytopenia, pulmonary hemorrhage, and recent prior corticosteroid use than

---

TABLE 12–3
Treatment of Scleroderma Renal Crisis

- Definition of renal crisis: Diastolic pressure of 110 or greater with at least two of the following: grade III or IV K-W funduscopic changes, seizures, proteinuria, hematuria, azotemia, microangiopathic hemolytic anemia, or rapidly changing renal function
- Patients should be hospitalized emergently and monitored closely
- Start a short-acting angiotensin-converting enzyme inhibitor, captopril, at 25 mg every 8 hours, increasing by 25 mg every 8–12 hours to control blood pressure; dosage and titration schedules should be adjusted to the level of renal insufficiency; maximum dosage of captopril is 450 mg daily.
- Toxicities: Hypotension, proteinuria, neutropenia, agranulocytosis, anemia, pancytopenia, dysgeusia, dermatitis, cough, and angioedema; hyperkalemia is common and should be carefully monitored

the hypertensive group. Although the mechanism in normotensive renal failure is unclear, some postulate that ACE inhibitors will improve outcome. In patients with scleroderma who present with increasing renal dysfunction and normal blood pressure, other causes of renal insufficiency should be investigated, particularly drug toxicities and prerenal causes. Nonsteroidal medications should be stopped and corticosteroid use curtailed if possible. If no other cause of the renal insufficiency is found, then judicious use of ACE inhibitors can be tried with careful monitoring of renal function and systemic blood pressure.

Management of Raynaud's Phenomenon in Scleroderma

Calcium channel blockers are the drugs most commonly used for the management of Raynaud's phenomenon, but they can be disappointing in patients with scleroderma. Despite the lack of objective improvement, most scleroderma patients will subjectively benefit and report fewer and less intense Raynaud's attacks. There has been no evidence to suggest that vasodilator therapy improves the primary vessel disease in scleroderma, but calcium channel blockers have been shown to improve blood flow to the lung and heart in patients with scleroderma.[71,96,97]

Patients with scleroderma who develop ischemic fingertip ulcers may benefit from vasodilator therapy, and all the recommendations in the general section on treatment of Raynaud's phenomenon can be followed (see Chapter 13 in this volume). In addition, all patients with new ischemic ulcerations or evidence of demarcation of a digit from ischemia should be put at rest and kept warm. Hospitalization may be necessary. The digital circulation in scleroderma, in fact, has some reserve and the capacity to vasodilate if external provoking stimuli are eliminated. When scleroderma patients are at rest in a warm ambient temperature, their skin surface temperature may return to normal without other therapy.[98]

All scleroderma patients, particularly those with digital ischemia, should be given low-dose aspirin (80 mg/d), inasmuch as platelet activation, fibrin deposition, and local thrombosis occurs in these patients. The calcium channel blockers have been shown to inhibit platelet activation in scleroderma.[99] Although fibrinolytic therapy has been suggested for the treatment of Raynaud's phenomenon and digital occlusion in scleroderma,[100] there are no good clinical trials to define the role for these agents. Anticoagulation is generally not recommended; however, the precise role of anticoagulation has not been studied. Patients with scleroderma and severe Raynaud's phenomenon or digital ischemic ulcers may benefit from prostaglandin therapy. These agents are currently given by the intravenous route. PGE_1 is available but requires placement of a central intravenous line for administration (see Raynaud's section). Prostacyclin and its analog, iloprost, have been shown to be of benefit to patients with scleroderma but are not available for use in the United States.[101,102] Oral prostaglandins are now being tested. Misoprostol is an oral PGE_1 analog marketed for the prevention of peptic ulceration secondary to nonsteroidal antiinflammatory drugs. It has not been tested in a clinical trial in scleroderma but was no better than placebo in reversing cold-induced Raynaud's phenomenon in patients with primary Raynaud's phenomenon.[103] Pentoxifylline (Trental) has been frequently used in scleroderma patients with ischemia.[104–106] However, there are no convincing studies to show that it improves local blood flow in these patients, and its use cannot be recommended.

Antiinflammatory or immunosuppressive therapy for ischemic ulcerations secondary to scleroderma is not recommended. There is no evidence of a vasculitis, and these agents may be counterproductive by inhibiting tissue healing. This is particularly true of corticosteroids.

Patients with scleroderma may develop occlusion of a major blood vessel, which could be reversed by surgical correction. One must consider other causes of major vessel disease, such as atherosclerosis in more proximal vessels. Relief of these lesions may improve peripheral blood flow. However, the most common situation involves severe peripheral vascular changes alone that do not provide surgical options. Noninvasive vascular studies should be considered in patients who have evidence of larger-vessel disease (decreased pulses). Angiographic studies are not recommended in patients with scleroderma unless the diagnosis of the vascular lesion is unclear or noninvasive studies show evidence of a surgically correctable lesion.

Management of Skin in Scleroderma

In early active scleroderma the skin, particularly over the forearm and hands, is often mildly erythematous with nonpitting edema and associated intense pruritus. This tends to disappear within weeks to months and is generally unresponsive to antiinflammatory agents or antihistamines. Topical corticosteroid (1% hydrocortisone or 0.1% triamcinolone cream applied one to two times daily) has been used with some success (personal experience) but should be limited to short-term treatment.

The natural lubrication of the skin is abnormal in scleroderma because of damage to sweat and eccrine glands. Drying causes pruritus, which leads to scratching, skin excoriation, and thus more skin damage. Topical care is essential. Frequent use of topical lubricants and emollients containing lanolin, silicone, or petroleum derivatives (Aquaphor, Eucerin, Lubriderm, Vaseline Dermatology lotion, Theraplex, or Lac-Hydrin 12% lotion) are helpful. Patients need to avoid excessive exposure to sun and water. Less frequent bathing, use of protective gloves, and avoidance of detergents and soaps that can dry the skin are important measures.

Patients may have telangiectasis over the face (not on the fingers or palms) removed by phototherapy (laser) for cosmetic reasons. Some patients will benefit from education about the use of cosmetic products that can cover areas of hypopigmentation or telangiectasis.

There are several types of digital lesions in scleroderma. Although all are aggravated by vascular disease, not all the lesions are ischemic in nature. Drying of the skin with fissuring and scaling is common, and the skin may ulcerate. Fissuring and drying of the fingertips can be decreased by nighttime application of petrolatum followed by the use of cotton gloves to cover the treated fingers. Paronychia can occur and can be complicated by secondary soft tissue infection or ulceration. Traumatic ulcerations over the proximal interphalangeal joints of the fingers or other sites, such as the elbow or ankle, are most problematic because these sites usually have thin atrophic overlying skin. Secondary infection of these traumatic ulcers can be severe and can threaten the viability of the digit. Digital ischemic ulcerations occur at the fingertip; they can be both superficial and deep infarctions with associated gangrene.

Theoretically, improving local blood flow with vasodilator therapy should improve healing of ischemic and other lesions (see management of Raynaud's phenomenon). Ulcerations are best treated with a topical antibiotic such as bacitracin and periodic cleansing by whirlpooling (two times daily) of the skin with soap and water or a warm povidone-iodine (Betadine) solution. Colloid dressings (Mitraflex) that reduce skin maceration caused by dressing tapes are now available. Signs of cellulitis or soft tissue infection should be treated aggressively with systemic antibiotics. Debridement may be necessary, but allowing the lesion to naturally demarcate generally prevents further loss of healthy tissue. Prevention of repeated trauma to an active lesion is helpful and can be accomplished by local padding or protective cages designed by the occupational therapist.

Pain control should be liberal during the acute phase of ischemic lesions, as uncontrolled paid may potentiate vasospasm. However, narcotics are also vasoconstrictors and therefore should be discontinued as soon as possible.

Surgical management of ulcerations in lesions of scleroderma should be conservative. However, digital gangrene usually will require surgical amputation. Surgical correction of finger contracture has improved digital function and prevented repeated trauma of the exposed joint. Large ankle ulcers have been successfully treated with skin grafting.

Subcutaneous calcinosis occurs in all subsets of scleroderma but is more prominent in limited scleroderma. It is caused by the deposition of amphorous calcium hydroxyapatite in connective tissue and tends to occur at sites of trauma (around the elbow or forearm) or in the tissues of the finger, probably a consequence of ischemia. The calcinosis may become superficial and rupture through the skin, leading to ulceration and secondary infection. Deposits may just become bothersome lumps, or they can be associated with recurrent local inflammatory episodes induced by the crystalline material. Crystal-induced inflammation can be treated with a nonsteroidal antiinflammatory drug or low doses of colchicine (0.6 mg twice daily).

Medical management of subcutaneous calcinosis has been disappointing. Treatment with low-dose warfarin (1 to 2 mg of Coumadin),[107] chelation therapy,[108] diphosphonates,[109] calcium channel blockers,[110] and probenecid[111] has been reported. However, there is no convincing evidence that any of these agents are effective. Management is limited to protection of these sites from trauma, aggressive treatment of infection and, if technically possible, surgical removal. Lesions on the fingers are usually associated with poor blood flow, and therefore there may be no surgical options other than amputation. Sites that have formed skin ulcerations or fistulas are particularly difficult to manage because the local skin thickening and calcinosis usually does not allow for usual surgical maneuvers and closure of the wound. Local padding and bandages may be the only option.

Management of the Musculoskeletal System

The musculoskeletal pain in scleroderma is often less responsive to antiinflammatory drugs, particularly when signs of an inflammatory arthritis are not present or if there is an associated tendon friction rub. It is reasonable to use a nonsteroidal antiinflammatory drug or low doses of corticosteroid (prednisone, 5 to 10 mg daily). Patients with an inflammatory polyarthritis can be treated with drugs used for rheumatoid arthritis (see Chapter 3). In the late stages of scleroderma, muscle wasting and contracture of the fingers and elbows are often major problems, particularly in diffuse scleroderma.

Almost every patient will benefit from a management program that includes exercise and, especially, hand therapy. Early consultation with an experienced physical or occupational therapist is recommended. Although not well studied, it is the general impression that digits or limbs that are immobilized are more likely to develop serious contracture and worse scleroderma. At the same time, range of motion may be limited by the overlying skin sclerosis; therefore forced exercise may be painful and counterproductive. Patients find that massage, local heat, and gentle stretching are soothing and reduce pain. An appropriate conditioning exercise program is helpful. Activities of daily living, such as dressing, personal hygiene, preparing meals, and mobilization, are often difficult for the patient and the family. A variety of devices are available to help improve the patient's ability to perform independent activities. Most scleroderma patients lose a percentage of hand function secondary to contracture or painful skin ulcerations. These patients in particular are helped by the occupational therapist. Assessment of the home environment and family education can be most helpful for patients with severe musculoskeletal disability.

Fatigue and a sense of weakness are common complaints of patients with scleroderma. The cause is multifactorial, including disease activity, the effects of drugs, malnutrition, and disuse from joint disease. A noninflammatory myopathy can occur secondary to local fibrosis of the connective tissue in muscle tissue. This process does not appear to respond to corticosteroid or immunosuppressive therapy and is best treated with exercise and supportive care. An inflammatory myositis can lead to rapid and profound weakness. Inflammatory myositis should be treated in the same manner as polymyositis or dermatomyositis alone (see Chapter 14).

Management of Cardiovascular Disease

Pericarditis is common in scleroderma, but usually it is clinically silent. When it causes symptoms, pericarditis can be treated with nonsteroidal antiinflammatory drugs or corticosteroids. Large pericardial effusions are uncommon and, when present, should be investigated by pericardiocentesis. Hemodynamic consequences of pericarditis, such as tamponade, are most uncommon.

It has been suggested that myocardial injury in scleroderma is a consequence of reperfusion injury following reversible vasospasm of myocardial vessels. Patchy tissue fibrosis leads to a cardiomyopathy, which can be complicated by heart failure or by ectopic atrial or ventricular beats and other serious arrhythmias. Studies have suggested that vasodilator therapy with a calcium channel blocker (nifedipine) might reverse cardiac vasospasm.[97] However, there are no data on which to make judgment on the benefit of long-term vasodilator therapy. The heart in the patient with scleroderma may be secondarily affected by multiple factors, including severe lung disease (cor pulmonale), associated metabolic disease (hypothyroidism), malnutrition, hypertension, or drugs. In particular, care should be taken not to overlook myocarditis associated with polymyositis. An endomyocardial biopsy may be helpful in a difficult diagnostic situation. Myocarditis should be treated with corticosteroids.

All patients with symptoms of cardiac compromise should be evaluated with 2-D ECHO to assess ventricular function and to noninvasively estimate pulmonary artery pressure. Since the presence of a cardiomyopathy is often underestimated and is a late complication in scleroderma, periodic objective testing to determine cardiac rhythm and function is prudent. Arrhythmias and heart failure are treated in the conventional manner, in conjunction with a cardiologist.

Management of Psychosocial Issues in Scleroderma

A recent survey of patients with scleroderma found that nearly half the patients have mild depressive symptoms and almost 20% have moderate to severe depression.[1] The degree of depression does not correlate with disease severity but is influenced by personality traits and the degree of supportive care available, both at home and professionally. Scleroderma can be demoralizing and both physically and emotionally stressful. Although usually not mentioned by the patient to the physician, loss of usual sexual relationships is common. Each patient with scleroderma should be evaluated for depression or other emotionally distressful issues. These emotional issues are often very responsive if appropriate support and management are instituted. Treatment of serious depression is best managed in conjunction with a psychiatrist.

Management of Other Issues

Impotence is a common problem among male patients with scleroderma. The cause is organic in most cases and is thought to be secondary to defects in neurovascular function. Patients can be helped by referral to a specialist (urologist) in male dysfunction. Neuropathy from carpal tunnel syndrome or trigeminal neuralgia may occur. Carpal tunnel syndrome may require surgical release, while neuralgia may respond to a tricyclic antidepressant or neuroleptic drugs (Tegretol, Dilantin). Anemia in scleroderma can be multifactorial; when it is present, careful assessment for chronic blood loss, malnutrition, and vitamin B_{12} deficiency must be done. Chronic pain is frequent in scleroderma.

It is best to avoid narcotics because they can affect bowel function and because narcotics are vasoconstrictors.

REFERENCES

1. Roca RP, Wigley FM, Needleman BW. Prevalence and correlates of depression in systemic sclerosis. Arthritis Rheum 1992;35:S206.
2. Seibold JR, Furst DE, Clements PJ. Why everything (or nothing) seems to work in the treatment of scleroderma. J Rheumatol 1992;19:673.
3. Torres MA, Furst DE. Treatment of generalized systemic sclerosis. Rheum Dis Clin North Am 1990;16:217.
4. Medsger TA Jr. Treatment of systemic sclerosis. Ann Rheum Dis 1991;50:877.
5. Steen VD, Medsger TA Jr, Rodnan GP. D-penicillamine therapy in progressive systemic sclerosis (scleroderma). Ann Intern Med 1982;97:652.
6. Jimenez SA, Sigal SH. A 15-year prospective study of treatment of rapidly progressive systemic sclerosis with D-penicillamine. J Rheumatol 1991;18:1496.
7. Steen VD, Blair S, Medsger TA Jr. The toxicity of D-penicillamine in systemic sclerosis. Ann Intern Med 1986;104:699.
8. Ntoso KA, Tomaszewski JE, Jimenez SA, et al. Penicillamine-induced rapidly progressive glomerulonephritis in patients with progressive systemic sclerosis: successful treatment of two patients and a review of the literature. Am J Kidney Dis 1986;8(3):159.
9. Fernandez-Herlihy L. Skin elasticity and colchicine in scleroderma. Arthritis Rheum 1976;19:832.
10. Guttadauria M, Diamond H, Kaplan D. Colchicine in the treatment of scleroderma. J Rheumatol 1977;4:272.
11. Alarcon-Segovia D, Ibañez G, Kershenobich D, et al. Treatment of scleroderma by modification of collagen metabolism: a double-blind trial with colchicine vs placebo. J Rheumatol 1974;1(suppl):97.
12. Alarcon-Segovia D, Ramos-Niembro F, Ibañez de Kasep G, et al. Long-term evaluation of colchicine in the treatment of scleroderma. J Rheumatol 1979;6:705.
13. Steigarwald JC. Colchicine vs. placebo in the treatment of progressive systemic sclerosis. In: Black CM, Myers AR. Systemic sclerosis (scleroderma). New York: Gower Medical Publishing, 1985:415.
14. Priestley GC, Brown JC. Effects of potassium para-aminobenzoate on growth and macromolecule synthesis in fibroblasts cultured from normal and sclerodermatous human skin and human synovial cells. J Invest Dermatol 1979;72:161.
15. Zarafonetis CJ, Dabich L, Shouronski JJ, et al. Retrospective studies in scleroderma: skin re-

sponse to potassium para-aminobenzoate therapy. Clin Exp Rheumatol 1988;6:261.

16. Clegg DO for the Aminobenzoate Study Group. Comparison of aminobenzoate and placebo in the treatment of scleroderma. Arthritis Rheum 1992;35:S205.

17. Scherbel AL. The effect of percutaneous dimethyl sulfoxide on cutaneous manifestations of systemic sclerosis. Ann NY Acad Sci 1983;411:120.

18. Binnick SA, Shore SS, Corman A, et al. Failure of dimethyl sulfoxide in the treatment of scleroderma. Arch Dermatol 1977;113:1398.

19. William HJ, Furst DE, Dahl SL, et al. Double-blind, multicenter controlled trial comparing topical dimethyl sulfoxide and normal saline for treatment of hand ulcers in patients with systemic sclerosis. Arthritis Rheum 1985;28(3):308.

20. MacKenzie AH. Prolonged alkylating drug therapy is beneficial in systemic sclerosis [Abstract]. Arthritis Rheum 1970;13:334.

21. Steigerwald JC. Chlorambucil in the treatment of progressive systemic sclerosis. In: Black CM, Myers AR. Systemic sclerosis (scleroderma). New York: Gower Medical Publishing 1985:423.

22. Furst DE, Clements PJ, Hillis S, et al. Immunosuppression with chlorambucil vs placebo, for scleroderma: results of a three-year, parallel, randomized, double-blind study. Arthritis Rheum 1989;32:584.

23. Jansen GT, Barraza DF, Ballard JL, et al. Generalized scleroderma: treatment with an immunosuppressive agent. Arch Dermatol 1968;97:690.

24. Casas JA, Subauste CP, Alarcon GS. A new promising treatment in systemic sclerosis: 5-fluorouracil. Ann Rheum Dis 1987;46:763.

25. Casas JA, Saway PA, Villarreal I, et al. 5-Fluorouracil in the treatment of scleroderma: a randomized, double-blind, placebo controlled international collaborative study. Ann Rheum Dis 1990;49:926.

26. Van den Hoogen PH, Boerbooms AM, van de Putte LB, et al. Low dose methotrexate treatment in systemic sclerosis. J Rheumatol 1991;18:1763.

27. Van den Hoogen FHJ, Boerbooms AMT, Henk JJ, et al. Methotrexate in systemic sclerosis: preliminary 24 week results of a placebo controlled double blind trial. Arthritis Rheum 1993;36(9):S217.

28. Gisslinger H, Burghuber OC, Stacher G, et al. Efficacy of cyclosporin A in systemic sclerosis. Clin Exp Rheumatol 1991;9:383.

29. Ruiz JO, Val F, de Francisco ALM, et al. Progressive systemic sclerosis and renal transplantation: a contraindication to the use of cyclosporin A? Transplant Proc 1991;23(4):2211.

30. Clements PJ, Lachenbruch PA, Sterz M, et al. Cyclosporin in systemic sclerosis: results of a 48-week open safety study in ten patients. Arthritis Rheum 1993;36:75.

31. O'Dell JR, Steigerwald JC, Kennaugh RC, et al. Lack of clinical benefit after treatment of systemic sclerosis with total lymphoid irradiation. J Rheumatol 1989;16:1050.

32. Balaban EP, Sheehan RG, Lipsky PE, et al. Treatment of cutaneous sclerosis and aplastic anemia with antithymocyte globulin. Ann Intern Med 1987;106:56.

33. Balaban EP, Zashin SJ, Geppert TD, et al. Treatment of systemic sclerosis with antithymocyte globulin [Letter]. Arthritis Rheum 1991;34(2):244.

34. Sinclair HD, Williams JD, Rahman MA, et al. Clinical efficacy of anti-thymocyte globulin in systemic sclerosis: results of a placebo controlled trial. Arthritis Rheum 1993;36(9):S217.

35. Yale J of Biol Med. November/December 1989;62(6).

36. Rook AH, Freundlich B, Jegasothy BV, et al. Treatment of systemic sclerosis with extracorporeal photochemotherapy: results of a multicenter trial. Arch Dermatol 1992;128:337.

37. Trentham DE. Photochemotherapy in systemic sclerosis: the stage is set. Arch Dermatol 1992;128:389.

38. Delbarre F, Godeau P, Thivolet J. Factor XIII treatment for scleroderma. Lancet 1981;2:204.

39. Guillevin L, Chouvet B, Mery C, et al. Treatment of progressive systemic sclerosis using factor XIII. Pharmatherapeutica 1985;4:76.

40. Stevens W, Vangheeswaren R, Black CM, et al. Alpha interferon-2a (Roferon-A) in the treatment of diffuse cutaneous systemic sclerosis: a pilot study. Br J Rheumatol 1992;31:683.

41. Kahan A, Amor B, Menkes CJ, et al. Recombinant interferon-γ in the treatment of systemic sclerosis. Am J Med 1989;87:273.

42. Maurice PDL, Bunker CB, Dowd PM. Isotretinoin in the treatment of systemic sclerosis. Br J Dermatol 1989;121:367.

43. Ferri C, Bernini L, Bombardieri S, et al. Long-term griseofulvin treatment for progressive systemic sclerosis. Scand J Rheumatol 1986;15:356.

44. Guillevin L, Leon A, Levy Y, et al. Treatment of progressive systemic sclerosis with plasma exchange: seven cases. Int J Artif Organs 1983;6(6):315.

45. Dau PC, Kahaleh MB, Sagebiel RW. Plasmapheresis and immunosuppressive drug therapy in scleroderma. Arthritis Rheum 1981;24:1128.

46. Mongan ES. The treatment of progressive systemic sclerosis with disodium edetate. Arthritis Rheum 1965;8:1145.

47. Fuleihan FJD, Kurban AK, Abboud RT, et al. An objective evaluation of the treatment of systemic scleroderma with disodium EDTA, pyridoxine and reserpine. Br J Dermatol 1968;80:184.

48. Furst DE, Clements PJ, Harris R, et al. Measurement of clinical change in progressive systemic sclerosis: a 1-year double-blind placebo-controlled trial of N-acetylcysteine. Ann Rheum Dis 1979;38:356.

49. Blom-Bülow B, Öberg K, Wollheim FA, et al. Cyclofenil vs placebo in progressive systemic sclerosis. Acta Med Scand 1981;210:419.

50. Kirk A, Dixon ASJ. Failure of low molecular weight dextran infusions in scleroderma. Ann Rheum Dis 1969;28:49.

51. Gruber BL, Kaufman LD. A double-blind randomized controlled trial of ketotifen vs placebo in early diffuse scleroderma. Arthritis Rheum 1991;34:362.

52. Border WA, Noble NA, Yamamoto T, et al. Natural inhibitor of transforming growth factor-β protects against scarring in experimental kidney disease. Nature 1992;360:361.

53. Clements P, Lachenbruch P, Furst D, et al. The course of skin involvement in systemic sclerosis over three years in a trial of chlorambucil vs placebo. Arthritis Rheum 1993;36:1575.

54. Giovanni AR, Bitterman PB, Rennard SI, et al. Evidence for chronic inflammation as a component of the interstitial lung disease associated with progressive systemic sclerosis. Am Rev Respir Dis 1985;131:612.

55. Strumpf JI, Feld MK, Cornelius MJ, et al. Safety of fiberoptic bronchoalveolar lavage in evaluation of interstitial lung disease. Chest 1981;80:268.

56. Silver RM, Miller KS, Kinsella MB, et al. Evaluation and management of scleroderma lung disease using bronchoalveolar lavage. Am J Med 1990;88:470.

57. Warrick JH, Bhalla M, Schabel SI, et al. High resolution computed tomography in early scleroderma lung disease. J Rheumatol 1991;18:1520.

58. Witt C, Romberg B, Brenke A, et al. Diagnostic and prognostic relevance of bronchoalveolar lavage in systemic sclerosis. Arthritis Rheum 1993;36:5132.

59. Wallaert B, Hatron PY, Grosbois JM, et al. Subclinical pulmonary involvement in collagen-vascular diseases assessed by bronchoalveolar lavage. Am Rev Respir Dis 1986;133:574.

60. Cess GM, Kallenberg MD, Henk MJ, et al. Steroid-responsive interstitial pulmonary disease in systemic sclerosis: monitoring by bronchoalveolar lavage. Chest 1984;86:489.

61. Keogh BA, Bernardo J, Hunninghake GW, et al. Effect of intermittent high dose parenteral corticosteroids on the alveolitis of idiopathic pulmonary fibrosis. Am Rev Respir Dis 1983;127:18.

62. Johnson MA, Kwan S, Snell JN, et al. Randomized controlled trial comparing prednisone alone with cyclophosphamide and low dose prednisolone in combination in cryptogenic fibrosing alveolitis. Thorax 1989;44:280.

63. Silver RM, Warrick JH, Kinsella MB, el al. Cyclophosphamide and low-dose prednisone therapy in patients with systemic sclerosis (scleroderma) with interstitial lung disease. J Rheumatol 1993;20:838.

64. Steen VD, Owens GR, Redmond C, et al. The effect of D-penicillamine on pulmonary findings in systemic sclerosis. Arthritis Rheum 1985;28(8):882.

65. DeClerck LS, Dequeker J, Francx L, et al. D-penicillamine therapy and interstitial lung disease in scleroderma. Arthritis Rheum 1987;30:643.

66. Steen VD, Graham G, Conte C, et al. Isolated diffusing capacity reduction in systemic sclerosis. Arthritis Rheum 1992;35:765.

67. Rubin LJ. Primary pulmonary hypertension. Chest 1993;104:236.

68. Morgan JM, Griffiths M, Du Bois RM, et al. Hypoxic pulmonary vasoconstriction in systemic sclerosis and primary pulmonary hypertension. Chest 1991;99:551.

69. Fuster V, Steele PM, Edwards WD, et al. Primary pulmonary hypertension: natural history and the importance of thrombosis. Circulation 1984;70:580.

70. Rich S, Kaufmann E, Levy PS. The effect of high doses of calcium-channel blockers on survival in primary pulmonary hypertension. N Engl J Med 1992;327:76.

71. Alpert MA, Pressly TA, Mukerji V, et al. Short and long-term effect of nifedipine on pulmonary and systemic hemodynamics in patients with pulmonary hypertension associated with diffuse systemic sclerosis, the CREST syndrome and mixed connective tissue disease. Am J Cardiol 1991;68:1687.

72. Alpert MA, Pressly TA, Mukerji W, et al. Short and long-term hemodynamic effects of captopril in patients with pulmonary hypertension and selected connective tissue disease. Chest 1992;102:1407.

73. Rubin LJ, Mendoza J, Hood M, et al. Treatment of primary pulmonary hypertension with continuous intravenous prostacyclin (epoprostenol): results of a randomized trial. Ann Intern Med 1990;112:485.

74. Thurm CA, Wigley FM, Dole WP, et al. Failure of vasodilator infusion to alter pulmonary diffusing capacity in systemic sclerosis. Am J Med 1991;90:547.

75. Zamost BJ, Hirschberg J, Ippoliti AF, et al. Esophagitis in scleroderma: prevalence and risk factors. Gastroenterology 1987;92:421.

76. Petrokubi RJ, Jeffries GH. Cimetidine vs antacid in scleroderma with reflux esophagitis: a randomized double-blind controlled study. Gastroenterology 1979;77:691.

77. Maton PN. Omeprazole. N Engl J Med 1991;324(14):965.

78. Johnson DA, Drane WE, Curran J. Metoclopramide response in patients with progressive systemic sclerosis. Arch Intern Med 1987;147:1597.

79. Horowitz M, Maddern GJ, Maddox A, et al. Effects of cisapride on gastric and esophageal emptying in progressive systemic sclerosis. Gastroenterology 1987;93:311.

80. Kahan A, Chaussade S, Gaudric M, et al. The effect of cisapride on gastroesophageal dysfunction in systemic sclerosis: a controlled

manometric study. Br J Clin Pharmacol 1991; 31:683.

81. Limburg AJ, Smit AJ, Kleibeuker JH. Effects of cisapride on the esophageal motor function of patients with progressive systemic sclerosis or mixed connective tissue disease. Digestion 1991; 49:156.

82. Kahan A, Chaussade S, Michopoulos S, et al. Erythromycin and esophageal abnormalities in systemic sclerosis [Abstract]. Arthritis Rheum 1991;34(suppl 52):116.

83. Mansour KA, Malone CE. Surgery for scleroderma of the esophagus: a 12-year experience. Ann Thorac Surg 1988;46:513.

84. Soudah HC, Hasler WL, Owyang C. Effect of octreotide on intestinal motility and bacterial overgrowth in scleroderma. N Engl J Med 1991;325(21):1461.

85. Mathias JR, Ferguson KL, Clench MH. Debilitating "functional" bowel disease controlled by leuprolide acetate, gonadotropin-releasing hormone (GnRH) analog. Dig Dis Sci 1989; 34:761.

86. Ng SC, Clements PJ, Berquist WE, et al. Home central venous hyperalimentation in fifteen patients with severe scleroderma bowel disease. Arthritis Rheum 1989;32(2):212.

87. Stafford-Brady FJ, Kahn HJ, Ross TM, et al. Advanced scleroderma bowel: complications and management. J Rheumatol 1988;15:869.

88. Sequeira W. Pneumatosis cystoides intestinalis in systemic sclerosis and other diseases. Semin Arthritis Rheum 1990;19(5):269.

89. Battle WM, Snape WJ, Wright S, et al. Abnormal colonic motility in progressive systemic sclerosis. Ann Intern Med 1981;94:749.

90. Whitehead WE, Taitelbaum G, Wigley FM, Schuster MM. Rectosigmoid mobility and myoelectric activity in progressive systemic sclerosis. Gastroenterology 1989;32(97):428.

91. Lopez-Ovejero JA, Saal SD, D'Angelo WA, et al. Reversal of vascular and renal crises of scleroderma by oral angiotensin-converting-enzyme blockade. N Engl J Med 1979;300(25): 1417.

92. Steen VD, Costantino JP, Shapiro AP. Outcome of renal crisis in systemic sclerosis: relation to availability of angiotensin converting enzyme (ACE) inhibitors. Ann Intern Med 1990;113:352.

93. Smith DC, Smith RD, Korn JH. Hypertensive crisis in systemic sclerosis: treatment with the new oral angiotensin converting enzyme inhibitor MK 421 (enalapril) in captopril-intolerant patients. Arthritis Rheum 1984;27:826.

94. Donohoe JF. Scleroderma and the kidney. Kidney Int 1992;41:462.

95. Helfrich DJ, Banner B, Steen VD, et al. Normotensive renal failure in systemic sclerosis. Arthritis Rheum 1989;32:1128.

96. Sfikakis PP, Pyriakidis MK, Vergos CG, et al. Cardiopulmonary hemodynamics in systemic sclerosis and response to nifedipine and captopril. Am J Med 1991;90:541.

97. Kahan A, Devaux JY, Amor B, et al. Nifedipine and thallium-201 myocardial perfusion in progressive systemic sclerosis. N Engl J Med 1986; 314:1397.

98. Gelber AC, Wigley FM, White B. Continuous ambulatory skin temperature (CAST) in patients with Raynaud's phenomenon (RP). Arthritis Rheum 1993;36:S217.

99. Rademaker M, Thomas RH, Kirby JD, et al. Anti-platelet effect of nifedipine in patients with systemic sclerosis. Clin Exp Rheumatol 1992;10:57.

100. Fritzler MJ, Hart DA. Prolonged improvement of Raynaud's phenomenon and scleroderma after recombinant tissue plasminogen activator therapy. Arthritis Rheum 1990;33:274.

101. Wigley FM, Seibold JR, Wise RA, et al. Intravenous iloprost treatment of Raynaud's phenomenon and ischemia ulcers secondary to systemic sclerosis. J Rheumatol 1992;19:1407.

102. Wigley FM, Wise RA, Seibold JR, et al. Intravenous iloprost infusion in patients with Raynaud's phenomenon secondary to systemic sclerosis: a multi-center placebo-controlled double-blind study. Ann Intern Med 1994;120: 199.

103. Wise RA, Wigley FM. Acute effects of misoprostol on digital circulation in patients with Raynaud's phenomenon. J Rheumatol 1994;21:80.

104. Neirotti M, Longo F, Molaschi M, et al. Functional vascular disorders: treatment with pentoxifylline. Angiology J Vas Dis 1987;38:575.

105. Arosio E, Montesi G, Zannoni M, et al. Comparative efficacy of ketanserin and pentoxiphylline in treatment of Raynaud's phenomenon. Angiology 1989;40:633.

106. Goodfield MJD, Rowell NR. Treatment of peripheral gangrene due to systemic sclerosis with intravenous pentoxifylline. Clin Exp Dermatol 1989;14:161.

107. Berger RG, Hadler NM. Treatment of cutaneous calcinosis of dermatomyositis or scleroderma with low dose narfarin. Arthritis Rheum 1985;28:539.

108. Klein R, Harris SB. Treatment of scleroderma, sclerodactylia and calcinosis by chelation (EDTA). Am J Med 1955;19:798.

109. Metzger AL, Singer FR, Bluestone R, et al. Failure of disodium etidronate in calcinosis due to dermatomyositis and scleroderma. N Engl J Med 1974;291:1294.

110. Farah MJ, Palmieri GMA, Sebes JI, et al. The effect of diltiazem on calcinosis in a patient with the crest syndrome. Arthritis Rheum 1990;33:1287.

111. Dent CE, Stamp TCB. Treatment of calcinosis circumscripta with probenecid. Br Med J 1972;1:216.

112. Kelley WN, Harris ED, Ruddy S, Sledge CB, eds. Textbook of rheumatology. 4th ed. Philadelphia: WB Saunders, 1993.

13

RAYNAUD'S PHENOMENON

Fredrick M. Wigley
Alan K. Matsumoto

DEFINITIONS

Patients who have Raynaud's phenomenon complain of abnormally cold hands and feet associated with episodes of digital cutaneous color changes.[1] These episodes are caused by closure of the muscular digital artery, precapillary arterioles, and arteriovenous shunts of the skin after exposure to cold temperatures or during periods of emotional stress. There is no "gold standard" for making a definite diagnosis, although it is now believed that a history of cold-induced digital pallor and cyanosis is necessary and sufficient to make a clinical diagnosis. A color chart containing actual photographs of fingers during an attack has been used to validate the clinical history. With the use of this method, it has been estimated that the prevalence of Raynaud's phenomenon is between 3% and 15% of the general population.[2] It is more common in women than in men (2:1). Unfortunately, there is no simple and reliable laboratory test that confirms a diagnosis of Raynaud's phenomenon, and laboratory testing such as an ice water cold challenge is not recommended.

After a diagnosis of Raynaud's phenomenon has been made, it should be determined whether the patient has primary Raynaud's phenomenon or Raynaud's phenomenon secondary to another disease process (see Seibold, Chapter 66, in Kelley et al., reference 64). In general, patients with primary Raynaud's phenomenon are more likely to respond to treatment and less likely to have complications than patients with secondary forms of Raynaud's phenomenon. Patients with the primary form have onset in their teens, are usually female,

have mild episodes, deny ischemic damage to the tissues, have no evidence of a secondary process on physical examination, and have normal laboratory data, including a negative antinuclear antibody test and Westergren sedimentation rate.[3] The natural history of primary Raynaud's phenomenon is not uniform in every patient; however, the episodes usually become less intense over time, particularly (in women) after menopause. In primary Raynaud's phenomenon, digital ulcerations do not occur and the patient should have no systemic complications related to the Raynaud's phenomenon. However, there is evidence that Raynaud's phenomenon may be the cutaneous manifestation of a generalized vasospastic disorder. For example, migraine headache, esophageal reflux, primary pulmonary hypertension, and atypical angina have all been associated with uncomplicated "primary" Raynaud's phenomenon.

In patients with secondary Raynaud's phenomenon, onset occurs in the third and fourth decades. The episodes are usually intense with often painful, ischemic lesions. The intensity of the Raynaud's attacks usually follows the course of the underlying cause. Secondary causes of Raynaud's phenomenon are frequently associated with both vasospasm and either intrinsic vessel disease or abnormalities of the physical properties of the blood flowing in these vessels. Treatment should be directed at both the vasospasm and, if possible, the underlying disease process that is causing the vascular defect. For example, vasculitis can damage blood vessels, causing abnormal vascular reactivity and Raynaud's phenomenon. Controlling the vasculitis with immunosuppressive therapy may cure the associated secondary Raynaud's phenomenon.

RECOMMENDED EVALUATION

The teenage patient who has cold sensitivity and typical Raynaud's episodes should have a thorough physical examination, including examination of the nailfold capillaries. If the examination findings are normal and the patient is otherwise in excellent health, then careful follow-up is all that is necessary. Laboratory studies can be done to confirm the diagnosis of primary Raynaud's phenomenon: the antinuclear antibody and Westergren sedimentation rate should be normal. Other special testing should be done only if clinical clues suggest that they are necessary. The most common rheumatic diseases associated with Raynaud's phenomenon are scleroderma, systemic lupus erythematosus, Sjögren's syndrome, and dermatopolymyositis. These diseases may occur with Raynaud's phenomenon as the first symptom.

The cutaneous capillaries can be examined by placing a drop of grade B immersion oil on the skin at the base of a fingernail. The nail fold capillaries can then be viewed by means of a stereozoom microscope or an ordinary ophthalmoscope set at 40 diopters. Normal capillaries will appear as orderly, delicate vascular loops (Fig. 13–1A). Patients with secondary Raynaud's phenomenon and a connective tissue disease frequently have abnormal nailfold capillaries characterized by enlargement of capillary loops, loss of capillaries, or distortion of normal capillary forms (Fig. 13–1B). Approximately, 80% of patients with scleroderma have abnormal nailfold capillaries, while less than 5% of SLE patients with Raynaud's phenomenon have abnormal capillary loops.

Patients with Raynaud's phenomenon may have abnormal nailfold capillaries, a positive antinuclear antibody test or both, without any other systemic features of a connective tissue disease. In approximately 15% to 20% of these patients, a definite connective tissue disease, usually scleroderma or scleroderma-like disease, will develop over the next few years of follow-up.[4] Therefore, if the patient has abnormal nail fold capillaries or the presence of autoantibodies, one should suspect that an early stage of an autoimmune disorder is present. Careful clinical follow-up is recommended. It is also recommended that patients with Raynaud's phenomenon and abnormal nailfold capillaries undergo pulmonary function testing to determine whether there is any parenchymal lung disease or evidence of pulmonary vascular abnormalities.

Patients over the age of 30 who have Raynaud's phenomenon for the first time are likely to have a defined secondary cause, particularly if the episodes are intense, painful, asymmetrical, or associated with ischemic skin lesions. These patients should have a complete evaluation with appropriate special testing dictated by the clinical clues and situation. Special testing may include noninvasive vascular studies to determine whether there is any evidence of larger-vessel occlusive disease.

NONDRUG MANAGEMENT OF RAYNAUD'S PHENOMENON

Patients with primary Raynaud's phenomenon usually can be managed without drugs, because these patients do not develop ischemic ulcers or evidence of systemic disease. Drug therapy can be helpful and should be considered if, despite the use of nondrug treatment, the patient has a poor quality of life because of frequent uncomfortable attacks and the annoying need to practice cold avoidance. Treatment begins in all cases with education. Raynaud's attacks are not only uncomfortable, but they

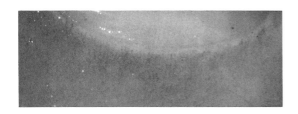
A

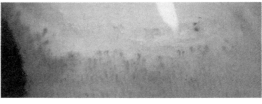
B

FIGURE 13–1
A, Normal capillaries at base of fingernail. **B,** Abnormal nailfold capillaries seen in secondary Raynaud's phenomenon.

can be frightening. Fear (emotional stress) not only can trigger an attack, but it can also enhance cold sensitivity. Patients need to understand how attacks occur, what specifically triggers the attacks, how to prevent attacks, and what to expect in the future. The patient should be supplied with educational material that supplements the physician's explanation. The patient can be asked to keep a diary of Raynaud's attacks and the specific events and situations that provoke the attacks. The information from the diary is useful in illustrating to the patient specific situations that aggravate the Raynaud's phenomenon. Patients also need to understand that, in addition to cold exposure of the hands and feet, rapid shifts in the ambient temperature or a general body chill will also provoke a Raynaud's attack. Warm, loose-fitting clothing, warm stockings, warm headwear, and gloves or mittens are useful to prevent an attack during cold weather exposure. In fact, avoidance of cold temperatures is the best way to prevent an episode of Raynaud's phenomenon. It seems that core body temperature cooling as well as extremity cold exposure will cause Raynaud's phenomenon.

Some patients will deny that emotional stress provokes a vasospastic episode in the absence of a cold stimulus. However, studies have suggested that Raynaud's phenomenon is more likely to occur if a sympathetic stimulus is coupled with cold exposure. In fact, both observational and experimental studies have demonstrated that peripheral vasoconstriction can be affected by emotional and behavioral factors,[5] suggesting that behavioral interventions may be helpful in the treatment of Raynaud's phenomenon.

Temperature biofeedback has frequently been used in combination with different relaxation techniques in the treatment of Raynaud's phenomenon. Autogenic training (the use of relaxation-inducing self-statements that suggest warmth and heaviness) have been used alone or in combination with biofeedback.[6,7] A controlled trial has suggested improvement in the number and intensity of Raynaud's symptoms over 1 year of follow-up.[7] Biofeedback studies have been difficult to control, however, and there remain questions about the role of these techniques in the treatment of Raynaud's phenomenon.

Conditioning treatment has also been advocated.[8,9] This involves pairing the unconditioned stimulus of warm water applied to the hands with a conditioned stimulus of exposure of the whole body to cold. After training, exposure to cold alone elicits vasodilation in the hands (the conditioned response). Using this or similar techniques, patients with Raynaud's have been shown to have increases in digital temperatures compared with untreated controls.

The combination of temperature biofeedback and cold exposure as used by Freedman et al.[5] is the nonpharmacologic treatment method of choice. The addition of other relaxation techniques appears unnecessary.[10] These techniques require a trained therapist and learning them takes approximately 10 training sessions over a 5-week period. Home reenforcement has been advocated to maintain these skills. Patients with Raynaud's phenomenon secondary to systemic lupus erythematosus and scleroderma have been reported to benefit, but the only controlled trial with scleroderma patients failed to show any benefit in either skin temperature responses or symptoms.[11] It is recommended that biofeedback be considered in patients with primary Raynaud's phenomenon if they are not doing well with cold-avoidance methods. It is expected that patients with secondary Raynaud's phenomenon will benefit little from biofeedback.

PHARMACOLOGIC TREATMENT OF RAYNAUD'S PHENOMENON

Currently no drug is approved in the United States for the treatment of Raynaud's phenomenon. A number of vasodilators have been used in the treatment of Raynaud's phenomenon, but there have been relatively few well-controlled studies to determine the efficacy of these drugs.

Several factors are important when one evaluates the literature on therapeutic intervention in Raynaud's phenomenon. It is important to determine whether the patient population studied had primary or secondary Raynaud's phenomenon. Primary patients are more likely to respond to vasodilators because of the absence of structural abnormalities of the blood vessels or other difficult-to-control factors.[12,13] It is also important to distinguish between clinical self-reported measures and laboratory hemodynamic measures of response to treatment. Several studies have reported subjective improvement in the frequency, duration, or severity of Raynaud's attacks after drug treatment but have been unable to objectively demonstrate a positive effect on laboratory measurements of digital blood flow.[13-18] Finally, the ideal therapeutic trial should have a double-blind randomized design that is placebo, temperature, and activity controlled.

Calcium Channel Blockers

Of the currently available drugs on the market, the calcium channel blockers, because of their vasodilating properties, are the most widely used agents for the treatment of Raynaud's phenomenon. Nifedipine has been the most widely studied of the available calcium channel blockers,[12,14-17,19-33] but nicardipine,[34,35] diltiazem,[36-38] verapamil,[39] isradipine,[40] and nisoldipine[41] have also been investigated.

Three studies with nifedipine have enrolled only patients with primary Raynaud's phenomenon,[21,31,33] and two studies have enrolled only patients with scleroderma.[22,32] The studies in patients with primary Raynaud's phenomenon have reported approximately a 50% reduction in frequency of attacks and a significant reduction in severity of attacks. In the two published studies on the evaluation of nifedipine for the treatment of Raynaud's phenomenon in patients with scleroderma, subjective improvement was documented with digital ulcer healing in one study[22] and improved finger temperature and finger blood flow in the other.[32] In contrast, other studies have failed to show a response in the subset of patients with severe secondary Raynaud's phenomenon.[12,19]

There have been no controlled clinical trials of the slow-release preparations of nifedipine (Procardia XL, Adalat CC). Despite the lack of data, most physicians use the slow-release preparations because of the ease of administration and the reported lower frequency of side effects compared with the short-acting preparations. Nifedipine side effects, while not serious, are frequent, with 30% to 100% of patients reporting problems.[12,19,21,33,41] The most common side effects are headache, tachycardia, flushing, light-headedness, and edema. During long-term nifedipine therapy, a trend toward diminished effectiveness was observed over time in patients with primary Raynaud's phenomenon.[21] However another study[17] demonstrated long-term benefit.

There are few published studies of the other available calcium channel blockers in the treatment of Raynaud's phenomenon. One study compared nicardipine and placebo therapy in 25 patients with primary and secondary Raynaud's phenomenon and failed to show a difference between the two treatment groups with respect to number and severity of attacks, character of the Raynaud's phenomenon, use of hands in the winter months, patient assessment of medication effectiveness, or objective measurements of finger systolic pressure and critical closing temperature.[34] Kahan et al.[35] reported that nicardipine reduced the frequency of attacks (mean 29.6 ± 13.6 attacks per 2 weeks on placebo versus 23.1 ± 17.0 attacks per 2 weeks on nicardipine; $p < 0.05$) and the severity of Raynaud's phenomenon (mean score 2.2 ± 0.4 on placebo versus 1.8 ± 0.07 on nicardipine; $p < 0.05$).[35]

The nondihydropyridine calcium channel blocker verapamil failed to show clinical benefit in the one published study of 16 patients with Raynaud's phenomenon.[39] Diltiazem has been reported to reduce frequency and severity of Raynaud's attack in three placebo-controlled studies.[36-38] However, one study reported that, although the improvement was striking in patients with primary Raynaud's phenomenon, it did not reach statistical significance in patients with associated systemic disease.[37] Felodipine and isradipine have been shown to be helpful in clinical trials conducted in Europe.

Other Drugs

Many agents other than calcium channel blockers have been used in the treatment of Raynaud's phenomenon, but few controlled studies have been done. In general, other agents have been disappointing in their clinical usefulness or they are not currently available in the United States.

Sympatholytic agents, including reserpine,[42,43] guanethidine,[44] methyldopa,[45] prazosin,[46] phenoxybenzamine,[47] phentolamine,[48] indoramin,[49] and tolazoline,[50] have been reported to be useful. Reserpine was popular in the treatment of Raynaud's phenomenon until a controlled trial demonstrated that intraarterial reserpine was no better than placebo.[43] Although the adrenergic α-1-receptor blocker, prazosin, has been shown to reduce symptoms, it is less effective in secondary Raynaud's phenomenon and the clinical improvement may not be sustained with prolonged treatment.

Other agents that have been reported in the treatment of Raynaud's phenomenon include angiotensin-converting enzyme inhibitors,[51,52] serotonin receptor blockade,[18,53] thromboxane synthetase inhibitors,[19] prostaglandin I_2 (prostacyclin),[54] PGE_1,[55,56] PGE_2,[57] evening primrose oil,[58] iloprost,[59,60] direct-acting vasodilating agents such as nitroglycerin[61] and hydralazine,[47] and calcitonin gene-related peptide.[62] The usefulness of most of these agents is hampered by the high frequency of side effects, the inconvenient route of administration, or the lack of demonstrated effectiveness in a placebo-controlled trial.

There have been few studies comparing other agents with calcium channel blockers.[22] Thus nifedipine remains the usual drug of choice in the treatment of Raynaud's phenomenon because of its availability, ease of administration, clinical benefit demonstrated in placebo-controlled studies, and reasonably low-toxicity profile (Table 13–1).

AUTHORS' APPROACH TO DRUG TREATMENT

Patients should be considered candidates for drug therapy if management without drugs has failed or if there is evidence of ischemic tissue injury. Patients who have secondary Raynaud's phenomenon are more likely to need drug treatment, but they are also less likely to respond to treatment. One must recognize that a high number (up to 30%) of patients will improve when given a placebo, that warm weather will reduce the attack rate, and that subjective symptoms are more likely to improve than objective measures of local blood flow. Therefore careful assessment of the chosen drug treatment is prudent; if possible, treatment is usually stopped in the warm months. Although Raynaud's attacks can be uncomfortable and unattractive, most patients have little disability or significant consequences of the attacks.

In uncomplicated cases, it is reasonable to start therapy with the slow-release nifedipine preparation. A dose of nifedipine XL 30 mg daily is started. If there is no response in a 1- to 2-week period, then the dose can be increased

to 60 mg daily. Nifedipine can be increased by 30 mg at 1- to 4-week intervals until the maximal tolerated dose is reached. Generally, patients who do not respond to nifedipine are unlikely to respond to other currently available vasodilators. However, if the extended-release nifedipine is not effective, it is reasonable to either try intermittent dosing with the short-acting nifedipine preparation or to try another calcium channel blocker. Diltiazem is the usual second choice, while nicardipine and verapamil have been disappointing in the treatment of Raynaud's phenomenon. Amlodipine is well tolerated but has not been tested in a controlled clinical trial. Combinations of calcium channel blockers have generally not been helpful.

Other classes of vasodilating drugs, including nitrates and sympatholytic agents, are usually of no greater value than the calcium channel blockers and may be poorly tolerated. Patients with Raynaud's phenomenon and severe ischemia who fail to respond to a calcium channel blocker can be tried on another vasodilator agent, either alone or in combination with a calcium channel blocker.

Topical nitrates have been reported to be helpful. Patients can be started on $1/4$ to $1/2$ inch of topical nitroglycerin ointment 2% applied two times daily—once in the morning on arising and repeated 6 hours later. A rest from nitrates for 10 to 12 hours is necessary to prevent a refractory state. Similar to antianginal therapy, the dose can be increased until a maximal tolerated dose is reached (maximal recommended dose, 2 inches). Alternatively, a nitrate patch can be used. Headaches are the most common reason that patients stop taking nitrates. Topical nitrates can be combined with a calcium channel blocker or with other vasodilators; however, combinations of these agents have not been studied in clinical trials.

Prasozin is the first choice among the sympatholytic agents. It can be started with a 1 mg test dose and then slowly increased to 2 to 5 mg by mouth three times daily (maximal daily dose, 20 mg). Most patients who benefit find prasozin is less effective over time. Other α-blocking agents have not been particularly useful for long-term therapy; however, uncontrolled experience has shown that intravenous phentolamine and phenoxybenzamine can be useful to reverse severe ischemia. These potent agents should be given only in an appropriate

TABLE 13–1
Summary of Pharmacological Treatment of Raynaud's Phenomenon

DRUG	CONTROLLED TRIAL	CLINICALLY EFFECTIVE	SIDE EFFECTS	COMMENTS
Calcium Channel Blockers				
Nifedipine TID or QID	+++	+++	++	Side-effects mild
Nifedipine (XL) QD	0	Unknown	+	
Nicardipine	++	±	++	
Diltiazem	++	++	+	
Verapamil	+	0	++	
Isradipine	0	+	+	Not FDA approved
Nisoldipine	+	0	++	Not FDA approved
Sympatholytic				
Guanethidine	+	±	+++	
Methyldopa	0	±	+++	
Phenoxybenzamine	+	+	+++	
Phentolamine	0	++	+	Intravenous only
Prasozin	++	++	++	Less efficacious in secondary RP, improvement not sustained
Reserpine	++	0	++	Intraarterial preparation not available
Tolazoline	0	±	++	Not available orally
ACE Inhibitors				
Captopril/Enalapril	+	±	+	
Serotonin Receptor Blockers				
Kentanserin	++	++	++	Not FDA approved
Prostaglandin				
Prostacyclin	+	++	+++	Intravenous only
Prostaglandin E$_1$	+	±	+++	Intravenous only
Prostaglandin E$_2$	+	+	+	Topical patch
Iloprost	++	++	+++	Intravenous only; not FDA approved
Thromboxane Inhibitors				
Dazoxiben	++	0	+	Not FDA approved
Direct Vasodilator				
Nitroglycerin	++	+	+++	Headache common
Hydralazine	0	+	++	
Other				
Pentoxifylline	0	±		

hospital setting for proper monitoring of cardiovascular parameters.

Intravenous prostaglandins have been shown to be helpful in patients with Raynaud's and in patients with scleroderma and ischemic ulcers. Prostaglandin E$_1$ (alprostadil) is available for maintaining a patent ductus arteriosus in neonates with congenital heart defects. It must be administered through a large central vein, and the patient must be in the hospital and appropriately monitored. The drug is infused at a starting dose of 0.1 µg/kg/min and increased if necessary to a maximum of 0.4 µg/kg/min. Intravenous prostacyclin and its analog, iloprost, have been shown to be effective in treating ischemia but are not available. Oral prostaglandins are now under study, but none now available have been shown to be effective for Raynaud's phenomenon. Misoprostol (oral PGE_1) is available; however, one investigation found it no better than placebo in preventing vasospasm from an acute cold challenge in patients with Raynaud's phenomenon.[63]

Since the risk of ischemic tissue damage is minimal in patients who have primary uncomplicated Raynaud's phenomenon, every effort should be made to avoid potentially toxic medication. Unfortunately, Raynaud's phenomenon due to secondary causes, which may have associated ischemic tissue damage, may not respond to currently available drug therapy. It is essential to maximize cold avoidance nondrug therapy, including rest (hospitalization if necessary) during a crisis. Aggressive care of ischemic ulcers will prevent complications and amputation.

SURGICAL TREATMENT OF RAYNAUD'S PHENOMENON

Severe Raynaud's phenomenon may be refractory to any drug treatment, particularly if it is complicated by prolonged ischemia and tissue ulceration. Surgical sympathectomy has been reported to be helpful in these cases; however, little controlled data are available for assessment of the role of these procedures. Cervical sympathectomy may provide transient relief but is rarely curative. However, lumbar sympathectomy has been quite helpful for lower-extremity vasospasm. A temporary lumbar, cervical, or digital sympathetic block can be attempted to determine whether sympathectomy will reverse acute vasospasm. If a temporary sympathectomy "breaks" the vasospasm, then an oral vasodilator can be started to control new vasospastic events. Failure of vasodilators to control the situation following a successful temporary block may suggest consideration of permanent sympathectomy. There is, however, little enthusiasm for permanent sympathectomy in the upper extremities because of the poor long-term outcome. Digital sympathectomy, alone or in combination with surgical repair of obstructed arteries, has been reported to be helpful, but no controlled trials or long-term follow-up has been reported. It is our experience that the usefulness of these radical procedures is very limited and clearly should be done only by skilled and experienced surgeons after careful selection of appropriate cases.

REFERENCES

1. Coffman JD. Raynaud's phenomenon. New York: Oxford University Press, 1989.
2. Maricq HR, Carpentier PH, Weinrich MC, et al. Geographic variation in the prevalence of Raynaud's phenomenon: Charleston, SC, USA, vs Tarentaise, Savoie, France. J Rheumatol 1993; 20:70.
3. LeRoy EC, Medsger TA Jr. Raynaud's phenomenon: a proposal for classification. Clin Exp Rheumatol 1992;10:485.
4. Kallenberg CGM. Early detection of connective tissue disease in patients with Raynaud's phenomenon. Rheum Dis Clin North Am 1990;16:11.
5. Freedman RR, Iaani P, Wenig P. Behavioral treatment of Raynaud's disease. J Consult Clin Psychol 1983;51:539.
6. Surwit RS, Pilon RN, Fenton CH. Behavioral treatment of Raynaud's disease. J Behav Med 1978;1:323.
7. Keefe FJ, Surwit RS, Pilon RN. A one-year follow-up of Raynaud's patients treated with behavioral therapy techniques. J Behav Med 1979; 2:385.
8. Jobe JB, Sampson JB, Roberts DE, et al. Comparison of behavioral treatments for Raynaud's disease. J Behav Med 1986;9:89.
9. Melin H, Fagerstrom K. Treatment of peripheral vasospasm. Scand J Behav Ther 1981;1097.
10. Rose GD, Carlson JG. The behavioral treatment of Raynaud's disease: a review. Biofeedback Self Regul 1987;12:257.
11. Freedman RR, Ianni P, Wenig P. Behavioral treatment of Raynaud's phenomenon in scleroderma. J Behav Med 1984;7:343.
12. Rodeheffer RJ, Rommer JA, Wigley FM, et al. Controlled double-blind trial of nifedipine in the treatment of Raynaud's phenomenon. N Engl J Med 1983;308:880.
13. Wigley FM, Wise RA, Mikdashi J, et al. The post-occlusive hyperemic response in patients with systemic sclerosis. Arthritis Rheum 1990; 33:1620.
14. Aldoori M, Bruce W, Dieppe PA. Nifedipine in the treatment of Raynaud's syndrome. Cardiovasc Res 1986;20:466.
15. Smith DC, McKendry RJR. Controlled trial of nifedipine in the treatment of Raynaud's phenomenon. Lancet 1982;2(8311):1299.
16. Sauza J, Kraus A, Gonzalez-Amaro R, et al. Effect of the calcium channel blocker nifedipine on Raynaud's phenomenon: a controlled double-blind trial. J. Rheumatol 1984;11:362.
17. Kallenberg CG, Woundra AA, Kuitert JJ, et al. Nifedipine in Raynaud's phenomenon: relationship between short term and long term effects. J Rheumatol 1987;14:284.

18. Coffman JD, Clement DL, Creager MA, et al. International study of ketanserin in Raynaud's phenomenon. Am J Med 1989;87:264.

19. Ettinger WH, Wise RA, Schaffhausser DA, et al. Controlled double-blind trial of dazoxiben and nifedipine in the treatment of Raynaud's phenomenon. Am J Med 1984;77:451.

20. White CJ, Phillips WA, Abrahams LA, et al. Objective benefit of nifedipine in the treatment of Raynaud's phenomenon: double-blinded controlled study. Am J Med 1986;80:623.

21. Sarzoki J, Blookman AM, Mahon W, et al. Nifedipine in the treatment of idiopathic Raynaud's syndrome. J Rheumatol 1986;13:331.

22. Rademaker M, Cooke ED, Almond NE, et al. Comparison of intravenous infusions of iloprost and oral nifedipien in the treatment of Raynaud's phenomenon in patients with systemic sclerosis: a double-blind randomized study. Br Med J 1989;298:561.

23. Vayssairat M, Capron L, Fiessinger JN, et al. Calcium channel blockers and Raynaud's disease. Ann Intern Med 1981;95:243.

24. Dale J, Landmark KR, Myhre E, et al. The effects of nifedipine, a calcium antagonist, on platelet function. Am Heart J 1983;105:103.

25. Kahan A, Weber S, Amor B, et al. Nifedipine and Raynaud's phenomenon. Ann Intern Med 1981;94:546.

26. Winston EL, Pariser KM, Miller KB, et al. Nifedipine as a therapeutic modality for Raynaud's phenomenon. Arthritis Rheum 1983;26:1177.

27. Nilsson H, Jonasson T, Ringqvist I, et al. Nifedipine in cold-induced vasospasm. Eur Heart J 1984;33(Abstract suppl):5.

28. Nilsson H, Jonasson T, Ringqvist I, et al. Treatment of digital vasospastic disease with the calcium-entry blocker nifedipine. Acta Med Scand 1984;215:135.

29. Wollersheim H, Thien TH, Van't Laar A, et al. Nifedipine in primary Raynaud's phenomenon and in scleroderma: oral vs sublingual hemodynamic effects. J Clin Pharmacol 1987;27:907.

30. Kirch W, Linder HR, Hutt HJ, et al. Ketanserin vs nifedipine in secondary Raynaud's phenomenon. Vasa 1987;16:77.

31. Gjorup T, Kelbaek J, Hartling OJ, et al. Controlled double-blind trial of the clinical effect of nifedipine in the treatment of idiopathic Raynaud's phenomenon. Am Heart J 1986;111:742.

32. Finch MB, Dawson J, Johnston GD, et al. The peripheral vascular effects of nifedipine in Raynaud's syndrome associated with scleroderma: a double-blind crossover study. Clin Rheumatol 1986;5:493.

33. Corbin DOC, Wood DA, Macintyre CC, et al. A randomized double-blind crossover trial of nifedipine in the treatment of primary Raynaud's phenomenon. Eur Heart J 1986;7:165.

34. Wigley FM, Wise RA, Malamet R, Scott T. Nicardipine in the treatment of Raynaud's phenomenon: dissociation of platelet activation from vasospasm. Arthritis Rheum 1987;39:281.

35. Kahan A, Amor B, Menkes CJ, et al. Nicardipine in the treatment of Raynaud's phenomenon: a randomized double-blind trial. Angiology 1987;38:333.

36. Rhedda A, McCans J, et al. A double-blind placebo controlled crossover randomized trial of diltiazem in Raynaud's phenomenon. J Rheumatol 1985;12:720.

37. Kahan A, Amor B, Menkes C. A randomized double-blind trial of diltiazem in the treatment of Raynaud's phenomenon. Ann Rheum Dis 1985;44:30.

38. Matoba T, Chiba M. Effects of diltiazem on occupational Raynaud's syndrome (vibration disease). Angiology 1985;36:850.

39. Kinney EL, Nicholas G, Gallo J, et al. The treatment of severe Raynaud's phenomenon with verapamil. J Clin Pharmacol 1982;22:74.

40. Leppert J, Jonasson T, Nilsson H, et al. The effect of isradipine, a new calcium-channel antagonist, in patients with primary Raynaud's phenomenon: a single-blind dose-response study. Cardiovasc Drugs Ther 1989;3:397.

41. Gjorup T, Hartling O, Kelbaek H, et al. Controlled double-blind trial of nisoldipine in the treatment of idiopathic Raynaud's phenomenon. Eur J Clin Pharmacol 1986;31:387.

42. Surwit RS, Gilgor RS, Duvic M, et al. Intra-arterial reserpine for Raynaud's syndrome. Arch Dermatol 1983;119:733.

43. McFadyen IJ, Housley E, Macherson AIS. Intra-arterial reserpine administration in Raynaud's syndrome. Arch Intern Med 1973;132:526.

44. LeRoy EC, Downey JA, Cannon PJ. Skin capillary blood flow in scleroderma. J Clin Invest 1971;50:930.

45. Varadi DP, Lawrence AM. Suppression of Raynaud's phenomenon by methyldopa. Arch Intern Med 1969;124:13.

46. Russell LJ, Lessard JA. Prazosin treatment of Raynaud's phenomenon: a double-blind single crossover study. J Rheumatol 1985;12:94.

47. Russell IJ, Walsh RA. Selection of vasodilator therapy for severe Raynaud's phenomenon by sequential arterial infusion. Ann Rheum Dis 1985;44(3):151.

48. Coffman JD, Cohen RA. Intra-arterial vasodilator agents to reverse finger vasoconstriction. Clin Pharmacol Ther 1987;41:574.

49. Robson P, Pearce V, Antcliff AC, et al. Double-blind trial of indoramin in digital artery disease. Br J Clin Pharmacol 1978;6:88.

50. Allegra C, Tonelli V, Ecari U, et al. Pharmacological treatment of Raynaud's phenomenon: a new therapeutic approach. Curr Ther Res 1986;40:303.

51. Miyazaki S, Miura K, Kasai Y, et al. Relief of digital vasospasm by treatment with captopril and its complete inhibition by serine proteinase inhibitors in Raynaud's phenomenon. Br J Med 1982;284:310.

52. Tosi SA, Marchesoni A, Messina K, et al. Treatment of Raynaud's phenomenon with captopril. Drugs Exp Clin Res 1987;13:37.

53. Seibold JR, Terregino CA. Selective antagonism of S_2-serotonergic receptors relieves but does not prevent cold-induced vasoconstriction in primary Raynaud's phenomenon. J Rheumatol 1986;13:337.

54. Belch JJF, Drury JK, Capell H, et al. Intermittent epoprostenol (prostacyclin) infusion in patients with Raynaud's phenomenon. Lancet 1983; 1(8320):313.

55. Morhland JS, Porter JM, Smith EA, et al. A multicenter placebo-controlled, double-blind study of prostaglandin E_1 in Raynaud's syndrome. Ann Rheum Dis 1985;44:754.

56. Langevitz P, Buskila D, Lee P, et al. Treatment of refractory ischemic skin ulcers in patients with Raynaud's phenomenon with PGE_1 infusions. J Rheum 1989;16:1433.

57. Belch JJF, Shaw B, Sturrock RD, et al. Double-blind trial of CLII5,347, a transdermally absorbed prostaglandin E_2 analogue, in treatment of Raynaud's phenomenon. Lancet 1985;1:1180.

58. Belch JJF, Shaw B, O'Dowd A, et al. Evening primrose oil (efamol) in the treatment of Raynaud's phenomenon: a double-blind study. Thromb Haemost 1985;54:490.

59. Kyle MV, Belcher G, Hazelman B. Placebo controlled study showing therapeutic benefit of iloprost in the treatment of Raynaud's phenomenon. J Rheumatol 1992;19:1403.

60. Wigley FM, Seibold JR, Wise RA, et al. Intravenous iloprost treatment of Raynaud's phenomenon and ischemic ulcers secondary to systemic sclerosis. J Rheumatol 1992;19:1407.

61. Franks AG Jr. Topical glyceryl trinitrate as adjunctive treatment in Raynaud's disease. Lancet 1982;1:76.

62. Bunker CB, Reavley C, O'Shaughnessy DJ, et al. Calcitonin gene-related peptide in treatment of severe peripheral vascular insufficiency in Raynaud's phenomenon. Lancet 1993;342:80.

63. Wise RA, Wigley FM. Acute effects of misoprostol on digital circulation in patients with Raynaud's phenomenon. J Rheumatol 1994;21:80.

64. Kelley WN, Harris ED Jr, Ruddy S, Sledge CB, eds. Textbook of rheumatology. 4th ed. Philadelphia: WB Saunders, 1993.

IDIOPATHIC INFLAMMATORY DISEASES OF MUSCLE

Robert L. Wortmann

The idiopathic inflammatory diseases of muscle are uncommon and poorly understood conditions. Patients with one of these diseases generally have (1) proximal muscle weakness, (2) elevated serum levels of enzymes derived from skeletal muscle, (3) myopathic electromyographic changes, and (4) muscle biopsy evidence of inflammation. Over time, the inflammatory myopathies have been classified in a variety of ways,[1-5] but in recent years the scheme proposed by Bohan and Peter[1] has been employed by most clinicians and investigators. Bohan and Peter proposed the first criteria for making a diagnosis of idiopathic myositis (Table 14–1) and divided patients who fulfilled those criteria into five groups: (1) primary idiopathic polymyositis, (2) primary idiopathic dermatomyositis, (3) dermatomyositis or polymyositis associated with cancer, (4) childhood dermatomyositis (or polymyositis) associated with vasculitis, and (5) polymyositis or dermatomyositis associated with another recognized collagen vascular disease. (For more information on pathogenesis and diagnosis, see Wortmann, in Kelley et al., reference 18.)

More recently, additional types of myositis have been recognized. Those groups have emerged from studies of patients who generally fulfill Bohan and Peter's criteria for polymyositis and include inclusion-body myositis and myopathy with circulating myositis-specific autoantibodies. Criteria for the diagnosis of inclusion-body myositis have been proposed and employed for the investigation of this group of patients (Table 14–2).[6] Discovery of myositis-specific autoantibodies has allowed further evolution of

TABLE 14–1

Criteria to Define Polymyositis-Dermatomyositis Proposed by Bohan and Peter

1. Symmetric weakness of limb-girdle muscles and anterior neck flexors, progressing over weeks to months, with or without dysphagia or respiratory muscle involvement.
2. Skeletal muscle histology showing evidence of necrosis of type 1 and 2 muscle fibers, phagocytosis, regeneration with basophilia, large sarcolemmal nuclei and prominent nucleoli, atrophy in a perifascicular distribution, variation in fiber size, and an inflammatory exudate.
3. Elevation of serum skeletal muscle enzymes (CK, aldolase, AST, ALT, and LDH).
4. Electromyographic triad of short, small, polyphasic motor units; fibrillations, positive waves, and insertional irritability; and bizarre high-frequency discharges.
5. Dermatologic features including lilac (heliotrope) discoloration of the eyelids with periorbital edema; scaly, erythematous dermatitis over the dorsa of the hands, especially over the metacarpophalangeal and proximal interphalangeal joints (Gottron's sign), and involvement of the knees, elbows, medial malleoli, face, neck, and upper torso.

Reprinted with permission from Bohan A, Peter JB. Polymyositis and dermatomyositis (first of two parts). N Engl J Med 1975;292:344. Copyright 1975, Massachusetts Medical Society.

our classification of these diseases (Table 14–3). Most myositis-specific autoantibodies are directed against cytoplasmic ribonucleoproteins, bind to evolutionary conserved epitopes, and inhibit the functions of the target autoantigen.[7,8] Eight specific autoantibodies have been recog-

TABLE 14–2
Diagnostic Criteria Proposed for Inclusion Body Myositis

Pathologic Criteria
Electron Microscopy
  1. Microtubular filaments in the inclusions
Light Microscopy
  1. Lined vacuoles
  2. Intranuclear or intracytoplasmic inclusions or both

Clinical Criteria
1. Proximal muscle weakness (insidious onset)
2. Distal muscle weakness
3. Electromyographic evidence of a generalized myopathy (inflammatory myopathy)
4. Elevation of muscle enzymes (CK or aldolase or both)
5. Failure of muscle weakness to improve on a high-dose corticosteroid regimen (at least 40–60 mg/d for 3–4 months)

Definite IBM = pathologic electron microscopy criterion I and clinical criterion I plus one other clinical criterion. Probable IBM = pathologic light microscopy criterion I and clinical criterion I plus three other clinical criteria. Possible IBM = pathologic light microscopy criterion 2 plus any three clinical criterion.

From Calabrese LH, Mitsumoto H, Chou SM. Inclusion body myositis presenting as treatment-resistant polymyositis. Arthritis Rheum 1987;30:397.

nized to date.[8–16] An individual patient will have only one of these. The presence of a particular autoantibody appears to define homogeneous groups of patients.[17]

Thus today one can apportion patients among seven different groups:

1. Polymyositis
2. Dermatomyositis
3. Myositis with myositis-specific autoantibodies
4. Inclusion-body myositis
5. Juvenile (childhood) dermatomyositis
6. Cancer-related myositis
7. Myositis with another recognized collagen vascular diseases

One must recognize that the differences among them are not always clear. The initial approach to therapy for any patient with an idiopathic inflammatory muscle disease may be the same. Nevertheless, one must define the diagnosis as accurately as possible because, despite similarities in initial therapeutic approach, the prognosis for each may differ significantly.

NATURAL HISTORY AND LONG-TERM EXPERIENCE

The true natural history of the inflammatory myopathies is difficult to determine for several reasons. The diseases are relatively rare. Most series report small numbers of patients who were evaluated retrospectively over a period of many years. Much uncertainty exists concerning the accuracy of diagnoses in studies before the middle 1970s. Furthermore, the classification schemes applied have varied widely over time.[1–6,17] Patients were not always divided among groups; when groups were identified, however, criteria were not employed consistently. Because of small numbers, different groups were often combined in the analysis.

TABLE 14–3
Myositis-Specific Autoantibodies

AUTOANTIBODY	ANTIGEN	CLINICAL FEATURES
Anti-synthetases	Aminoacyl-tRNA synthetases	Myositis with arthritis, fever, interstitial lung disease, and poor response to therapy
Anti-Jo-1	Histidyl-tRNA synthetase	
Anti-PL-7	Threonyl-tRNA synthetase	
Anti-EJ	Glycyl-tRNA synthetase	
Anti-PL-12	Alanyl-tRNA synthetase	
Anti-OJ	Isoleucyl-tRNA synthetase	
Anti-SRP	Signal recognition particle	Poor response to therapy
Anti-Mi-2	220 kD nuclear protein of unknown function	Dermatomyositis, good response to therapy
Anti-MAS	A common ~4S RNA of unknown function	Alcoholic rhabdomyolysis and good response to therapy

Serum enzymes, electrophysiologic studies, and autoantibody testing were less available and the diagnosis and treatment of neoplastic diseases, hypertension, and infections were quite different. Finally, since the 1950s almost every patient with a diagnosis of inflammatory muscle disease has been treated with corticosteroids. Many of these problems continue to plague investigations today. We will continue to have difficulty defining the best treatment for these diseases until we have a truly accurate classification scheme and can evaluate sufficient numbers of patients.

Because of the difficulties of studying adequate numbers of patients and the lack of controlled clinical trials, treatment of the inflammatory myopathies is largely empiric.[18-21] Corticosteroids have been the cornerstone of drug therapy for each of these diseases since their introduction to clinical medicine. Corticosteroid use has improved the prognosis for patients with idiopathic inflammatory myopathies, although some argue about the amount of that improvement.[22,23] Studies of adults indicate a 5-year survival of 60% in the precorticosteroid era, 68% between 1947 and 1968,[24] and 80% to 90% in more recent reports.[17] Survival still varies among the different groups (Fig. 14–1). The reasons for the improved survival are not clear but may relate to earlier and more accurate diagnoses, better treatments for associated medical problems, and the earlier use of immunosuppressive agents. Today determination of the appropriate clinical group and the time from disease onset to diagnosis of myositis provide the most useful information for predicted response to therapy.[17,25-28] It appears that the presence of a circulating myositis-specific autoantibody will be useful in this respect.[17,29] Other poor prognostic factors include more severe weakness at the time therapy is initiated, pharyngeal muscle weakness, aspiration, and interstitial pulmonary fibrosis.[30-34] White patients generally have a better prognosis than black patients.

Prognosis can be based on the classic clinical groups of Bohan and Peter or on the presence or absence of a circulating myositis-specific autoantibody. Children have a better prognosis than adults. Ninety percent of children with juvenile dermatomyositis who live 10 years lead normal lives. Mortality in children is attributable most often to myocarditis,

perforation of a viscus, or infection. Adults with myositis and cancer fare the worst and almost always die of the neoplasm. However, some with a treatable or curable cancer may do quite well. The prognosis for patients with associated connective tissue diseases is determined by the other manifestations of their underlying diagnosis. The myositis of patients in that clinical group typically responds very well to corticosteroids, often at low doses. The actual prognosis for patients with inclusion-body myositis appears to be good but is still unknown because of the recent discovery of the entity. Generally, the course is slow and prolonged. In most persons the weakness becomes fixed or progresses slowly. Less commonly, progression is relentless, leading to severe incapacitation and death.

Identification of a circulating myositis-specific autoantibody seems to predict the clinical characteristics and prognosis (Fig. 14–1).[17,29] According to the small number of observations to date, survival varies tremendously among the various autoantibody groups, with 5-year survival rates of 100% for patients with anti-Mi2 or anti-MAS, 70% for those with anti-synthetase, and 30% for persons with anti-SRP. Some caution should be exercised in accepting these data, because they were collected in a selected group of patients seen at the National Institutes of Health. Analysis of patients from rural community practices indicate that many may have a better prognosis.[35]

CONTROLLED CLINICAL TRIALS

For the treatment of any idiopathic inflammatory myopathy, the information available from controlled clinical trials is extremely limited because only three studies have been published.[36-38] In addition, each of these studies involved low numbers of patients, and previous therapies had failed in all patients included.

The first blinded, controlled trial evaluated the use of azathioprine.[36] Sixteen patients with polymyositis and dermatomyositis whose improvement had reached a plateau during treatment with prednisone alone were divided into two groups and randomized to continue taking prednisone alone or to receive prednisone plus azathioprine. Although no difference between the groups was apparent at 3 months, the azathioprine group showed significant improve-

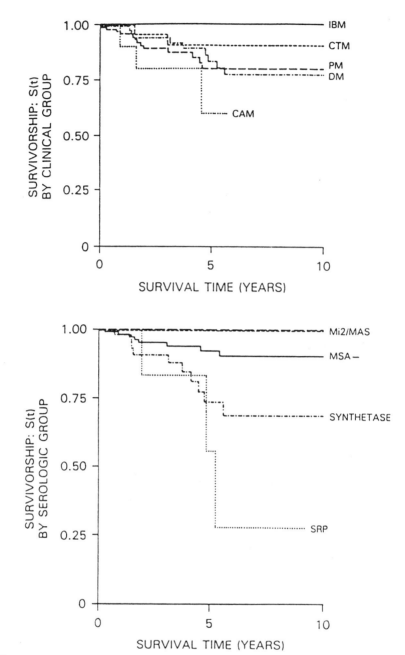

FIGURE 14–1

Classification of idiopathic inflammatory myopathy. Kaplan-Meier analysis of survival in the clinical *(top)* and serologic *(bottom)* groups of patients with idiopathic inflammatory myopathies. The data were analyzed by the Fisher Exact Test for significance with Bonferroni corrections for multiple comparisons. Patients with IBM had significantly prolonged survival from the time of diagnosis ($p \leq 0.05$) when compared to PM and DM patients. Although differences were noted between the CAM patients (all of whom died of cancer) and all the other clinical groups, these were not significant when corrected for multiple comparisons. Analysis of survival data in the serologic groups showed significantly increased mortality in the SRP group compared to those without SRP autoantibodies and in the synthetase-positive patients compared to patients with either Mi-2 or those without an MSA. PM = polymyositis, DM = dermatomyositis, CTM = myositis with another connective tissue disease, CAM = cancer-associated myositis, IBM = inclusion body myositis, Synthetase = autoantibodies to 1 of the 5 known aminoacyl-tRNA synthetases, SRP = autoantibodies to proteins of the signal recognition particle, Mi-2 = autoantibodies primarily directed against a 220 kDa nuclear protein of unknown function, MAS = sera precipitating a common ~4S RNA of unknown function, MSA– = no known myositis-specific autoantibodies. (From Love LA, Leff RL, Fraser DD, et al. A new approach to the classification of idiopathic inflammatory myopathy: myositis-specific autoantibodies define useful homogeneous patient groups. Medicine 1991;70:360.)

ment with respect to functional abilities at 1 and 3 years. In addition, the azathioprine group required less prednisone.

Plasmapheresis and leukapheresis were studied in a double-blind fashion and compared with a sham apheresis control group.[37] Corticosteroid therapy had failed in all 39 participants in that trial, and most of the patients had not responded to other agents. Patients who underwent plasma exchange did have significant reductions in serum levels of muscle enzymes, and those who had leukapheresis experienced significant decreases in lymphocyte counts. Nevertheless, only 3 of the 13 patients in each group showed improvement in strength and functional capacity. Deterioration occurred in three patients treated with leukapheresis and in one treated with plasma exchange. At the conclusion of the study, there were no significant differences in muscle strength or functional capacity among the three treatment groups. This study suggests that leukapheresis and plasma exchange are not effective in patients with inflammatory myopathy. However, 26 of the 39 patients (8 plasma exchange, 11 leukapheresis, and 7 sham apheresis) had antisynthetase or anti-SRP antibodies in their sera. It is now recognized that patients with these serologic markers generally respond poorly to treatment.[17,29] Consequently, it is difficult to extrapolate the results of this trial to patients with an inflammatory myopathy and no circulating myositis-specific antibody.

A double-blind, placebo-controlled trial of high-dose intravenous immune globulin has been performed in 15 adults with treatment-resistant dermatomyositis.[38] All patients had biopsy-proved disease and were unresponsive or poorly responsive to high-dose prednisone or therapeutic dosages of another immunosuppressive agent (azathioprine, methotrexate, or cyclophosphamide) for at least 4 months. The doses of prednisone and other immunosuppressive agents were kept constant, and the patients were randomly assigned to receive one infusion of immune globulin (2 g per kilogram of body weight) or placebo per month for 3 months, with the option of crossing over for 3 months. The eight patients assigned to receive immune globulin had a significant improvement in muscle strength and neuromuscular symptoms, whereas the seven who received placebo did not. With crossovers, a total of 12 patients received immune globulin. Of those, nine had major improvement to nearly normal function, two had mild improvement, and one had no change. Of 11 placebo-treated patients, none had major improvement, three had mild improvement, and five deteriorated. Thus high-dose intravenous immune globulin is effective for some patients with refractory dermatomyositis over a 3-month period. However, the positive effects of immune globulin remained for only 6 weeks. It appears that repeated treatment would be needed for long-term benefits.

AUTHOR'S APPROACH TO MANAGEMENT

Pretreatment Decisions

The first steps in the management of any inflammatory myopathy include assuring the accuracy of the diagnosis and assessing the patient's baseline status. Since there is no specific "diagnostic test" for these diseases, the diagnosis must be made by excluding other possible causes (Table 14–4). An objective baseline assessment is needed because the available outcome measures generally lack precision. It is difficult to determine the actual effects of therapy in some cases because some patients fail to respond to any treatment and others achieve only partial resolution of their symptoms.

Muscle strength should be evaluated before any medication is used. Objective testing of individual muscle group strength provides valuable information. This can be done manually by a trained examiner (physician, nurse, physical therapist) or with isokinetic dynamometry. A timed-stands test is also a simple and useful means of assessing lower-extremity weakness (Fig. 14–2).[39] Baseline measurements should be compared with those obtained during the course of therapy to help determine the effects of treatment.

Pretreatment assessment should also include measurements of serum levels of muscle enzymes, any tests that might be influenced by medications used in treatment, analysis of pulmonary status and swallowing, and screening for cancer. Muscle enzymes include the creatine kinase (CK), aldolase, alanine aminotransferase (ALT, SGPT), aspartate aminotransferase (AST, SGOT) and lactate dehydrogenase (LDH). Each

TABLE 14–4
Causes of Muscle Weakness That Could Be Confused With Polymyositis

Other Rheumatic Diseases
Giant cell arteritis/polymyalgia rheumatica
Wegener's granulomatosus
Polyarteritis nodosa
Systemic lupus erythematosus

Neurologic Disorders
Muscular dystrophies
  Becker's
  Limb-girdle
Myasthenia gravis
Amyotropic lateral sclerosis

Infections
Toxoplasmosis
Acquired immunodeficiency syndrome
Coxsackievirus
Influenza

Metabolic/Nutritional
Malabsorption
Electrolyte disorders
  Hyponatremia
  Hypokalemia
  Hypophosphatemia
  Hypomagnesemia
  Hypercalcemia

Cancer-related
Carcinomatous neuromyopathy
Eaton-Lambert syndrome

Toxic/Drug-related
Alcohol
Chloroquine/hydroxychloroquine
Clofibrate
Cimetidine
Cocaine
Corticosteroids
Colchicine
Cyclosporine
Gold salts
Lovastatin
Zidovudine (AZT)

Inborn Errors of Metabolism
Glycogen-storage diseases
  Myophosphorylase deficiency (McArdle's disease)
  Phosphofructokinase deficiency
Carnitine deficiency
Myoadenylate deaminase deficiency

should be measured at baseline, but only the most abnormal value(s) needs to be tested routinely. This is almost always the CK. Blood counts, serum electrolytes, creatinine, glucose, and other values that might be affected by therapeutic agents should be quantitated. Testing for antinuclear antibodies may prove useful if there is consideration of an associated collagen vascular disease. Today, testing for the presence or absence of a circulating myositis-specific autoantibody is of limited value. With the possible exception of anti-Jo-1, most laboratories do not perform these tests. Furthermore, the presence of fever, interstitial lung disease, or arthritis provides the same information regarding therapy and prognosis as the presence of an antisynthetase autoantibody. The practical value of testing for these antibodies is likely to improve in the future.

Blood pressure determination, chest examination, and chest x-ray should be done routinely. Pulmonary function testing, including diffusion capacity, may be indicated. Fluoroscopic swallowing studies with radiographic contrast material are important if the patient has difficulty swallowing, dysphagia, or dysphonia. Precautions that might prevent aspiration should be emphasized for patients at risk. These include swallowing education, elevation of the head of the bed on blocks, and use of antacids or H_2 blockers to neutralize gastric secretions. The recognized association between the inflammatory myopathies and cancer must always be considered. One should therefore do a careful history with systems review, physical examination, and cancer-screening procedures recommended on the basis of the patient's age and sex. Extensive evaluations in search of an occult neoplasm are not warranted.[40]

Nonpharmacologic Considerations

Physical therapists can prove invaluable in the treatment of patients with myositis. Not only are they able to assist in testing muscle group strength, but they can also design, assist, and instruct in an exercise program. Although exercise programs may be unnecessary in very

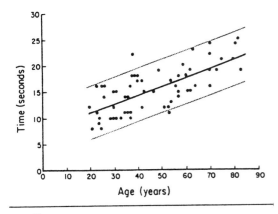

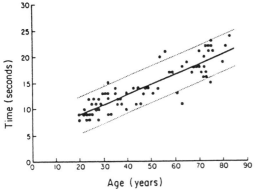

FIGURE 14–2

Timed-stands test as a function of age in 62 normal women *(top)* and in 77 normal men *(bottom)*. The mean and limits of normal (90 percent prediction region) are shown. (Reprinted from Csuka ME, McCarty DJ. Simple method for measurement of lower-extremity muscle strength. Am J Med 1985;78:77.)

mild cases, they may be important in others. Physical therapy should be used to preserve function, avoid disuse atrophy, and prevent contractures.[40,41] The patient's program must take into account the amount of inflammation. Initially bed rest may be very important for severely affected persons. Anecdotally, muscle strength and CK levels have improved dramatically from a disabled to a functioning status with bed rest as the only intervention in some patients who refused to take any medication. Unfortunately, these remissions were transient and rarely lasted more than 2 months. Passive motion is encouraged during periods of maximum inflammation in an effort to maintain normal range of motion and prevent contractures. Contractures are more often a problem in juvenile dermatomyositis, where residual contractures and calcinosis can contribute significantly to residual disability. However, these

complications can occur in other groups as well. With signs of improvement, the exercise program can include active-assisted exercises, then active exercises. Patients with active disease can perform resistive exercises without elevations in CK level and with improvement of muscle strength.[42] With recovery, active isometric or isotonic exercises are clearly recommended to increase strength and endurance.

Drug Therapies

Corticosteroids are the standard first-line medication for patients with any inflammatory myopathy. I prefer to begin with prednisone at a dose of approximately 1 mg/kg taken orally in a single morning dose. This preference is purely empirical, as are all programs proposed for treating inflammatory myopathies.[18–21] Once instituted, daily high-dose prednisone is continued until strength improves. Clinical improvement may be noted in the first weeks or gradually over a period of 3 to 6 months. This variability is related, at least in part, to the timing of treatment initiation.[27] The earlier in the course of the disease the prednisone is given, the faster and more effectively it will work.[29] Evaluations of muscle strength are performed at 3- to 6-week intervals. Ideally, the initial steroid dosage is maintained until both strength and CK values have returned to normal. Objective testing of strength is necessary to make certain that the patient's reported improvement is not simply due to a euphoric or "energizing" effect from the corticosteroids. Although it is reassuring to see strength improve and CK levels fall, strength is the more important measure.[43] Lowered CK values can be observed even when there is no improvement in strength because circulating CK inhibitors are present in some patients with active inflammation,[44] in some cases of myositis associated with cancer, or as a "nontherapeutic" result of treatments such as plasmapheresis or intravenous immune globulin. On the other hand, CK values may remain elevated after complete normalization of muscle strength because the disease process has resulted in damaged or "leaky" membranes.

At 6 weeks a decision is made. If the patient is strong or definitely improving, prednisone is continued at the initial dosage until strength and, it is hoped, CK values have returned to normal and have remained normal for 4 to 8 weeks. Once remission is apparent, the prednisone dosage is tapered by reducing the daily dosage by 10 mg each month. After a dosage of 10 mg/d has been taken for 1 month, the dosage is reduced to 5 mg/d. This dosage is maintained until the patient has remained in remission for 1 year. Control of a flare that occurs at any time during the taper requires raising the prednisone dosage, often to the level that brought about the initial remission.

Given the empiric nature of treatment for the inflammatory myopathies, other valid methods have been proposed for the use of corticosteroids. Starting doses range from a fixed dose of 60 mg/d up to 2 mg/kg/d.[45,46] Some begin with daily intravenous infusions of methylprednisolone.[47] Some prefer to divide the initial daily dosage. Although a divided schedule may provide greater antiinflammatory effect than a single-dose schedule, it may prove more toxic. With improvement, some authors would taper as much as 25% each month. Others would employ an alternate-day schedule toward the end of the taper. Alternate-day steroid therapy does result in fewer side effects, but if initiated too soon it may trigger a flare of the disease.

Corticosteroid therapy will lead to improvement in up to 90% of patients and complete remission in 50% to 75%.[25] However, if improvement is not obvious at 6 weeks or if the improvement has reached a plateau before complete remission is achieved, I add a second agent. Invariably, the choice of second agents is between azathioprine and methotrexate. Azathioprine, which has been tested in a blinded, controlled trial,[36] is favored as a second agent by some.[46] Azathioprine, 2 to 3 mg/kg/d, is usually effective given in a single oral dose. In adults I begin with 50 mg/d and check for results and potential side effects, primarily bone marrow depression, after 3 weeks. If there is no response, the dose is increased to 100 mg/d and the process is repeated. If response is still not adequate, the dose is increased again to a maximum of 150 mg/d.

Methotrexate, the other possible second agent, has been shown to be beneficial in adults and children with myositis.[48–50] Although methotrexate has not been tested in a blinded or controlled fashion, there is growing support for this agent.[19,29,51] Methotrexate is given in a single weekly dose, with the dosage selected somewhat arbitrarily. I prefer to start with 7.5 mg orally in most patients and increase the dose to 15 mg after 4 to 6 weeks if improvement has not occurred. Children are given oral methotrexate at a dosage of 20 mg/m².[50] In sicker adults, or those in whom compliance may be questioned, I prefer a dosage of 25 mg, escalating to 50 mg, given by intramuscular or intravenous injection.

Once the patient is in remission (is free of symptoms, has a normal CK level, and has been off medication for 3 to 9 months), the serum enzyme levels are checked infrequently unless recurrence is suggested by symptoms or changes on physical examination. Before remission the CK is monitored on a regular basis. If it becomes elevated but the patient has no symptoms, medication is not automatically prescribed. Rather, the patient is questioned about physical activity and other factors that might spuriously elevate the CK level and increase the frequency of checkups. Therapy should be reinstituted at the first sign of weakness and must be considered if the enzyme levels continue to rise. As a general rule, however, one should treat weakness, not laboratory results.

The general approach outlined above can be applied to all inflammatory myopathies. However, special consideration must be given to patients within certain clinical groups. The cutaneous lesions of dermatomyositis may respond to hydroxychloroquine at doses of up to 200 mg orally twice a day. This treatment may be effective even in patients with cancer.[52] Hydroxychloroquine, however, has no effect on the myositis. The primary focus of treatment for patients with myositis and cancer should be on the neoplasm. Removal (debulking) of the tumor or cure of the cancer may be accompanied by resolution of the myopathy. The myositis associated with another collagen vascular disease often is very sensitive to corticosteroid therapy. High doses may be necessary for only short intervals, and dosages of 10 to 30 mg per day may suffice in many cases.

Inclusion-body myositis and myopathy associated with myositis-specific autoantibodies represent the more challenging groups. When first described, inclusion-body myositis was thought to be refractory to treatment.[6] However, a small number of patients have had excellent response to therapy and there is now some evidence that treatment may retard progression in a percentage of patients.[51,53] Many patients with myositis and antisynthetase antibodies or anti-SRP antibodies also appear to be relatively resistant to treatment.[29] It is not clear whether this poor response correlates with the amount of interstitial pulmonary fibrosis encountered in these patients or to other factors. Nevertheless, therapeutic trials are warranted in each of these groups, and I begin as described above. If no improvement is observed at 6 weeks, I add a second agent as described. If no improvement is noted in the following 6 to 12 weeks, I discuss the option of adding a third agent versus discontinuing the medicines. It is bad enough to have treatment-resistant myositis. The additional problems of cost, inconvenience, and side effects that arise when potentially toxic medications are used should not be added to the situation unless the patient is fully aware of the alternatives.

When a patient is refractory to treatment with corticosteroids, especially if there is no response whatsoever, one should confirm the accuracy of the initial diagnosis. Patients with a wide variety of conditions that would not necessarily respond to corticosteroid therapy can satisfy some or all of the criteria for polymyositis (Table 14–2). When the diagnosis is confirmed or when patients must discontinue the above treatments because of serious side effects, one must weigh the potential risks and benefits of more experimental therapies listed below.

Pulmonary complications should be suspected when the patient complains of dyspnea or cough, auscultation of the chest reveals crackles or "Velcro" rales, or the chest x-ray is abnormal. These complications may include interstitial fibrosis, aspiration pneumonitis, or opportunistic infections. Each portends a poor prognosis, although some patients with interstitial fibrosis remain free of symptoms. Therapy often has little effect on interstitial fibrosis when it progresses. Aspiration usually occurs in severe disease with hypopharyngeal muscle involvement. Opportunistic infections are related to the degree of immunosuppression caused by corticosteroids or other agents.

No deviation from the above protocol for patients with interstitial lung disease is recommended unless their pulmonary status is deteriorating. Serial measurements of diffusing capacity are useful in assessing this decline. A gallium scan may also detect active inflammation in the lungs. Abnormal results in either of

these parameters may be an indication for use of higher-dose corticosteroid therapy (up to 2 mg/kg/d) and addition of another immunosuppressant agent, if one is not already being used. Maximum immunosuppressive therapy should also be considered when there is evidence of aspiration. Although the risk of complications from such therapy are great, that risk is outweighed by the potential good, as aspiration is almost always followed by death. If an opportunistic infection develops, the dose of corticosteroids should be reduced to one that would cover for stress (the lowest dose tolerated but no more than 40 mg of prednisone per day) and the dosage of other immunosuppressions should be lowered to that which allows a leukocytosis to develop. (This may require discontinuing these agents.)

Finally, the pulmonary complications of methotrexate must be considered for patients who are taking that medication. Methotrexate should be discontinued immediately in the presence of cough, dyspnea, or an abnormal chest x-ray and not reinstituted until the cause of the pulmonary problem is defined and determined not to be methotrexate.

Clinically significant cardiac complications are unusual, although conduction abnormalities may be seen on electrocardiograms and congestive heart failure can result from hypoxia or cardiomyopathy. Most cardiac problems should be managed as they would be if they developed in a patient who did not have myositis. An exception would be the patient with cardiomyopathy, who might benefit from a trial of higher-dose corticosteroid therapy and other immunosuppressive agents.

DRUG SIDE EFFECTS AND RECOMMENDED MONITORING SCHEDULES

The methods used to monitor for side effects of corticosteroids, azathioprine, or methotrexate are the same as when those agents are used to treat other rheumatic diseases. However, two potential side effects of corticosteroids—steroid myopathy and steroid-induced osteoporosis—warrant special consideration.

The possibility of steroid-induced myopathy poses a unique problem. The question of steroid myopathy is very difficult to deal with in patients with myositis, especially in those whose improvement has reached a plateau or those who have had a partial, if not gratifying, response to therapy and then become weaker. In those situations one must determine whether the decline in muscle strength is due to a flare of the inflammatory process or to steroid myopathy.[54,55] Unfortunately, no specific test will provide the answer. Even a muscle biopsy is of little value. Active inflammatory changes can be observed even when steroid myopathy is contributing to the weakness. Further complicating the situation, type 2 fiber atrophy, the typical histologic change of steroid myopathy, is a nonspecific finding and may be seen with disuse atrophy or as a change induced by inflammation. A provocative challenge with higher-dose corticosteroids or a trial of rapid tapering of the dose may be the only way to determine the cause of weakness in this situation.

The risk of corticosteroid-induced osteoporosis is significant for patients with myositis, especially if they are immobilized by weakness. Vertebral compression fractures are a significant long-term morbidity in these patients.[56] Thus weight-bearing exercises, such as walking, should be emphasized when possible, and the use of supplemental calcium (1000 to 1500 mg/d) should be encouraged. Vitamin D and estrogen may also be appropriate. Please see Chapter 22, this volume, for additional detailed information about management of osteoporosis.

Azathioprine can be used safely in most patients with inflammatory muscle disease. The major concern with this agent is bone marrow suppression. Initiating treatment with lower doses and monitoring blood counts before increasing the dose helps avoid problems. If anemia, leukopenia, or thrombocytopenia is encountered, azathioprine should be discontinued. It may be reinstituted after blood counts have returned to normal, but at a lower dose. Dosages as low as 25 mg every other day have been used safely and effectively in some patients who are very sensitive to azathioprine. Other rare side effects include hepatotoxicity and pancreatitis. A hypersensitivity reaction consisting of fever and hypotension may occur. The issue of azathioprine inducing cancer is of concern to some. Although reports of azathioprine-related neoplasia can be found in the renal transplant population, this relationship has not been established for patients with rheumatic diseases. The issue is further complicated because of the relationship between myositis and cancer. I do not believe the concern about cancer should be used as a reason to withhold azathioprine therapy from patients with myositis.

When methotrexate is selected, SGOT and SGPT levels should be measured and pulmonary function should be considered before the start of treatment in order to minimize confusion between changes in these parameters caused by the basic disease and the potential hepatic and pulmonary toxicities of the medication. The intramuscular route is usually avoided because of the resulting elevation in CK levels. However, if blood is sampled just before a dose (i.e., 6 or 7 days after the last injection), the elevation of CK due to the trauma of the injection is rarely a problem. This timing also avoids confusion due to transient elevations in transaminases that may develop immediately after a dose of methotrexate, regardless of the route of administration.

INVESTIGATIONAL DRUGS, ADDITIONAL APPROACHES, AND FUTURE DIRECTIONS

A number of therapies have been employed in an attempt to help the patient with refractory myositis. The approaches used include a variety of modalities and agents used singly or in combination. Each has been chosen in the hope of improving muscle strength and of avoiding the side effects of corticosteroids. In refractory cases, I prefer to add a third agent—azathioprine if methotrexate is the second agent or methotrexate if azathioprine is the second. The use of combinations is attractive. Theoretically, improved results may occur because the different agents act through different mechanisms and might work synergistically. The combination of methotrexate and azathioprine has been used successfully in a few patients with myositis[57] and is presently under investigation at the National Institutes of Health. Other combinations have been tried with some reported benefit, but numbers of patients treated to date are very small.[58]

Two alkylating agents, chlorambucil and cyclophosphamide, have been reported to be effective for some patients with myositis. Chlorambucil has been used in combination with prednisone and methotrexate in two patients with dermatomyositis[58,59] and has been successfully used in five others who had not responded to azathioprine and methotrexate.[60] The initial dosage of chlorambucil used is from 2 to 4 mg/d with adjustments up to a maximum of 8 mg/d as necessary to obtain a response. Leukopenia has been the only side effect encountered in these subjects, but more profound bone marrow suppression and seizures are potential complications of this treatment. The potential for development of cancer is higher for chlorambucil than for azathioprine or methotrexate. The risk of developing cancer with or after chlorambucil therapy increases with both duration of treatment and total dosage.[61]

Cyclophosphamide has been used orally on a daily schedule with anecdotal reports of success.[62,63] Recently, intravenous administration has received some attention. Advocates of intravenous administration believe it should be as effective, primarily on the basis of experience in treating lupus nephritis. Results have been mixed, however. Cyclophosphamide was ineffective in 10 of 11 corticosteroid-refractory patients at a monthly dose of 0.75 to 1.25 g/m^2.[64] The other patient had an unsustained improvement. In another study, four of seven patients with refractory polymyositis given intravenous cyclophosphamide at a dose of 500 mg/w were reported "recovered."[65] The patients in these reports had long-standing refractory disease. Perhaps earlier treatment would give better results and smaller, more frequent doses would prove more effective.

Cyclosporine is an immunosuppressive agent that inhibits calcium-dependent T cell activation and blocks transcription of genes that code for some cytokines, including interleukin 2. Through these actions, cyclosporine prevents proliferation of T helper cells and development of cytotoxic lymphocytes. Experience with cyclosporine in the treatment of myositis is quite limited, but more recent reports appear favorable.[66–70] Lower doses (2.5 to 5.0 mg/kg/d) may be as effective as higher doses (7.5 to 10 mg/kg/d) for treating myositis. Presumably, lower doses would be less toxic. Monitoring blood levels of cyclosporine helps keep toxicity to a minimum. Strength generally begins to improve within the first month to 6 weeks of treatment in those who respond to cyclosporine. More frequently encountered toxicities include tremors, hypertrichosis, gingival hyperplasia, hypertension, renal insufficiency, anemia and, very rarely, lymphoproliferative cancer. Cyclosporine can also cause a myopathy,[71] a side effect that may complicate its use in myositis. The reversibility of these side effects is controversial, especially with regard to renal insufficiency. Although the serum creatinine value may return to normal after the agent is discontinued, the creatinine clearance may not. The cost of this medication is approximately $500 per month for a 5 mg/kg/d dose in a 70 kg person.

Levamisole use has been reported in less than a dozen cases. This agent has been partially effective in some patients but led to rapid deterioration in at least two. Levamisole therapy is not recommended at this time.[72]

Perhaps validated by its effectiveness in Kawasaki's disease, intravenous immune globulin is now being touted as a therapeutic agent for multiple disorders, including the inflammatory myopathies. This has proved variably effective in a number of uncontrolled trials.[73–76] The largest of these studied 20 patients with disease duration ranging from 6 months to 14 years.[76] In all but one patient prior therapies had failed. Fifty percent had moderate or better improvement, 20% had no improvement, and one patient's condition worsened. Improvement usually occurred within 2 months, and better responses were observed in patients with shorter duration of disease. Intravenous immune globulin will surely be given stronger consideration now that a controlled trial has shown it to be effective over the short term for patients with dermatomyositis.[38] Intravenous immune globulin is associated with little toxicity, but the cost is nearly prohibitive. Patients commonly receive 1 to 2 g/kg each month at an approximate cost of $25 per gram. Interpreting the results from trials and understanding how best to use this therapy will be complicated because of variations in batches and preparations of immune globulin available from different manufacturers.

There is reason to believe that intravenous immune globulin therapy would be effective in dermatomyositis. The pathologic change in that form of inflammatory myopathy appears to be initiated by antibodies bound to microvascular components. With activation of the classic complement pathway, C5b-9 membranolytic attack complexes are deposited in capillaries bound to those antibodies.[77–79] Fiber damage is mediated by the membranolytic attack complex.[80] These processes eventuate in fiber necrosis and regeneration, inflammatory cell infiltration, perifascicular atrophy, capillary loss, and ischemia. A T cell–mediated and MHC-1–restricted cytotoxic process has also been implicated in dermatomyositis.[78] The mechanisms whereby immune globulin modulate the immune system are far from understood. Of the postulated mechanisms, immune globulins may block Fc receptors on vessel walls.[81,82] Immune globulin may also inhibit the effector functions of activated T cells [81–83] or decrease the expression of MHC-1 molecules.[84,85] High levels of immunoglobulin neutralize complement neoantigens[86] and inhibit formation of membrane attack complexes from activated C4b and C3b fragments.[87] Any of these actions would interfere with the pathogenesis of dermatomyositis. If those actions do contribute to the efficacy of immune globulin in dermatomyositis, then that therapy would likely also be effective in other forms of myositis in which the complement membrane attack complexes or MHC-1 restricted T cell cytotoxicity are involved in the pathogenesis.

Apheresis, predominantly plasmapheresis, has been advocated as a very effective therapy in refractory polymyositis. Until recently, all reports were uncontrolled, unblinded trials in which patients also received other therapies. Interestingly, many patients also received immune globulin or took cyclophosphamide as a routine component of the plasmapheresis protocol. A recent controlled trial showed that plasmapheresis was not effective.[37] Although that study does not prove total ineffectiveness of this expensive and time-consuming procedure, it does show that it is unlikely to help patients with circulating myositis-specific autoantibodies. The advantage of apheresis with intravenous immune globulin or cyclophosphamide over immune globulin or cyclophosphamide alone is yet to be demonstrated.

Total body or total nodal irradiation (TBI) has been used with varying results in patients with polymyositis.[88–90] The use of TBI has been reported in five patients. Two patients achieved remission; one patient responded, relapsed, and responded to repeat therapy; one patient did not respond; and one patient died of bone marrow suppression. The potential side effects of TBI are numerous and serious, causing lasting effects on the immune system. Death has occurred after this therapy.[88] Previous cytotoxic therapy may well potentiate the serious bone marrow–suppressive effects of TBI. This therapy can be effective in patients who have been refractory to multiple other treatments, but it should be reserved for the sickest of patients refractory to other modalities.

Selected Considerations

Today it is very difficult to determine the most appropriate treatment for inclusion-body myositis because there is simply too little information available. Although inclusion-body myositis may be responsible for perhaps 30% of the cases in some series of idiopathic inflammatory myopathy, many physicians still are unaware of its existence. Initially, patients with inclusion-body myositis were thought to be totally resistant to therapy. Two recent studies have added support to the position that treatment may be beneficial. Nevertheless, our expectations should probably be different when we are treating patients with inclusion-body myositis. The first report was a retrospective analysis of 32 patients.[51] Four patients received no therapy and their condition deteriorated, as would be predicted. Thirteen received prednisone alone. Of those, seven deteriorated, four seemed to stabilize, and two experienced temporary improvement. The remainder received prednisone in combination with methotrexate or azathioprine, with six deteriorating, one stabilizing, five experiencing transient improvement, and three achieving remission. Methotrexate appeared to provide better results than azathioprine. These results suggest that although remission is quite rare in inclusion-body myositis, one may stabilize the patient's weakness or slow the rate of progression of the disease with therapy. One still must balance the possible long-term benefits against the long-term toxicities and expense of treating this condition. Therefore it is essential that objective guides for determining efficacy are followed. The second study reported improvement in strength in three of four patients treated with two monthly infusions of high-dose intravenous immune globulin (2 g/kg/mo).[91] Greatest improvement was seen in the proximal and less atrophic muscles. CK levels fell after each treatment but rose again after the second infusion. No relationship was found between the fall in

CK levels and improvement. This probably means that the lowered enzyme levels were the consequence of an effect that had little influence on the underlying disease process. These data are very interesting because inclusion-body myositis has been ascribed such a futile prognosis. However, controlled trials with larger numbers must be performed before the appropriate use of immune globulin can be ascertained.

The treatment of children with recalcitrant myositis is of concern because of the potential long-term effects that therapy might have on developing systems. Methotrexate seems to be the preferred choice at this time for children whose disease is resistant to corticosteroids. Support for this view is provided by a study of 16 children with dermatomyositis who had failed to respond to prednisone.[50] Patients received methotrexate orally at a dosage of 20 mg/m². Twelve children who took the medication for more than 8 months achieved normal muscle strength at a median of 5 weeks after beginning treatment, and 11 of the 12 were able to decrease the daily prednisone dosage to 5 mg or less. As encouraging as those data appear, 31% of the patients in the study were unable to take methotrexate because of side effects, poor compliance, or complications. Furthermore, myositis recurred, as evidenced first by elevated CK levels and then by weakness, in all five patients in whom this agent was discontinued after achieving remission. Thus methotrexate appears to be useful in refractory childhood dermatomyositis. However, the drug cannot be used in all cases and may have only suppressive effects for those who can tolerate it.

Cyclosporine has been used in children with dermatomyositis at doses of 2.5 to 7.5 mg/kg/d with some beneficial results.[92–94] Strength improved in all patients. Similarly, CK levels fell, but not always to normal limits. Daily corticosteroid dosage was reduced in all and eventually discontinued in some. Side effects and toxicities were similar to those for adults, with the added occasional report of flulike symptoms.

Intravenous immune globulin has been suggested as a safe therapy for childhood dermatomyositis. An uncontrolled trial from two centers involving 11 patients indicated that this approach might be useful in corticosteroid-resistant patients.[95] Strength improved or was maintained in all patients. CK levels fell but not always to within normal limits. Prednisone

dosage was decreased or discontinued in all patients. As with other forms of myopathy, additional information will be necessary to determine the most appropriate role for this expensive therapy.

REFERENCES

1. Bohan A, Peter JB. Polymyositis and dermatomyositis (first of two parts). N Engl J Med 1975; 292:344.
2. Walton JN, Adams RD. Polymyositis. Baltimore: Williams & Wilkins, 1958.
3. Research Group Neuromuscular Diseases of the World Federation of Neurology. Classification of neuromuscular disorders. J Neurol Sci 1968; 6:165.
4. DeVere R, Bradley WG. Polymyositis: its presentations, morbidity and mortality. Brain 1975;98:637.
5. Banker BQ, Engel AG. The polymyositis and dermatomyositis syndromes. In: Engel AG, Banker BQ, eds. Myology. Vol 2. New York: McGraw-Hill, 1986.
6. Calabrese LH, Mitsumoto H, Chou SM. Inclusion body myositis presenting as treatment-resistant polymyositis. Arthritis Rheum 1987;30:397.
7. Targoff IN. Autoantibodies in polymyositis. Rheum Dis Clin North Am 1992;18:455.
8. Cronin ME, Plotz PH, Miller FW. Abnormalities of the immune system in the idiopathic inflammatory myopathies. In Vivo 1988;2:25.
9. Bunn CC, Bernstein RM, Mathews MB. Autoantibodies against alanyl-tRNA synthetase and tRNA(ALA) coexist and are associated with myositis. J Exp Med 1986;163:1281.
10. Mathews MB, Bernstein RM. Myositis autoantibodies inhibits histidyl-tRNA synthetase: a model for autoimmunity. Nature 1983;304:177.
11. Mathews MB, Reichlin M, Hughes GR, Bernstein RM. Anti-threonyl-tRNA synthetase, a second myositis-related autoantibody. J Exp Med 1984;160:420.
12. Targoff IN. Autoantibodies to amino-acyltransfer RNA synthetases for isoleucine and glycine: two addition synthetases are antigenic in myositis. J Immunol 1990;144:1737.
13. Bunn CC, Mathews MB. Autoreactive epitope defined as the anticodon region of alanine transfer RNA. Science 1987;238:1116.
14. Targoff IN, Arnett FC, Berman L, et al. Anti-KJ: a new antibody associated with the syndrome of polymyositis and interstitial lung disease. J Clin Invest 1989;84:162.
15. Targoff IN, Reichlin M. The association between Mi-2 antibodies and dermatomyositis. Arthritis Rheum 1985;28:796.
16. Targoff IN, Johnson AE, Miller FW. Antibody to signal recognition particle in polymyositis. Arthritis Rheum 1990;33:1361.
17. Love LA, Leff RL, Fraser DD, et al. A new approach to the classification of idiopathic inflam-

matory myopathy: myositis specific autoantibodies define useful homogeneous patient groups. Medicine 1991;70:360.

18. Wortmann RL. Inflammatory diseases of muscle. In: Kelley WN, Harris ED Jr, Ruddy S, Sledge CB, eds. Textbook of rheumatology. 4th ed. Philadelphia: WB Saunders, 1993.

19. Oddis, CV. Therapies for myositis. Curr Opin Rheumatol 1993;5:742.

20. Plotz PH, Dalakas M, Leff R, et al. Current concepts in the idiopathic inflammatory myopathies: polymyositis, dermatomyositis and related disorders. Ann Intern Med 1989;111:143.

21. Bunch TW. The therapy of polymyositis. Mt Sinai J Med 1988;55:483.

22. Tuffanelli DJ, Lavoie PE. Prognosis and therapy of polymyositis/dermatomyositis. Clin Dermatol 1988;6:93.

23. Vignos PJ Jr, Bowling GP, Watkins MP Jr. Polymyositis: effect of corticosteroids on final results. Arch Intern Med 1964;114:263.

24. Medsger TA, Robinson H, Masi AT. Factors affecting survivorship in polymyositis: a life-table study of 124 patients. Arthritis Rheum 1986;15:168.

25. Henriksson KG, Sandstedt P. Polymyositis-treatment and prognosis: a study of 107 patients. Acta Neurol Scand 1982;65:280.

26. Moyer RA, Phillips CA, Toretti D, Newman ED. Clinical features and outcome in inflammatory myopathy. Arthritis Rheum 1989;32(suppl):S32.

27. Fafalak RG, Peterson MGE, Kagen LJ. Strength in polymyositis and dermatomyositis: best outcome in patients treated early. J Rheumatol 1994;21:643.

28. Hochberg MC, Feldman D, Stevens MB. Adult onset polymyositis/dermatomyositis: an analysis of clinical and laboratory features and survival in 76 patients with a review of the literature. Semin Arthritis Rheum 1986;15:168.

29. Joffe MM, Love LA, Leff RL, et al. Drug therapy of the idiopathic inflammatory myopathies: predictors of response to prednisone, azathioprine, and methotrexate and a comparison of their efficacy. Am J Med 1993;94:379.

30. Arsura EL, Greenberg AS. Adverse impact of interstitial pulmonary fibrosis on prognosis in polymyositis and dermatomyositis. Semin Arthritis Rheum 1988;18:29.

31. Pearson CM. Patterns of polymyositis and their responses to therapy. Ann Intern Med 1963;59:827.

32. Hochberg MC, Lopez-Acuna D, Gittelsohn AM. Mortality from polymyositis and dermatomyositis in the United States, 1968–1978. Arthritis Rheum 1983;26:1465.

33. Benbassat J, Gefel D, Larholt K, et al. Prognostic factors in polymyositis/dermatomyositis: a computer-assisted analysis of ninety-two cases. Arthritis Rheum 1985;28:249.

34. McKendry RJR. Influence of age at onset on the duration of treatment in idiopathic adult polymyositis and dermatomyositis. Arch Intern Med 1987;147:1989.

35. Hoffman GS, Franck W, Raddatz DA, Stallons L. Presentation, treatment and prognosis of idiopathic inflammatory muscle disease in a rural hospital. Am J Med 1983;75:433.

36. Bunch TW. Prednisone and azathioprine for polymyositis: long-term follow up. Arthritis Rheum 1981;24:45.

37. Miller FW, Leitman SF, Cronin ME, et al. A randomized controlled trial of plasma exchange and leukapheresis in polymyositis and dermatomyositis. N Engl J Med 1992;326:1380.

38. Dalakas MC, Illa I, Dambrosia JM, et al. A controlled trial of high-dose intravenous immune globulin infusions as treatment for dermatomyositis. N Engl J Med 1993;329:1993.

39. Csuka ME, McCarty DJ. A rapid method for measurement of lower extremity muscle strength. Am J Med 1985;78:77.

40. Cox NH, Langtry JAA, Lawrence CM, Ive FA. Dermatomyositis and malignancy: an audit of the value of extensive investigations. Br J Dermatol 1989;121:47.

41. Hicks JE. Comprehensive rehabilitative management of patients with polymyositis and dermatomyositis. In: Dalakas MC, ed. Polymyositis and dermatomyositis. Boston: Butterworths, 1988:293.

42. Escalante A, Miller L, Beadmore, TD. An N-of-1 trial of resistive vs. non-resistive exercise in inflammatory muscle disease (IMD). Arthritis Rheum 1991;34(suppl):S173.

43. Oddis CV, Medsger TA Jr. Relationship between serum creatine kinase level and corticosteroid therapy in polymyositis-dermatomyositis. J Rheumatol 1988;15:807.

44. Kagan LJ, Aram S. Creatine kinase activity inhibitor in sera from patients with muscle disease. Arthritis Rheum 1987;30:213.

45. Oddis CV. Therapy for myositis. Curr Opin Rheumatol 1991;3:919.

46. Dalakas MC. Polymyositis, dermatomyositis, and inclusion-body myositis. N Engl J Med 1991;325:1486.

47. Yangisawa T, Sueshi M, Nawata Y, et al. Methylprednisolone pulse therapy in dermatomyositis. Dermatologica 1983;167:47.

48. Bookbinder SA, Espinoza LR, Fenske NA, et al. Methotrexate: its use in the rheumatic diseases. Clin Exp Rheumatol 1984;2:185.

49. Metzger AL, Bohan A, Goldberg LS, et al. Polymyositis and dermatomyositis: combined methotrexate and corticosteroid therapy. Ann Intern Med 1974;81:182.

50. Miller LC, Sisson BA, Tucker LB, et al. Methotrexate treatment of recalcitrant childhood dermatomyositis. Arthritis Rheum 1992;35:1143.

51. Sayers ME, Chou SM, Calabrese LH. Inclusion body myositis: analysis of 32 cases. J Rheumatol 1992;19:1385.

52. Woo TY, Callen JP, Voorhees JJ, et al. Cutaneous lesions of dermatomyositis are improved by hydroxychloroquine. J Am Acad Dermatol 1984;10:592.

53. Cohen MR, Sulaiman AR, Garancis JC, Wortmann RL. Clinical heterogeneity and treatment

response in inclusion body myositis. Arthritis Rheum 1989;32:734.

54. Afifi AK, Bergman RA, Harvey JC. Steroid myopathy: clinical, histologic, and cytologic observations. Johns Hopkins Med J 1968;123:158.

55. Askari A, Vignos PJ, Moskowitz RW. Steroid myopathy in connective tissue disease. Am J Med 1976;61:485.

56. Oddis CV, Hill P, Medsger TA Jr. Functional outcome in a national cohort of polymyositis-dermatomyositis (PM-DM) patients. Arthritis Rheum 1992;35(suppl):S88.

57. Trotter D, McCarty DJ, Csuka ME. Treatment of dermatomyositis/polymyositis with combination chemotherapy in early disease. Arthritis Rheum 1991;34(suppl):S149.

58. Wallace DJ, Metzger AL, White KK. Combination immunosuppressive treatment of steroid resistant dermatomyositis/polymyositis. Arthritis Rheum 1985;28:590.

59. Cagnoli M, Marchesoni A, Tosi S. Combined steroid, methotrexate, and chlorambucil therapy for steroid-resistant dermatomyositis. Clin Exp Rheumatol 1991;9:658.

60. Sinoway PA, Callen JP. Chlorambucil: an effective corticosteroid-sparing agent for patients with recalcitrant dermatomyositis. Arthritis Rheum 1993;36:319.

61. Cameron S. Chlorambucil and leukemia. N Engl J Med 1977;296:1065.

62. al-Janadi M, Smith CD, Karsh J. Cyclophosphamide treatment of interstitial pulmonary fibrosis in polymyositis/dermatomyositis. J Rheumatol 1989;16:1592.

63. Bombardieri S, Hughes GH, Neri R, et al. Cyclophosphamide in severe polymyositis [Letter]. Lancet 1989;1:1138.

64. Cronin ME, Miller FW, Hicks JE, et al. The failure of intravenous cyclophosphamide therapy in refractory idiopathic inflammatory myopathy. J Rheumatol 1989;16:1225.

65. Haga H, D'Cruz D, Asherson R, Hughes GRV. Short term effects of intravenous pulses of cyclophosphamide in the treatment of connective tissue disease crisis. Ann Rheum Dis 1992;51:885.

66. Lueck CJ, Trend P, Swash M. Cyclosporin in the management of polymyositis and dermatomyositis. J Neurol Neurosurg Psychiatry 1991;54:1007.

67. Correia O, Polonia J, Nunes JP, et al. Severe acute form of adult dermatomyositis treated with cyclosporine. Int J Dermatol 1992;31:517.

68. Pugh MT, Collins NA, Rai A, et al. Case of adult dermatomyositis treated with cyclosporine A. Br J Rheumatol 1992;31:855.

69. Mehregan DR, Su WPD. Cyclosporine treatment for dermatomyositis/polymyositis. Cutis 1993;51:59.

70. Jongen PJ, Joosten EM, Berden JM, Ter-Laak HJ. Cyclosporine therapy in chronic slowly progressive polymyositis—preliminary report of clinical results in three patients. Transplant Proc 1988;20(suppl):335.

71. Noppen M, Velkeniers B, Dierckx R, et al. Cyclosporine and myopathy. Ann Intern Med 1987;107:945.

72. Rovensky J, Lukac J, Tauchmannova H. Effect of levamisole treatment in polymyositis patients. J Rheumatol 1982;9:158.

73. Cherin P, Herson S, Wechsler B, et al. Intravenous immunoglobulin for polymyositis and dermatomyositis [Letter]. Lancet 1990;336(8707):116.

74. Roifman CM, Schaffer FM, Wachsmuth SE, et al. Reversal of chronic polymyositis following intravenous immune serum globulin therapy. JAMA 1987;258:513.

75. Lang BA, Laxer RM, Murphy G, et al. Treatment of dermatomyositis with intravenous gammaglobulin. Am J Med 1991;91:169.

76. Cherin P, Herson S, Wechsler B, et al. Efficacy of intravenous immunoglobulin G therapy on chronic refractory polymyositis and dermatomyositis: an open study with 20 adult patients. Am J Med 1991;91:162.

77. Kissel JT, Mendell JR, Rammohan KW. Microvascular deposition of complement membrane attack complex in dermatomyositis. N Engl J Med 1986;314:329.

78. Emslie-Smith AM, Engel AG. Microvascular changes in early and advanced dermatomyositis: a quantitative study. Ann Neurol 1990;27:343.

79. Stein DP, Jordan SC, Toyoda M, et al. Antiendothelial cell antibodies (AECA) in dermatomyositis (DM). Neurology 1993;43(suppl):356.

80. Engel AG, Biesecker G. Complement activation in muscle fiber necrosis: demonstration of the membrane attack complex of complement in necrotic fibers. Ann Neurol 1982;12:289.

81. Dwyer JM. Manipulating the immune system with immune globulin. N Engl J Med 1991;326:107.

82. Ballow M. Mechanisms of action of intravenous immunoglobulin therapy and potential use in autoimmune connective tissue diseases. Cancer 1991;68(suppl):1430.

83. Gelfand EW. Intervention in autoimmune disorders: creation of a niche for intravenous gammaglobulin therapy. Clin Immunol Immunopathol 1989;53:S1. (Erratum, Clin Immunol Immunopathol 1990;53:492.)

84. Blaszczyk R, Westhoff U, Grosse-Wilde H. Soluble CD4, CD8, and HLA molecules in commercial immunoglobulin preparations. Lancet 1993;341:789.

85. Dustin ML, Springer TA. Role of lymphocyte adhesion receptors in transient interactions and cell locomotion. Annu Rev Immunol 1991;9:27.

86. Bacchi VF, Maillet F, Berlan L, Kazatchkine MD. Neutralizing antibodies against C3NeF in intravenous immunoglobulin. Lancet 1992;340:63.

87. Basta M, Kisrshbom P, Frank MM, Fries LF. Mechanism of therapeutic effect of high-dose intravenous immunoglobulin: attenuation of acute, complement-dependent immune damage in a guinea pig model. J Clin Invest 1989;84:1974.

88. Morgan SH, Bernstein RM, Coppen J, et al. Total body irradiation and the course of polymyositis. Arthritis Rheum 1985;28:831.

89. Kelly JJ, Mudoc-Jones H, Adelman LS, et al. Response to total nodal irradiation in dermatomyositis. Muscle Nerve 1988;11:120.

90. Cherin P, Herson S, Coutellier A, et al. Failure of total body irradiation in polymyositis: report of three cases. Br J Rheumatol 1992;31:282.

91. Soueidan SA, Dalakas MC. Treatment of inclusion-body myositis with high-dose intravenous immunoglobulin. Neurology 1993;43:876.

92. Heckmatt J, Hasson N, Saunders C, et al. Cyclosporine in juvenile dermatomyositis. Lancet 1988;1:1063.

93. Pistola V, Buoncompagni A, Scribans R, et al. Cyclosporine A in the treatment of juvenile chronic arthritis and childhood polymyositis-dermatomyositis: results of a preliminary study. Clin Exp Rheumatol 1993;11:203.

94. Rawlings DJ, Herson S, Wechsler B, et al. Cyclosporine is safe and effective in refractory JRA and JDMS: results of an open clinical trial. Arthritis Rheum 1992;35:C130.

95. Barron KS, Sher MR, Silverman ED. Intravenous immunoglobulin therapy: magic or black magic. J Rheumatol 1992;19:94.

JUVENILE RHEUMATOID ARTHRITIS AND THE PEDIATRIC SPONDYLOARTHROPATHIES

Bernhard H. Singsen
Carlos D. Rosé

Juvenile rheumatoid arthritis (JRA) and the pediatric spondyloarthropathies are a heterogeneous group of clinically defined conditions. Onset subsets of JRA include systemic, polyarticular, and early- and late-onset pauciarticular. Ankylosing spondylitis, Reiter syndrome, psoriatic arthritis, and the gut-associated arthropathies are all described in children. The major differences from the same disorders in adults are the intermittence, absence, or late onset of clinical and radiologic abnormalities of the sacroiliac joints, a low frequency of spine and costochondral involvement, and the incomplete and/or late expression of diagnostic rashes. Children with an early spondyloarthritis often manifest only enthesitis, an asymmetric predominantly low-extremity arthritis, and a suggestive family history. Unexplained recurrent conjunctivitis, minimal dysuria, and/or diarrhea may also be present. In such patients, HLA-B27 testing can be a very helpful diagnostic adjunct.

During the past 15 years, pediatric rheumatologists have progressively treated JRA and the spondyloarthropathies of childhood earlier and more aggressively. Newer nonsteroidal antiinflammatory drugs (NSAIDs) have been replacing aspirin, NSAID dosages per body weight have slowly increased, and there has been a trend toward more rapid addition of disease-modifying antirheumatic drugs (DMARDs), starting with gold 15 years ago and now particularly involving methotrexate. Combination therapy that adds either hydroxychloroquine or sulfasalazine to an NSAID and a DMARD is increasingly common for children with active arthritis of longer than 6 to 12 months' duration. Although it was once the norm to add a DMARD only after the onset of erosions (e. g., after 1 to 3 years), the goal now is to avoid their occurrence. Similarly, early intervention clearly promotes more normal growth and development for children with arthritis. Since it is difficult to evaluate the long-term efficacy of any pediatric drug regimen, and since unpredictable improvement often occurs in children, pharmacotherapy is focused on helping to "control" synovitis, minimize joint destruction and deformities, and maximize age-appropriate activities of daily living until disease quiescence or spontaneous remission occurs. There are almost no prospective, multidimensional, long-term observations of disease outcomes related to drug therapy in children with arthritis. This is partly because of a paucity of health status assessment instruments available for children with chronic diseases[1] and partly because major efforts have been focused by the pediatric rheumatology community on important short-term dose findings, safety, and efficacy trials to increase the therapeutic alternatives available for children with arthritis.

Data from retrospective, one-center studies reveal that prognosis in JRA is highly dependent on type of disease onset.[2] One recent review of 147 JRA patients showed remission rates of (1) 50% for systemic-onset JRA at 5 years and 57%

at 10 years; (2) 0% for rheumatoid factor–positive, polyarticular-onset JRA at 10 years but 60% for seronegative, polyarticular-onset JRA; (3) 70% for early-onset pauciarticular JRA at 10 years but 55% for late-onset pauciarticular JRA.[3] The relative impact of specific drugs on outcome could not be established and in most studies is difficult because of the absence of control groups and of standardized long-term treatment protocols. Overall, synovitis may be adequately controlled in 50% of JRA patients receiving only NSAIDs.[4]

ASPIRIN

Aspirin is still the most widely known and least expensive of the NSAIDs. The analgesic action of the leaves, bark, and roots of the willow had been known since Hippocrates, its antipyretic action was confirmed in the eighteenth century, and the active ingredient (salicin) was identified in the nineteenth century. In 1876 Maclagan[5] used salicin to treat acute rheumatism. Aspirin was synthesized for manufacture by F. Hofman (from Bayer) in 1893 and was the only commercially available antiinflammatory compound until 1949.

Since 1980, the known association with Reye's syndrome has made both parents and physicians reluctant to use aspirin for arthritis in children. Nonetheless, aspirin remains a good choice if a child has already had definite chickenpox and is not currently exposed to influenza. Multiple enteric-coated, buffered, liquid, and nonacetylated preparations are now available. Some of these may result in lower serum levels, although buffering increases solubility and absorption.

Antiinflammatory doses of aspirin in children are 75 to 90 mg/kg/d in pauciarticular and polyarticular JRA and occasionally up to 100 to 110 mg/kg/d in systemic disease with marked fever, polyserositis, or both. It should be administered in four or five divided daily doses and should be given with food to minimize gastritis. Aspirin is rapidly absorbed in the proximal gastrointestinal (GI) tract but is optimally effective only when stable serum levels of 150 to 250 μg/L are achieved after 3 to 5 days of treatment. The maximal antiinflammatory action of aspirin is generally achieved within 2 to 4 weeks, with some further benefit occurring up to 3 months. Increasing of doses above 100

mg/kg/d (or 3 g/d for adolescents and adults) should be done carefully, since small changes may lead to significant elevation in blood levels of aspirin. Metabolism is by hepatic microsomal enzymes; aspirin is conjugated to glycine to form salicyluric acid, which then undergoes renal excretion. If the urine is alkylinized, clearance is enhanced and serum aspirin levels will be reduced.

Toxicity and Monitoring

During aspirin therapy, parents and children should be regularly questioned about eating habits, abdominal pain or diarrhea, tinnitus or subtle hearing loss, behavioral changes, bruising, and epistaxis. In small children, anorexia may herald the presence of gastritis or mild hepatotoxicity. Guaiac cards should be given to families if gastrointestinal symptoms are reported. Occult stool blood losses may be 2 to 10 ml/d in 50% to 70% of adults with arthritis and are not altered by giving aspirin with food. The prevalence and significance of stool blood loss in children with arthritis is not known. However, children with arthritis have multiple reasons to be anemic, and iron supplementation, if tolerated, will often raise the serum hemoglobin level by about 1 g/dl.

Patients with newly diagnosed JRA often have mild hepatic inflammation, and pretreatment transaminase values should be determined. Mild reversible hepatic toxicity caused by salicylates will occur at some time in 60% to 70% of JRA cases; this often appears as anorexia or nausea and may be exacerbated by intercurrent infection or dehydration.[6] A brief (3- or 4-day) stoppage of aspirin and then reintroduction at a 15% to 20% lower dose will usually permit continued treatment. To avoid the small risk of Reye's syndrome, aspirin should be discontinued for 3 to 5 days after exposure to influenza, and similarly after contact with varicella unless previous clinical chickenpox is certain. Increased shin bruising, related to altered platelet function, is common and benign; parents are often suspected of mistreating the child, however, and written materials to reassure others may be helpful. Recurrent epistaxis may require discontinuation of aspirin. If elective surgery is planned, a template bleeding time, prothrombin time, and partial thromboplastin time are needed. If impaired hemostasis is present, aspirin should be stopped, and low-dose corticosteroids may be required in the perioperative period.

Aspirin-induced peptic ulcer disease is rare, but gastritis is common and can be managed with antacids, sucralfate, cimetidine, or ranitidine and by attention to possible colonization with *Helicobacter* pylori. Regarding antacids, children are particular about flavor and about tablets versus liquids, and the purchase of several trial sizes is useful. Constipation and diarrhea are potential complications. Despite the perception that children prefer liquids, antacid tablets permit much greater social flexibility in patients over 7 to 8 years of age.

Other rare side effects of aspirin include severe bleeding, disseminated intravascular coagulation (mainly in systemic JRA), interstitial nephritis, urticaria, bronchospasm, and hypersensitivity pneumonitis. Severe salicylism may manifest as hyperpyrexia, hyperpnea, metabolic acidosis, central nervous system (CNS) stimulation or depression, and cardiovascular shock. When any child is at risk of dehydration, aspirin should be immediately discontinued. Salicylates are contraindicated in children with G6PD deficiency, pyruvate kinase deficiency, hemophilia, or von Willebrand disease and in children who are receiving anticoagulant therapy.

Among adults, aspirin compliance rates are 50%; the figures for children may be similar and are probably worse for adolescents. Serum aspirin levels can be checked after 5 to 10 days of treatment, and pill counts may be helpful. However, many compliance studies suggest that simply asking patient and parent whether the medication is being taken is less expensive and usually quite reliable.

NONSTEROIDAL ANTIINFLAMMATORY DRUGS

Until recently, salicylates were the most common beginning treatment for pediatric arthritis, but the NSAIDs are now much more frequently prescribed. Although only tolmetin and naproxen have received regulatory approval with specific indications for children, ibuprofen and indomethacin are also widely employed, and diclofenac and sulindac are occasionally used. Fenoprofen, ketoprofen, and sodium meclofenamate have also been studied by the Pediatric Rheumatology Collaborative Study Group (PRCSG) and Food and Drug Administration (FDA) approval is pending.

As a group, the NSAIDs have antipyretic, antiinflammatory, analgesic, and platelet-inhibitory properties. Although they differ chemically, in both pharmacokinetics and pharmacodynamics, the clinical consequences of these differences are not clear.[7] Most NSAIDs are weakly acidic, which may cause preferential concentration in the synovium, but those that are lipid soluble also appear to cause more CNS side effects, which can be subtle but important in children. Major mechanisms of actions of the NSAIDs include inhibition of cyclooxygenase and lipoxygenase enzymes with reduced production of prostaglandins, decreased leukocyte or synovial cell generation of leukotrienes, lowered proteoglycan synthesis, interference with cell membrane functions, and inhibition of some neutrophil actions, perhaps related to the uncoupling of protein-protein interactions within plasma membrane lipid bilayers.[8]

Generally, the NSAIDs are well absorbed, highly albumin bound (>95%), and not rapidly metabolized. NSAIDs may be grouped into those with half-lives <6 hours and those with half-lives >10 hours; however, relationships between dose and serum levels and both efficacy and toxicity are very often not linear. There is little to suggest that compliance with NSAIDs differs appreciably from aspirin. The NSAIDs are far more expensive, and hopes for significantly lower toxicity profiles have not been borne out. It is not possible to predict which NSAID will be best for a given child with arthritis. Simultaneous use of two NSAIDs may provide small additional clinical benefit but also can lead to increased risk of toxicity. Recent evidence suggests that NSAIDs are also helpful in controlling inflammatory eye disease in JRA.

The NSAIDs most commonly used by pediatric rheumatologists in the United States are reviewed below. However, all NSAIDs marketed in the United States and in Europe are occasionally employed in children when there is intolerance or lack of efficacy related to tolmetin, naproxen, or ibuprofen. Summaries of pediatric dosage (Table 15–1), toxicity monitoring (Table 15–2), side effects (Table 15–3), and approach to associated peptic disease (Table 15–4) for several NSAIDs are provided.

Tolmetin has been approved for use in children with JRA since 1979 and is widely used,

TABLE 15–1

Dosages of Antirheumatic Drugs in Children

DRUG	ROUTE	DOSAGE	COMMENT
Aspirin	PO, qid	75–100 mg/kg/d (8–12 325-mg tablets in older children >40 kg)	Inexpensive; can be initial treatment choice
Tolmetin	PO, tid	20–35 mg/kg/d Max: 1800 mg/d	May be initial treatment choice; expensive; low GI toxicity, occasional CNS effects
Indomethacin	PO, tid	2–4 mg/kg/d	Potential for headaches; GI toxicity common
Indomethacin	PO, qhs	0.5–1 mg/kg/d	Good to reduce AM gel; spondyloarthropathy
Ibuprofen	PO, tid–qid	30–40 mg/kg/d	Good initial treatment; no prescription required
Naproxen	PO, bid–tid	10–15 mg/kg/d	Good initial treatment; bid dosing helpful
Oral steroids	PO, qd or qod as AM dose	0.1–1 mg/kg/d	Therapeutic bridge; flare of systemic complications
Oral steroids	PO, tid/qid	1–2 mg/kg/d	Severe complications
IV Methylprednisolone	QD, for 1–3 d	30 mg/kg/dose Max: 1–1.5 g/d	Therapeutic bridge for systemic/visceral uncontrollable, severe complications
IA steroids (triamcinolone hexacetonide)		0.2–0.8 mg/kg/dose	Persistent, isolated disabling joint(s)
Methotrexate	PO, qwk	10–20 mg/m²/wk	Severe/progressive disease
Methotrexate	SQ/IM, qwk	0.5–1.0 mg/kg	Nonresponsive to oral MTX
Gold	IM, qwk	Max: 1 mg/kg/wk	Active, polyarticular JRA
Sulfasalazine	PO, bid	1–2.5 g/d	Progressive disease; add to NSAID or SAARD or both
Auranofin	PO, qd	0.1 mg/kg/d	Lower cost, convenient, limited efficacy
Hydroxychloroquine	PO, qd	5–7 mg/kg/d	Safe, adjunctive, mild activity
D-Penicillamine	PO, qd	5–10 mg/kg/d	Second-line DMARD; may use for combination therapy, or if have other DMARD toxicity
Gamma globulin	IV, q2–4wk	1.0–1.5 g/kg/dose	Systemic disease unresponsive to other treatments; very expensive

although it remains costly. It is well absorbed from the GI tract. Although tolmetin causes less CNS and GI toxicity than indomethacin, similar fatigue, dizziness, and gastritis can occur. It is equal to aspirin in the treatment of JRA, and is more effective for the spondyloarthropathies. At a dose of 20 to 30 mg/kg/d, it may be given three or four times a day. A false-positive sulfosalicylic urine test for protein can be seen in patients taking the drug.

TABLE 15–2

Laboratory Monitoring for Drug Toxicity in Children

DRUG	BASELINE TESTS	FOLLOW-UP TESTS
NSAIDs	CBC, AST, ALT, creatinine	Not needed if asymptomatic
Methotrexate	CBC, platelet count, AST, ALT, urinalysis, creatinine	CBC, platelet count, AST, ALT, urinalysis weekly for 3 wk; then monthly
IM gold	CBC, platelet count, urinalysis, creatinine	CBC, platelet count, urinalysis weekly for 6 mo
Hydroxychloroquine	Detailed eye examination	Same, q6mo
D-Penicillamine	CBC, platelet count, urinalysis, creatinine, ANA, immunoglobulins, CK	CBC, platelet count, urinalysis, CK monthly
Sulfasalazine	CBC, platelet count, AST, ALT	Same monthly

TABLE 15–3
Common Effects of NSAIDs

	GASTRITIS	CNS	TRANSAMINASE ELEVATIONS
Aspirin	+	+	++
Tolmetin	+	++	–
Naproxen	+	+	–
Ibuprofen	+	+	–
Indomethacin	+++	+++	++

Ibuprofen in a dose of 25 to 35 mg/kg/d is moderately effective for JRA and is usually given four times daily because of its short half-life.[9] It has little GI toxicity, and the liquid form is well liked by children. It has rarely been associated with white cell aplasia and hemolytic anemia. In school-aged children, giving doses at breakfast, after school with a snack, at dinner, and at bedtime will avoid the stigma of taking medication at school. Its low cost and over-the-counter availability can be an advantage, although some families feel that nonprescription drugs are "less potent" and will resist their use.

Naproxen safety, efficacy, and toxicity have been described in 10 published reports, as well as in several unpublished studies, in a total of 472 children with "juvenile arthritis," half of whom received the suspension.[10–12] It was approved by the FDA for children in 1987. Absorption, metabolism, and side effects are similar to those found in adults with rheumatoid arthritis (RA). Naproxen is given in doses of 15 to 20 mg/kg/d, and twice-daily administration, because of its longer half-life, may more effectively reduce morning stiffness and preclude the need for in-school administration. About 50% of children with JRA will respond well to naproxen, but a 3-month trial may be

required. Its tolerability, taste, and schedule make this drug a good choice for early-onset pauciarticular JRA, although its relatively high cost is a disadvantage. GI toxicity occurs in 5% to 10% of children; idiosyncratic reactions include a photosensitive rash, which is more common in light skinned patients. Rarely, pseudoporphyria may occur.[13]

Indomethacin is a very potent NSAID, but headaches, dizziness, fatigue, and gastric distress can be limiting factors. It is particularly useful for the pediatric spondyloarthropathies, the fever and/or pericarditis of systemic onset JRA, and as a single nighttime dose to ameliorate severe morning stiffness. In one study of indomethacin, 50% of the children had reduced symptoms of arthritis and 75% showed improved fever control, but the drug had to be discontinued in 40% of the cases because of adverse reactions.[14] The usual dose is 2 to 3 mg/kg/d or 0.5 to 1.0 mg/kg at bedtime, and it should always be taken with food or an antacid preparation. Initiation of therapy with 25% of the final calculated dose and increases by 25% increments every 4 to 5 days may avert the onset of headaches.

Diclofenac is widely used in Europe. An open-label, 8-month study of diclofenac, 2 mg/kg/d, in 50 children with JRA (no other NSAIDs and all slow-acting antirheumatic drugs [SAARDs] left unchanged) revealed 68% to be improved or in remission.[15] Forty-five of these patients were still receiving Voltaren after 2 years, with almost no toxicity. One randomized, double-blind study compared aspirin (50 to 100 mg/kg/d), diclofenac (2 to 3 mg/kg/d), and placebo, with 15 children in each treatment group; however, therapy lasted only 2 weeks.[16] Diclofenac was judged as effective as aspirin but had fewer side effects.

TABLE 15–4
Management of NSAID-induced Peptic Ulcer Disease

	TREATMENT	PREVENTION
Dietary measures	++	+++
Antacids	+++	–
Cimetidine	+++	–
Sucralfate	+*	+++

*For duodenal ulcers.

Adverse Reactions to NSAIDs in Children

The spectrum of adverse reactions to NSAIDs is broad, but full appreciation of toxicity in children may be delayed because of fewer and smaller studies, the often greater functional and reserve capabilities of young healthy organs involved in drug metabolism and elimination, the greater pain tolerance and limited communication skills of children, and less experience in both child and parent with what is "abnormal" or unacceptable.

Since most NSAIDs cause some degree of GI irritation in children, they are preferably given with food (i.e., with a snack or at the beginning of a meal); many parents incorrectly give NSAIDs at the end of a meal, which may increase the likelihood of gastritis. Gastrotoxicity is partly caused by prostaglandin inhibition, leading to increased gastric acid synthesis, and decreased esophageal sphincter tone; direct epithelial damage by the NSAID may also occur. Elevation of hepatic enzymes is less common than with aspirin, although hepatitis can occur during treatment with sulindac.[17] It is advisable to check serum liver enzyme levels every 6 months.

Among adults, reports of NSAID-related renal toxicity suggest a prevalence of 1% to 2%, but renal complications appear rare in children.[18] In a 4-year prospective study, Szer et al.[18] evaluated 226 children with JRA who received one or several NSAIDs for a median of 1.3 years (range, 0.5 to 8 years). One child had persistent, unexplained proteinuria, while 21 of 22 children with abnormal urinalyses had resolution of abnormalities without discontinuation of the NSAID. The overall prevalence of hematuria/proteinuria was no different than in normal schoolchildren. Renal parenchymal disease rarely occurs in JRA, although hematuria may be associated with fever. Thus all children should have a urinalysis prior to starting an NSAID. Although renal papillary necrosis is a rare complication, many NSAIDs have been implicated in its occurrence. It is important to emphasize sufficient fluid intake, especially in the summer or if the child is active in athletics. If cardiovascular complications or hypovolemia develop in a child, it is advisable to discontinue NSAIDs because of potential inhibition of prostaglandin-mediated renal function. The relationship of NSAID administration to the rare occurrence of renal tubular dysfunction in JRA is unclear.

Although the mechanisms are not known, increasing experience has shown that CNS side effects are quite common in children receiving NSAIDs. Manifestations include dizziness or light-headedness, mild headaches, tinnitus, behavioral changes such as confusion, euphoria, or depression, and difficulty in concentrating. Fatigue is also a common complaint and can be difficult to separate from underlying disease activity. Visual complaints may occur. CNS toxicity in children may become known only after prolonged NSAID administration for months to years. Since the NSAID has often greatly ameliorated the child's arthritis, the physician may be quite reluctant to stop the medication. Our practice is to regularly take a behavioral history and immediately discontinue NSAIDs if CNS abnormalities are noted. The number of children who rapidly improve, despite no evidence of other significant side effects, has been impressive. Most children tolerate another NSAID well, suggesting that at least some CNS side effects are idiosyncratic. There is no evidence to suggest an association between NSAIDs and Reye's syndrome.

Other rare NSAID-related complications that occur in children with arthritis include anaphylaxis, hypoplasia or aplasia of bone marrow cell lines, decreased platelet adhesiveness, fluid and electrolyte imbalance, edema, and a variety of rashes.

CORTICOSTEROIDS

General Principles

Earlier diagnosis and referral of patients with JRA, wide choice of NSAIDs, more rapid addition and prolonged use of methotrexate or SAARDs or both, and increased use of combination therapy during the past decade have led to much less dependence on corticosteroids to treat JRA. The potentially severe and lifelong negative effects of corticosteroids on growth and development are also now better appreciated. Systemic and local steroids should be given in the lowest possible doses, for minimal periods of time, and only to achieve specific objectives.[19] Indications include (1) a therapeutic "bridge" for early, disabling arthritis prior to achieving control with methotrexate (MTX) or other DMARDs; (2) uveitis that does not respond to topical treatment; (3) uncontrolled fever and/or visceral manifestations of systemic-onset JRA; (4) intraarticular injection to restore functional use in one or a few joints.

Dosage

Prednisone, prednisolone, and methylprednisolone are commonly used oral preparations. Recently, a randomized double-blind trial compared deflazacort with prednisone in JRA; deflazacort had a similar antiinflammatory effect and a better-maintained spinal bone mineral content.[20] Wherever possible, alternate-day steroid therapy should be tried first. However, in new or severely flaring patients who are experiencing loss of ambulation, intractable fever, or visceral manifestations, a brief 2- to 3-week course of oral prednisone, 1 to 2 mg/kg/d in divided doses, may be required. Alternatively, intravenous Solu-Medrol pulse therapy, 30 mg/m²/d (1 g maximum) for 3 days can lead to rapid improvement. In either case, appropriate doses of NSAIDs, DMARDs, and/or MTX should be started simultaneously. Plans for consolidation, provision of a tapering schedule, and education of child and family about possible consequences should begin immediately. Mild intercurrent exacerbations of JRA or spondyloarthropathy often respond to brief, low doses (0.25 to 0.5 mg/kg/d) of oral prednisone given daily or every other day. It is often difficult for families to accept that total control of JRA is usually accompanied by many unwanted steroid side effects.

When high divided doses of oral steroids are necessary, tapering begins with consolidation to a single daily dose; this can be associated with worsening of disease and may require a few days to implement (e.g., 10 mg three times daily, to 15 mg twice daily, to 30 mg every morning over a period of 10 to 15 days). Reductions of about 10% of the dose every 5 to 7 days should then be attempted. When one fourth of the original dose is reached, the rate of reduction should be slowed to 5% per week. After a total dose of 5 mg/d is achieved, weekly reductions of only 0.25 to 0.50 mg/d (or every other day) are often necessary. At low doses, for reasons that are not clear, children with JRA are exquisitely sensitive to small decremental changes. As much as 3 to 6 months may be needed to complete weaning, but this approach usually averts the cyclic need to treat recurrent disease exacerbations, and the total corticosteroid dosage over years is much lower.

Single daily doses of corticosteroids should be given in the early morning to minimize pituitary inhibition. Methylprednisolone bypasses hepatic activation by methylation, which may be useful in the presence of liver disease. Dexamethasone and other long-acting fluorinated oral preparations are contraindicated in JRA because of the high incidence of associated steroid myopathy. Tablets can be crushed and mixed with food; liquid preparations are available but more expensive. Restrictions of fat and caloric intake must be emphasized, and some parents report improved appetite control with high-bulk snacks.

Toxicity

Steroid side effects pose special problems for children and teenagers, often impairing school attendance and social development. These include (1) poor self-image because of acne, striae, cushingism, and hirsutism; (2) reduced growth velocity, in combination with inflammatory JRA, which also often limits ultimate height; (3) osteopenia leading to vertebral fractures; (4) increased likelihood of peptic ulceration and infections; (5) mood and behavioral disturbances, posterior subcapsular cataracts, and occasional myopathy. The development of toxicity is unpredictable, but there is a clear relationship to total dose and length of therapy. Hypertension, aseptic necrosis, pseudotumor cerebri, and glaucoma are now infrequent with the newer steroid treatment regimens.

As little as 5 mg/m² of prednisone daily for a month may affect linear growth. The likely mechanism is peripheral resistance to somatomedin-C. With short treatment courses, recovery from growth delay can be seen by 4 to 6 weeks after steroids are stopped. The ability to exhibit "catch-up" growth is inversely related to age; alternate-day regimens are associated with less growth retardation.

Intravenous Pulse Corticosteroids

Large intravenous doses of methylprednisolone (30 mg/kg/d; up to a 1 g maximum), given over 20 to 60 minutes, are often used for renal transplant (graft-versus-host) rejection, and for JRA, severe or life-threatening systemic lupus erythematosus (SLE), childhood dermatomyositis, vasculopathies, and other rheumatic conditions.[21] The goal is to achieve a rapid and profound antiinflammatory effect, with minimum toxicity. Various daily or every-other-day protocols, up to three total doses, have been employed. The efficacy of oral high-dose pulse therapy is not known.

In JRA, uncontrolled fever, disabling arthritis, myocarditis, pneumonitis, other systemic features, and disseminated intravascular coagulopathy are all potential indications for intravenous pulse corticosteroids. Although less toxic than long-term oral steroids, several rare complications are possible, including acute osteonecrosis, sudden hypokalemia, electrolyte imbalance, seizures or psychosis, and increased infections.[22] Many centers perform pulse therapy on an outpatient basis, although some authors prefer hospitalization. The antiinflammatory and pain-reducing actions of methylprednisolone may last only a few days or up to 4 to 8 weeks, thus allowing other interventions to become effective.

Intraarticular Corticosteroids

If one or a few inflamed joints are unresponsive to NSAIDs, or have caused severe disability in a patient with newly diagnosed JRA, intraarticular corticosteroids may be used. The rationale is to relieve pain, facilitate physical therapy and improve range in a stiff joint, and/or assist correction of joint deformity. While rapidly effective, improvement may last only a few days or may be sustained for months. Common preparations are triamcinolone hexacetonide and prednisone tertiary butyl acetate, which have high potency and a prolonged half-life. The dose is 0.5 mg/kg (10 to 20 mg) in small joints, and 1.0 mg/kg (20 to 40 mg) in large joints, depending on age. Mixing the steroid solution with an equal volume of a nonpreservative containing local anesthetic may reduce discomfort. The correct frequency of injections has not been established; recommendations range from once only, to monthly, up to three times. Children who respond well may be younger and have shorter disease durations; in one study 37% had joint relapse by 6 months after injection, and 50% by 1 year.[23]

The incidence of side effects is extremely low, although subcutaneous atrophy, infection, crystal-induced synovitis, calcification, avascular necrosis, and osteoporosis are known.[24] Good outcome following multiple injections has been reported in 51 joints among a total of 145 joints in 51 children.[24] However, general anesthesia with its associated risks was given to an unknown number of patients.

METHOTREXATE

Background and Efficacy

The efficacy of aminopterin, a folic acid antagonist, in controlling RA was first described by Gubner et al.[25] in 1951. By 1985 several placebo-controlled clinical trials, involving more than 200 RA patients, had demonstrated the benefits of MTX in suppressing manifestations of disease activity such as swelling, morning stiffness, and sedimentation rate.[26,27] However, one early controlled study could not show a reduction in radiologic evidence of joint destruction.[28] Recently, a randomized trial in adult RA has suggested that MTX alone, in comparison to auranofin alone, or in combination with auranofin leads to a "slowing" in the progression of erosions in RA.[29] In JRA, measurements of carpal bone length revealed limited radiologic evidence of progression among children who also had evidence of a positive clinical response.[30]

In 1986 MTX was first reported to be efficacious for JRA,[31] and other studies with similar findings quickly followed.[32–34] Subsequently, a double-blind placebo-controlled multicenter trial showed that MTX was effective for children with "resistant" JRA at either 5 mg/m^2/wk or 10 mg/m^2/wk dosage schedules.[35]

Mechanism of Action

MTX is a folic acid analog with potent inhibitory binding to the enzyme dihydrofolate reductase (DHFR). It appears to alter several folate-dependent pathways that affect immune response and the reactivity of inflammatory cells, but with relatively little cytotoxic effect. Although much of its toxicity seems related to DHFR inhibitions, whether such inhibition is responsible for the antiinflammatory and/or antiproliferative action(s) of MTX is not clear. In vitro, MTX is capable of affecting several metabolic pathways, including the following:

1. De novo synthesis of purines. The inhibition of DHFR limits the conversion of dihydrofolic to tetrahydrofolic acid, which in turn is the universal donor of one-carbon units involved in de novo manufacture of purines. This effect is mainly mediated by inhibiting AICAR (5-aminoimidazole-4-carboxamide ribonucleotide transformylase) and GAR (glycinamide ribonucleotide transformylase), both of which require one-carbon units in the purine synthesis pathway.
2. Thymidilate synthase also uses one-carbon units and is crucial for manufacture of thymidine.
3. Serine formation from methionine, which requires tetrahydrofolate as a donor of a one-carbon unit.

Although there are few studies that relate specific in vitro MTX effects to defined alterations in clinical outcomes, it is known that the binding of MTX to DHFR is easily reversed by low concentrations of dihydrofolic acid-FH2, which permits "rescue" therapy when significant clinical toxicity occurs.[36]

MTX selectively inhibits both peripheral blood mononuclear cell (PBMC) proliferation in RA patients[37] and T and B cell proliferative and mitogen responses, which may amplify its antiinflammatory activity.[38] Its suppression of rheumatoid factor production is striking.[39,40] MTX also exhibits folate-dependent inhibition of the actions of IL-1, a potent mediator of local and systemic inflammation, and markedly inhibits IL-1–induced IL-2 synthesis and proliferation of T cells in vitro when added to PBMC. This mechanism is reversible by the addition of leucovorin.[41–43]

Other observed methotrexate actions include (1) an effect on neutrophil LTB$_4$ production in the lipoxygenase pathway[44]; (2) diminished expression of Ia antigens on the surface of peritoneal macrophages of rats with adjuvant arthritis; (3) inhibition of the folate-dependent regeneration of methionine from homocysteine, leading to (a) an antiproliferative action on lymphocytes because of interference with the manufacture of polyamines, which are essential for the synthesis of DNA, and (b) reduced production of proteins such as immunoglobulins, rheumatoid factor, and interleukin 2.[45]

Kinetics

Data on the kinetics of MTX in children are limited. According to animal and adult human studies, oral MTX is effectively absorbed at a variable rate, with peak serum levels achieved 2 hours after ingestion. Its serum half-life is 6 hours, and its volume of distribution is 0.25 L/kg. Half of MTX is free in the serum, while the remaining 50% is protein bound and transported to the liver, where it is partially converted to 7-hydroxymethotrexate before being removed by active renal tubular secretion.[46] Biliary elimination of up to 30% of MTX occurs via the enterohepatic circulation[47]; this may act as a safety valve to reduce the risk of toxicity in patients with decreased renal function.

Bioavailability of MTX is similar after oral, subcutaneous, and intramuscular administration. However, uncontrolled observations in both adults and children suggest that selected patients receiving oral therapy who do not respond, reach a plateau after variable degrees of improvement, or experience an exacerbation after significant disease regression may benefit from switching to either the intramuscular or the subcutaneous route at a similar dose.[48–52] It is not clear whether changes in response are due to (1) delayed MTX absorption, (2) altered bioavailability, or (3) coincidental changes in disease activity.

Methotrexate is actively transported into cells and then polyglutamated, which increases its inhibitory action on DHFR and also prevents MTX from "escaping" from the cell. Polyglutamation may play an important role in conservation of MTX, since very low intracellular levels are required to be effective, and these are readily achieved with weekly oral pulses.[36,46,53]

In adults with RA, known MTX interactions with other drugs include salicylates, indomethacin, naproxen, ketoprofen, and phenylbutazone.[54] Although a recent investigation by Dupuis et al.[54] of children with arthritis showed that MTX half-life was prolonged by tolmetin, indomethacin, aspirin, and naproxen, no interactions were found by Skeith et al.[55] for ibuprofen or flurbiprofen. Whether clinically significant interactions of MTX with other medications occur in JRA is uncertain at present.

Toxicity

MTX is well tolerated by children with JRA. Giannini et al.[35] found that only 3% of patients had to discontinue the drug because of toxicity. Overall, as collated from five reports involving MTX treatment of 203 children with JRA, the most commonly observed side effects were upper gastrointestinal upset (9%), diarrhea (4.5%), and abdominal pain (4%).[31–35] Such reactions are usually self limited,[34] may be due to folic acid depletion,[56] and often will resolve if MTX is withheld for 1 week and then reinstituted at a 15% to 25% lower dose. MTX toxicity in adults with RA may also rarely include alopecia, gynecomastia, transient azospermia, impotence, and CNS disease, although these side effects have not been reported in children. MTX is potentially teratogenic and should be discontinued if pregnancy is being considered. Long-term studies of fertility among patients with JRA are not available.

Initial parental anxiety about MTX, often related to reproductive, teratogenic, or mutagenic issues, is often allayed by negotiating a 4- to 6-week trial of low-dose oral treatment. This allows families to make an informed risk-benefit decision by contrasting actual clinical improvement in a disabled child with an incompletely studied group of possible future complications. In our experience, this approach has been highly successful in initiating therapy.

Bone marrow suppression due to MTX has been reported, but it is rare and idiosyncratic[26]; megaloblastic changes are more common and are caused by a relative folic acid depletion. In adults with RA, studies suggest that folic acid supplementation does not reduce MTX efficacy but does decrease gastrointestinal toxicity.[38,56] Children with JRA have not been studied in detail. Oral folate dosage for children is 1 mg/d; folate is available in tablets but is rarely included in over-the-counter pediatric multivitamin preparations.

Among 117 children with JRA for whom data on liver enzymes were available, 9% demonstrated one or more episodes of enzyme elevations.[31-34] Persistent aspartate aminotransferase (AST) elevations usually precede development of liver fibrosis,[57,58] but their absence does not preclude asymptomatic fibrosis. Most serial liver biopsy studies of adults with RA indicate that significant liver fibrosis is not associated with MTX intake,[59-61] although one report using electron microscopy suggested that an unspecified subset of RA patients receiving MTX may be prone to progressive liver fibrosis.[58] Graham et al.[62] described liver biopsies in seven JRA patients after an average cumulative MTX dose of 1709 mg and found normal tissue in each child.[62] Clinical MTX-related liver fibrosis in JRA is rare.[63]

Although idiosyncratic interstitial pneumonitis is seen with antitumor doses of MTX, it is only rarely reported in patients with arthritis. Three retrospective clinical, radiographic, and pulmonary function studies, including two involving a total of 40 JRA patients[64,65] and one involving adults,[66] found no evidence of interstitial pneumonitis. One prospective follow-up of 200 cases of adult RA, over 41.5 months, revealed no MTX-related pulmonary toxicity.[38]

Methods of monitoring children receiving MTX for evidence of toxicity vary somewhat among practitioners. Early frequent follow-up, including detailed oral and written education and assessment of understanding, is particularly important for young, anxious parents. Compliance tends to be excellent, once clinical benefits are perceived. We perform the following laboratory studies: a complete blood count (CBC), mean corpuscular volume (MCV), liver enzyme determinations, renal function tests, and urinalysis at baseline. A CBC, AST, and alanine aminotransferase (ALT) are recommended weekly for 2 weeks, biweekly for 1 month, and then monthly. We are not aware of any pediatric rheumatologists who are regularly performing liver biopsies, except via study protocol or in special circumstances. Wallace et al.[32] have not found plasma MTX levels in children with JRA to correlate with efficacy or likelihood of liver abnormalities, and side effects have been observed even within the range of "safety."

In children receiving MTX, in the complete absence of clinical complaints, it is common for serum liver enzyme levels to rise and then stabilize at two to three times baseline values. In about 40% of these children, a further elevation of liver enzymes appears to develop after 6 to 9 months of therapy. In such cases MTX may be withheld for one or several weekly doses, depending on the degree and duration of rise in enzymes. Liver enzymes should then again be monitored weekly until they normalize. Normalization often occurs within 1 week, in which case the drug is often successfully restarted at the same dosage. If enzyme levels again rise after rechallenge at the same dose, MTX is once more withheld and then restarted after several weeks at a dose that is reduced by 15% to 25%. Mild gastrointestinal upset or a few oral mucosal ulcerations, each of 24 hours' duration, and a single episode of elevated liver enzymes are the most commonly observed adverse reactions.

Routes of Administration

Oral administration of MTX is the least expensive and most convenient for most children and their families. Rarely, where socioeconomic disruption suggests a high likelihood of noncompliance with an oral MTX regimen in a significantly involved patient with JRA, we will initiate weekly subcutaneous treatment. Parenteral therapy is often attempted if children do not respond, plateau, do not comply, or develop toxic reactions to oral MTX. In patients who have an initial favorable response but then develop a plateau or flare, larger parenteral doses of (0.5 to 1 mg/kg/wk) can also be tried. Because of pressures for cost containment or long travel distances, some families administer parenteral MTX at home, much as with insulin; a local laboratory can communicate toxicity monitoring results to the consulting rheumatologist.

Clinical Use

The most common pediatric candidate for MTX therapy is a child who has persistent or progressive polyarticular JRA despite an adequate trial of nonsteroidal antiinflammatory agents. Increasing physician experience and comfort with MTX has led to its earlier use, even in pauciarticular JRA, particularly if a child is nonambulatory, is developing significant bone growth disturbances, or has iridocyclitis that is unresponsive to topical therapy. Controversy remains as to whether to initiate MTX as early as 4 weeks after starting NSAIDs or only after a more prolonged trial of 6 to 12 months. In severely compromised patients, to avoid hospitalization, allow ambulation, or restore lost age-appropriate activities such as school attendance, a 3-day course of intravenous Solu-Medrol (30 mg/kg/d, up to a maximum of 1 g) may be an effective therapeutic "bridge" until MTX becomes effective.

INJECTABLE GOLD

Background and Efficacy

Gold was the first drug ever tested in a controlled clinical trial in adult RA, and it has long been an excellent option for treating progressive or severe polyarticular JRA. A total of 12 studies of intramuscular gold in 372 children with JRA were published between 1964 and 1988. Six were retrospective, four were open and compared gold with another SAARD, and three were randomized.[67] In only 56% was the type of JRA onset reported. Where noted, the usual dose was 1 mg/kg/d, and mean durations of treatment were 0.5 to 3.8 years, with a

range of 3 months to 8 years. Rates of remission, variously defined, ranged from 0% to 57%, with a cumulative rate of 16% among the 372 patients, when adjusted for study size. Similarly, "improvement" was found in 18% to 78% of cases, with a combined rate of 48%. Among the 10 reports that detailed gold toxicity, the rates were 20% to 52%, and the combined rate was 38%, while toxicity requiring drug termination occurred in 7% to 58% of patients (noted in 11 studies), with a combined rate of 23%.

In two other reports, Brewer et al.[68] showed that gold reduced the severity of disease in 63% and reduced joint counts in 49% of 51 patients with JRA, while Fink[19] suggested that a 50% rate of efficacy will occur, particularly in polyarthritis. Gold is generally not effective for the systemic manifestations of JRA and, indeed, may be associated with neutropenia or intravascular coagulation.

Mechanism

The mechanism of action of gold remains poorly understood, despite multiple studies. In vitro, gold inhibits the growth of some viruses and bacteria, alters classical and alternate complement pathway functions, may block T-lymphocyte activation by impairing monocyte function, can suppress mitogen-induced IgM and IgM-RF synthesis, alters the chemotactic response of human peripheral monocytes and neutrophils, and may reduce overactive phagocytosis in patients with RA. Gold compounds may also decrease the activity of endothelial leukocyte adhesion molecule 1 and thus reduce recruitment of leukocytes to sites of inflammation. In vitro inhibition of macrophage differentiation[69] and decreased HLA-DR expression after interferon-γ stimulation[70] have also recently been described. In animals and human beings gold inhibits many enzymes, including cathepsin, β-glucuronidase, acid phosphatase, and malic dehydrogenase. Thus gold may reduce inflammation by retarding the production or release of lysosomal enzymes.

Administration

Gold aurothioglucose and sodium thiomalate (GSTM) are the common injectable forms. The former is more viscous and is associated with rare hypersensitivity; thus GSTM is most often used. Gold salts are given by weekly intramuscular injection. In children an initial test dose of 0.25 to 0.33 mg/kg is administered and then increased weekly by 25% to 33% until a final weekly dose of 1 mg/kg is reached (maximum of 50 mg/wk). Beneficial effects usually occur after 6 to 12 weeks but may require 20 weeks, and optimal response may take 12 months. After 20 weeks, or a total cumulative dose of 500 to 1000 mg, the patient is reassessed and if there is no improvement the drug is discontinued.

In children who respond well, gold should be continued indefinitely, or at least until growth and development are complete; dosage is adjusted as the patients gain weight. After 20 weeks it may be possible to gradually decrease the frequency of injections to once a month at 1 mg/kg; if the arthritis worsens, however, weekly injections must be resumed. Occasionally, concomitant NSAIDs can be discontinued. Some physicians treat patients with monthly gold for several years after achieving remission. Recently, MTX has been displacing injectable gold because of the shorter time required to determine efficacy, fewer side effects, lower cost and less frequent monitoring, fewer office visits, and less discomfort. Nonetheless, for many children intramuscular gold remains an excellent first-line remittive agent.

Toxicity and Monitoring

Major side effects due to injectable gold involve the skin, kidneys, and bone marrow. Rashes are usually mildly red and maculopapular, they are pruritic in 15% of cases, they may be scaly, and they subside after drug discontinuation. Less common effects include alopecia, photosensitivity, urticarial, bullous, and severe exfoliative reactions, and chrysiasis (skin pigmentation). Stomatitis occurs in 5% to 10% of cases. Hematuria, proteinuria, or both may indicate an immune complex–mediated membranous glomerulonephritis (10% to 20% of cases). If toxicity develops, in some cases injections can be restarted at a lower dose after a 1-month interruption. Otherwise, termination of the drug is usually effective, although corticosteroids may be required. Of importance, some children with JRA have mild hematuria or proteinuria before any drug treatment, and NSAID administration can also be associated with renal abnormalities. These causes must be separated from those related to gold. Urine must be collected fresh and midstream, must not involve vigorous cleansing, and must be examined by an experienced observer. If gold therapy is started in the presence of unexplained urinary abnormalities, future therapeutic decisions are very difficult.

Hematologic toxicity is infrequent (1% to 2% of cases), except for eosinophilia. Thrombocytopenia, leukopenia, and aplastic anemia have all been described. In adults, bone marrow, skin, and renal toxicity are all increased in patients who have HLA-DR3. Other less common toxic effects include fever, postinjection arthralgias, chest pain or tachycardia, pneumonitis, GI distress, hematochezia, hepatitis, the nitritoid reaction, headaches, and various behavioral disturbances. These essentially all disappear on drug cessation.

Toxicity is monitored with a weekly urinalysis, CBC, and platelet count, although many practitioners reduce the frequency of testing to every 2 to 3 weeks if there is no evidence of side effects after 6 to 12 months. Regular evaluation must continue indefinitely. Although optimal compliance and monitoring may occur when treatment is performed by a rheumatologist, for family convenience it is common for laboratory tests and injections to be done by a local physician who is comfortable with the process. Increasingly, for reasons of cost and convenience, some families obtain local laboratory tests, FAX them to their rheumatologist, and then give the injections themselves at home.

ORAL GOLD (AURANOFIN)

Background and Efficacy

Before the advent of auranofin (triethylphosphine gold), oral preparations were poorly absorbed and ineffective. Auranofin is 29% gold by weight, and about 25% of that is absorbed, with serum levels stabilizing after about 3 months of daily administration. The first trial of auranofin was reported in adult RA in 1979, and several thousand patients have now been evaluated in open, placebo-controlled, comparative studies with most SAARDs.[71] Although auranofin is superior to placebo, dropouts because of lack of efficacy are higher when auranofin is compared with intramuscular GSTM. Auranofin may be more effective in patients with early disease; however, it has not been successful in sustaining remission in those who have switched to it after a good response to intramuscular GSTM. Auranofin produces a later response and more side effects than MTX.

Between 1983 and 1988, six open, noncontrolled, short- and long-term studies of auranofin for children with JRA were published.[72] At doses of 0.1 to 0.2 mg/kg/d almost all patients demonstrated some improvement by 6 months. However, in a 6-month double-blind, randomized, and placebo-controlled multicenter investigation, the Pediatric Rheumatology Collaborative Study Group evaluated 231 JRA patients for safety and 191 for efficacy.[4] Auranofin, at 0.15 mg/kg/d, showed only a modest, nonsignificant improvement over placebo among the primary study variables (66% versus 56%). In selected children, because of travel distances or social circumstances, auranofin may be an alternative to intramuscular GSTM. Total monthly costs, including laboratory tests, average $80 to $150.

Monitoring and Toxicity

Common adverse reactions with auranofin include diarrhea, dermatitis, stomatitis, and a metallic taste; renal complications are extremely rare. Intolerance causes only one fourth (5%) as many withdrawals as injectable gold (20%). Auranofin is not recommended for pregnant or nursing mothers. Monitoring includes an initial CBC, urinalysis, and chemistry profile, followed by CBC and urinalysis in 2 weeks and then monthly. A careful history and examination are mandatory. Diarrhea often subsides with dosage reduction or if dosage is skipped 1 or 2 days per week.

SULFASALAZINE

Sulfasalazine (SSZ) was developed in Sweden in the 1940s to treat RA, which was then thought to be caused by infection. Sulfapyridine (a sulfonamide) was linked to 5-aminosalicylic acid (an antiinflammatory agent) by an azo bond in order to effect delivery to the colon, where it undergoes bacterial cleavage. About one third of the 5-ASA is absorbed, but it does not achieve effective antiinflammatory levels. Almost 90% of the sulfapyridine is absorbed from the colon, but its mechanism of action is not understood. In controlled trials in adult RA, SSZ has been found to be superior to placebo and similar to gold and D-penicillamine.[73] It is also effective in ankylosing spondylitis,[74] the reactive arthropathies,[75] and inflammatory bowel disease.

In 1986, Ozdogan et al.[76] reported significant improvement in 12 of 18 patients in an open study of JRA treated with SSZ, although toxicity was a limiting factor. Joos et al.[77] employed enteric-coated SSZ (30 to 50 mg/kg; median dose 1 g/d) for 41 patients with JCA ≤16 years old who had been unsuccessfully treated for at least 3 months with NSAIDs. Remission was achieved in 21 patients and substantial improvement in 12; four were unchanged, and three worsened. A significant decrease in the number of swollen joints was observed after 3 months and then maintained, while the erythrocyte sedimentation rate (ESR) was significantly reduced after 6 months of therapy. Toxicity was observed in five children, of whom four stopped taking SSZ (one each because of GI intolerance, leukopenia, rash, and agitation), but all side effects were reversible on withdrawal of the drug.

In a retrospective study by Grondin et al.[67] of SAARD treatment in 43 children with JCA, 12 patients received SSZ. Improvement occurred in six, remission in one, no change in four, and worsening in one. Their review of the literature noted toxicity in 37% of patients, with 10% requiring discontinuation. Most recently, Jacobs[78] used SSZ in 18 patients with JRA for whom conventional therapy had failed; improvement occurred in 50% of the cases within 3 months[78]; in 20% of the children the SSZ was discontinued because of side effects.

Monitoring and Toxicity

Overall, SSZ causes reversible side effects in 37% of children, but only 10% require discontinuation.[79] The most common toxic effect is an allergic skin reaction, including maculopapular, urticarial, and multiforme rashes. Gastrointestinal toxicity may include nausea, vomiting, anorexia, or abdominal pain in up to 30% of children, while hematologic complications such as anemia, granulocytopenia, or hemolysis can develop in up to 23% of cases. Headaches, agitation, and depression are occasionally described, but renal toxicity is almost never seen. There may be idiosyncratic reactions, including serum sickness.[78] SSZ-related side effects almost always cease after drug discontinuation. Monthly monitoring of our patients includes history, examination, and complete blood cell counts.

Clinical Use

Clinical response to SSZ may occur as rapidly as several weeks, more often develops by 3 months, and in severe cases may require 12 months. The usual starting dose is 40 to 60 mg/kg/d, beginning with one fourth of the calculated dose and then increasing weekly by another one fourth, up to a maximum of 1 to 2 g/wk. The most frequent problem at the higher doses is GI upset. Administration with food can be helpful, and the enteric-coated preparation is often better tolerated.

SSZ is usually a third-line medication, which is added when initial NSAID treatment has not been sufficient and when either intramuscular gold or methotrexate (or both) has not controlled the disease process. One may add SSZ to a combination of NSAID and MTX in severe cases of JRA. SSZ is also very useful as secondary therapy for children with juvenile ankylosing spondylitis, nonspecific arthritis with enthesitis, or psoriatic arthritis or in the occasional teenager with aggressive Reiter syndrome.

HYDROXYCHLOROQUINE

Background and Efficacy

Antimalarial compounds have long been employed by pediatric rheumatologists as adjunctive therapy along with NSAIDs; their use in JRA varies widely from one center to another and may reflect success with hydroxychloroquine (HCQ) in other condition such as childhood systemic lupus erythematosus (SLE) and dermatomyositis. Early studies of HCQ in JRA suggested that it was effective and less toxic than D-penicillamine or gold.[80,81] A total of five trials (three retrospective, one open, and one prospective) have evaluated antimalarials (mostly HCQ) in 245 patients with JRA, including 76 with polyarticular, 74 with oligoarticular, and 35 with systemic onset. Overall, 41% (16% to 75%) showed improvement, and 28% (0% to 45%) achieved remission; rates of variously defined toxicity ranged from 8% to 61%, but the drug was stopped in only 6.5% of the cases. A recent double-blind, multicenter placebo-controlled study

of *severe* JRA suggested that HCQ alone is little better than placebo.[82]

Oral chloroquine and HCQ are rapidly absorbed and have a half-life of 3 to 12 days; serum levels plateau at 2 to 5 weeks. Tissue concentrations are much higher than plasma levels, particularly in fat, bone, cornea, and pigmented organs such as the iris and choroid. Proposed mechanisms of action for HCQ include direct intracellular enzyme inhibition, stabilization of lysosomal membranes, reduced immune complex formation, decreased function of lymphocytes, macrophages, and polymorphonuclear leukocytes, inhibition of DNA and RNA synthesis, and interference with prostaglandin manufacture.[83]

The starting dose of HCQ is 5 to 7 mg/kg/d, with a maximum of 200 mg in children under 40 kg and up to 400 mg in teenagers. HCQ has a delayed onset of action (3 to 6 months); 88% of the patients who respond do so by 6 months. Otherwise, the drug should usually be discontinued. Some authors recommend that HCQ should not be used in patients under the age of 8 years because of difficulties in ophthalmologic evaluation, although others will add HCQ to severely involved children as young as 3 to 4 years old. Therapy with HCQ should generally not exceed 2 to 3 years in duration, although in some cases treatment can be extended for longer periods.

Toxicity and Monitoring

The frequency of side effects with antimalarials is usually dose related and is generally lower than with other SAARDs, with only 8.5% dropouts because of toxicity in adults and 4% to 6% in children. The most common toxic reactions are lichenoid, urticarial, morbilliform, or maculopapular rashes. Photosensitivity and pruritus can also occur. GI toxicity may mimic that of concomitant NSAIDs but is usually milder and without hematochezia. Neurologic manifestations are usually minimal and easily reversible, but headaches, insomnia, nervousness, and loss of concentration may impair school performance. Questions about psychoneurologic performance should be asked at each visit. Hair and skin should also be monitored for depigmentation. Antimalarials have not been shown to be safe during pregnancy and must be safely stored; death due to respiratory suppression has occurred after a child ingested as few as four tablets (1 g) of chloroquine.

There are three types of ophthalmologic side effects, although their frequency is very low: (1) neurally mediated defects in convergence or accommodation, with blurred vision; (2) corneal deposits (keratopathy), which are reversible, appear to be dose related, and suggest a safe upper HCQ dose of 5 to 7 mg/kg/d[80]; and (3) retinopathy, which includes pigmentary stippling, mottling, clumping, central scotomata, or reduced peripheral fields. So-called "premaculopathy" is manifested by changes in red-green color vision or early pigmentary abnormalities and is usually reversible. More serious retinopathy, which often occurs in those who receive higher than recommended daily doses, may cause irreversible visual loss and can progress after HCQ is withdrawn.

At baseline and then every 6 months a pediatric ophthalmologist should (1) question children and parents about visual changes, (2) determine acuity, (3) assess red-green color vision, and (4) evaluate the retina for pigmentary changes.

PENICILLAMINE

Background and Efficacy

Since D-penicillamine (D-PEN) could dissociate human macroglobulins in vitro, Jaffee[84] hypothesized that adults with RA and high-titer RF might benefit. Early studies suggested that it was as effective as gold, had similar therapeutic indications, and was a little more toxic. When first introduced, there was much enthusiasm about D-PEN as a potential alternative for patients who had not shown a satisfactory response to gold. There have been nine trials of D-PEN in children (three retrospective, four open/randomized and compared with gold, and two double-blind placebo-controlled). Among a total of 505 patients, most received doses ranging from 10 to 30 mg/kg/d; disease subtype at onset was often not specified. Overall, although operational definitions of levels of disease activity either were not given or varied widely, 14 (2.8%) achieved remission, while 308 (61%) were "improved." Total toxicity was 92/415 (20%), while toxicity requiring drug termination was 68/495 (13.7%).[67]

A 1986 prospective, placebo-controlled, double-blind, randomized parallel study of HCQ and D-PEN in 162 children with active, poorly controlled JRA who had not responded adequately to NSAIDs did not show significant differences from placebo for either drug.[82] This well-designed study chose 30% clinical change as its arbitrary level for significance. These findings coincided with recognition of the efficacy of oral MTX for JRA, and the use of D-PEN declined rapidly thereafter, although it may retain a role in combination therapy. D-PEN can be useful in ameliorating the skin and internal organ complications of scleroderma and may contribute to reduction in the associated arthritis as well.

Mechanism and Dosage

The mechanisms of action of D-PEN on the inflammatory and/or immune systems remain poorly understood. The three major biochemical effects are (1) inhibition of disulfide bond formation by exchange or oxidative reactions, (2) prevention of posttranslational steps in collagen synthesis and dissociation of macroglobulins, and (3) chelation or complex formation with metals such as copper to interfere with the activity of such enzymes as carboxypeptidase, superoxide dismutase, and angiotensin-converting enzyme. Oral D-PEN is absorbed well on an empty stomach and achieves peak blood levels at 1 hour; a single dose is completely eliminated by 48 hours. Treatment is 10 to 20 mg/kg/d in one or two doses, which should be taken on an empty stomach. Dosage is increased slowly by 62.5 mg/wk in children <40 kg and by 125 mg/wk in larger patients to minimize GI intolerance. Maximum doses rarely exceed 750 mg/d. To combat vitamin B_6 deficiency, 25 mg/d of pyridoxine may be given simultaneously. Efficacy appears slowly, but D-PEN should be discontinued if there is no clear benefit in 9 to 12 months.

Monitoring and Toxicity

Adverse reactions include thrombocytopenia, agranulocytosis, aplastic anemia, membranous nephropathy, rashes, and cholestatic hepatitis. Autoimmune toxicity includes SLE-like syndrome, thyroiditis, polymyositis, myasthenia, and Goodpasture syndrome. Nausea, vomiting, diarrhea, alterations in taste, headache, and dizziness have also been described in children[67]; there are no noticeable clinical effects consistent with heavy metal chelation. Urinalysis, CBC, platelet counts, and liver enzyme studies should be performed initially and then monthly; antinuclear antibodies (ANA) and immunoglobulin levels may be obtained annually. Idiosyncratic allergic reactions are fairly common and occur more often in certain HLA types, such as Dw3, and in those with penicillin allergies. One recent study of 718 RA patients treated with D-PEN showed that HLA DR-2 was increased among those who developed myositis.[18] Some patients who experience toxic reactions to gold may also manifest allergies to D-PEN.

IMMUNOSUPPRESSIVE AGENTS

Immunosuppressive and cytotoxic agents should be used only for severe or life-threatening disease that has not responded to NSAIDs and SAARDs. Severe uveitis and amyloidosis may be specific indications.[85] Major concerns include late mutagenic and oncogenic potential, sterility, bone marrow suppression, and high rates of infection. Azathioprine has been used in 12 controlled trials in adult RA,[86] is similar in efficacy to SAARDs, but is not remittive. Anecdotally, it has been widely used for small numbers of severely involved children, but most pediatricians are not enthusiastic. At 1 to 2 mg/kg/d orally, it may be effective in up to 50% of cases, in comparison with placebo, for controlling arthritis.[87] Azathioprine is associated with frequent infections, particularly herpes zoster. Leukopenia, biochemical hepatitis, rash, and GI intolerance are other complications.

Chlorambucil is an effective but toxic alkylating agent whose side effects may be cumulative and delayed; it carries significant risks of thrombocytopenia, leukopenia, infections in 10%, herpes zoster in 15%, acute monoblastic leukemia in children with JRA, and other late malignant diseases. The dose is 0.1 to 0.3 mg/kg/d orally. Since it does not cause hair loss or bladder complications, it may be more acceptable than cyclophosphamide for some families and teenagers, particularly for uncontrollable uveitis, aortitis, vasculitis, or other complications of far advanced JRA.

Because of severe alopecia and bladder complications oral cyclophosphamide is now rarely used to treat JRA, although intravenous pulses (500 mg/m²/mo) are occasionally employed every 2 to 4 weeks for the same indications as chlorambucil. There have been nine clinical trials of cyclophosphamide in adult RA which indicate that it may decrease the rate of formation of new bone erosions. Its major role may be in the treatment of severe, unresponsive vasculitis.

Cyclosporine has been used to treat a broad range of autoimmune disorders, and several studies have shown efficacy in adult RA; experience in children with JRA is limited. Its postulated mechanism of action is an inhibition of IL-2 transcription; the absence of generalized bone marrow suppression is notable.[88] However, GI intolerance, hirsutism, hypertension, and renal toxicity are major complications. Cyclosporine, at a dose of 4 to 15 mg/kg/d, has been studied in 14 children with severe JRA; there were 11 withdrawals, four for lack of efficacy and seven because of side effects.[89]

BIOLOGIC AGENTS

Most of the newer biologic agents have not yet been evaluated in JRA and in other forms of arthritis in children.[90] Several pilot studies have used intravenous gamma globulin (IVGG) to treat systemic-onset JRA.[91] In one, five of six children who received IVGG, 2 g/kg/mo for 6 months, showed resolution of fever and reduction in morning stiffness from 2 hours to <30 minutes; arthritis improved in three cases. Our experience with five patients has been similar, with poor response of active synovitis being the limiting factor. The PRCSG is currently evaluating IVGG in a multicenter trial. Overall, IVGG therapy is extremely expensive, and its efficacy seems likely to be limited.

PRACTICAL MANAGEMENT STRATEGIES

The five cases that follow illustrate our approach to common patient care problems in children with arthritis.

CASE 1:   An 18-month-old white girl has a 3-month history of right knee swelling, a 5-degree flexion contracture, and morning toe-walking (e.g., morning stiffness); review of systems and family history are noncontributory. The following laboratory values should be obtained: CBC, urinalysis, ESR, liver enzyme studies, and ANA. The ESR is elevated at 21 mm/h (anything >15 is abnormal), and the ANA is positive at 1:160

(speckled). The most likely diagnosis is pauciarticular JRA, and regular ophthalmologic evaluation is mandatory. At present this girl has no evidence of uveitis on slit lamp examination, but in view of the positive ANA, she should have evaluations every 3 to 4 months for at least 5 years, since iridocyclitis in children is usually asymptomatic and young patients rarely complain of changes in visual acuity. ANA should be repeated annually.

Physical therapy evaluation reveals muscle wasting, with a 1 cm decrease in both thigh and gastrocnemius circumference; the child is given a home physical therapy program, and a night splint will be added if the knee is not straight within 3 weeks (the normal 18-month-old knee will hyperextend to –15 degrees). The parents are encouraged to allow full athletic activities to tolerance. Detailed, written education pamphlets about JRA are provided.

Radiographs of involved joints, and new ones as they become affected, should be obtained. This child demonstrated mild epiphyseal overgrowth at the femur, suggesting more chronic inflammation, and the potential need for aggressive management if initial therapy is not optimally beneficial. Follow-up radiographs should be performed annually.

PHARMACOLOGIC MANAGEMENT. Liquid or crushed-tablet NSAIDs are good initial choices. We use naproxen at 10 to 15 mg/kg/d, which for a 10 kg child will be 2 to 3 ml of naproxen (25 mg/ml suspension) twice daily. Ibuprofen may be given at 30 mg/kg/d; therefore, in this case, 5 ml (1 tsp) of the 20 mg/ml suspension three times daily will be a good starting dose. Aspirin and tolmetin sodium are alternatives, although the latter is expensive. Renal and liver function should be checked at baseline only. Further laboratory testing should depend on symptoms. If after 3 months and one NSAID switch the inflammation continues, one should consider intraarticular injection of triamcinolone hexacetonide (may be injected up to twice per year). One can expect this patient to need uninterrupted medical therapy for at least 2 years. Children complain little of, and rapidly adapt to, joint pain and also may have only subtle persistent synovitis. Nonetheless, the potential for major growth abnormalities is high, and thus parents should be prepared for a 2-year course of treatment. If deformity progresses, or if growth and development are impaired, this child is a candidate for methotrexate. Ophthalmologic follow-up continues even after articular remission. Evidence of gastritis may include declining appetite or epigastric discomfort. Mood changes may reflect medication toxicity or advancing arthritis.

CASE 2: Over a period of 2 months, a 6-year-old Hispanic girl develops an additive pattern of joints involvement, which includes both knees, one ankle, and a proximal interphalangeal joint. She has severe morning stiffness and cannot attend school. A paternal aunt has psoriasis, and a grandmother has classic rheumatoid arthritis. A diagnosis of extended pauciarticular JRA is most likely, although an atypical early presentation of psoriatic arthritis is possible. The ESR is 35 mm/h, the hemoglobin level is 11.9 g/dl, rheumatoid factor is absent, and the ANA is 1:160 (homogenous).

The principles of radiologic investigation, physical therapy evaluation, and treatment (e.g., home program), ophthalmologic assessment and follow-up, patient indifference to pain, and family education are the same as in Case 1. The prognosis for ultimate number of joints involved is guarded and should be clearly communicated to the family.

MANAGEMENT. Initial pharmacologic management is the same as in Case 1, but early preparation of the parents about the potential need for DMARDs should be added. If there is no or little visible improvement in the child's joints after 2 months of therapy, one may try azulfidine while remembering that this drug is safe but may have limited efficacy. We use 50 mg/kg/d in two divided doses. We like to start with one half of the dose during the first week and watch for skin rashes. We obtain a CBC with a platelet count after 2 weeks of therapy. In our example, if the weight is 20 kg we would start with one tablet per day (500 mg) and, if the girl tolerates this, move up to one tablet twice a day. We have had disappointing experience with the taste of the suspensions; however, the tablets are "crushable." One should remember not to order the enteric-coated tablets if there is need for tablet crushing. Some physicians will add hydroxychloroquine at this point, but improvement may then require another 6 to 12 months of observation. Our preference is to start oral methotrexate if there has been no improvement after the first 8 weeks. This child's body surface will be approximately 0.8 m^2. We start methotrexate at 10 mg/m^2/wk;

therefore an appropriate starting dose will be 7.5 mg (three tablets) per week. The total dose can be given at once or divided in two with a 12-hour interval. Morning baths are effective for morning gel but often disrupt busy family routines. We advise the use of an electric blanket set on medium-high and plugged into an electric timer that is set to actuate 1 hour before the child arises.

CASE 3: A 13-year-old girl has a 6-month history of prominent swelling in 10 joints, including one elbow, both wrists, knees, and ankles, and 4 proximal interphalangeal joints; she also has limitation and discomfort at the neck. Her mother notes 45 minutes of morning stiffness and progressive withdrawal from physical activities, both of which the teenager denies. There has been no height or weight gain for 6 to 9 months, and school performance has been deteriorating. There is no family history of systemic lupus erythematosus, and no butterfly facial rash, mucosal ulcerations, or alopecia. Laboratory evaluation reveals an ESR of 45 mm/h, a hemoglobin level 10 g/dl, and a white blood cell count of 6300 with normal differential; the urinalysis is normal. The patient most likely has polyarticular JRA, but a gut-associated arthropathy or psoriatic arthritis are possible.

MANAGEMENT. In this setting of progressive, disabling JRA we immediately start both an NSAID and oral MTX, 10 mg/m^2/wk, with an expected response time of 4 to 6 weeks. If, at the time of initial presentation, the patient cannot attend school, is experiencing severe fatigue, or cannot adequately ambulate, a 3-day course of intravenous pulse prednisolone or methylprednisolone, 30 mg/kg/d (up to a maximum of 1 g) for three consecutive or alternate days is also indicated. After the usual 7- to 21-day poststeroid "honeymoon period," if there is insufficient systemic and articular response, one may switch to the same dose of MTX administered subcutaneously or intramuscularly. Often, these patients inexorably develop more joint involvement, and the *addition* of azulfidine or hydroxychloroquine or both may become necessary. Such children commonly also have interval disease flares which respond only to brief courses of oral prednisone. It is highly preferable to start with alternate-day prednisone, and the patient and parents should clearly be given a firm stopping date in order to avoid the long-term consequences of steroid dependence, such as irreversible growth fail-

ure. Some practitioners would increase either oral or parenteral MTX to 15 mg/m^2/wk before adding any corticosteroids. A single bedtime dose of indomethacin, 25 to 50 mg (one or two 25 mg capsules), can help alleviate morning stiffness.

CASE 4: A 5-year-old boy develops a hectic fever, inanition, arthralgias, and lymphadenopathy. After 1 week of unsuccessful treatment with antibiotics, a faint salmon-colored rash and splenomegaly are detected. Viral titers are negative, the white blood cell count is 14,600 but with normal differential, the ESR is 96 mm/h, and the hemoglobin level has progressively fallen to 7.6 g/dl; the platelet count is 900,000. There is no family history of rheumatic disease, and no unusual infectious disease exposure. Both rheumatoid factor and ANA are absent. Although the patient does not yet have synovitis, the most likely diagnosis is systemic-onset JRA.

This child will not presently benefit from a radiologic arthritis survey or physical therapy evaluation, but both should be done with the advent of synovitis. A chest radiograph and an electrocardiogram, or an echocardiogram or both should be obtained if there is any suspicion of pericarditis or myocarditis. Ophthalmologic assessment may be done annually.

MANAGEMENT. Although most NSAIDs will be beneficial in patients with arthralgias, aspirin and indomethacin are the most effective antipyretics. Indomethacin is also an excellent choice for the pain and inflammation of pericarditis. A "therapeutic bridge" of oral prednisone, 1 to 2 mg/kg/d, two or three times daily, is often needed for several days or weeks to ameliorate systemic symptoms, and occasionally the severely compromised child will require intravenous pulse steroids as outlined above. The use of steroids should be tailored to severity of illness and the organs involved, particularly if vasculitis is present. It is essential to outline the therapeutic approach in detail to the parents, including alternative "what if . . ." strategies, intermediate- or long-term timelines, and events that might lead to changes. Oral MTX should be introduced early if articular involvement occurs. Although both remain investigational, immunosuppressive agents and/or intravenous immunoglobulin may be needed for uncontrollable systemic features.

Essentially, pediatric ankylosing spondylitis, Reiter's syndrome, psoriatic arthritis, and the limited enthesopathic syndromes can be managed like polyarticular JRA, although many practitioners favor tolmetin sodium or indomethacin among the NSAIDs. We have found that the early addition of oral MTX is also very useful in this group of illnesses. Psoriatic arthritis can be treated early with azulfidine, while the protean weight loss and fever of some children with Reiter's syndrome will respond to management similar to that of systemic-onset JRA. The principles of radiographic and physical therapy and laboratory evaluation are essentially the same. We have found HLA-B27 testing useful for family counseling, particularly because siblings often develop enthesitis-like symptoms, and parents desire early intervention.

Throughout the management of childhood arthritis it is important to be positive and optimistic about prognosis and to emphasize physical activity, independence, and athletic participation to **the child's** perception of tolerance. In this manner, the patient learns about self-efficacy and appropriate setting of limits. The parents, and progressively the child, should be encouraged to undertake a primary role in making decisions regarding school, family, social, vocational, and other aspects of life which relate to the illness.

THERAPEUTIC HINTS

Pain and Morning Stiffness

Children and parents should be questioned closely at each visit regarding joint pain, morning stiffness, limping, and fatigue. Older children will often deny discomfort, and it is well known that children acclimate to "pain," and have fewer complaints. This may occur to avoid perceived risk of physician- or parent-mandated limitations of activities (e.g., school, sports, family, or play). In young patients irritability, frequent crying, and reduction or change in play routines may be nonverbal indicators of significant inflammation or inadequate response to therapy.

Physical measures for morning stiffness, such as the use of a sleeping bag, can be helpful, but evening baths are not helpful and morning baths often conflict with hectic family routines. We recommend connecting an electric blanket, preset at medium to high, to a plug-in timer, which is set to activate 1 hour before arising. Thus the child is not too hot while sleeping but, after 1 hour of concentrated warmth, is easier to arouse and requires less assistance from the busy parent. Setting an alarm 1 hour before arising and supervising the child to awake briefly and take the first morning dose of medication from the bedside table can also be helpful.

Better quality and greater breadth of **written** patient-family education materials about arthritis in children have contributed to improved acceptance, compliance, and outcomes. A spectrum of high-quality, comprehensive take-home brochures concerning the common pediatric rheumatic disorders are now available from many centers. Important functions include the following:

1. Validation of disease presence and type
2. Clarification of disease severity, despite the child's often appearing "active and well"
3. Ease of brochure reproduction to achieve uniform knowledge among relatives, absent parents, school personnel, etc.
4. Stating of rationales for laboratory testing and possible alternative treatments
5. Discussion of prognosis.

It is important that education handouts be distributed to all new children with rheumatic diseases and their families. The Arthritis Foundation and the Arthritis Information Clearinghouse are excellent resources for these materials.

Patients with JRA usually wish to be physically active and tolerate exercise and sports surprisingly well, and their parents welcome loosening of restrictions in this area, particularly because enforcement is difficult and leads to family conflict. Although children with JRA often exhibit prolonged exercise recovery and are deconditioned relative to age- and sex-matched normals, fitness levels in JRA do not correlate with disease-severity scores.[92] Often, poor fitness in JRA is related to activity restrictions by concerned physicians, teachers and parents, leading to unfamiliarity with many physical skill activities. It has been shown that aerobic conditioning programs are safe, effective, and enjoyed in JRA, as in many other chronic childhood illnesses (e.g., cystic fibrosis, Down syndrome, asthma, and spina bifida).[93] Conditioning or sports in JRA can be accomplished in community settings, monitored with validated and age-normed tests, administered by nonhealth professionals, and may have a beneficial impact on social activities, school attendance, and self-efficacy. Similarly, summer camps for patients with JRA are widely enjoyed and promote social and physical growth and development.

When to Stop Treatment

Most pediatric rheumatologists continue treatment of all patients with any evidence of persistent disease activity, particularly if epiphyses are open and there is still growth potential. About 20% of children with JRA will exhibit synovial swelling, even with a normal ESR, and thus a normal ESR alone should not lead to discontinuation of treatment. Although parents are very perceptive about when their children are "normal," patients with JRA subtly but constantly alter their physical behaviors to accommodate joint involvement. Parents dislike the presence of arthritis and the costs and risks of medications; thus the physician may need to urge continued treatment to maximize outcome, despite variable levels of family resistance.

Conversely, some rheumatologists will elect not to treat some patients with low disease activity and no current "morbidity." These patients are often the children who deny pain and whose range of motion and growth are nearly normal but who have persistent pauciarticular or polyarticular joint bogginess (mild) without erosions. The decision to stop, or not start, treatment despite mild ongoing inflammation may be justified if the patient and family have strong feelings against taking medication(s) or if they perceive no discernible benefit. However, the potential for long-term impairment of normal growth and development must be clearly explained.

In the patient who achieves complete laboratory and clinical remission, various physicians suggest that the child be sustained on medication for another 3 to 6 to 12 months. Treatment is then usually slowly tapered over several weeks to months.

Compliance

Cost, denial of illness, drug side effects, poor understanding of treatment goals, unrealistic expectations, guilt about causality, desire to avoid drug "addiction," equating absence of pain with wellness, and familial pressures to try alternative remedies are just a few of the reasons for noncompliance that we regularly encounter. Numerous studies of adult RA estimate compliance with NSAIDs at about 50%. In general pediatrics, 50% to 54% rates of compliance have been reported,[94] while two retrospective studies of aspirin in JRA both yielded 55% values for compliance in teenagers as well as younger children.[95] Children will both over- and undermedicate themselves; they exhibit negative reactions to medications in 43%, to exercise regimens in 60%, and to splints in 43%.[96] Direct refusal of treatment by a child is a frequent problem, and yet, it often is not directly addressed by physicians. One investigation showed that 70% of JRA patients used unconventional remedies. Often, acknowledging that we all forget medications occasionally, and empowering patients and parents about catching up with missed doses, altering schedules to fit social situations, and being positive despite suboptimal compliance will actually improve future behaviors.

Patients with Arthritis in the Operating Room

All children with rheumatic diseases who undergo surgery should have a CBC because anemia is common, a platelet count, PT and PTT, and a template bleeding time to assess in vivo platelet function. NSAIDs may be stopped 3 to 4 days before surgery if the operation is expected to be associated with significant bleeding. Bleeding times may need to be checked more than once, and this should not be delayed until the day of hospitalization. If NSAIDs are discontinued, a short course of steroids may be necessary to control disease activity. Patients undergoing long-term corticosteroid therapy (>15 mg/d for 1 week, or >7.5 to 15 mg for 1 month) should receive 30 mg/m^2 of intramuscular hydrocortisone every 6 hours during the 12 to 24 hours preceding surgery (dependent on dose and duration of prior oral treatment). Some surgeons administer intravenous hydrocortisone during surgery to all such patients, whereas others use it only if complications develop. Another intramuscular dose of hydrocortisone should be given 1 hour later in the recovery room. While receiving nothing by mouth, children should be given the parenteral equivalent of any regularly prescribed preoperative steroid. In our experience, MTX has been continued without difficulty. The potential to develop or exacerbate immunosuppressive-induced bone marrow depression should be closely monitored in the postoperative period.

CONCLUSION

Therapeutic interventions for JRA and the pediatric spondyloarthropathies have gradually become more aggressive during the past 15 years. This may be attributed to the following:

1. Earlier and more accurate diagnosis
2. Availability of well-studied, relatively safe, and effective NSAIDs
3. Recognition of the potential for arrested growth and development and severe late disability if remittive therapy is delayed
4. Earlier use of SAARDs, often in combinations
5. The advent of MTX as a major treatment modality

Other important advances include the following:

1. Improved patient and parent education
2. Emphasis on family self-efficacy
3. Use of both individual and group support techniques
4. Less external setting of limits by parents, physicians, and schools
5. Greater patient participation in exercise and athletics

Such changes may contribute to better compliance, more age-appropriate social roles, and better scholastic performance in children with arthritis. Parents and patients have become more active participants in decision making, and the global impact on functional outcomes appears to be positive.

Exciting research in pediatric rheumatology continues and is developing the following:

1. Better understanding of the relationship between genetics and treatment responses
2. New protocols for combination therapy
3. Safer corticosteroids
4. Immunotherapy and other biologic treatments
5. Permissible limits of exercise and physical conditioning for the child with arthritis

REFERENCES

1. Singsen BH. Health status (arthritis impact) in children with chronic rheumatic diseases. Arthritis Care Res 1991;4:87.
2. Schaller JG. Juvenile rheumatoid arthritis: series I. Arthritis Rheum 1977;20(suppl 2):165.
3. Ansell BM. Juvenile chronic arthritis. Scand J Rheumatol 1987;66(suppl):47.
4. Giannini EH, Brewer EJ, Kuzmina N, et al. Auranofin in the treatment of juvenile rheumatoid arthritis. Arthritis Rheum 1990;33:466.
5. Maclagan TJ. The treatment of acute rheumatism with salicin. Lancet 1876;1:342.
6. Athreya BH, Moser G, Cecil HS, et al. Aspirin-induced hepatotoxicity in juvenile rheumatoid arthritis: a prospective study. Arthritis Rheum 1975;18:347.
7. Brooks PM, Day RO. Nonsteroidal antiinflammatory drugs—differences and similarities. N Engl J Med 1991;324:1716.
8. Abramson SB, Weissman G. The mechanism of action of nonsteroidal anti-inflammatory drugs. Arthritis Rheum 1989;32:1.
9. Price T, Venning H, Ansell BM. Ibuprofen in juvenile chronic arthritis. Clin Exp Rheumatol 1985;3:59.
10. Ansell BM, Hanna B, Moran H, et al. Naproxen in juvenile chronic polyarthritis. Eur J Rheumatol Inflamm 1979;2:79.
11. Makela AL. Naproxen in the treatment of juvenile rheumatoid arthritis. Scand J Rheumatol 1977;6:193.
12. Kvien TK. Naproxen and acetylsalicylic acid in the treatment of pauciarticular and polyarticular juvenile rheumatoid arthritis. Scand J Rheumatol 1984;13:342.
13. Suarez SM, Cohen PR, DeLeo V. Bullous photosensitivity to naproxen: "pseudoporphyria." Arthritis Rheum 1990;33:903.
14. Brewer EJ. A comparative evaluation of indomethacin, acetaminophen and placebo as antipyretic agents in children. Arthritis Rheum 1968;11:645.
15. Sanger L. Long-term treatment of juvenile chronic arthritis (juvenile rheumatoid arthritis) and systemic juvenile chronic arthritis (Still's syndrome) with diclofenac. Aktuel Rheum 1978;3:5.
16. Haapasaari J, Wuolijoki E, Ylijoki H. Treatment of juvenile rheumatoid arthritis with diclofenac sodium. Scand J Rheumatol 1983;12:325.
17. Kaul A, Reddy JC, Fagman E, Smith G. Hepatitis associated with use of sulindac in a child. J Pediatr 1981;99:650.
18. Szer IS, Goldenstein-Schainberg C, Kurtin P. Paucity of renal complications associated with nonsteroidal antiinflammatory drugs in children with chronic arthritis. J Pediatr 1991;119:815.
19. Fink CW. Medical treatment of juvenile arthritis. Clin Orthop 1990;259:60.
20. Loftus J, Allen R, Hesp R, et al. Randomized, double-blind trial of deflazacort versus prednisone in juvenile chronic (or rheumatoid) arthri-

tis: a relatively bone-sparing effect of deflazacort. Pediatrics 1991;88:428.

21. Miller JJ. Prolonged use of large intravenous steroid pulses in the rheumatic diseases of children. Pediatrics 1980;65:989.

22. Cassidy JT, Petty RE. Basic concepts of drug therapy. In: Textbook of pediatric rheumatology. 2nd ed. New York: Churchill Livingstone, 1990:55.

23. Allen RC, Gross KR, Laxer RM, et al. Intraarticular triamcinolone hexacetonide in the management of chronic arthritis in children. Arthritis Rheum 1986;29:997.

24. Sparling M, Malleson P, Wood B, Petty R. Radiographic followup of joints injected with triamcinolone hexacetonide for the management of childhood arthritis. Arthritis Rheum 1990; 33:821.

25. Gubner R, August S, Ginsberg V. Therapeutic suppression of tissue reactivity: effects of aminopterin in rheumatoid arthritis and psoriasis. Am J Med Sci 1951;221:176.

26. Weinblatt ME, Coblyn JS, Fox DA, et al. Efficacy of low-dose methotrexate in rheumatoid arthritis. N Engl J Med 1985;312:818.

27. Williams HJ, Wikens RF, Samuelson CO, et al. Comparison of low-dose oral pulse methotrexate and placebo in the treatment of rheumatoid arthritis. Arthritis Rheum 1985;28:721.

28. Nordstrom DM, West SG, Andersen PA, Sharp JT. Pulse methotrexate therapy in rheumatoid arthritis: a controlled prospective roentgenographic study. Ann Intern Med 1987;107:797.

29. Lopez-Mendez A, Daniel WW, Reading JC, et al. Radiographic assessment of disease progression in rheumatoid arthritis patients enrolled in the cooperative systematic studies of the rheumatic diseases program randomized clinical trial of methotrexate, auranofin, or a combination of the two. Arthritis Rheum 1993;36:1364.

30. Harel L, Wagner-Weiner L, Poznanski AK, et al. Effects of methotrexate on radiologic progression in juvenile rheumatoid arthritis. Arthritis Rheum 1993;36:1370.

31. Truckenbrodt H, Hafner R. Methotrexate therapy in juvenile rheumatoid arthritis. Arthritis Rheum 1986;29:801.

32. Wallace CA, Bleyer WA, Sherry DD, et al. Toxicity and serum levels of methotrexate in children with juvenile rheumatoid arthritis. Arthritis Rheum 1989;32:677.

33. Danao T, Steinbrunner J, Medendorp S, et al. Methotrexate in juvenile rheumatoid arthritis. Arthritis Rheum 1989;32:S28.

34. Rose CD, Singsen BH, Eichenfield, et al. Safety and efficacy of methotrexate therapy in juvenile rheumatoid arthritis. J Pediatr 1990;117:653.

35. Giannini EH, Brewer EJ, Kuzmina N, et al. Methotrexate in resistant juvenile rheumatoid arthritis. N Engl J Med 1992;346:1043.

36. White C. Reversal of methotrexate binding to dihydrofolate reductase by dihydrofolate. J Biol Chem 1979;254:10889.

37. Olsen NJ, Murray LM. Antiproliferative effects of methotrexate on peripheral blood mononuclear cells. Arthritis Rheum 1989;32:378.

38. Stewart KA, Mackenzie AH, Clough JD, Wilke WS. Folate supplementation in methotrexate-treated rheumatoid arthritis patients. Semin Arthritis Rheum 1991;20:1.

39. Olsen NJ, Callahan LF, Pincus T. Immunologic studies of rheumatoid arthritis patients treated with methotrexate. Arthritis Rheum 1987;30:481.

40. Alarcon G, Schrohenlocher RE, Bartolucci AA, et al. Suppression of rheumatoid factor production by methotrexate in patients with rheumatoid arthritis. Arthritis Rheum 1990;33:1156.

41. Segal R, Mozes E, Yaron M, Tartakovsky B. The effects of methotrexate on the production and activity of interleukin-1. Arthritis Rheum 1989;32:370.

42. Segal R, Yaron M, Tartakovsky B. Rescue of interleukin-1 activity by leucovorin following inhibition by methotrexate in a murine in vitro system. Arthritis Rheum 1990;33:1745.

43. Hine RJ, Everson MP, Hardin JM, et al. Methotrexate therapy in rheumatoid arthritis patients diminishes lectin-induced mononuclear cell proliferation. Rheumatol Int 1990;10:165.

44. Sperling RI, Coblyn JS, Larkin JK, et al. Inhibition of leukotriene B4 synthesis in neutrophils from patients with rheumatoid arthritis by a single oral dose of methotrexate. Arthritis Rheum 1990;33:1149.

45. Nesher G, Moore T. The in vitro effects of methotrexate on peripheral blood mononuclear cells. Arthritis Rheum 1990;33:954.

46. Furst DE, Kremer JM. Methotrexate in rheumatoid arthritis. Arthritis Rheum 1988;31:305.

47. Nuernberg B, Koehnke R, Solsky M, et al. Biliary elimination of low-dose methotrexate in humans. Arthritis Rheum 1990;33:898.

48. Gabriel S, Creagan EC, O'Fallon WM, et al. Treatment of rheumatoid arthritis with higher dose intravenous methotrexate. J Rheumatol 1990;17:460.

49. Shiroky JB, Neville C, Skelton JD. High dose intravenous methotrexate for refractory rheumatoid arthritis. J Rheumatol 1992;19:247.

50. Wallace CA, Sherry DD. Preliminary report of higher dose methotrexate treatment in juvenile rheumatoid arthritis. J Rheumatol 1992;19:1604.

51. Singsen BH, Rose CD. Parenteral methotrexate for juvenile rheumatoid arthritis. Arthritis Rheum 1993;36:S137.

52. Onel KB, Lehman TJA. High dose intramuscular methotrexate for juvenile rheumatoid arthritis. Arthritis Rheum 1993;36:S122.

53. Goldman D, Matherly LH. The cellular pharmacology of methotrexate. Pharmacol Ther 1985;28:77.

54. Dupuis LL, Koren G, Shore A, et al. Methotrexate-nonsteroidal antiinflammatory drug interaction in children with arthritis. J Rheumatol 1990; 17:1469.

55. Skeith KJ, Russell AS, Fakkreddin J, et al. Lack of significant interaction between low dose methotrexate and ibuprofen or flurbiprofen in patients with arthritis. J Rheumatol 1990;17:1008.

56. Morgan SL, Baggot JE, Vaughn WH, et al. The effect of folic acid supplementation on the toxicity of low-dose methotrexate in patients with rheumatoid arthritis. Arthritis Rheum 1990;33:98.

57. Walker AM, Funch D, Dreyer NA. Determinants of serious liver disease among patients receiving low-dose methotrexate for rheumatoid arthritis. Arthritis Rheum 1993;36:329.

58. Bjorkman DJ, Boschert M, Tolman KG, et al. The effect of long-term methotrexate therapy on hepatic fibrosis in rheumatoid arthritis. Arthritis Rheum 1993;36:1697.

59. Aponte J, Petrelli M. Histopathologic findings in the liver of rheumatoid arthritis patients treated with long-term bolus methotrexate. Arthritis Rheum 1988;31:1457.

60. Kremer JM, Lee RG, Tolman KG. Liver histology in rheumatoid arthritis patients receiving long-term methotrexate therapy. Arthritis Rheum 1989;32:121.

61. Rau R, Karger T, Herborn G, Frenzel H. Liver biopsy findings in patients with rheumatoid arthritis undergoing long-term treatment with methotrexate. J Rheumatol 1989;16:489.

62. Graham LD, Rivas-Chacon RF, Myones BL. Lack of hepatotoxicity with chronic administration of methotrexate in juvenile rheumatoid arthritis. Arthritis Rheum 1990;33:S144.

63. Keim D, Ragsdale C, Heilderberger K, Sullivan D. Hepatic fibrosis with the use of methotrexate for juvenile rheumatoid arthritis. J Rheumatol 1990;17:846.

64. Rose CD. Padman R, Wesdock KA, Singsen BH. Methotrexate safety in juvenile rheumatoid arthritis (JRA). Arthritis Rheum 1990;33:S95.

65. Graham LD, Myones BL, Rivas-Chacon RF, Pachman LM. Morbidity associated with long-term methotrexate therapy in juvenile rheumatoid arthritis. J Pediatr 1992;120:468.

66. Croock AD, Furst DE, Helmers RA, et al. Methotrexate dose does not alter pulmonary function in patients with rheumatoid arthritis. Arthritis Rheum 1989;32:S60.

67. Grondin C, Malleson P, Petty RE. Slow acting anti-rheumatic drugs in chronic arthritis of childhood. Semin Arthritis Rheum 1988;18:38.

68. Brewer EJ, Giannini EH, Barkley E. Gold therapy in the management of juvenile rheumatoid arthritis. Arthritis Rheum 1980;23:404.

69. Littman BH, Carlson PL, Loose LD, Sanders KM. Effects of gold sodium thiomalate and tenidap sodium (CP-66,2482-2) on a model of macrophage differentiation using HL-60 cells. Arthritis Rheum 1990;33:29.

70. Kawakami A, Eguchi K, Migita K, et al. Inhibitory effects of gold sodium thiomalate on proliferation and interferon-g induced HLA-DR expression in human endothelial cells. J Rheumatol 1990;17:430.

71. Abruzzo JL. Auranofin: a new drug for rheumatoid arthritis. Ann Intern Med 1986;105:274.

72. Marcolongo R, Mathieu A, Pala R, et al. The efficacy and safety of auranofin in the treatment of juvenile rheumatoid arthritis. Arthritis Rheum 1988;31:979.

73. Pinals RS. Sulfasalazine in the rheumatic diseases. Semin Arthritis Rheum 1988;17:246.

74. Nissila M, Lehtinen K, Leirisalo-Repo M, et al. Sulfasalazine in the treatment of ankylosing spondylitis. Arthritis Rheum 1988;31:1111.

75. Nordstrom DM, West SG, Freeman S, Reddy V. HLA-B27 positive enterogenic reactive arthritis: response of arthritis and microscopic colitis to sulfasalazine. Arthritis Rheum 1987;30:S24.

76. Ozdogan H, Turunc M, Deringol B, et al. Sulphasalazine in the treatment of juvenile rheumatoid arthritis: a preliminary open trial. J Rheumatol 1986;13:124.

77. Joos R, Veys EM, Mielants H, et al. Sulfasalazine treatment in juvenile chronic arthritis. J Rheumatol 1991;18:880.

78. Jacobs J. Sulfasalazine in the treatment of childhood arthritis: a preliminary report. Pediatr Res 1990;27:157A.

79. Furst DE. Toxicity of antirheumatic medications in children with juvenile arthritis. J Rheumatol 1992;19(suppl 33):11.

80. Laaksonen A, Koskiahde V, Juka K. Dosage of antimalarial drugs for children with juvenile rheumatoid arthritis and systemic lupus erythematosus: a clinical study with determination of serum concentration of chloroquine and hydroxychloroquine. Scand J Rheumatol 1974;3:103.

81. Stillman S. Antimalarials. In: Moore TD, ed. Arthritis in childhood: report of the 80th Ross Conference on Pediatric Research. Columbus, Ohio: Ross Laboratories, 1981:125.

82. Brewer EJ, Giannini EH, Kuzmina N, Alekseev L. Penicillamine and hydroxychloroquine in the treatment of severe juvenile rheumatoid arthritis. N Engl J Med 1986;314:1269.

83. van Kerckhove C, Giannini EH, Lovell DJ. Temporal patterns of response to D-penicillamine. hydroxychloroquine and placebo in juvenile rheumatoid arthritis. Arthritis Rheum 1988;31:1252.

84. Jaffee IA. Penicillamine treatment of rheumatoid arthritis: rationale, pattern of clinical response, and clinical pharmacology and toxicology. In: Munthe E, ed. Penicillamine research in rheumatoid disease. Oslo, Norway: Fabritius, 1976:11.

85. Ansell BM, Eghtedari A, Bywaters EGL. Chlorambucil in the management of juvenile chronic arthritis complicated by amyloidosis. Ann Rheum Dis 1971;30:331.

86. Arnold M, Schrieber L, Brooks PM. Immunosuppressive drugs and corticosteroids in the treatment of rheumatoid arthritis. Drugs 1988;36:340.

87. Kvien TK, Hoyeraal HM, Standstad B. Azathioprine versus placebo in patients with juvenile rheumatoid arthritis. J Rheumatol 1986;13:118.
88. Kahan BD. Cyclosporin. N Engl J Med 1989; 321:1725.
89. Ostensen M, Hoyeraal HM, Kass E. Tolerance of cyclosporine A in children with refractory juvenile rheumatoid arthritis. J Rheumatol 1988; 15:1536.
90. Rosenberg AM. Advanced drug therapy for juvenile rheumatoid arthritis. J Pediatr 1989;114: 171.
91. Silverman ED, Laxer RM, Greenward M, et al. Intravenous gamma globulin therapy in systemic juvenile rheumatoid arthritis. Arthritis Rheum 1990;33:1015.
92. Jasso-Giannini M, Protas EJ. Aerobic capacity in juvenile rheumatoid arthritis patients and healthy children. Arthritis Care Res 1991;4: 131.
93. Klepper SE, Darbee J, Effgen SK, Singsen BH. Physical fitness levels in children with polyarticular juvenile rheumatoid arthritis. Arthritis Care Res 1992;5:93.
94. Jay S, Litt IF, Durant RH. Compliance with therapeutic regimens. J Adolesc Health Care 1984;5:124.
95. Litt IR, Cuskey WR, Rosenberg BA. Role of self-esteem and autonomy in determining medication compliance among adolescents with juvenile rheumatoid arthritis. Pediatrics 1982; 69:15.
96. Rapoff MA. Compliance with treatment regimens for pediatric rheumatic diseases. Arthritis Care Res 1989;2:S40.

THE RHEUMATIC DISEASES OF CHILDHOOD

Bracha Shaham
Bram H. Bernstein

The clinician treating children with rheumatic diseases is faced with major challenges. These include fostering normal physical and emotional development while preventing organ damage. A long-term focus is necessary, since a prime goal in treating children is to achieve a life span measured in decades rather than in years.

Treatment of both inflammatory and noninflammatory rheumatic diseases of childhood will be described. The inflammatory diseases include systemic lupus erythematosus, neonatal lupus, dermatomyositis, poststreptococcal reactive arthritis, Henoch-Schönlein purpura, Kawasaki disease, polyarteritis nodosa, Wegener's granulomatosis, and limited scleroderma. Noninflammatory conditions include reflex neurovascular dystrophy and fibromyalgia. (For an in-depth discussion of current concepts of pathogenesis and clinical features of childhood rheumatic diseases, see Kelley et al., Chapter 72 [reference 216].)

SYSTEMIC LUPUS ERYTHEMATOSUS

Systemic lupus erythematosus (SLE) is an autoimmune, multisystem inflammatory disease that can affect children at all ages. Untreated, the disease can be fulminant, resulting in death within months from renal, cardiovascular, or other organ failure or from complicating sepsis.[1] Advances in supportive therapies, such as antibiotics and antihypertensive drugs, critical care and dialysis, and better means of identifying children at high risk of organ involvement or life-threatening complications, have improved the prognosis. With the survival rate now better than 80% at 10 years,[2,3] the course of the disease and its ultimate prognosis are no longer worse in childhood than in adults.[4,5] The episodic nature of the disease, with spontaneous exacerbations not always predictable before organ damage, and the effects of chronic illness and potentially toxic medications on emotional as well as physical growth and development, make the therapy of lupus particularly challenging in children.

The goal of therapy in childhood SLE is to control disease symptoms and prevent organ damage. Side effects must be avoided, while normal growth, development, and age-appropriate functioning are promoted. In the absence of a known cause, therapy is nonspecific. Milder symptoms may be treated conservatively with nonsteroidal antiinflammatory drugs (NSAIDs) and antimalarials. When disease manifestations are potentially damaging to organs, disabling, or life threatening, aggressive antiinflammatory and immunosuppressive therapies may be needed. Specialized treatment, such as anticoagulation, intravenous immunoglobulin (IVIG), or psychotropic drugs, may be required to treat such features as thromboses, uncontrolled thrombocytopenia, or psychosis.

A tendency toward more severe disease often requires more aggressive treatment in children than in adults. At the same time, emphasis must be placed on minimizing corticosteroid doses, so as to foster normal growth and avoid severe changes in appearance. The latter can lead to serious depressive reactions and to noncompliance, eventually resulting in death, especially in the teenage group.[3,4]

At this time, lupus continues to be a lifelong, incurable illness, with the potential for serious morbidity or death from the disease or from complications of treatment. The aim of therapy is to maintain as normal a lifestyle as possible while preventing organ damage. It is essential to support the child and the family through initial and subsequent anxiety, anger, and guilt and to help them establish support systems and effective coping mechanisms. A team approach, in which child and family are seen by a designated physician (pediatric rheumatologist) and specialized allied health personnel, is important in enhancing trust and communication. In our unit, patients and families are encouraged to participate in a support group. School liaison is provided by the team nurse or social worker. Since understanding should improve compliance, instruction about the disease process and its therapy is begun at the first visit and continues throughout follow-up.

General Therapeutic Measures

Supportive measures include management of nutritional status, blood pressure, fluid and electrolyte balance, and superimposed infections.

Easy fatigability, a common feature of active disease, may require adjustment of the child's schedule to provide rest periods and adequate sleep at night. Although the school schedule and physical education program may need to be altered initially, return to normal school activities as soon as possible is encouraged.

Children are taught to use sunscreens and to avoid direct sun exposure. Daily application of sunscreen carrying an SPF (sun protection factor) number of 15 or higher is recommended. Waterproof preparations are preferred for younger children. Local reactions such as erythema or stinging can occur, so patients establish a personal choice of product by trial and error. For the adolescents, makeup can be applied over the sunscreen.

Lupus dermatitis occurs in more than two thirds of children with SLE at presentation, with malar rash present in at least one third.[6] Antimalarials may be effective.[7] Most of the time the rash responds well to systemic steroids started for other disease manifestations. Topical steroids

are used for persistent rashes but should be used cautiously, since prolonged application can cause local side effects such as skin atrophy and depigmentation. This is a particular hazard with the high-potency fluorinated products. For facial lesions, we start with hydrocortisone 1% cream, increasing to 2.5% strength or changing to 0.1% betamethasone cream (Valisone) if necessary. Lesions in other areas can be treated with high-potency preparations, especially betamethasone dipropionate 0.05% (Diprolene) or fluocinonide 0.05% (Lidex). Long-term topical therapy should be avoided.

Discoid lupus, which is very rare in childhood, can be disfiguring. In addition to potent topical steroid preparations, systemic antimalarials or intralesional injections with steroids are prescribed.[8] Azathioprine has been reported to be effective for severe discoid lesions in uncontrolled trials.[9,10]

Mucosal ulcers are common with active disease. If symptomatic, sucralfate suspension applied topically or local application of a steroid such as triamcinolone acetonide 0.1%[11] (Kenalog in Orabase) every 2 to 3 hours may be helpful. Severe mucositis is treated with systemic steroids.

Salicylates and NSAIDs

Indications: Fever, Arthralgia, Myalgia, Arthritis, Mild Serositis

When disease symptoms are relatively mild, children can be treated with aspirin (ASA) or NSAIDs, often in combination with an antimalarial (see below). If ASA is chosen, monitoring for liver toxicity (frequent in children)[12,13] as well as for gastritis and bleeding is necessary. The need for frequent dosing often makes compliance with an ASA regimen difficult in the pediatric age group. The nonacetylated salicylates are better tolerated by the gastrointestinal tract and have less effect on platelet aggregation, but efficacy may be less and hepatotoxicity is still possible. Used concomitantly with corticosteroids, clearance of all salicylates is accelerated. Therefore the salicylate serum level may rise significantly as steroids are reduced,[14] increasing the risk of salicylism.

Because of these difficulties, we favor the use of NSAIDs over salicylates. At this time, only ibuprofen (40 to 45 mg/kg/d in four divided doses), tolmetin (35 to 40 mg/kg/d in three to four divided doses) and naprosyn (15 mg/kg/d in two divided doses) are approved for children. Efficacy is roughly equivalent in all. Compliance, particularly in teenagers, may be better with NSAIDs that require less frequent administration.

ASA in low dosage has a definite role in children with the lupus anticoagulant (antiphospholipid syndrome).[15] These children are at high risk of developing thrombotic complications. One baby aspirin (81 mg) daily is prescribed to inhibit platelet aggregation.

Side Effects

- *Gastritis, peptic ulcer, gastrointestinal (GI) bleeding.*[16] Concomitant steroids increase this risk.[17] Sucralfate, 0.5 to 1 g 30 minutes prior to NSAID, may provide protection.
- *Hepatic.* Mild elevation of transaminases is most common with ASA[12] but can occur with all NSAIDs.[18] It usually resolves with dose adjustment or withdrawal of medication. Mild to moderate elevation of liver enzyme levels is a frequent manifestation of lupus before treatment, possibly increasing the risk of additional hepatic insult from NSAIDs. Rarely, progression to parenchymal necrosis or pancreatitis develops, particularly with sulindac.[19] Since these drugs are highly protein bound, low levels of serum albumin (a common feature of lupus) may expose patients to high levels of potentially toxic unbound drug. Relatively low NSAID doses are advisable.
- *Renal.* Decreased renal blood flow and glomerular filtration rate (GFR) occur but usually stabilize with continued treatment. Patients taking diuretics or on a sodium-restricted diet may be especially sensitive. Further deterioration of renal function can result from the complex effects of NSAIDs on glomerular filtration rate (GFR) and aldosterone metabolism in lupus patients with glomerulonephritis, congestive heart failure, or ascites. Indomethacin is more commonly associated with these toxic effects,[20] while nonacetylated salicylates are safer. Although sulindac was initially reported to be less nephrotoxic than other NSAIDs,[21] subsequent studies demonstrated a potential for similar renal side effects.[22]

Interstitial nephritis, manifested by proteinuria without cellular casts, can occur as an idiosyncratic reaction related to NSAIDs.[23]

This is usually reversible with discontinuation of the offending drug but may require steroid therapy or even dialysis on rare occasions. Differentiation from active lupus nephritis is necessary.

- *Central nervous system.* Episodes of aseptic meningitis and nonspecific febrile reactions have been described with many NSAIDs, particularly ibuprofen, tolmetin, and sulindac.[19,24]
- *Other.* Skin rashes and ocular dryness, reversible on discontinuation of the NSAID, may confuse the clinical picture.[25] Pseudoporphyria has been described in children receiving naproxen.[26] Cytopenia may be aggravated by drug effect on the bone marrow. NSAIDs potentiate the anticoagulation effect of coumarin and should not be used concomitantly.[19]

Antimalarials

Indications: Cutaneous Manifestations, Arthritis, Steroid-Sparing Effect

Antimalarials have been used in the treatment of SLE for the past 100 years. Recent studies continue to demonstrate their effectiveness.[27] their mechanism of action is complex and is not fully understood. It includes blocking of ultraviolet rays, stabilization of lysosomal membranes, cyclooxygenase blockade, and immune modulation.[7]

Hydroxychloroquine (HCQ, Plaquenil) is the most commonly used antimalarial for childhood lupus. In our practice a major indication for starting HCQ is to provide a steroid-sparing effect. HCQ (5 to 6.5 mg/kg/d) has a slow onset of action (2 to 4 months) with peak effect at 6 to 12 months.[7]

Quinacrine (Atabrine) is prescribed less frequently than HCQ because of its toxicity (see below). It may have certain advantages, however. Its onset of action (3 to 4 weeks) is shorter, with maximal beneficial effect usually achieved by 6 to 8 weeks. There is no retinal toxicity, and it has a stronger effect in alleviating fatigue.[28] Its most common indication is the presence of severe cutaneous manifestations, especially in children with subacute cutaneous lupus who are not responding to combined HCQ and low- to moderate-dose steroids. The dose is 1 to 2 mg/kg/d, to a maximum of 100 mg/d. HCQ and quinacrine may even be synergistic and show less individual toxicity when combined at lower doses.[28]

HCQ Side Effects

- *Ocular.* HCQ accumulates slowly, over years, in the retinal cells, particularly the cones and rods of the macula. In the early, asymptomatic stages, retinal pigmentation can be detected. Macular pigmentation and edema, arteriolar constriction, pallor of the optical disk and corneal deposits with deterioration of visual acuity, scotoma, night blindness, and loss of color vision may be late developments. Such changes have been described only in patients who received more than 6.5 mg/kg/d or had concurrent conditions that could lead to elevated levels and in a few cases in which the drug was taken for more than 10 years.[7,29,30] We recommend that patients have a baseline ophthalmologic evaluation within a month of starting HCQ therapy and then at 4- to 6-month intervals, depending on dosage and length of therapy. Evaluation should include assessment of visual acuity, the fundus, and color vision.
- *Gastrointestinal.* Nausea, abdominal bloating, cramps, and diarrhea occur infrequently.[7]
- *Cutaneous.* A variety of rashes, including urticaria, can occur. These are reversible.[7]
- *Central nervous system.* A stimulatory effect, which may actually be beneficial in patients with fatigue, can also produce nervousness, insomnia, confusion, migrainelike headaches, tinnitus, nerve deafness, and vestibular dysfunction. Overdosage has been associated with convulsions, coma, and sudden death.[7,31]

Quinacrine Side Effects[28]

- *Cutaneous.* Quinacrine binds to melanin, causing yellowish skin in one third of patients. Dark pigmentation of nails and pretibial skin, resembling ecchymoses, is also reported.
- *Hematologic.* Bone marrow suppression with leukopenia or agranulocytosis is a major concern. A lichenoid skin rash is noted in most cases before the development of cytopenia; hence the drug must be discontinued immediately if a rash occurs. A complete blood count (CBC) should be obtained at least every 6 weeks.

Although bone marrow suppression can occur with either antimalarial, it is far more common with quinacrine. In addition, since antimalarials have oxidant properties, they are contraindicated in G6PD-deficient patients.

In the absence of side effects, tapering of either antimalarial should be gradual and slow, since disease flare has been associated with discontinuation.[27] The unit dose or the number of days per week the drug is taken is reduced every 2 to 3 months.

Guidelines for Minimizing Antimalarial Toxicity

- Do not exceed the recommended dosage. Retinopathy with HCQ and agranulocytosis with quinacrine are associated with higher doses.
- Stop HCQ at 6 to 9 months and quinacrine at 8 weeks if no beneficial effects have been noted.
- Stop either drug if *any* rash occurs. This is especially important in case of a lichenoid rash with quinacrine.
- Obtain a baseline ophthalmologic examination and follow-up every 4 to 6 months for patients who are taking HCQ.
- Check CBC at least every 6 weeks when quinacrine is used, or at 3-month intervals with HCQ. Discontinue the drug if significant cytopenia or anemia develops.
- Decrease the dose by one half if significant gastrointestinal symptoms occur. Antacids and antigas products may be given.
- When maximal beneficial effect has been achieved and disease control on minimal steroid doses is good, taper gradually to a lower maintenance dose.

Steroids

Indications: Major Organ Involvement or Significant Anemia, Thrombocytopenia, or Pancytopenia; Inadequate Response to NSAIDs and Antimalarials; Serologic Evidence of Increasing Disease Activity

The most potent of antiinflammatory agents, the glucocorticoids, control many manifestations of SLE. Their mechanism of action is complex and includes effects on leukocyte movement, number, and function; on reticuloendothelial clearance of antibody-coated cells; and on vascular endothelium.[32] The short-acting preparations, prednisone and prednisolone (oral) and methylprednisolone (Solu-Medrol, intravenous), are most frequently used. These drugs are protein bound in the plasma, and only the small unbound fraction is active. Metabolic deactivation occurs mainly in the liver, so such drugs as phenobarbital or such conditions as hyperthyroidism may hasten deactivation by enhancing hepatic microsomal enzyme activity.[19]

Low-dose, High-dose, and Intravenous Pulse Steroid Therapy

Even with relatively mild symptoms and without major organ involvement, many children do not respond adequately to NSAIDs and antimalarials alone but will improve when given low-dose prednisone. Such a regimen may also be used in selected patients in whom a drop in complement levels and a rise in anti-DNA antibodies signifies exacerbation, even in the absence of clinical symptoms.[33] A dose of 0.25 to 0.5 mg/kg/d, initially divided into two to four daily doses to increase the therapeutic effect, is prescribed. With good clinical and laboratory response, the drug is gradually consolidated to a single daily dose and then tapered to the minimum effective dose. Another option, when the disease is well controlled with a single daily dose, is to switch to alternate-day therapy with more than twice the previous daily dose.[34] Alternatively, the amount taken every other day may be slowly reduced until alternate-day dosing is reached. The exact extent and rate of steroid reduction are individualized as determined by the patient's condition, the quality of clinical and serologic response, and the severity of side effects. In lupus the general rule is *taper slowly!*

Steroid therapy for renal disease varies according to the particular type of renal lesion. An unusual lesion in children is pure membranous glomerulonephritis without a proliferative component. This lesion may not show much response to steroids or cytotoxic drugs. Fortunately, progression to chronic renal failure is not very common. Treatment is with intermediate doses of steroids: 1 mg/kg/d for 6 to 12 weeks, followed by gradual tapering.[35]

With more serious renal or other internal organ disease, or when anemia, thrombocytopenia, or pancytopenia is significant, prednisone or methylprednisolone (Solu-Medrol) is administered at up to 2 mg/kg/d in divided doses.[36] Initial intravenous treatment for 3 to 5 days or longer may be needed for the acutely ill child. With improvement, parenteral therapy can be converted to oral. Since prednisone is four-fifths as potent as methylprednisolone and since not all the drug may be enterally absorbed, the switch from intravenous to oral therapy at the same dose may represent a significant taper. The oral doses are then gradually consolidated and further reduced as discussed above.

Intravenous methylprednisolone pulse therapy has been administered to patients with very severe or life-threatening manifestations whose conditions continue to deteriorate on high-dose steroids.[19,37,38] This strategy may be particularly useful for lupus cerebritis.[37,39] Although there are reports of beneficial results from this treatment in acute lupus nephritis,[40,41] experience in our center with several patients who developed worsening renal failure and anasarca after pulse methylprednisolone suggests that caution be exercised in this situation. A dose of 30 mg/kg/d, up to 1 g per dose, is infused over $1/2$ to 1 hour on three consecutive days at monthly intervals. Following the pulse treatment, patients receive low-dose or no steroids, according to their condition. Pulse methylprednisolone treatment may be associated with potentially serious side effects, such as arrhythmias, sudden death, seizures, and anaphylaxis[19,42]; hence vital signs and general condition must be closely monitored. Opportunistic infections, avascular necrosis of bone, and glucose intolerance are potential risks.[43] Those patients who respond well, however, may benefit by avoiding the side effects of prolonged high-dose steroids.

Steroid Side Effects

In general, the different glucocorticoid preparations do not differ significantly in adverse effects. Major concerns *in children* are as follows:

1. *Stunted linear growth.*[44] Most children with SLE have not reached normal adult height at onset. If the child reaches puberty before steroid doses are lowered enough to allow "catch-up" growth, growth retardation becomes permanent, sometimes leading to serious difficulty with social and psychological development and adjustment. In general, linear growth is delayed with prednisone doses of more than 5 mg/d. Strategies to help in steroid-dose reduction include the use of antimalarials and cytotoxic drugs. A new synthetic glucocorticoid, deflazacort, may produce less growth delay[45,46] and provide

significant bone mineral sparing. This drug has not yet been approved by the Food and Drug Administration (FDA).

2. *Changes in appearance.* Cushingoid features, obesity, hirsutism, striae, acne, bruising, thin fragile skin. Body image and appearance are of extreme importance to adolescents, the age group that includes most juveniles with SLE. Anger, feelings of desperation, and a sense of social isolation can lead to noncompliance with treatment, depression, and even suicide.[1,3,47] Dietary advice, patient and family education, and support by the treatment team are essential to limit weight gain and to help the teenager cope with unavoidable changes. Hirsutism can be treated cosmetically by blanching and depilation; acne at times responds to topical benzoyl peroxide, or it can be treated with tretinoic acid.

3. *Avascular necrosis of bone and pathologic fractures.*[44,48] These cause significant morbidity, with pain and limited ambulation in children who are already struggling to carry on normal activities in the face of a serious chronic illness.

4. *Emotional lability.*[44] The psychological turmoil associated with diagnosis or flare-up can be further aggravated by steroid-induced mood changes. Reduction in steroid dose, if possible, while providing emotional support to the child and family, is the main strategy used to minimize this effect.

5. *Steroid-induced hypertension.*[19,44] This may necessitate higher doses of antihypertensive drugs, especially in children with renal disease.

6. *Interaction with other drugs*[19]:
   - The incidence of gastritis increases significantly with concomitant use of steroids and NSAIDs. Barrier agents, such as sucralfate, H_2 receptor blockers such as ranitidine, or antacids, can be given. Children should be questioned about epigastric discomfort or the presence of melena. Stool should be checked for occult blood if symptoms exist or if there is an unexplained drop in hemoglobin level.
   - Hypokalemic alkalosis may develop when thiazide diuretics are added. Electrolytes should be monitored.
   - Accelerated deactivation due to concomitant use of barbiturates, phenytoin, or rifampin may lead to higher steroid dose requirements.[19,49,50]

Cytotoxic Drugs

Alkylating agents and purine analogs are added to steroid therapy when severe organ or life-threatening disease develops, or when steroid dose must be reduced because of unacceptable side effects. Cyclophosphamide (Cytoxan) and azathioprine (Imuran) are most commonly used, with nitrogen mustard and methotrexate reserved for exceptional circumstances.

Cytoxan

Cytoxan, a synthetic derivative of nitrogen mustard, is used in the following situations: severe nephritis, vasculitis, neurologic disease, pulmonary disease, uncontrolled autoimmune thrombocytopenia, hemolytic anemia.[1,51–54] Cytoxan is an alkylating agent, which acts throughout the cell cycle and inhibits DNA replication. It is toxic to rapidly proliferating lymphoid tissues, causing a prolonged decrease in T cells and a transient decrease in B cells.[55] T cell function and antibody production are inhibited, and immunologic tolerance is induced. The drug has a short serum half-life (2 to 10 hours). It is mainly metabolized in the liver into compounds that are themselves alkylating agents.

Cytoxan Therapy in Lupus Nephritis. Studies suggest that many children with end-stage renal disease due to lupus do poorly.[56] For this reason, aggressive treatment is needed to prevent or delay progression in high-risk patients. In view of controlled studies from the National Institutes of Health (NIH) that concluded that parenteral use of Cytoxan was superior to steroids alone in preventing irreversible renal damage and end-stage renal disease,[57–60] a protocol has been adapted for use in children.[1,61] To provide adequate monitoring, hydration, and control of nausea, patients receiving Cytoxan are hospitalized for 16 to 24 hours (Fig. 16–2). Treatments are begun with a dose of 500 mg/m², increased to 750 mg/m² the following month and to a maintenance dose of 1000 mg/m² by the third month, leukocyte count permitting. If the white blood cell count is under 3000/mm³ at the nadir or under 4000/mm³ at month's end, the dose is adjusted downward. Treatment is continued at monthly intervals for the first 6 months. With satisfactory response to six monthly infusions, Cytoxan is continued at 3-month intervals for an additional 10 treatments. After a total of 36 months of therapy many patients show no evidence of active renal disease and the drug can be discontinued.

Improvement with Cytoxan is usually apparent by 3 to 6 months of treatment. If there has been no improvement by 6 months, the drug can be discontinued. A renal biopsy showing evidence of high chronicity at this point would suggest that no further cytotoxic treatment be given.[53] Children who show an initial response but relapse while receiving Cytoxan at 3-month intervals are given three monthly doses and then returned to the trimonthly maintenance schedule. A few patients experience relapse after completion of the full treatment course.[62] These children can be considered for resumption of therapy. Children who respond well to monthly Cytoxan but experience relapse whenever the interval increases pose a difficult management problem. Currently, most continue on treatment at intervals of 1, $1\frac{1}{2}$, or 2 months. Other approaches might include combining Cytoxan every 3 months with intravenous bolus methylprednisolone, with weekly low-dose methotrexate,[63] or with intermittent intravenous methotrexate at 300 mg/m[2].[53] Citrovorum rescue, using low intermittent doses of folinic acid after methotrexate, should be considered.[64] Selected children with lupus nephrotic syndrome have responded well to one or more injections of nitrogen mustard during the course of Cytoxan therapy. In this case, resumption of Cytoxan administration would be postponed so as to avoid additive bone marrow depression.

Cytoxan Therapy for Other Disease Manifestations[52–54] (Generalized Vasculitis, Central Nervous System [CNS] Lupus, Transverse Myelitis, Peripheral Neuritis, Pneumonitis or Pulmonary Hemorrhage, Uncontrolled Hemolytic Anemia, or Thrombocytopenia)

INTRAVENOUS THERAPY: In our experience, intravenous Cytoxan at 10 mg/kg every 2 weeks has been lifesaving in some children in whom high-dose steroid therapy alone had failed. Precautions and monitoring are similar to those of the renal protocol, although less hydration is needed. Nausea and vomiting are usually less severe. Response may be apparent within 2 weeks. Ongoing bimonthly Cytoxan can be given in the outpatient setting if the patient's condition permits. In this case, children are instructed to drink at least four cups of liquid (one sports bottle) prior to the appointment and to continue high fluid intake and frequent bladder evacuation throughout the day. CBC and urinalysis are checked, and the patient is evaluated before drug administration. The length of such treatment must be individualized. As the child responds, the dose may be reduced or the interval between doses prolonged.

ORAL THERAPY: Daily Cytoxan carries a higher risk of hemorrhagic cystitis and, perhaps, of eventual malignant disease. Nevertheless, some children whose response to intermittent intravenous Cytoxan has been inadequate, may benefit from daily oral therapy (1 to 2 mg/kg/d). This can also be considered for children whose quality of life with intermittent intravenous therapy is poor because of frequent hospitalizations or side effects. With good response, conversion to intermittent treatment (3 to 5 days per week) may be acceptable as a means of reducing toxicity. Patients are instructed to increase fluid intake and to evacuate the bladder frequently, as well as to report promptly any sign of infection. CBC, urinalysis, and clinical assessment are performed at 2- to 4-week intervals.

Adverse Effects[51,52]

1. *Nausea and vomiting.* These may occur within a few hours of treatment and are dose related. Hence, patients are usually premedicated intravenously with ondansetron hydrochloride (Zofran), 0.15 mg/kg, 30 minutes before Cytoxan administration and at 4 and 8 hours after infusion.[65] Other antiemetics (e.g., metoclopramide [Reglan]) may be prescribed for delayed nausea. New antinausea drugs are in the pipeline.

2. *Hair loss.* Significant alopecia occurs during monthly treatments, but hair usually regrows when frequency of administration is reduced. Although benefit has not been proved, use of an ice cap during the infusion can be considered. The team provides support to the child and the family. Wigs and head coverings are used creatively.

3. *Bone marrow suppression.* This is usually transient, since stem cells are spared.[66] Maximum leukopenia is expected 7 to 14 days after Cytoxan administration and resolves by 21 to 25 days. Anemia can accompany the leukopenia, but severe thrombocytopenia is rare. A CBC should be obtained before Cytoxan administration and 7 to 14 days after

each treatment. In the event that leukocyte, hemoglobin or thrombocyte levels drop significantly, the next Cytoxan dose should be adjusted accordingly.

4. *Hemorrhagic cystitis.*[67] The metabolite acrolein is toxic to bladder transitional cell epithelium and may cause severe hemorrhagic cystitis. This is usually preventable with vigorous hydration. Mesna (sodium 2-mercaptoethanosulfonate),[68] a chelating agent, binds acrolein to form a nontoxic compound without interfering with the desired Cytoxan effect. Our practice is to administer mesna to children receiving intermittent intravenous Cytoxan who cannot tolerate intravenous hydration or who have developed microscopic hematuria. Mesna (60% to 100%, [mg/mg] of the Cytoxan dose) is divided into three or four portions. It is administered intravenously before Cytoxan and repeated at 4- and 8-hour intervals.

5. *Infection.* Immunosuppression may lead to opportunistic bacterial or fungal infections.[56,69] These are difficult to differentiate from active lupus and can be life threatening. Maintaining the absolute granulocyte count above 2000/mm³ minimizes this risk. Immunoglobulin levels should be monitored, and prophylactic gamma globulin should be considered if hypogammaglobulinemia is severe. Patients are instructed to report fever, chills, dysuria, exposure to varicella, or other signs of infection immediately. Children exposed to varicella who do not have prior immunity should receive varicella zoster immunoglobulin (VZIG) within 96 hours.

6. *Sterility.* Although some adults and children who receive Cytoxan for malignant disease develop gonadal dysfunction,[70] normal fertility can occur.[71] Since Cytoxan doses for lupus are usually lower, impairment of gonadal function is less likely. We advise patients and parents that there is a risk of sterility. In older boys, consideration should be given to pre-Cytoxan sperm banking.

7. *Teratogenicity.*[72] A teratogenic effect may occur during the first trimester of pregnancy. However, a recent report comparing the outcome of pregnancy in lupus patients who received cytotoxic treatment during pregnancy with those who did not failed to show any difference in pregnancy outcome.[73] Nevertheless, counseling about the need to avoid pregnancy during Cytoxan treatment should be provided. Sexually active girls should have a negative pregnancy test before starting therapy.

8. *Late malignant disease.* This has been reported in adults treated with oral Cytoxan.[74] Although not reported in children, this complication remains a concern.

Summary. In summary, all patients undergoing Cytoxan treatment require careful clinical and laboratory monitoring. Vigorous hydration and use of mesna should protect them from hemorrhagic cystitis. Premedication with antiemetics controls nausea and vomiting in most patients. Blood counts at the nadir point and at frequent intervals are used to assess marrow suppression. The treatment team and the family maintain vigilance in monitoring for infection and other side effects. Although Cytoxan remains controversial as a therapy for lupus in children because of the possibility of long-term side effects, we believe its potential organ- and lifesaving effects outweigh its risks in appropriate patients.

Azathioprine

Azathioprine (AZA, Imuran) is a purine analog of hypoxanthine that suppresses the antibody response and reduces B cell numbers.[51] Indications include active generalized disease and severe nephritis requiring prolonged use of high-dose steroids. Studies in adults show a steroid-sparing effect,[75] improvement in generalized active lupus, efficacy in combination with prednisone alone or with both prednisone and Cytoxan in nephritis,[57] and improvement in severe cutaneous lesions.[9,10]

Side effects. These are generally similar to those described above but are less severe. Hemorrhagic cystitis does not occur. An increased incidence of infections, especially herpes zoster, is of concern.[76]

AZA is given in a dose of 1.5 to 2.5 mg/kg/d, with benefit usually apparent by 6 to 8 weeks. If no effect has been observed after 12 weeks, the drug should be discontinued. When maximal beneficial effect has been achieved, the dose may be gradually reduced to the lowest effective maintenance dose.

Monitoring includes frequent clinical and laboratory evaluations. Attention is given to loss of appetite or nausea, diarrhea, abdominal pain, malaise, rash, oral lesions, and signs of bleeding and of infection. A CBC is obtained at initiation of therapy, after 1 to 2 weeks, and then at monthly intervals.

Methotrexate

Methotrexate (MTX) is a folic acid antagonist whose mechanism of action in inflammatory illnesses is not yet fully understood. Failure of folinic acid to reduce MTX efficacy in rheumatoid arthritis[64] suggests that its effect is achieved via mechanisms other than inhibition of dihydrofolate reductase. An antiinflammatory effect is suggested by a relatively rapid onset of action, as well as by studies demonstrating an effect on IL-1 function, a reduction of polymorphonuclear chemotaxis, and a decrease in production of leukotriene B_4 5-lipoxygenase and superoxide.[77,78] Immunosuppressive mechanisms are suggested by MTX effect on antibody production and on T cells.[77,78] Thus various actions at multiple cellular levels may be operative. Small controlled studies in adults demonstrate a steroid-sparing effect and improvement in arthritis, myositis, rash, pleurisy, and nephritis when administered in low weekly doses.[79] Similar favorable results with minimal toxicity have recently been reported in 10 children with SLE.[63] In contrast, others have reported a lack of efficacy.[80] Children with diffuse proliferative lupus nephritis who have flare-ups when taking maintenance Cytoxan can be considered for weekly oral or intravenous MTX in combination with intravenous Cytoxan.[53]

Side effects include nausea, vomiting, and abdominal discomfort, reported in 30% of children receiving MTX for arthritis; transient elevation of liver transaminases, which usually resolves with dose reduction or discontinuation; susceptibility to infection; reversible leukopenia; and oral mucosal lesions.[81] Severe bone marrow suppression is rare, as are severe stomatitis, confusion, seizures, and idiosyncratic pneumonitis. Carcinogenicity and infertility have not been reported.

Monitoring includes determination of CBC and transaminase levels at monthly intervals. Careful evaluation of renal status in children with nephritis is essential, since MTX is primarily cleared by the kidney and a creatinine clearance less than 60 ml/min may be associated with increased risk of toxicity.

Nitrogen Mustard

Nitrogen mustard (HN_2) is an alkylating agent, toxic to rapidly proliferating cells. Several clinical studies have documented efficacy and a steroid-sparing effect in rapidly progressive nephrotic syndrome in adults with SLE.[82–84] In our center, the drug is used cautiously in selected children with life-threatening progressive lupus nephritis and nephrosis that has been unresponsive to steroids and Cytoxan. Although treatment can be repeated subsequently, our experience with acquired irreversible agammaglobulinemia in one patient has led us to exercise extreme caution in repetitive usage. A dose of 0.4 mg/kg is given in the hospital as a single infusion or may be split into two daily doses. Nitrogen mustard is a powerful vesicant and causes vein irritation or, with extravasation, local necrosis. Contact with skin or mucosal membranes must be avoided. Therefore, a secure peripheral or, preferably, central intravenous line should be used. Methylprednisolone is flushed through that line at a concentration of 1 mg/ml during the nitrogen mustard infusion to prevent phlebitis. Because the drug is unstable in solution, the crystals should be dissolved immediately prior to administration and slowly infused as an intravenous "push" by a physician who wears protective gloves.

Side Effects

1. Local irritation or necrosis.
2. Nausea and vomiting, expected within 1 to 3 hours of the infusion and lasting up to 24 hours. Antiemetics are given as with Cytoxan.
3. Predictable granulocytopenia (and occasional thrombocytopenia) within 6 to 8 days usually resolves in 10 to 21 days. Uncommonly, bone marrow depression may be prolonged or, rarely, progress to aplasia.
4. Infection related to granulocytopenia.
5. Risk of infertility and of malignancy.

In summary, cytotoxic drugs offer the possibility of improved survival and quality of life for selected children with lupus who might otherwise die or have to endure dialysis or disabling steroid side effects. Careful monitoring of clinical and laboratory parameters is indispensable to their use.

Investigational Treatments

Plasmapheresis. Plasma is selectively removed from blood and replaced with albumin, saline solution, or fresh frozen plasma, while all other blood components are returned to the patient. Plasmapheresis removes circulating immune complexes, reduces serum IgG and autoantibody levels, and restores normal phagocytic activity of reticuloendothelial cells.[85] Case reports describe benefit to adult lupus patients with thrombotic thrombocytopenic purpura and in CNS lupus.[86,87] A recent controlled, randomized study comparing prednisone plus Cytoxan and plasmapheresis to prednisone with Cytoxan alone for lupus nephritis showed a lack of benefit from plasmapheresis in that condition.[88] Plasmapheresis without cytotoxic therapy is associated with an antibody rebound phenomenon a few days after initial decline, presumably due to lack of negative feedback to B cells because of IgG removal. It is suggested, therefore, that Cytoxan be administered a few days after plasmapheresis to eliminate the most active autoimmune clones.[51] This approach is currently the focus of an international controlled trial.[85]

We use plasmapheresis in selected children whose lives are in imminent danger because of rapidly progressive lupus, especially if there is evidence of acute vasculitis or circulating immune complex disease with inadequate response to steroids and Cytoxan. Included are children with severe generalized disease, pulmonary hemorrhage, and CNS involvement. The frequency and duration of treatment are individualized. We usually start with 5 days per week, then 3, and subsequently taper as tolerated. The usual course of plasmapheresis lasts 3 months.

Complications. Plasmapheresis is an invasive procedure, usually requiring surgical insertion of a venous catheter. Removal of some red cells, platelets, and leukocytes occurs, resulting in varying degrees of anemia, thrombocytopenia, and leukopenia, as well as hypogammaglobulinemia. Because of manipulation of intravascular volume, hypotension and hemodynamic instability are possible.

The procedure is performed in the dialysis or critical care unit. Patients are closely monitored for stability of vital signs, fluid balance, change in serum mineral and electrolyte levels, and any evidence of bleeding, cytopenia, anemia, or infection.

Intravenous Immunoglobulin. Although effective in the treatment of some inflammatory diseases, IVIG remains controversial in SLE. Studies in adults show improvement of autoimmune thrombocytopenia, with faster response if used in combination with steroids, but no effect on lupus serology.[89] Improvement in serious manifestations of SLE (nephritis, pneumonitis, cerebritis) with prolonged monthly treatments has been noted in case reports.[90] A recent study involving children, however, found exacerbation of renal disease as well as new onset nephritis after 3 months of treatment.[91] We have used short-term IVIG for lupus thrombocytopenia in a few patients as a means of avoiding high-dose steroid therapy. A single dose of 2 g/kg is infused over 10 hours. Patients are monitored for fluid intolerance and for allergic reactions.

Cyclosporine A (CSA). CSA, a cyclic endecapeptide derived from fungi, inhibits T cell activation. This leads to a failure to activate the transcription of early genes, such as those encoding the cytokines.[92] High doses of this drug have been shown to control the clinical and serologic manifestations of SLE in mouse models of the disease.[93] Children and adults receiving low doses of CSA in combination with steroids showed improvement in renal and extrarenal manifestations of lupus, as well as a steroid-sparing effect.[94,95] Efficacy was apparent 6 months after the start of therapy. Although renal toxicity (hypertension, creatinine elevation) was noted in the majority of patients, CSA-related damage was not seen in renal biopsies. Disease reactivation occurred in most cases after discontinuation of CSA. In contrast, other studies failed to demonstrate improvement with CSA.[51]

Nephrotoxicity is the most troublesome of the adverse effects. The dose of CSA should be reduced if creatinine levels increase, even while they are still in the normal range. Hypertension is reported to occur independently of serum creatinine elevation. Hirsutism, facial swelling, skin flushing, dyspepsia, nausea, and anorexia, as well as laboratory evidence of hepatotoxicity, may develop.[93–95] All are usually reversible with withdrawal of the drug. Bone marrow suppression does not occur.

CSA may have a place in the treatment of children with severe lupus in whom steroids have failed. Therapy should begin with a dose of 2.5 mg/kg/d and should not exceed 5 mg/kg/d. However, uncertainty about the influence of this agent on immune regulation in SLE requires that further studies be carried out before general use is recommended.

Antiphospholipid Syndrome (Lupus Anticoagulant Syndrome)

This syndrome is characterized by the presence of circulating antibodies to phospholipids in association with clinical hypercoagulability (venous and arterial thromboses, stroke, fetal loss, myocardial infarction) and with thrombocytopenia and livedo reticularis.[96] Although most patients with this phenomenon have SLE, some may have no other manifestations of lupus and their condition is referred to as "the antiphospholipid syndrome."[96] Patients may demonstrate false-positive tests for syphilis (VDRL or RPR), prolonged activated partial thromboplastin time (aPTT) and specific anticardiolipin antibodies as measured by enzyme-linked immunosorbent assay (ELISA).[97] Although the mechanisms leading to clinical hypercoagulability in this syndrome are not fully understood, patients with the condition are clearly at risk of thromboembolic complications and may benefit from antithrombotic therapy.[97] In our institution, children who have a cerebrovascular accident or other thromboembolic event due to the antiphospholipid syndrome are managed with anticoagulation: heparin intravenously, followed by conversion to oral warfarin. Patients with circulating antiphospholipid antibodies but without thrombotic manifestations are given daily low-dose aspirin for platelet antagonist effect.

Putting It All Together (Algorithms 1 and 2)

Management of the child or adolescent with SLE requires use of clinical and laboratory guidelines, attention to detail, and individualization of therapy. General measures include the provision of adequate rest, sun protection, symptomatic therapy and appropriate immunizations. Disease education, emotional support, and coordination with the school by the multidisciplinary treatment team represent important components of helping the child and the family to normalize their lifestyle.

NEONATAL LUPUS

This rare syndrome is characterized by at least one of the following clinical manifestations: discoid skin lesions, thrombocytopenia, hemolytic anemia, hepatic inflammation, and congenital heart block, in association with placentally transmitted anti SS-A or SS-B (anti Ro or anti La) antibodies.[98,99,100] Mothers may not be identified as having an autoimmune illness at the time of birth of an affected infant. They are, however, at high risk of eventually developing SLE, Sjögren's syndrome, or rheumatoid arthritis.[98,101]

Noncardiac manifestations usually resolve spontaneously and completely. Hematologic and hepatic manifestations resolve within weeks to months and discoid skin lesions within 1 year.[98,101] Thrombocytopenia or anemia may require platelet or red blood cell transfusions. Steroids have been used successfully in infants with serious or persistent hematologic or hepatic manifestations.[100] The most serious manifestation of neonatal lupus erythematosus (NLE) is congenital complete heart block (CCHB), which occurs in approximately one half of affected babies[101] and is associated with 30% mortality.[99,102,103] Maternal-fetal transplacental transfer of anti SS-A or SS-B antibodies is thought to initiate cardiac inflammation, resulting in severe damage to the fetal conduction system and other cardiac tissue.[104-106] Attempts at early intervention, aimed at reducing the offending antibody load in the pregnant mother (high-dose steroids and plasmapheresis)[107,108] or at controlling fetal or newborn cardiac inflammation (steroid therapy for the fetus; postnatal plasma exchange, methylprednisolone, and IVIG)[100] have so far not succeeded in preventing CCHB and death from associated hydrops fetalis.[99] Further research to determine the mechanism and timing of cardiac damage is essential to resolve the controversy regarding aggressive treatment of the mother or the fetus.[99]

Early detection of fetal cardiac involvement might permit earlier supportive therapy. Pregnant women at risk (women known to have anti SS-A/SS-B antibodies or a history of previous babies with NLE) should be screened with fetal echocardiography every 2 to 4 weeks, starting at 16 weeks of gestation.[99] Currently, treatment of babies with cardiac NLE is supportive only. It consists of installation of a permanent pacemaker and control of congestive heart failure or pericardial effusion. There have

Algorithm 1. Treatment of Childhood Lupus Erythematosus

*For Renal Involvement see Algorithm 2.

been a few reports of NLE patients who eventually developed SLE.[109-111] Therefore, we recommend long-term follow-up of these babies.

JUVENILE DERMATOMYOSITIS

Juvenile dermatomyositis (JDMS) is an autoimmune multisystem inflammatory illness that primarily affects skin and skeletal muscle. Smooth muscle of the gastrointestinal tract, as well as myocardium, can also be involved. Small-vessel vasculitis is a prominent feature of

the disease in childhood. It can involve the CNS, peripheral nerves, and other internal organs. Calcinosis of cutaneous and subcutaneous tissues, muscles, tendons, and ligaments is a late manifestation that can develop while inflammation is still active or even years after resolution of active disease.

Although spontaneous recovery sometimes occurs, without treatment the disease is fatal in more than one third of the affected children and results in serious morbidity in another third. Treatment with corticosteroids and

Algorithm 2. Treatment of Proliferative Lupus Nephritis in Childhood

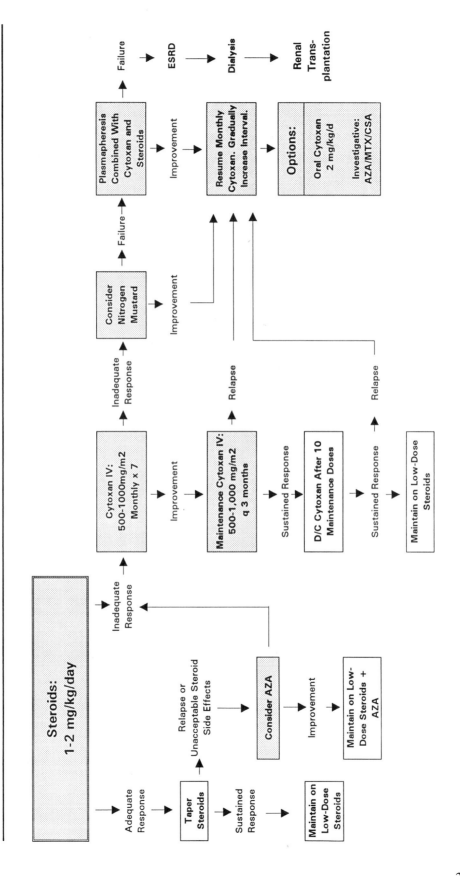

other drugs has greatly improved both survival and outcome in JDMS. Most children recover completely, with residual disability in less than one third. Nevertheless, early respiratory failure and complications of severe vasculitis continue to be leading causes of death in 5% to 10% of patients.[112,113]

Mild-to-Moderate Disease

A few children have minimal skin and muscle disease and no systemic involvement. They usually recover fully without treatment.

Corticosteroids are the mainstay of therapy in most patients.[114] Doses of 1 to 2 mg/kg/d are given during the acute phase. Maximal therapeutic effect is achieved by administration of steroids in divided doses at 6- to 8-hour intervals.[115] With clinical improvement and decreasing muscle enzyme levels, usually by 3 to 6 weeks, gradual tapering of steroids is instituted while the divided daily dose schedule is maintained. Once muscle enzymes have returned to normal and strength has shown consistent improvement, steroids can be consolidated to a single daily dose and slowly tapered. Total duration of steroid therapy is usually months to years.

Electron microscopic studies of muscle biopsy specimens show that fibrin microthrombi are a frequent finding in the early phase of the disease.[116] For this reason, we recommend that patients take low-dose aspirin (one 81 mg tablet daily) early in the course of the disease. The rationale is that thrombotic and ischemic phenomena due to underlying necrotizing vasculitis may thus be prevented. We also recommend the addition of hydroxychloroquine, 6 mg/kg/d, in patients whose dermatitis continues to be a problem even though myositis is controlled.[117]

More recently, we and others have been adding MTX, similar to the regimen used in JRA, to the therapy described above.[118–120] MTX in doses of 0.3 to 0.5 mg/kg once weekly by mouth is well tolerated and appears to provide a steroid-sparing effect and better disease control. Patients receive leucovorin 24 hours after each dose of MTX to reduce potential toxicity.[64] With clinical and laboratory evidence of improvement, steroids are gradually tapered, followed by slow reduction of MTX dosage over months to years.

Severe Disease

A variety of treatments have been used for children with progressive disease whose response to corticosteroids has been inadequate or in whom steroid side effects have been unacceptable:

Methotrexate. Oral doses of 0.6 to 1 mg/kg/wk, 20 mg/m^2,[121] or parenteral administration of 1 to 10 mg/kg every 3 weeks with leucovorin rescue, have resulted in improved muscle strength with decreasing muscle enzyme levels within a few weeks from the start of therapy.[112,122] Steroid sparing has also been noted.

Azathioprine (Imuran). The only therapy for dermatomyositis or polymyositis tested versus prednisone alone in a blinded controlled study,[123] this purine analog may be effective in controlling severe and prolonged disease, as well as in providing a steroid-sparing effect.[124] Onset of action is slow—at least 3 months. The dose is 1 to 2.5 mg/kg/d.

Cyclosporine A. This anti-T cell drug emerges as a promising treatment for children with severe and difficult to control disease.[120,125,126] Added to steroids alone or in combination with MTX, CSA is started at 2 to 5 mg/kg/d. Every effort should be made to keep the dose under 5 mg/kg/d to minimize renal toxicity. Onset of action may take a few weeks. Our experience has been that the drug is effective and usually well tolerated, but careful monitoring of renal function is essential. Pneumocystis carinii in one girl who received combined prednisone, MTX, and CSA treatment for extremely severe disease has led us to carefully monitor such patients for complicating opportunistic infections.

Summary. As disease control is achieved with MTX, AZA, or CSA, steroids are slowly tapered. The duration of therapy with these agents after complete disease control and discontinuation of steroids is still unknown. Our practice is to individualize length of therapy according to prior disease severity, response to treatment, and tolerance of the drug(s). In all cases, tapering should be carried out slowly while patients are monitored for clinical and laboratory evidence of JDMS activity.

Intravenous Immunoglobulin. Recent studies in adults and children have shown that

IVIG might be effective in controlling muscle, skin, and systemic manifestations, as well as in providing a steroid-sparing effect in JDMS.[91,127] Others have been unable to duplicate these results.[128] In our experience, a few children show temporary improvement, while others show little or no benefit. Patients who are deficient in IgA should receive preparations without IgA to prevent anaphylaxis. Possible adverse reactions include fluid overload, allergic reactions, aseptic meningitis, acquired viral infections, and temporary interference with response to vaccination against measles. The latter is due to the presence of antimeasles antibodies in the preparation.[91]

Chlorambucil. A prospective study as well as case reports demonstrated this alkylating drug to be an effective and steroid-sparing agent in adult patients with recalcitrant dermatomyositis in whom other immunosuppressive or cytotoxic therapies failed.[129–131] Oral doses of 0.1 to 0.2 mg/kg/d were used, and a beneficial effect was reported at 4 to 6 weeks. Frequent monitoring for leukopenia and bone marrow suppression, which are reversible, is required. Other potential side effects include azoospermia, teratogenicity, development of malignant disease (lymphoma, leukemia), gastrointestinal irritation, transaminase elevation, CNS irritability, and interstitial pneumonia.[131,132]

Life-threatening Disease

Severe vasculitis of the gastrointestinal tract, heart, lungs, or CNS may lead to potentially fatal complications, such as gastrointestinal perforation, arrhythmias, pulmonary alveolitis, pneumothorax, and neurologic disease. Cyclophosphamide (Cytoxan) may be effective in these situations when administered intravenously in a dose of 10 mg/kg every 2 weeks.[114,133] With consistent control of vasculitis, the interval between doses may be gradually increased. Other approaches include the use of intravenous pulse steroids: a 30 mg/kg dose of methylprednisolone (up to 1 g) daily for 3 days,[134] azathioprine at 2.5 mg/kg/d,[124] or IVIG.[127] Patients who fail to respond adequately to such treatment are at great risk and may benefit from plasmapheresis in combination with steroids and Cytoxan. Although we have seen several instances of desperately ill children who recovered with this treat-

ment, a recent controlled trial in adults with dermatomyositis or polymyositis failed to show efficacy with either leukopheresis or plasmapheresis.[135]

Supportive Measures

Patients with progressive or severe disease are at risk of aspiration, respiratory failure, dehydration, malnutrition, skin sores, and limb contractures due to weakness and debilitation. Supportive measures include elevation of the head, suction, cardiorespiratory monitoring, intravenous fluids, soft foods or parenteral feeding, stool softeners, skin care, and positioning. Psychological support to the child and the family and information about the disease and treatment are provided by the rheumatology team.

Calcinosis

Calcium deposits in the skin, subcutaneous tissue, fat, and fascia occur in more than 40% of children with JDMS within 6 months to years from the onset of disease.[136,137] Superficial masses of calcium may extrude spontaneously. Deep tumorous calcium deposits may liquefy and produce painful sterile abscesses, which frequently require surgical drainage. Deep, chronic ulceration of skin with bacterial superinfection may occur and can cause severe morbidity. These are treated much like full-thickness burns, with whirlpool, debridement, topical or systemic antibiotics, possibly skin grafting, pain control, fluids, and nutritional support. Sheets of calcium may limit mobility of joints or even chest expansion, leading to serious morbidity. Further muscle atrophy and loss of function in the face of well-controlled JDMS may occur as a result of limitation of motion caused by calcinosis.

No effective treatment for calcinosis is known. Warfarin in a low dose (1 mg/d) has been reported to be effective when given early,[138,139] but this has not been confirmed. Many other therapies, including calcitonin, diphosphonates, and chelating agents, have been tried, but none has proved effective. Fortunately, calcinosis spontaneously undergoes complete or partial remission in up to 50% of patients after 5 or more years.[112,114] Since improvement of calcinosis is associated with increased mobility, physical and occupational therapy should be strongly emphasized to prevent or correct contractures and maintain strength and range of motion.

Rehabilitation

Children with JDMS are at risk of long-term morbidity, with limited mobility and loss of independence in activities of daily living (ADL), even in the face of a good response to drug therapy. Prolonged muscle weakness with eventual scarring and development of calcinosis may lead to limited joint motion and loss of function. Physical and occupational therapy should be included in the treatment regimen of JDMS from onset. In the initial phase of acute muscle inflammation, proper positioning of the extremities is essential to avoid development of contractures. This may involve the use of resting splints as well as gentle passive stretching. When inflammation subsides, active exercises are introduced gradually to facilitate strengthening and to increase range of motion, function, and endurance. In addition, specific methods to stretch tight muscle groups or tendons (hamstrings, quadriceps, and gastrocnemius muscles) and to reduce flexion contractures (prolonged prone position on a firm, flat surface or traction for hips, serial casting for knees or elbows, special abduction splints for shoulders) may be used. The overall aim of the rehabilitative effort is to reverse the process of muscle deterioration, reduce contractures, and improve strength so as to enable these children to achieve optimal functioning.

POSTSTREPTOCOCCAL REACTIVE ARTHRITIS

Poststreptococcal reactive arthritis (PSRA) is the most common of a group of arthritides that can follow bacterial or viral infections in children. As initially described by Goldsmith and Long[140] in 1982, it is characterized by mostly symmetrical arthritis and arthralgias associated with fever and sometimes rash after a group A β-hemolytic streptococcal infection. It is distinguished from classic rheumatic fever (ARF) by longer duration of arthritis with involvement of small as well as large joints in a nonmigratory pattern and less dramatic response to aspirin. Resolution in 2 to 12 months can be expected. Recurrent episodes may occur.[141] In addition, there have been reports of some children with

apparent PSRA later developing signs of carditis, including valvular disease.[142-144]

Initial intervention includes administration of antibiotics to eradicate acute streptococcal infection. NSAIDs, such as ibuprofen, 35 to 45 mg/kg/d in three to four doses, or naproxen, 15 to 20 mg/kg/d in two doses (the mechanism of action and potential adverse effects are described earlier) are prescribed. As symptoms resolve, these drugs are gradually discontinued.

The issue of prophylactic treatment for prevention of further streptococcal infections is controversial, even in our own unit.[141,144] If prophylaxis is decided upon, monthly intramuscular injections of long-acting penicillin are the most reliable mode of prophylaxis: 0.6 million units for patients who weigh less than 27 kg and 1.2 million units for those weighing more than 27 kg. Alternatively, if good compliance is assured, oral penicillin (Pen•Vee K, 250 mg twice a day) may be used on a daily basis. Children who are allergic to penicillin receive erythromycin.

CHILDHOOD VASCULITIC SYNDROMES

Idiopathic inflammation of blood vessels characterizes a few syndromes that were traditionally classified according to affected vessel size, major organs involved, and histopathology of damaged vessel wall.[145] The recent discovery of antibodies to specific cytoplasmic antigens in neutrophils (antineutrophil cytoplasmic antibodies [ANCAs]) has revolutionized this classification, shed light on possible pathogenic mechanisms responsible for some vasculitides, and enhanced the ability to diagnose, treat, and follow ANCA-associated vasculitic conditions such as Wegener's granulomatosis.[146]

Henoch-Schönlein purpura and Kawasaki disease are the most common idiopathic vasculitides occurring before the age of 20 and are mostly unique to this age group. Their management, as well as that of the more rare forms of vasculitis in childhood, will be discussed in the following section.

Henoch-Schönlein Purpura

A wide spectrum of clinical manifestations, including nonthrombocytopenic purpura, gastrointestinal pain and bleeding, and large-joint arthritis, may occur in Henoch-Schönlein purpura (HSP) because of IgA-mediated necrotizing inflammation of small vessels. This vasculitis can also involve the CNS, scrotum, testes, and lungs.[147–149] The severity and extent of vasculitis determine the severity of the acute-phase manifestations as well as the long-term outcome. About half of the patients experience occult or frank gastrointestinal bleeding, which in 2% leads to intussusception. Acute hematuria develops in half of the children but progresses to end-stage disease in fewer than 1%.[147,148] Death occurs in 2% of cases during the acute phase, usually as a result of rapidly progressive glomerulonephritis or bowel obstruction.[150,151] Long-term morbidity and mortality are determined by the extent and progression of renal involvement.[147,152] In spite of the potential for serious manifestations and complications, HSP usually follows a self-limited course, with complete resolution in 4 to 6 weeks. This fact and the lack of controlled studies contribute to the controversy regarding efficacy of the various treatment modalities that are currently used.

Mild Disease. Patients with mild manifestations, such as rash, arthritis, abdominal pain, and malaise, are treated with supportive measures (hydration, pain control, nutritional support) and reassurance while being monitored for evidence of GI, renal, or other major organ involvement. Although NSAIDs may be effective for the joint manifestations, these drugs should be used with caution since they may confuse and aggravate the clinical picture if disease-related gastrointestinal bleeding or glomerulonephritis develops.[152] Discomfort may result from the purpuric rash and its underlying edema. Steroid therapy is effective but should be reserved for exceptionally severe symptoms.[153] Monitoring for evidence of renal disease with urinalyses and periodic blood pressure checks should continue for 1 year after resolution of illness. Since persistence of hematuria is a poor prognostic sign, such patients require more prolonged monitoring of renal function.

Moderate-to-Severe Disease

Gastrointestinal Bleeding or Severe Pain. Although most patients respond well to steroids at 1 to 2 mg/kg/d in divided doses,[153] controversy exists about their use, with two recent studies report-

ing no advantage over supportive measures alone.[154,155] In one controlled study, factor XIII, which reportedly is decreased in severe abdominal vasculitis, was used as effective therapy.[156] Complicating intussusception may respond to reduction by barium enema. Persistent intussusception or perforation requires surgical intervention.

Renal Involvement. The debate over whether steroids administered prophylactically or early in the course of nephritis will prevent development or progression of kidney disease is ongoing. One prospective study found prophylactic treatment with steroids to be effective in preventing renal disease,[157] while a more recent study concluded no such benefit.[158] Patients at increased risk of glomerulonephritis (onset over age 9, persistent rash, bloody stools) and those at risk of progression to end-stage renal disease (proteinuria or nephrotic syndrome)[152] should probably receive a trial of steroid therapy at 1 to 2 mg/kg/d in divided doses, with slow taper on improvement.

Treatment regimens for HSP glomerulonephritis can be difficult to evaluate because of the high rate of spontaneous resolution and the lack of randomized controlled trials. Furthermore, clean and definite efficacy has not been documented with any of the currently described therapies for persistent or progressive disease. These include steroids, cyclophosphamide, azathioprine, cyclosporine, plasmapheresis, and anticoagulation.[159] Patients who progress to renal failure may benefit from kidney transplantation.

CNS Vasculitis or Vasculitis in Other Organs. Steroids (daily divided doses of 1 to 2 mg/kg or pulses) are the mainstay of therapy.[153] Cyclophosphamide, plasmapheresis, and other cytotoxic agents may be used for progressive disease but are rarely required.

Kawasaki Disease

Kawasaki disease (KD) is an acute vasculitis of young children, involving small and medium-sized arteries in multiple organs. In spite of intensive research, the cause of KD is still unknown. Infantile polyarteritis nodosa, a serious and often fatal arteritis initially thought to be an early-age form of polyarteritis nodosa, is now recognized as identical to KD.[160] KD, like the adult form of polyarteritis nodosa, has been shown to be associated with ANCAs. In KD, however, clinical correlation of ANCAs with phase of the disease, severity, or outcome has not been shown.[161,162] Recently, superantigens have been implicated in the severe immune activation characteristic of KD.[163]

Most of the acute inflammatory manifestations of this disease follow a self-limited course and resolve without sequelae, even if untreated.[164] The most serious manifestation, which largely determines the long-term outlook, is coronary artery involvement. Without treatment, coronary aneurysms develop in 15% to 20% of patients.[148,164] Giant aneurysms, larger than 8 mm in diameter, are especially dangerous, since they do not undergo spontaneous regression and may result in stenosis and thrombosis, with resulting cardiac ischemia.[165,166] Aspirin, one of the first drugs used for KD was shown in a few retrospective studies to reduce the length of the febrile phase as well as the rate of coronary aneurysm formation.[167,168] Steroids, initially reported to produce encouraging results,[169] were later found to be associated with increased risk of coronary involvement.[170] For this reason, steroids are now avoided in KD except for certain life-threatening manifestations, such as nonischemic myocarditis.[164,171]

High-dose IVIG, in conjunction with ASA, became the cornerstone of KD treatment in the early 1980s. At that time, multicenter controlled clinical trials documented that early treatment reduced the incidence and severity of coronary aneurysms (from 20% to 8%) as well as the length of the febrile and acute inflammatory phase.[166,172] Studies followed to compare the efficacy of various single-dose regimens (always in conjunction with antiinflammatory doses of ASA) with the initial protocol of four daily doses of 400 mg/kg of IVIG in order to define the most efficient way of administering this expensive therapy.[173] A recent large controlled study showed that a single dose of 2 gm/kg of IVIG significantly reduced the incidence of coronary artery aneurysms and hastened resolution of fever and other inflammatory manifestations, without greater risk of adverse effects.[174] The importance of administration of IVIG within the first 10 to 12 days of illness in preventing formation of large aneurysms and fostering resolution of smaller ones is emphasized in all studies. Recent studies

demonstrating that antibodies in IVIG block superantigen-mediated T cell activation[175] or react against ANCA[176] suggest these as possible mechanisms of IVIG action.

The authors recommend the following for treatment of KD:

1. Admission of patients to hospital for monitoring of acute inflammatory symptoms in multiple organs, especially the cardiovascular, CNS, and gastrointestinal systems. Inpatient monitoring for defervescence of fever and subsidence of acute inflammatory manifestations, as well as for disease complications and treatment side effects is continued for 1 to 2 days after therapy.

2. Initiation of antiinflammatory doses of ASA and general supportive measures. IVIG, in a single dose of 2 gm/kg, is infused as a 5% solution over 10 to 12 hours. Patients are treated with IVIG, provided that the diagnosis has been made within 10 days of the onset of fever or that symptoms and laboratory signs of inflammation persist. This may be repeated once if fever recurs 48 hours or more after the initial dose.

3. Continuation of ASA in antiinflammatory doses (80 to 100 mg/kg/d, in four divided doses) until fever and acute inflammatory symptoms have resolved (usually 10 to 14 days).

4. Reduction of ASA dose to 3 to 5 mg/kg/d for an antithrombotic effect after resolution of fever. If coronary abnormalities are not detected, aspirin is discontinued when the platelet count and sedimentation rate have returned to normal (usually 7 to 8 weeks). In patients in whom coronary artery disease develops low-dose ASA therapy is continued.

5. Cardiac follow-up. A second echocardiogram is performed at 5 to 9 days after IVIG. Normal coronary appearance within 14 days after treatment is associated with virtually no risk of aneurysms later developing.[177] These patients are allowed to return gradually to normal levels of physical activity and school participation and are followed clinically. An echocardiogram is repeated once, 1 year after onset, to verify normal cardiac structure and function. Further echocardiograms are not indicated unless symptoms are present. Children with coronary artery disease require close cardiologic follow-up.

6. Treatment of persistent arthralgia or arthritis within the first 2 months of illness with NSAIDs (ibuprofen, 40 mg/kg/d or naproxen, 15 to 20 mg/kg/d).

7. Recurrence of acute KD after complete resolution of the initial episode is reported in 2% of patients.[178] Treatment is identical.

Polyarteritis Nodosa

Polyarteritis nodosa (PAN) is a rare disease in childhood in which necrotizing vasculitis of unknown origin involves small and medium-sized arteries in multiple sites, especially in the mesenteric, hepatic, renal, coronary, cutaneous, central, and peripheral nervous systems. Diversity of clinical manifestations is characteristic. These include fever, myalgia, skin lesions, abdominal symptoms, hypertension, glomerulonephritis, central or peripheral neurologic abnormalities, lung and cardiac findings, as well as laboratory evidence of acute-phase reactants.[179,180] Group A streptococcal infection is sometimes associated with onset or exacerbation of childhood PAN.[141] The spectrum of disease severity in childhood ranges from a limited cutaneous form to progressive organ involvement. Although attempts have been made to define clinical diagnostic criteria for childhood PAN,[180] definite diagnosis still requires typical biopsy or angiographic findings. In the future ANCA determination may permit earlier diagnosis and more reliable prediction of outcome. These antibodies, especially those directed against myeloperoxidase, are detected in 10% to 40% of adult patients with severe systemic involvement.[146,181]

The extent and reversibility of organ involvement determines the outcome of PAN. Hence, early diagnosis and prompt institution of therapy are essential. Renal impairment and CNS or severe gastrointestinal involvement are indications of poor prognosis.[180] Before steroids came into use, most children succumbed to these complications within the first year of disease.[182] Survival increased markedly with the introduction of corticosteroids in the 1960s.[183] Recently, a prospective randomized clinical trial in adults[184] showed that combined steroid and cyclophosphamide therapy improved the clinical response and reduced the number of disease episodes. Unfortunately, combined therapy did not appear to alter the survival rate (75% at 10 years with steroids alone). Similarly, another randomized trial cited better than 75% survival at 4 years.[185] This study, involving small numbers of patients, was unable to demonstrate any significant difference between treatment results with steroids alone or in combination with cytotoxic agents.

The Authors' Approach to Treatment. A few children have very limited cutaneous disease and may respond to NSAIDs. In general, however, steroids are the keystone of therapy.[180,183,186]

PAN Without Organ or Life-threatening Involvement. Steroids are administered intravenously or orally at 1 to 2 mg/kg/d in divided doses. With adequate response, usually in a few weeks, steroids are tapered. Patients are continued on low daily or alternate-day therapy until there is no evidence of active disease. Patients are closely monitored thereafter.

Organ- or Life-threatening Disease. Methylprednisolone pulse therapy (30 mg/kg up to 1 g per dose daily for 3 days) may be beneficial for CNS vasculitis.[186] Central or peripheral nervous system disease that does not respond to pulse steroids, as well as other severe disease manifestations such as significant gastrointestinal vasculitis, progressive glomerulonephritis, and pulmonary hemorrhage, are treated with a combination of steroids (1 to 2 mg/kg/d in divided doses) and cyclophosphamide[180,183,187] (10 mg/kg intravenously every 2 weeks). As previously discussed, mesna may be administered with Cytoxan (milligram for milligram) to prevent bladder complications. With adequate response, the interval between Cytoxan doses may be gradually increased. If necessary, efficacy may be enhanced by oral administration of Cytoxan (daily doses of 1 to 2 mg/kg); however, risk of infections and other adverse reactions increases. To minimize these risks, the frequency of Cytoxan administration may be reduced to 3 to 4 days per week, once improvement has begun.

• • •

Although efficacy of plasmapheresis in PAN is a subject of ongoing debate,[184,185] patients with pulmonary bleeding, rapidly progressive glomerulonephritis, or other life-threatening complications who respond inadequately to steroids and Cytoxan may benefit from the addition of plasmapheresis.

General supportive measures in all patients include control of hypertension, maintenance of normal hemodynamic status, and treatment of infection.

Wegener's Granulomatosis

Wegener's granulomatosis (WG) is a rare form of necrotizing granulomatous vasculitis in which the upper and lower respiratory systems and the kidneys are primarily involved. Clinical manifestations range from limited disease (only nasal sinus, ear, or upper airways affected) to the more generalized form (multiple systems involved, especially lungs and kidneys). Fever, arthralgia, and myalgia are common.[188,189] Untreated, the disease progresses rapidly and is often fatal. Daily steroid and Cytoxan therapy has greatly improved the course and survival of this illness. Outcome still depends on early diagnosis and prompt institution of therapy before the development of irreversible organ damage. Antibodies to proteinase 3 (c-ANCA), which are highly sensitive and specific to this condition, are used to hasten diagnosis and onset of therapy.[190] Recent evidence that a fourfold rise in ANCA frequently precedes relapse leads to the use of c-ANCA titers as a guide to therapy.[191,192] Standard treatment of WG combines daily oral Cytoxan at 2 mg/kg with daily steroids at 1 mg/kg.[193] As initial symptoms resolve, usually in 3 to 12 months, steroids are gradually tapered. Cytoxan is usually maintained for at least 1 year after complete remission and then gradually tapered while patients are monitored for evidence of clinical or laboratory reactivation. This treatment regimen was recently shown to result in complete remission in 75% of patients and marked improvement in 91% after a median of 12 months. Remissions lasted longer than 5 years in a significant number of patients. However, more than half have experienced one or more relapses within 3 months to 16 years from remission. Thirteen percent mortality due to complications of disease as well as of therapy was found.[188] A higher rate of disease relapse was associated with pulse Cytoxan therapy in two studies.[188,194] Although a favorable response to trimethoprim sulfamethoxazole was reported in selected patients,[195–197] this was not confirmed

in a prospective NIH trial.[188] A novel approach to the treatment of WG is the use of weekly oral methotrexate in low doses (as for rheumatoid arthritis) after initial induction of remission with steroids and Cytoxan.[188] This requires further study.

LIMITED SCLERODERMA

Localized scleroderma is the most common form of scleroderma in childhood. The disease may be limited to one or a few patches of sclerotic skin, also termed morphea, or it may occur as a linear sclerotic band (linear scleroderma). When linear lesions affect the face or scalp, they may resemble a sabre scar, termed *en coup de sabre*. Although the disease is not life threatening, linear bands may result in atrophy of the face or extremities, joint contractures, and failure of limbs to grow and develop. In addition, there may be localized involvement of adjacent internal organs, including brain, subcutaneous structures, muscle, bone, synovium, and blood vessels.[198,199] Unlike localized morphea lesions, linear lesions seldom regress spontaneously. The functional and cosmetic effects may lead to serious emotional difficulties.

A major impediment to treating this disease has been the lack of any laboratory parameter that indicates disease activity.[200] Since the clinical condition changes very slowly in many cases, it is often difficult to determine which patients need treatment. Recently, serum levels of soluble interleukin-2 receptor were shown to correlate with disease activity in limited scleroderma.[201] Further studies will be needed to confirm the use of this test as a marker of disease activity and a guide to therapy.

In very early stages of the disease clinical signs of inflammation, including erythema and swelling, are sometimes seen. In such patients a short course of steroids may be prescribed. For children with more chronic, slowly progressive disease, steroids are not effective and should not be used.

D-Penicillamine (D-PEN) has been the major agent used to treat this condition in our unit.[202,203] Our experience with this treatment is that it may prevent further progression of disease but does not reverse the restriction of limb growth. A recent long-term prospective study in adults[204] confirmed regression of sclerosis and induration, as well as increased softening and pliability of skin with D-PEN treatment, perhaps by interference with molecular cross-linking of collagen.[205]

Potential toxicities of this drug include the following[204,206–209]:

1. Nausea, vomiting, dysgeusia (loss of taste), dermatitis, and pruritus
2. Proteinuria progressing to nephrotic syndrome
3. Cytopenia; hypogammaglobulinemia
4. Autoimmune diseases, such as myasthenia gravis, lupus, Goodpasture's syndrome, and polymyositis.

We recommend D-PEN for children whose disease appears to be progressive and likely to produce severe disfigurement or limb shortening. The dose used is 3 to 10 mg/kg/d, not to exceed 750 mg. Treatment starts at the lower dose and is advanced at monthly intervals. The drug should always be taken on an empty stomach without other medications. Laboratory monitoring includes monthly blood counts and urinalyses with liver function tests and immunoglobulin levels at longer intervals.

More effective agents are clearly needed. Immune modulation by drugs such as cyclosporine and methotrexate is currently being investigated.[210–212]

Surgical release of scar tissue and skin grafting may improve range of motion, even though the grafted area may become involved in the disease process. When limb shortening is severe, a surgical approach to limit growth of the uninvolved extremity, such as epiphysiodesis, can be considered. Timing is critical, since this procedure is beneficial only when the normal limb is still growing. In rare cases, amputation of a severely deformed distal extremity that is interfering with function may be necessary.

As in other chronic rheumatic diseases, we use a team approach to treat these children. Physical and occupational therapists, a nurse, and a social worker work together to enable these children to function with minimal physical and emotional disability.

REFLEX NEUROVASCULAR DYSTROPHY

Reflex neurovascular dystrophy (RND) is a noninflammatory musculoskeletal pain syndrome characterized by severe extremity pain, tenderness to light touch, and changes in vasomotor instability. Underrecognized in children, it is most commonly seen in adolescent girls, but it can occur in younger children and in either sex. Although the outlook is better in children than in adults, RND can produce long-term disability and trophic changes, with eventual permanent damage to the affected extremity.[213]

Personality factors may be important in predisposing to this disease. Characteristically, children with RND tend to be overachievers. They *seem* to be "perfect children from perfect families." Secondary gain (a respite from responsibilities?) is often operative.

The goal of treatment is to improve function, rather than to relieve pain. In RND pain is generally not amenable to direct therapeutic intervention. Furthermore, our experience has demonstrated that pain tends to resolve as function improves. Accordingly, when the patient complains of pain we listen, but we move on to other issues as soon as possible. The basic therapeutic approach is to treat with a combination of physical therapy, aimed at fostering use of the involved extremity, and psychological counseling to help the child deal with underlying feelings and conflicts in more appropriate ways. We make it clear to patients that the more they use the involved extremity, the quicker it is going to get better; whereas disuse will worsen the condition.

Although there are reports in the literature of some adult patients benefitting from corticosteroids, ganglionic blocking agents, and chemical sympathetic blocks, experience in our unit has been that these modes of treatment generally produce short-lived or no benefit and may be associated with toxic effects. Furthermore, they may divert the patient from dealing with the underlying psychological issues. Except for the rare patient in whom emotional factors do not seem important, our tendency has been to avoid these forms of therapy.

Treatment begins with a clear, straightforward discussion of the diagnosis and its implications with the child and parents. As soon as the diagnosis is established, the child and parents should be so informed in definite terms. The important role that emotional factors may play in causing the disease should be explained. The fact that, with treatment, the prognosis is good can be emphasized. This is the time to set the stage for ongoing psychotherapy. In our experience, it has been crucial for the family to deal with the emotional aspects of the disease in order to ultimately achieve an excellent outcome. Although the prognosis for short-term improvement with physical therapy alone is good, without psychological intervention there is likely to eventually be a relapse of RND or other psychosomatic illness.

In mild cases outpatient management may suffice. When symptoms are more severe and long-standing, however, admission to a rehabilitation center is indicated.

Management in the Rehabilitation Center

The initial approach is crucial. If not yet done, the diagnosis and its implications, both physical and emotional, must be explained to the patient and the family. At this time the discharge goal is set up. A typical goal for a child with lower-extremity involvement might be ambulation for a reasonable distance, wearing shoes and socks, with no more than a minimal limp. Prosthetic devices and aids, such as wheelchairs, crutches, and braces, are quickly withdrawn. Patients are permitted mild analgesics, such as acetaminophen, but they are advised that drugs are not likely to provide major pain relief.

A weekly conference of multidisciplinary team members is held to review the patient's progress and to set a series of objectives for the week. These objectives, usually exercises involving use of the involved extremity, must be quantifiable and sufficiently challenging that the patient will have to work hard to accomplish them by the end of the week. At the same time, they must be realistic and attainable. We tell the patient and the family that the week begins on Monday and ends on Sunday. If the weekly objective is achieved earlier (e.g., Friday) the child may have a weekend pass. If not, "That is OK! But of course, the work must continue until the objective is met," so no pass is given. In this way, we attempt to avoid having the child interpret not getting a pass as punishment.

Role of the Therapeutic Team Members

Physician (Pediatric Rheumatologist). The physician sets the overall direction of the patient's management, determines the discharge goal, conducts team meetings, communicates with parents, and regularly evaluates the patient. He or she must be prepared to play the role of the "bad guy" when appropriate.

Nurse. The registered nurse plays a central role in the day-to-day coordination of the patient's care. Coordinating tasks include scheduling weekly team meetings; presenting and explaining weekly objectives to the patient; and checking on the patient's progress in meeting these objectives and his or her eligibility for weekend pass. The nurse is responsible for reporting 24-hour daily nursing observations of patient actions and interactions to the team members. Most important, the nurse has a special role to play in establishing a relationship of trust with the patient. He or she provides emotional support by encouraging the patient to talk about feelings and express anger appropriately. The nurse listens to the patient's complaints of pain but does not dwell on them and, at the same time, provides support to the family.

Physical Therapist. The physical therapist provides weight-bearing exercises for the involved extremity. Desensitization techniques, such as vigorous toweling or immersion in contrast baths, are applied. Atrophied muscles and endurance are improved. Throughout this process, choices are permitted within limits. That is, a "win-win" situation is set up so that the child attains his or her objectives while at the same time being allowed a certain amount of control over the treatment regimen. For example, the patient may be given the choice of vigorously toweling the involved extremity himself for a longer period or having the therapist do it for a shorter period. This fosters assertiveness, a trait frequently lacking in these children. Throughout the process, the therapist uses a firm but nonpunitive approach.

Occupational Therapist. Characteristically, children with RND are overachievers. Clearly, being an overachiever carries with it a psychological price. Therefore, the occupational therapist evaluates the patient's capabilities and the psychological costs involved in reaching his or her own or the family's expectations. If the expectations are not appropriate, the team works with the family to modify them. The occupational therapist's role also extends to facilitation of age-appropriate activities and interactions. He or she provides opportunities for the child to make choices and to exercise age-appropriate independence.

In childhood RND the upper extremity is involved less commonly than the lower extremity. When upper-extremity involvement is present, however, the occupational therapist provides tasks that require hand and arm use in much the same way the physical therapist does for the lower extremity.

The Parents. The parents form a vital component of the therapeutic team. Without their active participation, recovery tends to be slower and relapses more common. Mother and father should be enlisted as full members of the team. We encourage both to participate with the child in the exercise program. We instruct the parents to "cheer the child on" and to avoid negative statements about the activity. For example, when the child is working out on the stationary bicycle, the parent might do the same on another bicycle.

Social Worker or Psychologist. The role of this team member (in our unit, the social worker) is crucial in terms of the long-term outlook. The social worker's first task is to evaluate patient and family psychosocial dynamics. His or her experience in dealing with many RND cases has proved to be an extremely valuable asset, since a number of these patients, when previously evaluated elsewhere, had been informed that there were no psychological problems. Our studies, in contrast, have established a high frequency of subtle family conflict, difficulty in expressing anger, and enmeshment with the mother. The father, on the other hand, is frequently viewed by patient and the mother as being powerful but remote, and sometimes the mother appears to have a vested interest in keeping him that way.

Although the patient is the one with the symptoms, RND is frequently a family disorder—and family therapy may be highly desirable. The social worker, often using a psychiatrist as a consultant, provides both family and individual therapy during the inpatient phase of treatment. He or she usually refers the family for outpatient counseling after discharge.

The treatment program outlined above has evolved in our institution over many years. It has proved to be highly effective in returning the great majority of patients to normal life, with a very low rate of disease recurrence.

FIBROMYALGIA

Childhood fibromyalgia (FMS), another "noninflammatory pain syndrome," is more common than RND and also is underrecognized in children. It is characterized by chronic musculoskeletal pain, fatigue, and the presence of characteristic tender points.[214] There is often an associated sleep disturbance. In contrast to RND, objective physical changes are not seen. Emotional factors, especially related to family dysfunction, play a role in many childhood cases. Many of these patients are referred to the pediatric rheumatologist to rule out juvenile rheumatoid arthritis or SLE, sometimes because of a false-positive antinuclear antibody (ANA) test.

With a few exceptions, treatment is usually carried out in the outpatient setting. The treatment program addresses the emotional as well as the somatic aspects of the condition by combining the efforts of physician, nurse, physical and occupational therapists, and social worker. First, the child and the family are reassured that this is not a destructive chronic disease and that the long-term outlook is good.

The patient is evaluated by the social worker, physical therapist, occupational therapist, and rheumatology nurse. After carrying out a nursing assessment, the team nurse teaches the child and family about FMS. The social worker fully evaluates the child and family to assess possible psychological stress factors or disorders. He or she provides the patient and family support or counseling and arranges for community mental health referral if indicated. Both nurse and social worker emphasize the importance of participation in normal activities and advise the parents on how to avoid situations in which secondary gain may result from the child's complaints of pain.

Since children with FMS are deconditioned because of physical inactivity, the physical therapist develops a graduated reconditioning exercise program to be followed daily at home. Strengthening and flexibility exercises are prescribed. The exercise program stresses postural awareness and correction of poor posture, as well as activities aimed at improving endurance.

The occupational therapist assesses the impact of FMS on the child's daily life. The child's use of body mechanics during typical activities is evaluated and modified if necessary. The child is instructed on the use of relaxation techniques. Myofascial release is used to relieve trigger points, and children (as well as parents) are taught to use these releases at home so that they may take an active role in their treatment and reduce dependence on the medical team. With these various modalities, muscle stress and pain can be decreased and overall function and sense of well-being improved. Most important, the child will begin to develop a sense of having some control over the disease.

Amitriptyline (Elavil) may be useful when sleep disturbance is present.[215] We prescribe 10 to 25 mg at bedtime. The drug has an atropine-like effect and, therefore, may cause dryness of the mouth and other mucous membranes. We have not seen urinary retention or increased intraocular pressure in any of our patients. The drug should not be used in combination with cimetidine, which delays its elimination and may enhance toxicity. It should be used with caution in patients who are taking antihypertensive agents. Uncommon adverse effects include arrhythmias and nonspecific changes in the electrocardiogram, various CNS effects and anticholinergic effects, including paralytic ileus. In addition, this drug is known to be teratogenic and to be excreted in breast milk. Elavil has not been approved by the FDA for use in children under the age of 12. In our experience, however, the small doses prescribed (much lower than those used to treat depression) are well tolerated.

REFERENCES

1. Lehman TJA. Long term outcome of systemic lupus erythematosus in childhood. Rheum Dis Clin North Am 1991;17:921.
2. Glidden RS, Mantzouranis EC, Borel Y. Systemic lupus erythematosus in childhood: clinical manifestations and improved survival in fifty-five patients. Clin Immunol Immunopathol 1983;29:196.
3. Platt JL, Burke BA, Fish AJ, et al. Systemic lupus erythematosus in the first two decades of life. Am J Kidney Dis 1982;2(S1):212.
4. White PH. Pediatric systemic lupus erythematosus and neonatal lupus. Rheum Dis Clin North Am 1994;20:119.
5. Lehman TJA, McCurdy DK, Bernstein BH, et al. Systemic lupus erythematosus in the first decade of life. Pediatrics 1989;83:235.
6. King KK, Kornreich HK, Bernstein BH, et al. The clinical spectrum of systemic lupus erythematosus in childhood. Arthritis Rheum 1977;20:287.
7. Wallace DJ. Antimalarial agents and lupus. Rheum Dis Clin North Am 1994;20:243.
8. Callen JP. Intralesional triamcinolone is effective for discoid lupus erythematosus of the palms and soles. J Rheumatol 1985;12:630.
9. Shehade S. Successful treatment of generalized discoid skin lesions with azathioprine (Letter). Arch Dermatol 1986;122:376.
10. Tsokos GC, Caughman SW, Klippel JH. Successful treatment of generalized discoid skin lesions with azathioprine. Its use in patients with systemic lupus erythematosus. Arch Dermatol 1985;121:1323.
11. Wallace DJ. Principles of therapy and local measures. In: Wallace DJ, Hahn BH, eds. Dubois' Lupus Erythematosus. Philadelphia: Lea & Febiger, 1993.
12. Bernstein BH, Singsen BH, King KK, et al. Aspirin induced hepatotoxicity and its effect on juvenile rheumatoid arthritis. Am J Dis Child 1977;131:659.
13. Schaller JG. Chronic salicylate administration in juvenile rheumatoid arthritis. Aspirin "hepatitis" and its clinical significance. Pediatrics 1978;62:916.
14. Klinenberg JR, Miller F. Effect of corticosteroids on blood salicylate concentration. JAMA 1965;194:131.
15. Lockshin MD. Antiphospholipid antibody syndrome. Rheum Dis Clin North Am 1994;20:45.
16. Somerville K, Faulkner G, Langman M. Nonsteroidal antiinflammatory drugs and bleeding peptic ulcer. Lancet 1986;1:462.
17. Brater DC. Drug-drug and drug-disease interactions with nonsteroidal antiinflammatory drugs. Am J Med 1986;80(suppl 1A):62.
18. Katz LM, Love PY. Hepatic dysfunction in association with NSAIDs. In: Famaey JP, Paulus HE, eds. Nonsteroidal antiinflammatory drugs: subpopulation therapy and drug delivery systems. New York: Marcel Dekker, 1991.
19. Kimberly RP. Corticosteroids and antiinflammatory drugs. Rheum Dis Clin North Am 1988;14:203.
20. Walsh JJ, Venuto RC. Acute oliguric renal failure induced by indomethacin: possible mechanisms. Ann Intern Med 1979;91:47.
21. Erikkson LO, Sturfelt G, Thysell H, Wollheim FA. Effects of sulindac and naproxen on prostaglandin excretion in patients with impaired renal function and rheumatoid arthritis. Am J Med 1990;89:313.
22. Brater DC, Anderson S, Baird B, Campbell WB. Sulindac does not spare the kidney. Clin Pharmacol Ther 1984;35:269.
23. Blackshear JL, Napier JS, Davidman M, Stillman MT. Renal complications of nonsteroidal antiinflammatory drugs: identification and monitoring of those at risk. Semin Arthritis Rheum 1985;14:163.

24. Samuelson CO, Williams HJ. Ibuprofen associated aseptic meningitis in systemic lupus erythematosus. West J Med 1979;131:57.
25. O'Brian WM, Bagby GF. Rare adverse reactions to nonsteroidal antiinflammatory drugs. J Rheumatol 1985;12:13, 347, 562, 785.
26. Levy ML, Barron KS, Eichenfield A, Honig PJ. Naproxen induced pseudoporphyria: a distinctive photodermatitis. J Pediatr 1990;117:660.
27. The Canadian Hydroxychloroquine Study Group. A randomized study of the effect of withdrawing hydroxychloroquine sulfate in systemic lupus erythematosus. N Engl J Med 1991;324:150.
28. Wallace DJ. The use of quinacrine (Atabrine) in rheumatic disease: a reexamination. Semin Arthritis Rheum 1989;18:282.
29. Rynes RI, Bernstein HN. Ophthalmologic safety profile of antimalarial drugs. Lupus 1993;2:17.
30. Morsman CD, Livsey SJ, Richards IM, et al. Screening for hydroxychloroquine retinal toxicity: is it necessary? Eye 1990;4:672.
31. Evans RL, Khalid S, Kinney JL. Antimalarial psychosis revisited. Arch Dermatol 1984;120:765.
32. Parillo JE, Fauci AS. Mechanisms of glucocorticoid action on the immune processes. Ann Rev Pharmacol Toxicol 1979;19:179.
33. Szer IS. The diagnosis and management of systemic lupus erythematosus in childhood. Pediatr Ann 1986;15:596.
34. Jacobs JC. Pediatric rheumatology for the practitioner. New York: Springer-Verlag, 1982.
35. Hahn BH. Lupus nephritis: therapeutic decisions. Hosp Pract 1990;25(3A):89.
36. Pollak VE, Dosekun AK. Evaluation of treatment in lupus nephritis: effect of prednisone. Am J Kidney Dis 1982;2(suppl 2):170.
37. Evanson S, Passo MH, Aldo-Benson MA, et al. Methyl prednisolone pulse therapy for non renal lupus erythematosus. Ann Rheum Dis 1980;39:377.
38. Ballou SP, Khan MA, Kushner I. Intravenous pulse methylprednisolone in lupus erythematosus: a prospective evaluation. J Rheumatol 1985;12:944.
39. Hanmer O, Saltissi D. Response of acute cerebral lupus in childhood to pulse methylprednisolone in reduced dosage. Ann Rheum Dis 1986;45:606.
40. Barron KS, Person DA, Brewer EJ, et al. Pulse methylprednisolone therapy in diffuse proliferative lupus nephritis. J Pediatr 1982;101:137.
41. Kimberly RP, Lockshin MD, Sherman RL, et al. Reversible "end-stage" lupus nephritis: analysis of patients able to discontinue dialysis. Am J Med 1983;74:361.
42. McDougal BA, Whittier FC, Cross DE. Sudden death after bolus steroid therapy for acute rejection. Transplant Proc 1976;8:493.
43. Kimberly RP. Pulse methylprednisolone in SLE. Clin Rheum Dis 1982;8:261.
44. Melo-Gomes JA. Problems related to systemic glucocorticoid therapy in children. J Rheumatol 1993;20(suppl 37):35.
45. David J, Loftus J, Hesp R, et al. Spinal and somatic growth in patients with juvenile chronic arthritis treated for up to 2 years with deflazacort. Clin Exp Rheumatol 1992;10:621.
46. Loftus JK, Reeve J, Hesp R, et al. Deflazacort in juvenile chronic arthritis. J Rheumatol 1993;20(suppl 37):40.
47. Urowitz MB, Gladman DD. Late mortality in SLE: "The price we pay for control" J Rheumatol 1980;7:412.
48. Ansell BM. Overview of the side effects of corticosteroid therapy. Clin Exp Rheumatol 1991;9:19.
49. Stjernholm MR, Katz FH. Effects of diphenylhydantoin, phenobarbital, and diazepam on the metabolism of methylprednisolone and its sodium succinate. J Clin Endocrinol Metab 1975;41:877.
50. Buffington GA, Dominguez JH, Piering WF, et al. Interaction of rifampin and glucocorticoids, adverse effects on renal allograft function. JAMA 1976;236:1958.
51. Fox DA, McCune WJ. Immunosuppressive drug therapy of systemic lupus erythematosus. Rheum Dis Clin North Am 1994;20:265.
52. Haga HJ, D'Cruz D, Asherson R, Hughes GRV. Short term effects of intravenous pulse of cyclophosphamide in the treatment of connective tissue disease crisis. Ann Rheum Dis 1992;51:885.
53. Lehman TJA. Current concepts in immunosuppressive drug therapy of systemic lupus erythematosus. J Rheumatol 1992;19(suppl 33):20.
54. De Jesus A, Talal N. Practical use of immunosuppressive drugs in autoimmune disease. Crit Care Med 1990;18:S132.
55. McCune WJ, Globus J, Zeldes W, et al. Clinical and immunologic effects of monthly administration of intravenous cyclophosphamide in severe lupus erythematosus. N Engl J Med 1988;318:1423.
56. McCurdy DK, Lehman TJA, Bernstein BH, et al. Lupus nephritis: controlled trial of prednisone and cytotoxic drugs. Pediatrics 1992;89:240.
57. Austin HA, Klippel JH, Balow JE, et al. Therapy of lupus nephritis: controlled trial of prednisone and cytotoxic drugs. N Engl J Med 1986;314:614.
58. Balow JE, Austin HA, Tsokos GC, et al. NIH Conference: lupus nephritis. Ann Intern Med 1987;106:79.
59. Klippel JH, Austin HA, Balow JE, et al. Studies of immunosuppressive drugs in the treatment of lupus nephritis. Rheum Dis Clin North Am 1987;13:47.
60. Felson DT, Anderson J. Evidence for the superiority of immunosuppressive drugs and prednisone over prednisone alone in lupus nephritis: results of pooled analysis. N Engl J Med 1984;311:1528.

61. Lehman TJA, Sherry DD, Wagner-Weiner L, et al. Intermittent intravenous cyclophosphamide therapy for lupus nephritis. J Pediatr 1990; 114:1055.

62. Wagner-Weiner L, Magilavy DB, Emery HM. Flare of childhood lupus nephritis after discontinuing treatment with intravenous pulse cyclophosphamide (IVCY). Arthritis Rheum 1988; 31(suppl):S117.

63. Abud-Mendoza C, Sturbaum AK, Vasquez-Compean R, Gonzales-Amaro R. Methotrexate therapy in childhood systemic lupus erythematosus. J Rheumatol 1993;20:731.

64. Shiroky JB, Neville C, Easdaile JM, et al. Low dose methotrexate with leukovorin (folinic acid) in the management of rheumatoid arthritis. Arthritis Rheum 1993;36:796.

65. Levitt M, Warr D, Yelle L, et al. Odansteron compared with dexamethasone and metoclopramide as antiemetics in the chemotherapy of breast cancer with cyclophosphamide, methotrexate, and fluorouracil. N Engl J Med 1993; 328:1081.

66. Calabresi P, Parks RE. Alkylating agents, antimetabolites, hormones and other antiproliferative agents. In: Goodman LS, Gilman A, eds. The pharmacological basis of therapeutics. New York: Macmillan, 1975.

67. Plotz PH, Klippel JH, Decker JL, et al. Bladder complications in patients receiving cyclophosphamide for systemic lupus erythematosus or rheumatoid arthritis. Ann Intern Med 1979;91:221.

68. Hows JM, Mehta A, Ward L, et al. Comparison of mesna with forced diuresis to prevent cyclophosphamide-included haemorrhagic cystitis in marrow transplantation: a prospective randomized study. Br J Cancer 1984;50:753.

69. Hellman DB, Petri M, Whiting-O'Keefe Q. Fatal infections in systemic lupus erythematosus: the role of opportunistic organisms. Medicine (Baltimore) 1987;66:341.

70. Averette HE, Boike GM, Jarell MA. Effects of cancer chemotherapy on gonadal function and reproductive capacity. Cancer 1990;40:199.

71. Byrne J, Mulvihill JJ, Myers MH, et al. Effects of treatment on fertility in long term survivors of childhood or adolescent cancer. N Engl J Med 1987;317:1315.

72. Kirshon B, Wasserstrum N, Willis R, et al. Teratogenic effects of first trimester cyclophosphamide therapy. Obstet Gynecol 1988;72:462.

73. Ramsey-Goldman R, Mientus JM, Kutzer JE, Mulvihill JJ, Medsger TA Jr. Pregnancy outcome in women with systemic lupus erythematosus treated with immunosuppressive drugs. J Rheumatol 1993;20:1152.

74. Baker GL, Kahl LE, Zee BC, et al. Malignancy following treatment of rheumatoid arthritis with cyclophosphamide: long term case control follow-up study. Am J Med 1987;83:1.

75. Sztenbok M, Stewart A, Diamond H, Kaplan D. Azathioprine in the treatment of systemic lupus erythematosus: a controlled study. Arthritis Rheum 1971;14:639.

76. Balow JS. Lupus as a renal disease. Hosp Pract. October 15, 1988.

77. Kremer JM. The mechanism of action of methotrexate in rheumatoid arthritis: the search continues [Editorial]. J Rheumatol 1994;21:1.

78. Olsen N. Low dose methotrexate: antiinflammatory or immunosuppressive? [Editorial]. Cleve Clin J Med 1990;57:245.

79. Rothenberg RJ, Graziano FM, Grandote JT, et al. The use of methotrexate in steroid resistant systemic lupus erythematosus. Arthritis Rheum 1988;31:612.

80. Wilke WS, Krall PL, Scheetz RJ, et al. Methotrexate for systemic lupus erythematosus: a retrospective analysis of 17 unselected cases. Clin Exp Rheumatol 1991;9:581.

81. Graham LD, Myones BL, Rivas-Chacon RF, Pachman LM. Morbidity associated with long term methotrexate therapy in juvenile rheumatoid arthritis. J Pediatr 1992;120:468.

82. Dubois EL. Systemic lupus erythematosus: recent advances in its diagnosis and treatment. Ann Intern Med 1956;45:163.

83. Wallace DJ, Podell TE, Weiner JM, et al. Lupus nephritis: experience with 230 patients in a private practice from 1950 to 1980. Am J Med 1982;72:209.

84. Dillard MG, Dujovne I, Pollak VE, et al. The effect of treatment with prednisone and nitrogen mustard on the renal lesions and life span of patients with lupus glomerulonephritis. Nephron 1973;10:273.

85. Lupus Plasmapheresis Study Group. Plasmapheresis and subsequent pulse cyclophosphamide versus pulse cyclophosphamide alone in severe lupus: design of the LPSG trial. J Clin Apheresis 1991;6:40.

86. Hess DC, Kapil S, Awad E. Thrombotic thrombocytopenic purpura in systemic lupus erythematosus and antiphospholipid antibodies: effective treatment with plasma exchange and immunosuppression. J Rheumatol 1992;19: 1474.

87. Smith GM, Leyland MJ. Plasma exchange for cerebral lupus erythematosus [Letter]. Lancet 1987;1:103.

88. Lewis EJ and the Lupus Nephritis Collaborative Study Group. Plasmapheresis therapy is ineffective in SLE. J Clin Apheresis 1992;7: 153.

89. Borg EJT, Kallenberg CGM. Treatment of severe thrombocytopenia in systemic lupus erythematosus with intravenous gammaglobulin. Ann Rheum Dis 1992;51:1149.

90. Winder A, Molad Y, Ostfeld I, et al. Treatment of systemic lupus erythematosus by prolonged administration of high dose immunoglobulin: report of 2 cases. J Rheumatol 1993;20:495.

91. Barron KS, Sher MR, Silverman ED. Intravenous immunoglobulin therapy: magic or black magic. J Rheumatol 1992;19(suppl 33):94.

92. Schreiber SL, Crabtree GR. The mechanism of action of cyclosporin A and FK506. Immunol Today 1992;13:136.

93. Feutren G, Querin S, Noel LH, et al. Effects of cyclosporine in severe systemic lupus erythematosus. J Pediatr 1992;111(6 Pt 2):1063.

94. Favre H, Miescher PA, Huang YP, et al. Cyclosporin in the treatment of lupus nephritis. Am J Nephrol 1989;9(suppl 1):57.

95. Tokuda M, Kurata N, Mizoguchi A, et al. Effect of low dose cyclosporin A on systemic lupus erythematosus disease activity. Arthritis Rheum 1994;37:551.

96. Panush RS, Greer JM, Morshedian KK. What is lupus? What is not lupus? Rheum Dis Clin North Am 1993;19:223.

97. Lockshin MD. Which patients with antiphospholipid antibody should be treated and how? Rheum Dis Clin North Am 1993;19:235.

98. Olsen NY, Lindsley CB. Neonatal lupus syndrome. Am J Dis Child 1987;141:908.

99. Silverman ED. Congenital heart block and neonatal lupus erythematosus: prevention is the goal [editorial]. J Rheumatol 1993;20:1101.

100. Rider LG, Buyon JP, Rutledge J, Sherry DD. Treatment of neonatal lupus: case report and review of the literature. J Rheumatol 1993;20:1208.

101. McCune AB, Weston WL, Lee LA. Maternal and fetal outcome in neonatal lupus erythematosus. Ann Intern Med 1987;106:518.

102. Hardy JD, Solomon S, Banwell GS, et al. Congenital heart block in the newborn associated with maternal systemic lupus erythematosus and other connective tissue disorders. Arch Dis Child 1979;54:7.

103. Waltruk J, Buyon JP. Neonatal and maternal outcome incomplete heart block (CHB). Arthritis Rheum 1992;35:560.

104. Silverman ED, Mamula M, Hardin JA, Laxer R. Importance of the immune response to the Ro/La particle in the development of congenital heart block and neonatal lupus. J Rheumatol 1991;18:120.

105. Taylor PV, Taylor KF, Norman A, et al. Prevalence of maternal Ro (SS-A) and La (SS-B) autoantibodies in relation to congenital heart block. Br J Rheumatol 1988;27:128.

106. Deng JS, Blair LW Jr, Shen-Schwarz S, et al. Localization of Ro (SS-A) antigen in the cardiac conduction system. Arthritis Rheum 1987;30:1232.

107. Buyon JP, Swersky SH, Fox HE, et al. Intrauterine therapy for presumptive fetal myocarditis with acquired heart block due to systemic lupus erythematosus. Arthritis Rheum 1987;30:44.

108. Carreira PE, Gutierrez-Larraya F, Gomez-Reino JJ. Successful intrauterine therapy with dexamethasone for fetal myocarditis and heart block in a woman with systemic lupus erythematosus. J Rheumatol 1993;20:1204.

109. Fox JR, McCuistion CH, Schock EP Jr. Systemic lupus erythematosus: association with previous neonatal lupus erythematosus. Arch Dermatol 1979;115:340.

110. Jackson R, Gulliver M. Neonatal lupus erythematosus progressing into systemic lupus erythematosus. Br J Dermatol 1979;101:81.

111. Lanham JG, Walport MJ, Hughes GV. Congenital heart block and familial connective tissue disease. J Rheumatol 1983;10:823.

112. Spencer CH, Hanson V, Singsen BH, et al. Course of treated juvenile dermatomyositis. J Pediatr 1984;105:399.

113. Ansell BM. Juvenile dermatomyositis. Rev Int Rheum 1989;19:75.

114. Ansell BM. Juvenile dermatomyositis. Rheum Dis Clin North Am 1991;17:931.

115. Pachman LM. Juvenile dermatomyositis: natural history and susceptibility factors. In: Woo P, White P, Ansell, BM, eds. Paediatric rheumatology update. Oxford: Oxford University Press, 1990.

116. Wortmann RL. Inflammatory diseases of muscle. In: Kelley WM, Harris ED, Ruddy S, Sledge CB, eds. Textbook of rheumatology. 4th ed. Philadelphia: WB Saunders, 1993.

117. Olson NY, Lindsley CB. Adjunctive use of hydroxychloroquine in childhood dermatomyositis. J Rheumatol 1989;16:1545.

118. Schnabel A, Gross WL. Low dose methotrexate in rheumatic diseases: efficacy, side effects, and risk factors for side effects. Semin Arthritis Rheum 1994;23:310.

119. Newman ED, Scott DW. The use of low dose oral methotrexate in polymyositis and dermatomyositis. Arthritis Rheum 1993;36:S119.

120. Plotz PH, Dalakas M, Leff R, et al. NIH conference: current concepts in the idiopathic inflammatory myopathies: polymyositis, dermatomyositis, and related disorders. Ann Intern Med 1989;111:143.

121. Miller LC, Sisson BA, Tucker LB, DeNardo BA, Schaller JG. Methotrexate treatment of recalcitrant childhood dermatomyositis. Arthritis Rheum 1992;35:143.

122. Jacobs JC. Methotrexate and azathioprine treatment of childhood dermatomyositis. Pediatrics 1977;59:212.

123. Bunch TW, Worthington JW, Comb JJ, et al. Azathioprine with prednisone for polymyositis: a controlled clinical trial. Ann Intern Med 1980;92:365.

124. Bunch TW. Prednisone and azathioprine for polymyositis: long term follow up. Arthritis Rheum 1981;24:45.

125. Heckmatt J, Saunders C, Peters AM, et al. Cyclosporin in juvenile dermatomyositis. Lancet 1989;1:1063.

126. Pistoia V, Buoncompagni A, Scribanis R, et al. Cyclosporin A in the treatment of juvenile chronic arthritis and childhood polymyositis-dermatomyositis. Clin Exp Rheumatol 1993;11:203.

127. Lang BA, Laxer RM, Murphy G, et al. Treatment of dermatomyositis with intravenous gammaglobulin. Am J Med 1991;91:169.

128. Libman BS, Miller L, Beardmore TD. Controlled N of 1 trials of intravenous gammaglobulin in

resistant polymyositis and dermatomyositis (poster): 21st Western Region Conference, American College of Rheumatology, 1994:28.

129. Sinoway PA, Callen JP. Chlorambucil, an effective corticosteroid-sparing agent for patients with recalcitrant dermatomyositis. Arthritis Rheum 1993;36:319.

130. Cagnoli M, Marchesoni A, Tosi S. Combined steroid, methotrexate and chlorambucil therapy for steroid-resistant dermatomyositis. Clin Exp Rheumatol 1991;9:658.

131. Callen JP. Immunosuppressive and cytotoxic drugs: uses in the dermatology patient. Adv Dermatol 1990;5:3.

132. Rapini RP, Jordon RE, Wolverton SE. Cytotoxic agents. In: Wolverton SE, Wilkin JK, eds. Systemic drugs for skin diseases. Philadelphia: WB Saunders, 1991.

133. Ansell BM. Inflammatory disorders of muscle. Clin Rheum Dis 1984;10:205.

134. Laxer RM, Stein LD, Petty RE. Intravenous pulse methylprednisolone treatment for juvenile dermatomyositis. Arthritis Rheum 1987; 30:329.

135. Miller FW, Leitman SF, Cronin ME, et al. Controlled trial of plasma exchange and leukapheresis in polymyositis and dermatomyositis. N Engl J Med 1992;326:1380.

136. Bowyer SL, Clark RAF, Ragsdale CG, et al. Juvenile dermatomyositis: histological findings and pathogenic hypothesis for the associated skin changes. J Rheumatol 1986;13:753.

137. Blane CE, White SJ, Braunstein EM, et al. Patterns of calcification in childhood dermatomyositis. Am J Radiol 1984;142:397.

138. Berger RG, Featherstone GS, Raasch RH, et al. Treatment of calcinosis universalis with low dose warfarin. Am J Med 1987;83:72.

139. Yoshida S, Torikai K. The effects of warfarin on calcinosis in a patient with systemic sclerosis. J Rheumatol 1993;20:1235.

140. Goldsmith DP, Long SS. Post-streptococcal disease of childhood—a changing syndrome. Arthritis Rheum 1982;25(suppl 4):S18.

141. Fink CW. The role of the streptococcus in post-streptococcal reactive arthritis and childhood polyarteritis nodosa. J Rheumatol 1991;18 (suppl 29):14.

142. Emery H, Wagner-Weiner L, Magilavy D. Resurgence of childhood post-streptococcal rheumatic syndromes. Arthritis Rheum 1987; 30:S80.

143. Hicks R, Yim G. Post-streptococcal reactive arthritis (PSRA)—a manifestation of acute rheumatic fever. Arthritis Rheum 1990;33(suppl 9):S145.

144. Merino-Munoz R, Viota-Losada F, Sanch-Madrid B, et al. Rheumatic fever and post-streptococcal arthritis: clinical review. An Esp Pediatr 1991;35:239.

145. Michel BA. Classification of vasculitis. Curr Opin Rheumatol 1992;4:3.

146. Jeannette JC, Falk RJ. Disease associations and pathogenic role of antineutrophil cytoplasmic autoantibodies in vasculitis. Curr Opin Rheumatol 1992;4:9.

147. Lanzkowsky S, Lanzkowsky L, Lanzkowsky P. Henoch-Schönlein purpura. Pediatr Rev 1992; 13:130.

148. Reimer SS, Sanchez RL. Vasculitis in children. Semin Dermatol 1992;11:48.

149. Belman AL, Leicher CR, Moshe SL, Mezey AP. Neurologic manifestations of Schönlein-Henoch purpura: report of three cases and review of the literature. Pediatrics 1985;75:687.

150. Emery H. Henoch-Schönlein purpura. In: Hicks RV, ed. Vasculopathies in childhood. Littleton, Massachusetts: PSG Publishing Co., 1986.

151. Emery H, Carter W, Schaler SG. Henoch-Schönlein vasculitis. Arthritis Rheum 1977;20: 385.

152. Szer IS. Henoch-Schönlein purpura. Curr Opin Rheumatol 1994;6:25.

153. Allen DM, Diamond LK, Howell DA. Anaphylactoid purpura in children (Schönlein-Henoch syndrome): review with a follow up of the renal complications. Am J Dis Child 1960;99:833.

154. Rosenblum HD, Winter HS. Steroid effects on the course of abdominal pain in children with Henoch-Schönlein purpura. Pediatrics 1987; 79:1018.

155. Tramontano G, Pondrano M, Buyonaqura G, et al. Schönlein-Henoch syndrome: clinico-statistical analysis of 60 cases (1978–1984). Pediatr Med Chir 1985;7:563.

156. Fukui H, Kamitsuji H, Nagao T, et al. Clinical evaluation of a pasteurized factor XIII concentrate administration in Henoch-Schönlein purpura. Thromb Res 1989;56:667.

157. Mollica F, Li Volti S, Garozzo R, Russo G. Effectiveness of early prednisone treatment in preventing the development of nephropathy in anaphylactoid purpura. Eur J Pediatr 1992; 151:140.

158. Salisbury FT. Corticosteroid therapy does not prevent nephritis in Henoch-Schönlein purpura. Pediatr Nephrol 1993;7:69.

159. Jardin MP, Leake J, Ridson RA, Barratt TM, Dillon MJ. Crescentic glomerulonephritis in children. Pediatr Nephrol 1992;6:231.

160. Landing BH, Larson EJ. Are infantile periarteritis nodosa with coronary involvement and fatal mucocutaneous lymph node syndrome the same? Comparison of 20 patients from North America with patients from Hawaii and Japan. Pediatrics 1977;59:651.

161. Soppi E, Salo E, Pelkonen P. Antibodies against neutrophil cytoplasmic components in Kawasaki disease. APMIS 1992;100:269.

162. Rider LG, Wener MH, French J, et al. Autoantibody production in Kawasaki syndrome. Clin Exp Rheumatol 1993;11:445.

163. Melish ME. Kawasaki syndrome: a 1992 update. Pediatr Dermatol 1992;9:335.

164. Barron KS. Kawasaki disease: epidemiology, late prognosis, and therapy. Rheum Dis Clin North Am 1991;17:907.

165. Takahashi M, Mason W, Lewis AB. Regression of coronary aneurysms in patients with Kawasaki syndrome. Circulation 1987;75:387.

166. Akagi T, Rose V, Benson LN, et al. Outcome of coronary artery aneurysms after Kawasaki disease. J Pediatr 1992;121:689.

167. Daniels SR, Specker B, Capannari TE, et al. Correlates of coronary artery aneurysm formation and prevention in patients with Kawasaki disease. Pediatr Res 1986;20:169A.

168. Koren G, Rose V, Levi S. Probable efficacy of high dose salicylates in reducing coronary involvement in Kawasaki disease. JAMA 1985; 254:767.

169. Kato H, Ichinose E, Yoshioka F, et al. Fate of coronary aneurysms in Kawasaki disease: serial coronary angiography and long term follow up study. Am J Cardiol 1982;49:1758.

170. Kato H, Koike S, Yokoyama T. Kawasaki disease: effect of treatment on coronary artery involvement. Pediatrics 1979;63:175.

171. Bierman FZ, Gersony WM. Kawasaki disease: clinical perspective. J Pediatr 1987;111:789.

172. Newburger JW, Takahashi M, Burns JC, et al. The treatment of Kawasaki syndrome with intravenous gamma globulin. N Engl J Med 1986;315:342.

173. Barron KS, Murphy DJ Jr, Silverman ED, et al. Treatment of Kawasaki syndrome: a comparison of two dosage regimens of intravenously administered immune globulin. J Pediatr 1990; 117:638.

174. Newburger JW, Takahashi M, Beiser AS, et al. A single intravenous infusion of gamma globulin as compared with four infusions in the treatment of acute Kawasaki syndrome. N Engl J Med 1991;324:1633.

175. Takei S, Arora YK, Walker SM. Intravenous immunoglobulin contains specific antibodies inhibitory to activation of T cells by staphylococcal toxin superantigens. J Clin Invest 1993; 91:602.

176. Jayne DR, Lockwood CM. Pooled intravenous immunoglobulin in the management of systemic vasculitis. Adv Exper Med Biol 1993;336:469.

177. Gersony WM. Long-term issues in Kawasaki disease [Editorial]. J Pediatr 1992;121:731.

178. Dajani AS, Taubert KA, Gerber MA, et al. Diagnosis and therapy of kawasaki disease in children. Circulation 1993;87(5):1776.

179. Fink CW. Polyarteritis and other diseases with necrotizing vasculitis in childhood. Arthritis Rheum 1977;20:378.

180. Ozen S, Besbas N, Saatci U, Bakkaloglu A. Diagnostic criteria for polyarteritis nodosa in childhood. J Pediatr 1992;120:206.

181. Bacon PA. Systemic vasculitic syndromes. Curr Opin Rheumatol 1993;5:5.

182. Fink CW. Childhood polyarteritis. In: Hicks RV, ed. Vasculopathies of childhood. Littleton, Massachusetts: PSG Publishing Co., 1988.

183. Reinold EW, Weinberg AG, Fink CW, Battles ND. Polyarteritis in children. Am J Dis Child 1976;130:534.

184. Guillevin L, Jarrousse B, Lok C, et al. Long term follow-up after treatment of polyarteritis nodosa and Churg-Strauss angiitis with comparison of steroids, plasma exchange and cyclophosphamide to steroids and plasma exchange: a prospective randomized trial of 71 patients. J Rheumatol 1991;18:567.

185. Guillevin L, Fain O. Lhote F, et al. Lack of superiority of steroids plus plasma exchange to steroids alone in the treatment of polyarteritis nodosa and Churg-Strauss syndrome: a prospective, randomized trial in 78 patients. Arthritis Rheum 1992;35:208.

186. Blau EB, Morris RF, Yunis EJ. Polyarteritis nodosa in older children. Pediatrics 1977;60:227.

187. Magilavy DB, Petty RE, Cassidy JT, Sullivan DB. A syndrome of childhood polyarteritis. J Pediatr 1977;91:25.

188. Hoffman GS, Kerr GS, Leavitt RY, et al. Wegener's granulomatosis: an analysis of 158 patients. Ann Intern Med 1992;116:488.

189. Leavitt RY, Fauci AS. Less common manifestations and presentations of Wegener's granulomatosis. Curr Opin Rheumatol 1992;4:16.

190. Niles JL. Value of tests for antineutrophil cytoplasmic autoantibodies in the diagnosis and treatment of vasculitis. Curr Opin Rheumatol 1993;5:18.

191. Falk RJ, Hogan S, Cary TS, Jennette JC. Clinical course of anti-neutrophil cytoplasmic antibody-associated glomerulonephritis and systemic vasculitis. Ann Intern Med 1990;113:656.

192. Cohen Tervaert JW, Huitema MG, Hene RJ, et al. Prevention of relapse in Wegener's granulomatosis by treatment based on antineutrophil cytoplasmic antibody titre. Lancet 1990;336: 709.

193. Fauci AS, Haynes BF, Katz P, Wolf SM. Wegener's granulomatosis: prospective clinical and therapeutic experience with 85 patients for 21 years. Ann Intern Med 1983;98:76.

194. Hoffman GS, Leavitt RY, Fleisher TA, Minor JR, Fauci AS. Treatment of Wegener's granulomatosis with intermittent high dose intravenous cyclophosphamide. Am J Med 1990; 89:403.

195. De Remee RA, McDonald TJ, Weiland LH. Wegener's granulomatosis: observations on treatment with antimicrobial agents. Mayo Clin Proc 1985;60:27.

196. West BC, Todd JR, King JW. Wegener's granulomatosis and trimethoprim-sulfamethoxazole: complete remission after a twenty year course. Ann Intern Med 1987;106:840.

197. Yuasa K, Tokitsu M, Goto H, et al. Wegener's granulomatosis: diagnosis by transbronchial lung biopsy, evaluation by gallium scintigraphy and treatment with sulfamethoxazole/trimethoprim. Am J Med 1988;84:371.

198. Kornreich HK, King KK, Bernstein BH, Singsen BH, Hanson V. Scleroderma in childhood. Arthritis Rheum 1977;20:343.

199. Falanga V, Medsger TA Jr, Reichlin M, Rodnan GP. Linear scleroderma: clinical spectrum,

prognosis, and laboratory abnormalities. Ann Intern Med 1986;104:849.

200. Uziel Y, Krafchik BR, Silverman ED, et al. Localized scleroderma in childhood: a report of 30 cases. Semin Arthritis Rheum 1994;23:328.

201. Uziel Y, Krafchik BR, Feldman B, et al. Serum soluble interleukin-2 receptor (S-IL2R) levels in localized scleroderma. Arthritis Rheum 1993; 36(suppl):S54.

202. Curley RK, MacFarlane AW, Evans S, et al. The treatment of linear morphea with D-penicillamine. Clin Exp Dermatol 1987;12:56.

203. Falanga V, Medsger TA Jr. D-penicillamine in the treatment of localized scleroderma. Arch Dermatol 1990;126:609.

204. Jimenez SA, Sigal SH. A 15 year prospective study of treatment of rapidly progressive systemic sclerosis with D-penicillamine. J Rheumatol 1991;18:1496.

205. Nimni ME. A defect in the intramolecular and intermolecular crosslinking of collagen caused by penicillamine. I. Metabolic and functional abnormalities in soft tissues. J Biol Chem 1968; 243:1457.

206. Cassidy JT, Petty RE, eds. Basic concepts of drug therapy. In: Textbook of pediatric rheumatology. New York: Churchill Livingstone, 1993.

207. Forre O, Munthe E, Kass E. Side effects and autoimmunogenicity of D-penicillamine treatment in rheumatic diseases. Adv Inflam Res 1984;6:251.

208. Takahashi K, Ogita T, Okudaira H, et al. D-penicillamine-induced polymyositis in patients with rheumatoid arthritis. Arthritis Rheum 1986;29:560.

209. Kunkle RW, Restronk A, Drachman DB, et al. The pathophysiology of penicillamine-induced myasthenia gravis. Ann Neurol 1986;20:740.

210. Van Den Hoogen FH, Boerbooms AM, Van Der Putte LB, et al. Low dose methotrexate treatment in systemic sclerosis [Letter]. J Rheumatol 1991;18:1763.

211. Gisslinger H, Burghuber OC, Stacher G, et al. Efficacy of cyclosporin A in systemic sclerosis. Clin Exp Rheumatol 1991;9:383.

212. Clements PJ, Paulus HE, Sterz MG. Cyclosporin in systemic sclerosis (SSc): analysis of 48-week open study. Arthritis Rheum 1991; 34:S52.

213. Bernstein BH, Singsen BH, Kent JT, et al. Reflex neurovascular dystrophy in childhood. J Pediatrics 1978;93:211.

214. Wolfe F, Smythe HA, Yunus MB, et al. The American College of Rheumatology 1990 criteria for the classification of fibromyalgia. Arthritis Rheum 1990;33:16.

215. Goldenberg DL. Treatment of fibromyalgia syndrome. Rheum Dis Clin North Am 1989; 15:61.

216. Kelley WM, Harris ED, Ruddy S, Sledge CB, eds. Textbook of rheumatology. 4th ed., chap. 72. Philadelphia: WB Saunders, 1993.

CRYSTAL DEPOSITION DISEASES

Carlos A. Agudelo

Since McCarty and Hollander,[1] in 1961, first used polarized light microscopy to identify monosodium urate (MSU) crystals in synovial fluids of patients with acute gout, other crystals have been found to induce a similar inflammatory synovial reaction (Table 17–1).

The pathophysiology of the synovitis induced by these crystals is not completely understood, and asymptomatic crystalline deposits frequently occur. Although acute self-limited attacks of monoarthritis or polyarthritis are the most common presentation, chronic and at times destructive arthropathy may also occur. In the present chapter, we will review a practical approach to the management of patients with the different crystal-associated disorders, drug side effects, recommended monitoring schedules, risk factors, pertinent clinical pharmacology, and drug interactions. For a comprehensive review regarding pathophysiology and diagnosis of these conditions, the reader is referred to Kelley et al.[2–4]

GOUT

Gout is a syndrome that results from tissue deposition of MSU crystals. Chronic hyperuricemia is considered necessary for its development. In some persons, chronic hyperuricemia leads to MSU deposits in or around the joints. These deposits may remain unnoticed and asymptomatic, or they may be associated with the typical recurrent attacks of acute self-limited arthritis. If untreated, gout may progress to a destructive polyarticular process with joint or bone destruction. In about 20% of patients, uric acid urolithiasis and renal disease may occur.[5] Gout or MSU deposition disease clinical spectrum includes the following:

- Chronic hyperuricemia
- Tophaceous deposits
- Acute and chronic arthritis
- Renal: urolithiasis, urate nephropathy

Uric acid is the final product of purine metabolism in human beings. Most other animals produce uricase, which breaks down uric acid into alantoin and CO_2 resulting in much lower uric acid values. Human beings do not produce uricase in significant amounts and have acquired a propensity toward hyperuricemia. In vitro studies have shown that uric acid behaves as a powerful antioxidant and the higher levels found in human beings may be protective against degenerative and other diseases.[6,7] At 37° C, the saturation value of urate in plasma is ~7.0 mg/100 ml. Hyperuricemia is defined as a serum urate level >7.0 mg/100 ml by the uricase method or 7.5 to 8 mg/100 ml by automated analysis. This common biochemical abnormality has been described in 13.2% of hospitalized men in the United States.[8] During childhood, serum urate levels in both sexes average ~3.6 mg/100 ml. At puberty, levels are ~1 mg higher in males than in females, and this difference is thought to be mediated by an estrogen renal effect. After menopause, female levels approach those of men. Although chronic hyperuricemia is considered necessary for the development of gout, most persons with this common biochemical abnormality do not develop gout. Hyperuricemia alone, per se, is not a disease. Although its persistence as a chronic abnormality confers an increased risk of gout and renal stones, asymptomatic hyperuricemia should not be treated. In most patients, the physician should be able to ascertain

TABLE 17–1

Potentially Phlogistic Crystals Found In or Around Joints and Associated Diseases

CRYSTAL	ASSOCIATED DISEASE(S)

Monosodium urate (MSU)	Monosodium urate deposition disease: Gout
	    Asymptomatic tophaceous deposits
	    Symptomatic—acute arthritis, chronic arthritis
	Urate nephropathy

Calcium pyrophosphate dihydrate (CPPD)	CPPD deposition disease or pseudogout
	    Asymptomatic chondrocalcinosis
	    Acute arthritis and chronic arthritis

Basic calcium phosphate (BCP) (hydroxyapatite, octacalcium phosphate, tricalcium phosphate)	Subcutaneous calcifications Calcific periarthritis Acute arthritis Chronic arthritis
Calcium oxalate	Arthritis (patients with chronic renal failure, oxalosis) Acute and chronic arthritis
Lipid liquid	Acute and chronic arthritis
Long-acting microcrystalline corticosteroids	Postinjection (iatrogenic synovitis)

its cause and decide on the course of action to be taken. Thus the evaluation of the patient with chronic hyperuricemia requires that the evaluating physician have a good understanding of the multiple events leading to this biochemical abnormality (Fig. 17–1).[2] (For more detail, see Kelley et al., reference 3).

Although gout is one of the better understood and treated of the rheumatic diseases, there are still many questions regarding the events leading to crystal formation, inflammation, and the self-limited nature of the acute attack. In some persons, usually after years of uncontrolled asymptomatic hyperuricemia, deposits of urate begin to appear in or around the joints. Occasional patients, particularly among the elderly, may first present with visible tophaceous deposits in the absence of acute attacks,[9] and synovial membrane microtophaceous deposits may be present in every patient with acute gout, as they are frequently found even during first attacks.[10]

The acute attack of MSU-induced synovitis is quite characteristic, with exquisite and severe pain, swelling, redness, and functional impairment developing within a few hours. Early attacks are usually monoarticular, in lower-extremity joints, with ~60% of first attacks involving the first metatarsophalangeal joint. Most often, the attack lasts from a few days to a couple of weeks, with gradual resolution of

all inflammatory signs and a return to apparent normalcy. Weeks to months may elapse before a new attack occurs in the same or another joint. A few patients may have no further attacks. As the disease progresses if untreated, attacks occur more frequently; they may be polyarticular and associated with fever and with constitutional symptoms.[11] In the chronic polyarticular stage, the disease may be confused with either rheumatoid arthritis or degenerative joint disease.

Synovial fluid analysis, including a careful search for crystals, is a required step in evaluating patients with acute arthritis. The demonstration of intracellular, strongly negative, birefringent crystals with polarized light microscopy establishes the diagnosis. Concomitant infection should be excluded. Normal serum urate levels are seen in 20% to 30% of patients during the acute attack.

Acute Gout in Uncomplicated Patients or Without Comorbidities

The management of patients with acute gout and no other aggravating factor or comorbid condition (renal failure, liver disease, peptic ulcer, postoperative, etc.) is usually straightforward and poses no dilemma for the treating physician. For better results, the diagnosis should be established as soon as possible, since

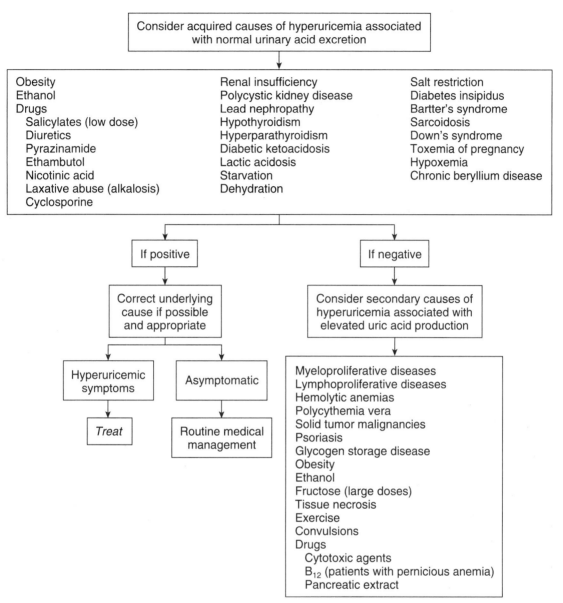

FIGURE 17–1

Evaluation of patient with hyperuricemia. (Modified from Kelley WN. Hyperuricemia. In: Kelley WN, Harris ED, Ruddy S, Sledge CB, eds. Textbook of rheumatology. 4th ed. vol. I. Philadelphia: WB Saunders, 1993:498.)

institution of treatment early during the attack is associated with faster improvement. Rest of the inflamed joint(s) is considered important in the management of acute gout, inasmuch as clinical experience and experimental results suggest that exercise may increase the inflammatory reaction to crystals. Several therapeutic options, listed in our order of preference, are indicated in Table 17–2.

Colchicine.   Colchicine is a derivative of *Colchicum autumnale* (meadow saffron). Extracts of

TABLE 17–2

Treatment of Acute Gout in Uncomplicated Patients

Therapeutic Options in Order of Preference
- Rest inflamed joint(s)
- NSAIDs
- Intraarticular microcrystalline corticosteroid
- IM corticosteroid
- ACTH
- Oral corticosteroid
- Colchicine (see text)

TABLE 17–3
Treatment of Gout in Uncomplicated Patients: Prophylaxis

FIRST ATTACK	FIRST ATTACK	TOPHACEOUS
NRF, <800 mg uric acid excreted in urine per day	NRF + stones and/or >800 mg uric acid excreted in urine per day	NRF + stones and/or >800 mg uric acid excreted in urine per day
↓	↓	↓
Lifestyle modifications: medications, diuretics, diet, alcohol	Allopurinol + colchicine or NSAIDs	Allopurinol + colchicine or NSAIDs
↓		
Watch		
↓		
Recurrent attacks		
↓		
Uricosurics or allopurinol + colchicine		

NRF = Normal renal function.

this plant, as a cathartic, were introduced for the treatment of acute gout in AD 600. The alkaloid colchicine was isolated in 1820 by Pelletier and Caventon.[12,13] Because of its selective antiinflammatory properties and effectiveness in the management of patients with acute gout, colchicine was the drug of choice for many years in managing patients with acute gout, and the striking improvement noted with its use also served diagnostic purposes. Because of its poor therapeutic benefit/toxicity ratio, and since many other effective drugs have become available, colchicine use in this setting has decreased. However, the medication continues to be useful and quite safe if used according to established guidelines.[14]

In the absence of comorbid conditions or risk factors (Table 17–3), colchicine is administered orally at a dose of one 0.5 or 0.6 mg tablet every hour or two tablets every 2 hours until improvement occurs or toxic effects are noted (usually diarrhea and nausea or vomiting, which may be severe in some patients) or until about 6 mg has been given. Unfortunately, >50% of the patients will experience toxic effects coincident with improvement or before improvement is noted. In a controlled study of 45 patients with acute gout, all of the 22 subjects given oral colchicine developed diarrhea or vomiting at a median time of 24 hours or after a mean dose of 6.6 mg.[15] To avoid or minimize gastrointestinal

(GI) toxicity, intravenous (IV) colchicine has been used. One to 2 mg diluted in ~20 ml of normal saline solution is slowly administered (over several minutes), preferably through an established IV line to avoid extravasation, since colchicine can be very irritating and tissue damage may occur. A smaller dose (0.5 to 1 mg) may be repeated every 6 hours without giving more than 4 mg as a total IV dose for acute attacks. No more colchicine by any route should be given for 1 week. Wallace and Singer[14] have reviewed the systemic toxicity associated with IV colchicine administration, reflecting on the appropriate use of the drug. They considered the following to be absolute contraindications to IV colchicine therapy: combined renal and hepatic disease, creatinine clearances <10 ml/min, and extrahepatic biliary obstruction (Table 17–4).

TABLE 17–4
Risk Factors for Colchicine Toxicity

Sepsis
Bone marrow depression
Decreased renal function
Hepatic disease or biliary obstruction
Prior maintenance colchicine
Older patient
Medications—cimetidine, tolbutamide, cyclosporine

Since many other therapeutic options exist (see Table 17–2 and 17–5), we believe it is best to avoid colchicine (at the doses used to treat the acute attack) in the management of patients with acute gout.

In recent years, the main use of colchicine in gout has been to prevent a rebound of the acute attack or as prophylaxis; in those patients treated with corticosteroids (intraarticular, intramuscular, or oral) or ACTH, we begin concomitant colchicine administration. Unless contraindicated, oral doses of 0.5 to 1.2 mg daily are quite effective. Higher doses are usually not well tolerated because of GI toxicity. Those treated with nonsteroidal antiinflammatory drugs (NSAIDs) may begin immediate colchicine prophylaxis or wait until the attack is under good control. Again, risk factors for its use must be considered, as chronic colchicine therapy may lead to toxic reactions (see Toxicity, below). In the patient without comorbid conditions and with no visible tophaceous deposits, colchicine may be given as prophylaxis for several months to years, depending on the individual case and whether or not urate-lowering drugs are used. In patients with a single first attack, education, modifications in lifestyle, diet, and alcohol intake, or changes in medications—such as avoidance of diuretics—may be enough to prevent further attacks. In patients with tophaceous gout, several years of colchicine prophylaxis may be required.

Metabolism. Colchicine is rapidly absorbed after oral administration, with peak concentrations of 0.3 µg/ml after 30 to 120 minutes; it concentrates in leukocytes, and ~50% is bound to plasma proteins. The drug is deacetylated in the liver and is excreted in the bile, feces, and urine. The frequency of intestinal toxicity is partly explained by the presence of large concentrations of the drug in bile and intestinal secretions. Colchicine affects rapidly dividing cells, most notably those of the bone marrow and intestinal mucosa. It is still detectable in white blood cells and in the urine 10 days after a single dose.[16]

Colchicine interferes with steps of the inflammatory reaction mediated by neutrophils. Its interference with microtubular systems may lead to decreased neutrophil motility, chemotaxis, formation of digestive vacuoles, degranulation, and suppression of a chemotactic factor released by neutrophils during phagocytosis of urate.[17–19]

Toxicity. The frequency and severity of side effects associated with colchicine administration depend on multiple factors, including dose, route of administration, presence of comorbid conditions (such as liver or renal dysfunction), previous maintenance doses, old age, and drug interactions (Table 17–4). The most common and longest-recognized side effects are GI ef-

---

TABLE 17–5
Treatment of Gout in Complicated Patients

ACUTE ATTACK	PROPHYLAXIS	
Exclude infection	First attack(s)	Chronic, tophaceous ARF
Rest inflamed joint(s)	↓	↓
Intraarticular corticosteroid		
IM corticosteroid	Nontophaceous	Allopurinol*
ACTH	↓	Colchicine*
Oral corticosteroid		
Analgesics	Do not prescribe	
	prophylactic medication	
	↓	
	Lifestyle modification: diet,	
	medications, alcohol	
	↓	
	Watch/follow	

ARF = Abnormal renal function.
*See text.

TABLE 17–6

Manifestations of Colchicine Toxicity

Gastrointestinal: abdominal pain; nausea/vomiting, diarrhea, paralytic ileus, hepatocellular damage, pancreatitis
Respiratory: respiratory distress, ARDS
Hematologic: leukocytosis (first stage), bone marrow hypoplasia, coagulopathy, hemolytic anemia
Skin: rash, alopecia
Cardiovascular: hypovolemia, hypotension, depressed myocardial contractility, peripheral vasodilation, arrhythmias, myocarditis
Renal: proteinuria/hematuria, acute renal failure
Metabolic: metabolic acidosis, hyponatremia, hypocalcemia, hypophosphatemia, hypomagnesemia
Neuromuscular: mental status changes, coma, ascending paralysis, seizures, peripheral neuropathy, rhabdomyolysis
Fertility: azoospermia, sterility
Miscellaneous: fever, hypothermia

From Putterman C, Ben-Chetrit E, Caraco Y, et al. Colchicine intoxication: clinical pharmacology, risk factors, features, and management. Semin Arthritis Rheum 1991;21:143.

fects, with most patients experiencing diarrhea and/or vomiting at the doses used to treat the acute attacks. The main circumstances in which severe toxicity occurs are suicide attempts and inappropriate therapeutic overdoses. The correlation between amount ingested, severity of toxicity, and prognosis is not straightforward, inasmuch as fatalities have been reported after oral doses of 7 mg over 3 days and single doses of 7.5, 8, and 11 mg, and survival has been reported after ingestion of >300 mg.[13] Many manifestations have been associated with colchicine toxicity (Table 17–6).

Hematologic manifestations include disseminated intravascular coagulation and bone marrow depression. In some patients, severe diarrhea and leukopenia may lead to hypotension, sepsis, and death. A colchicine-induced myoneuropathy mimicking polymyositis has been described in a study in which all 12 patients had decreased renal function and were receiving long-term colchicine prophylaxis (1.2 mg/d).[20] Muscle weakness, distal arreflexia, and elevation of creatine kinase were noted. Electromyography showed myopathic changes, and muscle biopsy revealed a distinctive vacuolar myopathy with no apparent inflammatory changes. Prompt recovery followed colchicine discontinuation or dose reduction.

The treatment of severe colchicine toxicosis is supportive. The drug's short half-life and its ability to bind to tissues makes hemodialysis and exchange transfusions useless.[13,21] It may be useful to administer gastric lavage, emetics, activated charcoal, or cathartics in the absence of diarrhea. Recent experimental work suggests that immunotherapy with colchicine monoclonal antibodies may be useful in managing patients with colchicine toxicity.[22]

Nonsteroidal Antiinflammatory Drugs. The term *NSAID* was first applied to phenylbutazone in 1949. Since that time, many other NSAIDs have been introduced, all having in common the suppression of prostaglandin synthesis. This suppression explains in part some of their antiinflammatory potential and side effects. NSAIDs have also been shown to interfere with neutrophil activation and the release of cytotoxic substances, including free radicals, lysosomal enzymes, and lipooxygenase products.[17] Although they may differ by chemical class, plasma half-life, and dosage, they have similar antiinflammatory properties and potential for toxicity.

In the absence of comorbid conditions or risk factors (Table 17–7), NSAIDs are an excellent alternative to colchicine. Indomethacin in doses of 100 to 200 mg during the first 2 or 3 days of the acute attack is highly effective. As the inflammatory process subsides, the dose is reduced to 75 mg/d. Unfortunately, many patients—particularly the elderly—are unable to tolerate the high doses required because of toxic effects such as headaches, problems with mentation, fluid retention, hyperkalemia, etc. (Table 17–8). Examples of available NSAIDs are naproxen in doses of 375 to 500 mg three times a day, gradually reduced to maintenance doses of 375 to 500 mg twice a day; ibuprofen 800 mg three times daily; sulindac, 200 mg twice daily; piroxicam, 20 mg/day, or ketopro-

TABLE 17–7
NSAID-induced Toxicity: Potential Risk Factors

Decreased renal function
Liver disease
Peptic ulcer disease
Congestive heart failure
Elderly persons
Allergic, hypersensitive: asthma, rhinitis, nasal polyps
Drug interactions: anticoagulants (avoid combination), lithium (monitor carefully), oral hypoglycemics (monitor), potassium-sparing diuretics (avoid combination), digoxin (avoid combination if possible in patients with renal insufficiency), cyclosporine (avoid combination). Probenecid increases NSAID levels by up to 50%.

fen, 100 mg three times a day. As the attack is controlled, maintenance doses of the NSAID can be used for prophylaxis if necessary. If it is not well tolerated, one may try other NSAIDs or colchicine in the doses previously discussed. GI, renal, and, in the elderly, central nervous system toxicity play a significant role in limiting the usefulness of NSAIDs in managing the acute attack.[23,24]

Corticosteroids. In cases in which one or two large joints are involved, an intraarticular microcrystalline corticosteroid injection (such as 40 to 80 mg methylprednisolone acetate or triamcinolone acetonide) is quite effective, with control of the pain and the inflammatory signs within a few hours. In the absence of infection and under strict aseptic techniques, the joint is

TABLE 17–8
Adverse Reactions to NSAIDs

Gastrointestinal: dyspepsia, erosive gastritis, peptic ulcer disease, diarrhea, liver dysfunction, small-bowel ulceration
Renal: decreased renal function, acute renal failure, interstitial nephritis, papillary necrosis, hyperkalemia, chronic renal failure?
Central nervous system: headache, dizziness, aseptic meningitis (ibuprofen, sulindac, tolmetin), decreased mentation, psychosis
Skin: fixed drug reaction, erythema multiforme, urticaria, pseudoporphyria (naproxen)
Other unusual reactions: pneumonitis, aplastic anemia, bone marrow depression

aspirated, diagnosis is confirmed, and the injection is performed. Smaller joints may be injected with one third or one half of the dose used for larger joints. Although well tolerated by most patients, in rare cases intraarticular injections lead to infectious arthritis, and careful follow-up of the patient, with specific instructions, must be recorded. Tendon rupture, local hypopigmentation, and skin atrophy may occur. Since the preparations for intraarticular injections are microcrystalline, an occasional patient may experience a brief flare-up beginning a few hours after the injection. Repeated, frequent injections into the same joint may lead to joint damage.

Single intramuscular IM injections of 60 mg of triamcinolone acetonide have been found effective and comparable to indomethacin. A few patients may require a second injection.[25] However, significant tissue atrophy may occur. We have used 40 to 80 mg IM methylprednisolone acetate with similar good results. Oral or parenteral courses of corticosteroids have been used in selected cases, primarily in patients with polyarticular gout or in those in whom NSAIDs or colchicine were contraindicated. Initial doses of 20 to 50 mg were used and necessitated 10 to 15 days of therapy because of slow resolution of symptoms. No significant side effects were noted, except for mild hyperglycemia in one of 12 patients so treated.[26] Because of the longer therapy required and the experience with transplant patients receiving maintenance corticosteroid therapy and developing acute gout we favor other options for treatment of acute polyarticular gout, such as parenteral synthetic adrenocorticotropic hormone (ACTH). Wolfson et al.[27] first reported the use of ACTH in acute gout. Axelrod and Preston compared IM ACTH injection to oral indomethacin in 76 patients.[28] Results favored ACTH as, in the 36 patients who received ACTH, pain relief was noted within a few hours and there were no apparent side effects; in contrast, of 40 patients who received indomethacin, 12 had problems with mentation and pain relief was delayed. A single injection of 40 IU, if given early in the attack, may be effective for monarticular attacks. Polyarticular attacks may require two or three injections at 8-hour intervals to achieve control. Oral or systemic corticosteroid therapy, as well as parenteral ACTH, should be accompanied by oral colchicine, 0.5 to 1.2 mg daily, for prophylaxis and to avoid a rebound of the attack.

Acute Gout in Complicated Patients or With Comorbid Conditions

The management of acute gout is often complicated by the coexistence of other medical conditions that the physician must consider in deciding on therapeutic options (Tables 17–4, 17–5, and 17–7). Many of these complications occur in older patients, who may be more prone to toxic reactions. Concomitant medications must be reviewed. In the absence of infection, the best choices appear to be an intraarticular corticosteroid preparation, as previously discussed, or an injection of ACTH.[29] Colchicine may be used for prophylaxis. Maintenance doses of colchicine in patients with chronic renal insufficiency may lead to neuromyopathy or bone marrow depression; therefore careful monitoring must be the rule. In some patients who are unable to tolerate higher doses, primarily those with renal insufficiency, one colchicine tablet daily or even less often may be effective. An alternative to colchicine prophylaxis will be low-dose NSAIDs with careful follow-up of renal function, particularly in the elderly. In an occasional patient whose multiple medical problems may contraindicate the medications previously discussed, analgesics may be used until stabilization makes their use safer (Table 17–5). The physician must recognize that, although dramatic in its clinical presentation, acute gout is a benign condition.

The management of gout in transplant patients taking cyclosporine poses another dilemma for the clinician. Studies are needed to evaluate the safety and efficacy of therapy in this setting. For some patients with acute gout, colchicine and NSAIDs should be avoided (Tables 17–4 and 17–5). Since most of these patients are receiving long-term corticosteroid therapy with adrenal suppression, it is likely that ACTH will be ineffective. For larger joints, and once infection is excluded, an intraarticular microcrystalline corticosteroid injection appears to be the best choice. Other options include an increase in the daily oral corticosteroid dose or an IM injection. If required, analgesics may be added. The long-term management is also difficult, as similar restrictions apply to colchicine and NSAIDs for prophylaxis, and no data are available regarding safety. To lower the serum urate level, uricosurics should be avoided because of the renal dysfunction often present (renal transplant or cyclosporine-in-duced). Small doses of allopurinol (i.e., 50 mg daily) may be given with close observation for possible toxicity (see under Allopurinol) and, if tolerated, after 1 or 2 months the dose may be gradually increased. Patients receiving concurrent azathioprine are at increased risk of toxic effects (allopurinol inhibits xanthine oxidase, which is required in azathioprine degradation) and their azathioprine dose must be reduced.

Control of Hyperuricemia and Urate Deposits

The aim of therapy is to control hyperuricemia, reverse urate deposition (thus avoiding or arresting joint damage), and prevent further gouty attacks. The uric acid excreted in urine derives from exogenous and endogenous purines. We believe that strict measurement of urinary uric acid is impractical, as it requires 4 to 7 days of a purine-free diet. Under these conditions, normal male subjects excrete about 400 mg/d. With elimination of purine-rich foods only, urinary uric acid values range from 400 to ~600 mg/d. Since even this control is difficult to achieve in clinical practice, a urinary uric acid excretion >750 mg/d on a regular diet has been considered an indication of overproduction and overexcretion and will identify most patients who will require further study for possible genetic or enzymatic abnormalities or lymphoproliferative disorders. The great majority of gouty patients will have normal urinary uric acid excretion.[30] Therefore measurement of urinary uric acid is primarily indicated in the evaluation of the young patient with persistent hyperuricemia.

There has been a recent trend toward a conservative approach to hypouricemic therapy, with the suggestion that the presence of tophi can be used as an indication for treatment.[31] Since chronic gouty arthritis and visible tophaceous deposits in most patients take years to develop, unnecessary or premature medication may be avoided.[3] In some patients, a second attack may never occur; in others, recurrence may take several months to years. Those patients with a single or a few gouty attacks, normal renal function, no history of renal stones, no apparent tophaceous deposits, and <800 mg of uric acid in 24-hour urine may be managed conservatively with education, lifestyle modifications, avoidance of diuretics, weight control, reduction in alcohol consumption, and, if necessary, maintenance colchicine. Should this approach fail and the patient experience more frequent attacks, a uricosuric or allopurinol may be used. As seen in Table 17–5, the presence of chronic arthritis, tophaceous deposits, kidney stones, or >800 mg of uric acid in 24-hour urine require urate-lowering measures with allopurinol.

In general, it is best to start antihyperuricemic therapy after the attack is well controlled and the patient is free of symptoms which is usually ~2 weeks after the attack. Urate-lowering medication begun while the patient has symptoms may delay the antiinflammatory response or lead to a rebound of the attack. (However, urate-lowering medications are not stopped in patients who develop acute gout while taking them.) For patients in whom urate-lowering medications are indicated, concomitant maintenance colchicine or low-dose NSAIDs should be added for prophylaxis. The length of this prophylactic therapy must be individualized; in some patients, a few months to a year may be sufficient, whereas those with tophaceous gout may require years of such therapy.

Allopurinol. Allopurinol was first developed as a chemotherapeutic agent but had little or no effect on experimental tumors. As an inhibitor of xanthine-oxidase, allopurinol was first given to human patients in 1963 to achieve reduced values in both serum and urinary uric acid.[32,33] Uric acid is the final product of purine metabolism in human beings. In the final steps, hypoxanthine is oxidized to xanthine and xanthine to uric acid; these reactions are catalyzed by xanthine-oxidase. Allopurinol is metabolized to oxipurinol, and this reaction is also catalyzed by xanthine-oxidase. Both allopurinol and oxipurinol inhibit xanthine-oxidase, thus decreasing uric acid production and resulting in increased xanthine and hypoxanthine. Allopurinol also inhibits de novo purine synthesis, decreasing total urinary purine excretion.[34]

Allopurinol is well absorbed after oral administration, reaching peak levels within 30 to 60 minutes and having a plasma half-life of 2 to 3 hours. Some is excreted in the feces and urine; however, most is converted to oxipurinol, which has a much longer half-life of up to 20 hours in patients with normal renal function. Most of the oxipurinol is excreted by the kidney. Therefore, a decrease in renal function may markedly in-

crease its half-life. A similar increase may occur with a low-protein diet in malnourished persons, thus increasing the risk of toxicity. The long half-life of oxipurinol may be responsible for most of the urate-lowering effect and toxicity of allopurinol. Although allopurinol increases the half-life of probenecid and uricosurics increase the clearance of oxipurinol, these interactions have minimal practical consequences and both medications have been used together without altering their usual doses.[34]

The administration of allopurinol is followed by a decrease in serum and urinary uric acid values within 24 to 48 hours. Maximal reductions are reached within 2 weeks and then remain relatively constant over prolonged periods of time.[32] Optimally, serum urate levels should be reduced to below saturation of ~6 mg/100 ml or less if possible. In patients with normal renal function, 200 to 300 mg/d in one dose should be started in combination with prophylactic doses of colchicine or low-dose NSAIDs. The allopurinol dose may be gradually increased if necessary. An occasional patient may require 600 to 800 mg daily. Patients should be informed that, during the initial months of treatment, they may experience an increase in the frequency of attacks. This is thought to be due to increased mobilization of urates from tophaceous deposits and shedding of crystals into joints. Good control of the hyperuricemia should lead to gradual resolution of tophaceous deposits, control of arthritis, and preservation of joint and renal function. In patients with decreased renal function, where allopurinol therapy is firmly indicated (Table 17–9), the medication should be started

---

TABLE 17–9

Main Indications for Allopurinol Therapy in Patients With Hyperuricemia and Gout

1. Urinary uric acid excretion of ≥800 mg in 24 hours
2. Hypoxanthine-guanine-phosphoribosyltransferase deficiency
3. PP-ribose-P synthetase overactivity
4. Uric acid nephropathy
5. Nephrolithiasis
6. Allergy to uricosurics
7. Tophaceous gout
8. Severe gout with renal insufficiency (see text)

Other: As prophylaxis before cytolytic therapy to avoid tumor lysis syndrome

TABLE 17–10

Protocol for Maintenance of Allopurinol Based on Creatinine Clearance

CREATININE CLEARANCE (ML/MIN)	ALLOPURINOL DOSE
0	100 mg every 3 days
10	100 mg every 2 days
20	100 mg daily
40	150 mg daily
60	200 mg daily
80	250 mg daily
100	300 mg daily

at a much lower dose and based on renal function. Hande et al.[35] have suggested the protocol in Table 17–10 for maintenance of allopurinol based on creatinine clearance.

In patients with mild renal insufficiency (creatinine clearance 60 to 80 ml/min), we prefer initial therapy at low doses beginning with only 100 mg daily. If the medication is tolerated and there are no side effects, the dose is gradually increased.

Toxicity.   After 25 years of clinical use, allopurinol continues to be a standard therapy for most patients with chronic tophaceous gout, urate nephropathy, and nephrolithiasis and in cases of gout and renal insufficiency. Although uricosurics may be of value in controlling hyperuricemia in patients with mild renal insufficiency (unless contraindicated by urate nephropathy, nephrolithiasis, and overexcretors), allopurinol is mainly indicated in cases of significant renal insufficiency (GFR <60 ml/min) and severe gout. However, the medication should be used very cautiously in these patients, with initial low doses of 50 to 100 mg only (see above listing) and a gradual increase if necessary to avoid toxic effects. Renal and liver function should be carefully monitored. Although most patients tolerate allopurinol without toxic reactions, some may experience significant side effects. There is ample evidence that allopurinol is given inappropriately to many patients. It should not be given initially at full doses to patients with renal insufficiency. Hande et al.[35] and Singer and Wallace[36] have described a life-threatening allopurinol hypersensitivity syndrome in 158 patients. High fever, severe dermatitis in >90% of patients (erythema multiforme, toxic epidermal necrolysis, or exfo-

liative rash), hepatitis, eosinophilia, and worsening of renal function were noted, and 38 (24%) of the 158 patients died. Postmortem examination revealed diffuse vasculitis. The syndrome tended to occur early in therapy (within a few days to weeks), and most patients were receiving full doses of allopurinol despite renal insufficiency. In the Singer and Wallace series, 33 of 59 patients had been given allopurinol for asymptomatic hyperuricemia.[36] Risk factors for this syndrome are the presence of renal insufficiency, concomitant diuretic therapy, and perhaps the use of full loading doses of allopurinol (300 mg). Since allopurinol metabolizes to oxipurinol, and the half-life of the latter substance is very prolonged in the presence of renal insufficiency, accumulation of oxipurinol occurs.[35] Oxipurinol has been implicated in allopurinol-induced toxicity.

Allopurinol may induce milder rashes that do not require discontinuation of the medication; however these patients must be very carefully monitored, and a dose reduction should be instituted. The presence of fever, worsening dermatitis, decreased renal function, abnormal liver enzymes, or eosinophilia should prompt discontinuation of the drug. Bone marrow suppression, aplastic anemia, agranulocytosis, granulomatous hepatitis, and jaundice have been described. Drug interactions include increased incidence of rashes in combination with ampicillin therapy, the need to decrease the dose of azathioprine or mercaptopurine to about one third of the usual dose if given with allopurinol (they are inactivated by xanthine-oxidase), and the need to avoid cyclophosphamide because the combination may lead to bone marrow suppression. Allopurinol prolongs the half-life of dicumarol, warfarin, and theophylline.[34] Rarely in patients with uric acid overproduction and excretion, such as those with enzyme deficiencies or undergoing cytolytic therapy, allopurinol may induce xanthinuria or xanthine stone formation.

Oxipurinol (not available in the United States) has been tried as an alternative in allopurinol-sensitive patients. Although toxic events similar to their allopurinol allergy occurred in 40% of the patients, slow incremental doses were tolerated by 60% of patients with complicated hyperuricemia.[37] Patients sensitive to allopurinol and requiring the same medication as those with severe tophaceous gout may need a desensitization trial. Oral and IV desensitization has been successful in a few patients.[38,39,39a] Close monitoring is necessary, as serious toxicity has occurred. Patients should be fully informed of the potential for severe reactions, even at low doses. Oral desensitization should be tried first, as it may be safer. Gradually increasing doses of an oral solution, beginning on the first day at 0.008 mg and increasing by 0.008 mg each day for 10 days, reaching 20 mg at day 20 and 300 mg at 1 month, have been successful in a few cases.[39] An alternative regimen for slow, oral desensitization has been published by Fam et al.[39a] Walz-LeBlanc et al.[38] have used IV desensitization after failure of the oral route.[38] After a negative skin test with 0.1 µg, they arbitrarily gave IV doses of 1, 10, 50, 100, and 500 µg at 15-minute intervals followed by 1, 2, 5, 10, 20, and 50 mg at 30-minute intervals; 100 mg was given 1 hour later with no apparent problem (200 mg of allopurinol was diluted in 500 mg of 5% dextrose in water).

Uricosuric Agents.

Uric acid is almost completely freely filtered at the glomerulus. More than 90% undergoes tubular reabsorption and then tubular secretion, reabsorption, and excretion; this explains the final product in the urine. Uricosurics compete with urate for the tubular brush border transporter, thus inhibiting urate reabsorption. The net result is increased uric acid excretion and decreased serum urate levels. The uricosurics available in the United States are probenecid, sulfinpyrazone, and salicylates.

Probenecid was initially developed to sustain high levels of penicillin and para-aminosalicylic acid by interfering with their renal excretion. Probenecid is well absorbed from the GI tract with a half-life ranging from 6 to 12 hours. It is highly bound to plasma proteins and is excreted in the urine.[34] Gutman and Yu[40] and Talbott et al.[41] noted increased urinary uric acid excretion and normalization of serum urate in patients treated with different doses of probenecid ranging from 0.5 to 2 g/d. A precipitous drop in serum urate levels was noted in a few days. As with allopurinol, an increase in acute gouty attacks was seen, and 2 of 18 patients on 2 g/d of probenecid in the Gutman and Yu study experienced a recurrence of renal colic. Since uricosurics increase urine uric acid excretion, they may precipitate—primarily in uric acid overproducers—uric acid crystals or lead to uric

acid stones when given initially at high doses. It is advisable to begin therapy at low doses to prevent crystallization. Precipitation is unusual in the normal producer of uric acid. Initial doses of 0.5 to 1 g/d are given and may be increased to 1.5 to 2 g/d in divided doses. Higher doses may be needed. Uricosurics are highly effective for most gouty patients. However, they should not be used in such patients with uric acid overproduction and overexcretion or in those with urate nephropathy or nephrolithiasis because of the propensity to crystal precipitation and stone formation. To minimize the risk of crystalluria and stone formation, fluid intake should be increased, particularly at the beginning of therapy when larger quantities of uric acid are excreted. Urine alkalinization increases uric acid solubility, thus decreasing the chance of crystallization. It has been suggested that patients be given 2 to 6 g of sodium bicarbonate during the first days of therapy, but this is impractical in clinical practice. Acetazolamide, 200 mg taken at night during the first 7 to 10 days, will help alkalinize the urine throughout the night. Uricosurics are ineffective in patients with impaired renal function (glomerular filtration rate <30 to 40 ml/min).

In long-term studies, ~20% of probenecid-treated patients developed side effects, mostly GI and dermatologic: GI intolerance, fever, hypersensitivity reactions, rashes. Probenecid decreases the renal excretion of salicylates, acetazolamide, dapsone, indomethacin, ampicillin, penicillin, cephradine, and methotrexate. It delays heparin metabolism, which may lead to increased anticoagulation.[34]

Sulfinpyrazone is a derivative of a phenylbutazone metabolite. It lacks antiinflammatory properties but is a strong uricosuric. It is rapidly absorbed from the GI tract. It is highly bound to plasma proteins and has a half-life of 1 to 3 hours.[42] Most of the drug is excreted in the urine. An added advantage is its antiplatelet effect. This medication is administered in divided doses of 200 to 800 mg/d. GI intolerance of sulfinpyrazone is similar to that of probenecid. Occasional bone marrow toxicity has been observed. Because of its strong uricosuric effect, sulfinpyrazone should not be given to patients with overexcretion of uric acid, urate nephropathy, or a history of uric acid stones.

Aspirin or salicylates in doses 4 to 6 g/d are effective uricosurics. Most patients are unable to tolerate such high doses, however, and there are other options. Low doses (<2.4 g/d) of aspirin or salicylates appear to inhibit the renal tubular secretion of uric acid, leading to hyperuricemia. At any dose, they inhibit the uricosuric effect of probenecid and sulfinpyrazone and should not be used together.

In most cases, gout is a very treatable disease and good control can be achieved. However, some patients with severe disease have comorbid conditions that make therapeutic decisions very difficult. As previously discussed, colchicine and NSAIDs are often contraindicated for acute attacks. Uricosurics cannot be used for long-term control, and patients may not tolerate allopurinol. Desensitization may work in some cases. A solution may be provided by the development of new medications such as uricase. This enzyme degrades uric acid into allantoin and carbon dioxide; in injectable form, it has shown significant reduction of serum urate.[43]

Other useful general measures in long-term management of gout include education of the patient regarding hyperuricemia and gout medications, liberal ingestion of fluids to maintain good urinary output (particularly in overexcretors), slow weight reduction in overweight individuals, avoidance of excessive alcohol consumption (leads to increased lactic acid, which interferes with uric acid excretion and increased purine production), and finally dietary measures to control or decrease purine intake.

PSEUDOGOUT OR CPPD DEPOSITION DISEASE

Calcium pyrophosphate dihydrate (CPPD) deposition disease or pseudogout was first described in 1962.[44] The term *pseudogout* was used to characterize acute arthropathy similar to gout, with calcifications in cartilage (chondrocalcinosis) and CPPD crystals in the synovial fluid. Other clinical presentations have since been described. The acute variety may be monoarticular or polyarticular and febrile. Tophaceous deposits in tendons and periarticular tissues have been described. Like gout, the disease may be chronic, destructive, and incapacitating with different patterns: pseudorheumatoid with symmetric disease, pseudoosteoarthritis, pseudoneurotrophic and lanthanic (asymptomatic) disorder. Joints commonly involved include the knees, wrist, shoulders, hips, and ankles. The disease has been associated with hyperparathyroidism, hemochromatosis, hypophosphatasia, and hypomagnesemia and is more common in the elderly. The diagnosis is established by the clinical presentation, roentgenographic features, and demonstration of intracellular weakly positive birefringent crystals under polarized light microscopy. Careful search for these crystals is necessary, as they are often missed by laboratories. The pathophysiologic mechanism by which CPPD deposition disease develops is uncertain, and the events leading to the inflammatory reaction are likely similar to MSU (gout) and other crystals.[4] (For more detail on pathogenesis, see Kelley et al, Chapter 77, pp. 1337 to 1348 [reference 4].)

Management. Treatment is symptomatic. Since there is no therapy to remove CPPD deposits or retard joint damage, the aim is to control pain and inflammation. In acute attacks, drainage of the joint with removal of the inflammatory fluid may be sufficient. Other options include the intraarticular injection of microcrystalline corticosteroids (as previously discussed for acute gout) or any one of the NSAIDs, including salicylates, unless contraindicated (Table 17–7). An ACTH injection or IM corticosteroid (see under Gout) may be useful. We prefer not to use colchicine in acute CPPD disease or in acute crystal-induced synovitis because of its toxicity at the dosage required to control the acute inflammatory process and because other options are available (see under Gout). In the setting of chronic disease, colchicine in doses of 0.6 to 1.2 mg/day is helpful for prophylaxis against recurrent attacks,[45] and NSAIDs or analgesics are appropriate for other forms of the disease that require treatment.

BASIC CALCIUM PHOSPHATE CRYSTAL DEPOSITION DISEASE

Similar to MSU and CPPD crystal deposition diseases, a number of articular syndromes may be associated with basic calcium phosphate crystals and primarily with hydroxyapatite (Table 17–1). (For more detail, see Kelley et al., Chapter 77, pp. 1349 to 1354 [reference 4].) Deposits may be asymptomatic or associated with acute inflammation, acute calcific periarthritis, and acute arthritis or with chronic destructive arthropathy as seen in the Milwaukee syndrome with shoulder or knee involvement. Acute calcific periarthritis is common and may be seen in patients undergoing chronic hemodialysis. Periarticular calcifications are roentgenographically evident. An acute arthritis involving the first metatarsophalangeal joint in young women, and mimicking acute gout, has been described.[46] Periarticular calcification was noted, with partial to complete dissolution of these deposits occurring weeks after the attack. The synovial fluid is inflammatory, and crystals can be seen on electron microscopy or x-ray diffraction. Identification with light microscopy is difficult, but shiny nonbirefringent intracellular cytoplasmic inclusions may be seen.[4] The management of this crystal-induced process is symptomatic. There is no specific therapy. Local microcrystalline corticosteroid injections or NSAIDs are the treatments of choice. For acute attacks, marked improvement within 5 days was noted with NSAIDs, and mean duration of the treated attack was 10 days with no recurrence in the follow-up period ranging from 9 months to 14 years.[46] For those with chronic disease, NSAIDs or analgesics may be tried. As in other forms of subacute or chronic arthritis, it is important to pay appropriate attention to physical therapy programs to maintain and preserve joint and muscle function. Surgery may occasionally be required to remove large symptomatic calcific deposits.[4]

CALCIUM OXALATE DEPOSITION DISEASE

Patients with primary or secondary oxalosis caused by end-stage renal disease may present with acute or chronic arthropathy involving small joints of the hands, knees, elbow, and ankles. Calcific deposits of digits or subcutaneous tissues may be noted, and synovial fluid shows mild inflammation and oxalate crystals. Roentgenograms may reveal chondrocalcinosis. There is no specific therapy, and clinical response to colchicine, NSAIDs, or intraarticular corticosteroids has been poor.[47]

LIPID LIQUID CRYSTALS

Intracellular and extracellular birefringent lipid microspherules (appearing as Maltese crosses) have been found in inflammatory fluids of patients presenting primarily with acute monoarthritis. Only a few cases have been described, including two in association with pigmented villonodular synovitis.[47,48] Either NSAIDs or colchicine have been successful in controlling the attack. It is not clear what, if any, role such crystals play in the inflammatory reaction; nor has the nature of their origin been clarified.[47,48]

REFERENCES

1. McCarty DJ Jr, Hollander JL. Identification of urate crystals in gouty synovial fluids. Ann Intern Med 1961;54:452.
2. Kelley WN. Hyperuricemia. In: Kelley WN, Harris ED, Ruddy S, Sledge CB, eds. Textbook of rheumatology, 4th ed., vol I. Philadelphia: WB Saunders, 1993:498.
3. Kelley WN, Schumacher HR. Gout. In: Kelley WN, Harris ED, Ruddy S, Sledge CB, eds. Textbook of rheumatology. 4th ed., vol II. Philadelphia: WB Saunders, 1993:1291.
4. Moskowitz RW. Diseases associated with the deposition of calcium pyrophosphate or hydroxyapatite. In: Kelley WN, Harris ED, Ruddy S, Sledge CB, eds. Textbook of rheumatology. 4th ed., vol I. Philadelphia: WB Saunders, 1993: 1337.
5. Agudelo CA. Gout and hyperuricemia. Curr Opin Rheum 1989;1:286.
6. Ames BN, Cathcart R, Schwiers E, et al. Uric acid provides an antioxidant defense in humans against oxidant- and radical-cause aging and cancer: a hypothesis. Proc Natl Acad Sci USA 1981; 78:6858.
7. Agudelo CA, Turner RA, Panetti M, et al. Does hyperuricemia protect from rheumatoid inflammation? A clinical study. Arthritis Rheum 1984; 27:443.
8. Paulas HE, Coutts A, Calabro JJ, et al. Clinical significance of hyperuricemia in routinely screened hospitalized men. JAMA 1970;211:277.
9. Shmerling RH, Stern SH, Gravellese EM, et al. Tophaceous deposition in the finger pads without gouty arthritis. Arch Intern Med 1988;148: 1830.
10. Agudelo CA, Schumacher HR. The synovitis of acute gouty arthritis. Hum Pathol 1973;4:265.
11. Lawry GV, Fan PT, Bluestine R. Polyarticular versus monoarticular gout: a prospective, comparative analysis of clinical features. Medicine (Baltimore) 1988;67:335.
12. Wyngarden JB, Kelley WN. An abbreviated history of gout. In: Wyngarden JB, Kelley WN, eds. Gout and hyperuricemia. New York: Grune & Stratton, 1976:3.
13. Putterman C, Ben-Chetrit E, Caraco Y, et al. Colchicine intoxication: clinical pharmacology, risk factors, features, and management. Semin Arthritis Rheum 1991;21:143.

14. Wallace SL, Singer JZ. Review: systemic toxicity associated with the intravenous administration of colchicine-guidelines for use. J Rheumatol 1988;15:495.

15. Ahern MJ, Reid C, Gordon TP, et al. Does colchicine work? The results of the first controlled study in acute gout. Austr NZ J Med 1987;17:301.

16. Wyngarden JB, Kelley WN. Pharmacology of colchicine, indomethacin, and phenylbutazone. In: Wyngarden JB, Kelley WN, eds. Gout and hyperuricemia. New York: Grune & Stratton, 1976:421.

17. Clements PJ, Paulus HE. Nonsteroidal anti-inflammatory drugs (NSAIDs). In: Kelley WN, Harris ED, Ruddy S, Sledge CB, eds. Textbook of rheumatology. 4th ed. vol I. Philadelphia: WB Saunders, 1993:700.

18. Phelps P. Appearance of chemotactic activity following intraarticular injection of monosodium urate crystals: effect of colchicine. J Lab Clin Med 1970;76:622.

19. Spillberg I, Mandell B, Mehta J, et al. Mechanism of action of colchicine in acute urate-induced arthritis. J Clin Invest 1979;64:775.

20. Kuncl RW, Duncan G, Watson D, et al. Colchicine myopathy and neuropathy. N Engl J Med 1987;316:1562.

21. Elwood MG, Robb HJ. Self-poisoning with colchicine. Postgrad Med 1971;47:129.

22. Edmond-Rouan SK, Otterness IG, Cunningham AC, et al. Reversal of colchicine-induced mitotic arrest in Chinese hamster cells with a colchicine-specific monoclonal antibody. Am J Pathol 1990;137:779.

23. Brooks PM, Day RO. Nonsteroidal antiinflammatory drugs: differences and similarities. N Engl J Med 1991;324:1716.

24. Altman RD, Honig S, Levin JM, et al. Ketoprophen versus indomethacin in patients with acute gouty arthritis: a multicenter double-blind comparative study. J Rheumatol 1988;15:1422.

25. Alloway JA, Moriarty MJ, Hoogland YT, et al. Comparison of triamcinolone acetonide with indomethacin in the treatment of acute gouty arthritis. J Rheumatol 1993;20:111.

26. Groff GD, Franck WA, Raddatz DA. Systemic steroid therapy for acute gout: a clinical trial and review of the literature. Semin Arthritis Rheum 1990;19:329.

27. Wolfson WQ, Cohn C, Levine R. Rapid treatment of acute gouty arthritis by concurrent administration of pituitary adrenocorticotropic hormone (ACTH) and colchicine. J Lab Clin Med 1949;34:1766.

28. Axelrod D, Preston S. Comparison of parenteral adrenocorticotropic hormone with oral indomethacin in the treatment of acute gout. Arthritis Rheum 1988;31:803.

29. Hill GL, Agudelo CA, Semble EL. Parenteral adrenocorticotropic hormone (ACTH) in the treatment of acute gout. Arthritis Rheum 1991;34:S145.

30. Wyngarden JB, Kelley WN. The workup of the hyperuricemic patient. In: Wyngarden JB, Kelley WN, eds. Gout and hyperuricemia. New York: Grune & Stratton, 1976:284.

31. Diamond HS. Control of crystal-induced arthropathies. Rheum Dis Clin North Am 1989;15:557.

32. Wyngarden JB, Kelley WN. Pharmacology of xanthine oxidase inhibitors. In: Wyngarden JB, Kelley WN, eds. Gout and hyperuricemia. New York: Grune & Stratton, 1976:439.

33. Rundles RW, Wyngarden JB, Hitchings GH, et al. Effects of a xanthine oxidase inhibitor on thiopurine metabolism, hyperuricemia, and gout. Trans Assoc Am Physicians 1963;76:126.

34. Fox IH. Antihyperuricemic drugs. In: Kelley WN, Harris ED, Ruddy S, Sledge CB, eds. Textbook of rheumatology. 4th ed. vol I. Philadelphia: WB Saunders, 1993:822.

35. Hande KR, Noone RM, Stone WJ. Severe allopurinol toxicity: description and guidelines for prevention in patients with renal insufficiency. Am J Med 1984;76:47.

36. Singer JZ, Wallace SL. The allopurinol hypersensitivity syndrome: unnecessary morbidity and mortality. Arthritis Rheum 1986;29:82.

37. O'Duffy JD. Oxipurinol therapy in allopurinol-sensitive patients. Arthritis Rheum 1993;36:S159.

38. Waltz-LeBlanc B, Reynolds WJ, MacFadden DK. Allopurinol sensitivity in a patient with chronic tophaceous gout: success of intravenous desensitization after failure of oral desensitization. Arthritis Rheum 1991;34:1329.

39. Webster E, Panush RS. Allopurinol hypersensitivity in a patient with severe chronic tophaceous gout. Arthritis Rheum 1985;78:707.

39a. Fam AG, Lewtas J, Stein J, et al. Desensitization to allopurinol in patients with gout and cutaneous reactions. Am J Med 1992;93:299.

40. Gutman AB, Yu TF. Benemid (p-di-n-propylsulfamyl)-benzoic acid as uricosuric agent in chronic gouty arthritis. Trans Assoc Am Physicians 1951;64:279.

41. Talbott JM, Bishop C, Norcross BM, et al. The clinical and metabolic effects of benemid in patients with gout. Trans Assoc Am Physicians 1951;64:372.

42. Wyngarden JB, Kelley WN. Pharmacology of uricosuric agents. In: Wyngarden JB, Kelley WN, eds. Gout and hyperuricemia. New York: Grune & Stratton, 1976:430.

43. Chua CC, Greenberg ML, Viau AT. Use of polyethylene glycol-modified uricase (PEG-urisase) to treat hyperuricemia in a patient with non-Hodgkin lymphoma. Ann Intern Med 1988;109:114.

44. McCarty DJ, Kohn NN, Faires JS. The significance of calcium phosphate crystals in the synovial fluid of arthritis patients: the "pseudogout syndrome." 1. Clinical aspects. Ann Intern Med 1962;56:711.

45. Alvarellos A, Spilberg I. Colchicine prophylaxis in pseudogout. J Rheumatol 1986;13:804.

46. Fam AG, Rubenstein J. Hydroxyapatite pseudopodagra: a syndrome of young women. Arthritis Rheum 1989;32:741.

47. Reginato AJ, Kurnik B. Calcium oxalate and other crystals associated with kidney diseases and arthritis. Semin Arthritis Rheum 1989;18:198.

48. Kazuhiro U, Masohiro K, Hirohata K. Lipid microspherules in synovial fluid of patients with pigmented villonodular synovitis. Arthritis Rheum 1988;31:1442.

OSTEOARTHRITIS

Deirdre A. Gramas
Nancy E. Lane

Osteoarthritis (OA) is a slowly evolving articular disease of cartilage degeneration characterized by the gradual development of joint pain, stiffness, and limitation of motion. Osteoarthritis is common if one accepts the radiographic definition of the disease, more than 75% of persons over 70 years of age showing some radiographic evidence.[1] It affects the joints of the hands, including the distal interphalangeal joints, the proximal interphalangeal joints, and the carpometacarpal joint of the thumb. Other joints involved include the cervical spine, the lumbosacral spine, the hip, the knee, and the first metatarsophalangeal, with much less frequent involvement of the ankle, wrist, elbow, and shoulder. There are known inconsistencies between findings on radiographs and clinical symptoms, with only 50% to 60% of persons with radiographic evidence of OA having clinical symptoms.[2]

A number of factors have been implicated in the pathogenesis of OA: the genetic predisposition of the individual, previous trauma, inflammation, exercise, and biochemical and metabolic abnormalities.[2,3] Put in another way, investigators have suggested that theories of pathogenesis fit into one of two categories: either a primary role for chondrocyte failure to maintain normal homeostasis or an initiating role for physical forces associated with a primary biomechanical failure of cartilage and subchondral bone.[3] OA probably begins in the articular cartilage, but it eventually involves the surrounding bone and synovium. When cartilage is absent from the articular surface, the underlying bone is subjected to greater local stress. Wolff's law of bone remodeling predicts new bone formation in these

areas, resulting in bony sclerosis that is often seen on radiographs.[4] Subarticular bone cysts are also commonly seen on radiographs and generally exist only in the absence of overlying cartilage. Bone cysts are the result of the transmission of intraarticular pressure onto the marrow spaces of the subchondral bone. Cysts increase in size until the pressure in the cyst is equal to the intraarticular pressure. If the joint becomes covered with reparative cartilage, the cysts regress.[5] Finally, the breakdown of both cartilage and bone produces a chronic inflammatory response in the synovium of the joint.[2,3,6] For a more in-depth discussion of the pathogenesis and clinical features of OA, please refer to Kelley et al. (reference 141), Chapters 78 and 79.

CLASSIFICATION OF OSTEOARTHRITIS

Osteoarthritis is not a single disease but one with multiple, diverse causes that result in a well-recognized clinical pattern. In July 1985 a workshop on the classification and etiopathogenesis of osteoarthritis was held.[7] In this classification system, OA is divided into either an idiopathic or a secondary form. The idiopathic form may be either *localized* or *generalized*. The localized form includes isolated joint involvement or involvement of groups of joints (for example, the hip, knee, hands, feet, spine, or other single joints). The generalized form involves three or more sites of OA.[7]

Idiopathic OA

Numerous investigators have confirmed the existence of distinct groups of patients who have

OA in three or more joints. These patients are referred to as having generalized, idiopathic OA.[8–10] Although no common pathologic abnormalities have been discovered in these patients, the recent finding of a polymorphic genetic error in type II collagen in a family with primary osteoarthritis may lead to an understanding of the pathogenesis of this disease.[11] Further epidemiologic and molecular genetic studies are necessary to further the understanding of this form of osteoarthritis.

Idiopathic osteoarthritis may also be localized and can affect isolated joints or groups of similar joints, such as the distal interphalangeal joints. Frequently all of the interphalangeal joints of the hands or feet will be involved and are called Heberden's and Bouchard's nodes. Although there appear to be no distinct pathologic or biochemical characteristics, Heberden's and Bouchard's nodes occur more frequently in women, may be familial, and develop around the age of menopause.[12] As we begin to study the genetics of this group of patients, we may begin to understand the pathogenesis of this type of OA.

Secondary Osteoarthritis

The secondary causes of OA are numerous and, except for those related to trauma, are infrequently seen in clinical practice. The secondary form of OA may result from a congenital abnormality (Perthes' disease, congenital dislocation of the hip, slipped capital femoral epiphysis, and bone dysplasias), metabolic abnormalities (ochronosis, hemochromatosis, calcium pyrophosphate dihydrate disease, and gout), endocrine abnormalities (acromegaly and obesity), other bone and joint diseases (osteonecrosis, prior infection and Charcot's arthropathy), and diseases of obscure etiology (such as Kashin-Beck disease, Mseleni disease).[7] Both acute and chronic trauma to the axial or appendicular skeleton and injury that results in malalignment of the joint can develop into OA. These patients develop osteoarthritis that is indistinguishable from the idiopathic forms.

Although it is important for classification purposes to subdivide OA, it appears that there is a final common pathway of the disease that is similar for all etiologic factors. Since osteoarthritis emanates from a degeneration of articular cartilage, an understanding of the biochemical events of osteoarthritis is important. We will begin with a discussion of normal articular cartilage.

NORMAL ADULT ARTICULAR CARTILAGE

The articular cartilage surface of the joint is avascular, aneural, hypocellular, and alymphatic. Cartilage is composed of chondrocytes within a complex extracellular matrix. Chondrocytes are metabolically very active cells that produce collagen and proteoglycan, the primary elements of the extracellular matrix. Chondrocytes also produce the enzymes necessary for the synthesis, maintenance, and degradation of cartilage. They are nested as single cells within lacunae and account for less than 5% of the volume of the articular cartilage. The extracellular matrix provides articular cartilage with structural and biomechanical properties. Although articular cartilage has little ability to repair itself, it functions well for a lifetime if the physical demands on it are not excessive.[2,3,6]

Cartilage is a biphasic material composed of 80% water and 20% organic solid. The extracellular matrix is composed of type II collagen, proteoglycans, noncollagenous proteins, and water. Collagen molecules are composed of three polypeptide chains bound in a triple-helix conformation. The amino acid sequence of collagen imparts a unique three-dimensional stability to the triple helix. Type II cartilage makes up 95% of the fibrillar network of the articular cartilage and is secreted by chondrocytes as a precursor procollagen molecule that forms microfibrils and, subsequently, fibrils. Interfibrillar cross-linking is thought to be facilitated by the minor collagen types IX and XI.[3,6] Other types of collagen, such as V and VI, may be responsible for the control of fibril diameter, fibrillogenesis, and fibril cross-linking. Collagen cross-linking determines the tensile strength of the extracellular matrix.

Proteoglycans account for 5% to 10% of the wet weight of articular cartilage. They are complex anionic glycoproteins that, in concert with the collagenous network, determine the load-bearing ability of the joint surface. Proteoglycans are composed of glycosaminoglycans chondroitin-4-sulfate, chondroitin-6-sulfate, and keratan sulfate, which combine with a core protein to form a monomer. These are then bound to hyaluronic acid by a link protein to form the proteoglycan aggregate. This macromolecular structure is responsible for the compressive properties of the articular cartilage.

The third major component of the extracellular matrix consists of noncollagenous proteins and glycoproteins. Some of these proteins, such as chondronectin, anchorin, and link protein, assist in the aggregation and stabilization of macromolecules and may participate in the prevention of neovascularization and proteolysis.

Extracellular matrix homeostasis is mediated by the chondrocyte. In addition to synthesizing and secreting the synthetic elements of the matrix, chondrocytes synthesize and secrete the enzymes necessary for matrix degradation. The metalloproteases collagenase and stromelysin degrade both proteoglycans and collagen.[13,14] Some metalloproteases may be neutral proteases that, when secreted, are activated by an acidic environment to degrade intraarticular proteins. In addition, chondrocytes and synovial tissue produce protease inhibitors. These inhibitors, known as tissue inhibitors of metalloprotease (TIMP-1 and -2), are normally found in excess in synovial fluid and articular cartilage and inhibit the proteolytic properties of collagenase and stromelysin. Investigators have postulated that specific events and conditions may independently trigger the release of each of these seemingly conflicting agents. For a discussion of the biology and biomechanics of diarthrodial joints, please see Kelley et al. (reference 141), Chapters 1 and 99.

PATHOPHYSIOLOGY OF OSTEOARTHRITIS

Although there may be different precipitating factors in osteoarthritis, there are similar biochemical changes. These changes affect the joints in OA in two major matrix components: proteoglycan and type II collagen. There is a progressive depletion of cartilage proteoglycan, which parallels the severity of the disease.[13] At a certain stage, the chondrocytes appear unable to fully compensate for the proteoglycan depletion, resulting in a net loss of matrix. The structural changes of the proteoglycan macromolecules include a decrease in hyaluronic acid content, a diminution in the size of the proteoglycan aggregates to monomers, and a decrease in the size and aggregation of monomers.[13–15] The latter

changes are probably related to the enzymatic cleavage of the proteoglycan monomer core protein in several areas, including the hyaluronic acid binding region.[16]

Although the content of type II collagen remains unchanged in OA, increased cartilage hydration and ultrastructural changes of the collagen fibers represent important alterations in the collagen fiber network.[17] The increase in minor collagen types such as type I collagen, particularly in the pericellular area, suggests a change in chondrocyte metabolism. Together with the damaged collagen structure, changes in the proteoglycan content of the matrix lead to a functional deterioration of the cartilage. This makes the cartilage less resistant to compression or mechanical stress and leads to the appearance of cartilage loss.

Cartilage loss in OA occurs by enzymatic and mechanical degradation.[18] The enzymatic process appears to be a cascade of events. Whereas in rheumatoid arthritis the synovium is the most important source of degradative enzymes, the chondrocytes appear to be the most significant source of enzyme responsible for OA cartilage matrix catabolism.[19,20] The two main metalloprotease enzymes responsible for cartilage matrix degradation are collagenase and stromelysin.[21,22] Collagenase appears to be responsible for the breakdown of the collagen network in OA cartilage, as increased collagenase level has been detected both in experimental OA and in human OA cartilage.[17,21] The collagenase level was also found to correlate with the severity of OA cartilage lesions. Likewise, stromelysin has been identified in human articular cartilage, and its level correlates with the severity of the OA lesions.[23,24]

The biologic activity of metalloproteases is controlled by both physiologic inhibitors and activators. At least two tissue inhibitors of metalloproteases (TIMP-1 and -2) are known to exist in human beings. In OA cartilage, there is an imbalance between synthesis of TIMP and metalloproteases. A relative deficiency in the amount of the inhibitor[25,26] favors an increased level of active metalloproteases and, secondarily, matrix degradation.

Early changes in OA—cartilage swelling and increased hydration—can be attributed to a breakdown of the collagenous framework that allows further hydration of the matrix.[2,13] Synthesis of proteoglycans (especially those richer in chondroitin sulfate) increases early in OA, presumably as attempted repair mechanisms are overwhelmed, and then overall proteoglycan degradation of the aggregate to monomers ensues. With further breakdown of the collagen framework and depletion of matrix proteins, structural changes, such as blistering, fibrillation, and fissuring, appear. There are concomitant changes in the subchondral bone, and eventually the articular surface is denuded.[2,13] For an in-depth discussion of collagen, elastin, matrix glycoproteins, proteoglycous, proteinosea and matrix degeneration, please see Kelley et al. (reference 141), Chapters 2, 3, and 14.

After the initial stages of cartilage degeneration, which may have resulted from an injury, there may be a delay of many years before the person feels any joint pain or a radiograph shows evidence of cartilage degeneration (joint space narrowing or osteophyte formation). This delay in the appearance of symptoms is due in part to the lack of innervation of the cartilage. There is a rich nerve supply to the surrounding structures, including the periosteum, subchondral bone, and the joint capsule.[2,3] Therefore significant and irreversible cartilage damage has occurred before inflammation and attendant joint pain appear.

Currently, no therapy has been shown or proven to arrest the progression of OA. The challenge for the clinician is to find a way to best preserve joint function, manage pain, and treat concurrent inflammation. The remainder of this chapter will cover the current therapeutic approaches for osteoarthritis.

GENERAL PRINCIPLES AND DEFINITIONS

The key to the effective management of osteoarthritis is an accurate and appropriate diagnosis. As noted above, osteoarthritis has a long asymptomatic period, and there is little justification for its treatment during this stage. Radiographic evidence of joint space narrowing, subchondral sclerosis, and osteophytosis may be an incidental finding in someone with musculoskeletal pain from another cause. A careful history and physical examination, radiographs, and well-directed laboratory tests are required. When the diagnosis of osteoarthritis is secure, therapeutic decisions are made on the basis of the patient's pain, discomfort, level of disability, and to some extent degree of radiographic damage. Finally, although the principles of etiopathogenesis may be the same for all areas of the body that are affected by OA, treatment strategies are directed by location of the problem to specific areas such as the hand, knee, and hip (to be discussed in detail later). A general discussion of the overall management of OA is found in Kelley et al. (reference 141), Chapter 80.

Simple, noninvasive measures should be used initially in the treatment of osteoarthritis. If the problem suggests a "mechanical" component, such as pain developing during the day or after activity, therapy should be directed toward reduction of stress or load onto that joint and promotion of muscle strengthening aimed toward optimal biomechanical alignment. If the appropriate physical therapy has not improved pain or disability, other modalities should be considered. These include analgesics, intraarticular glucocorticoids, and nonsteroidal antiinflammatory agents.

Nonsteroidal antiinflammatory drugs (NSAIDs) and analgesics are the most widely prescribed therapeutic agents for the symptomatic relief of pain in OA. Other measures must be taken to avoid further mechanical damage, and they include the use of assistive devices, muscle-strengthening techniques, and avoidance of previously destructive habits. Strategies used to prevent excessive use and reduce mechanical strain to the hands, knees, and hips are simple and straightforward. Following are some suggested measures to prevent mechanical stress, reduce pain and decrease joint damage in the hands, knees, and hips:

1. Use light-weight utensils rather than those that are heavy.
2. Wrap utensils with foam rubber for grip.
3. Use a ring or loop on the zipper to pull up and down.
4. Use electric appliances whenever possible.
5. Use Velcro fasteners and zippers instead of buttons.
6. Use a single-lever faucet.
7. Avoid lifting heavy objects; get help.
8. If you must lift heavy items, use both hands or forearms, and place them under the object.
9. Avoid standing for prolonged periods.

Poor body mechanics and improper posture may be a leading factor in the causation and exacerbation of pain in osteoarthritis. Numerous epidemiologic studies have taught us that obesity is commonly associated with OA and causes abnormal stresses on the articular cartilage in weight-bearing joints. Therefore weight loss may provide additional symptomatic relief of pain as well as the theoretical ability to reduce mechanical joint damage.[27] To best maintain independent and active living, collaboration and close contact with the patient's family, the physical therapist, and the occupational therapist are important. Education of the patient and the family about factors that cause excessive joint loading is essential to achieve compliance and effective rehabilitation. Self-help classes based on patient education and ability to gain control over one's disease have been shown to reduce pain and improve function in OA patients.[28]

PRINCIPLES OF PHARMACEUTICAL THERAPY IN OSTEOARTHRITIS

OA is a chronic disease with intermittent exacerbations and disease flares that often resolve without intervention. The natural history of OA makes it difficult to demonstrate a difference between the investigational drug and placebo in clinical trials. In addition, there are no standardized radiographic or histologic parameters that have been used for the measurement of progression of disease. Without standardized disease definitions and study designs, it is difficult to compare the efficacy of different treatments.[28]

Nevertheless, many studies focusing on drug efficacy in OA have been performed.[28] These studies use outcome measures such as pain relief, joint mobility, walk time, quality of life, time lost from work, and global patient and physician assessment. Other studies use radiographic or histologic end points, determined by serial radiographs, arthroscopic scores, and cartilage or synovial specimens. Reviews of common outcome measurements for OA have been recommended and appear in other publications.[29,30]

In the next sections of this chapter, we will discuss the most common medications used to treat the pain and inflammation of OA, recommend guidelines for prescribing them, and discuss clinically important side effects.

Analgesia

The patient's degree of pain, amount of functional disability, and lack of improvement with nonpharmaceutical therapies should be the basis for consideration of medications for relief of pain. For a single joint, therapy is directed locally. When multiple joints are involved, systemic therapy should be considered. Treatment of OA is multifactorial and consists of a combination of analgesics and antiinflammatory agents.[28]

Analgesics, such as acetaminophen, may be the initial and sole therapy for some persons with osteoarthritis. Acetaminophen is generally safe if doses are kept under 4000 mg/d (eight tablets of 500 mg/d or 12 tablets of 325 mg/d), except in persons with preexisting liver disease, which may limit full therapeutic dosages.[31]

Surprisingly, there is a paucity of scientific information on the use of analgesics in osteoarthritis. Some studies compare analgesics with NSAIDs in the treatment of pain, and the results are varied. In 1981, Doyle et al.[32] compared ketoprofen with propoxyphene-acetaminophen in the treatment of OA. In this double-blind, crossover study of 44 patients with osteoarthritis, there were no observed differences in the relief of pain. However, the articular index score and the "patient preference" scale favored ketoprofen as the drug of choice. In a second randomized, double-blind study of 864 patients with OA of the hip, knee, wrist, or ankle, there was a significant decrease in pain with slow-release diclofenac as compared with propoxyphene/acetaminophen.[33] Finally, in a small, double-blind, crossover study comparing flurbiprofen with nefopam (an analgesic) for the treatment of pain in 30 patients with osteoarthritis of the knee, no differences were found between the study agents.[34]

Bradley et al.[35] recently compared two doses of ibuprofen with high-dose acetaminophen in the treatment of a flare of mild to moderate osteoarthritis of the knee. In this study, 195 subjects were randomly assigned to three treatment groups: low or analgesic dosage of ibuprofen (1200 mg/d), high or antiinflammatory levels of ibuprofen (2400 mg/d), and acetaminophen (4000 mg/d). Baseline characteristics for these persons with OA of the knee were similar. After 4 weeks of therapy, change in pain and disability score,[36] walking pain score, walking distance, 50-foot walk time, and physician assessment were comparable between groups. There was a statistically significant improvement in rest pain in the ibuprofen-treated groups compared with the acetaminophen-treated group (p = 0.05). This suggests but does not prove that high-dose acetaminophen may be equivalent to high- and low-dose ibuprofen for a flare of knee OA. However, in this study there was no placebo group to assess the degree of spontaneous improvement as compared to drug effect. Therapeutic trials longer than 4 weeks are needed to assess the efficacy and clinical importance of acetaminophen in OA.

The most recent study comparing the relative safety and efficacy of NSAIDs with analgesics compared naproxen and acetaminophen in a 2-year, double-blind, multicenter parallel trial performed by the Cooperative Systematic Studies of Rheumatic Disease (CSSRD) group.[37] In that study, 178 patients with OA of the knee were followed for up to 2 years. The primary end point of the study was radiographic progression of osteoarthritis and withdrawal of the drug because of lack of efficacy. Although only 62 patients completed the 2-year study, the efficacy of acetaminophen and naproxen was similar. The reason for withdrawal from acetaminophen was lack of response and noncompliance, while the naproxen group withdrew from the study because of gastrointestinal side effects, lack of efficacy, and noncompliance. The toxicity rate of acetaminophen was slightly lower than that of naproxen and was reversible. Because of the high dropout rate and other problems related to study design, it is not possible to draw definite conclusions from this ambitious study comparing safety and efficacy of NSAIDs and analgesics.

Nonsteroidal Antiinflammatory Drugs

Nonsteroidal antiinflammatory agents are widely used in OA based upon the concept that in low doses, NSAIDs are effective analgesics; in higher doses, they have antiinflammatory activity. Low doses provide an analgesic effect by inhibiting prostaglandin sensitization of peripheral pain receptors.[38] In higher doses, they exert their antiinflammatory actions potentially through a number of biologic systems:

- Prostaglandin production
- Leukotriene function
- Lymphocyte function
- Neutrophil aggregation and granule release
- Rheumatoid factor production
- Alteration of membrane viscosity
- Superoxide generation
- Lysosomal enzyme release
- Cell membrane function
- Inhibition of diacylglycerol production

First, NSAIDs inhibit the production of the enzyme cyclooxygenase, which catalyzes the formation of prostaglandins from arachidonic acid (Fig. 18–1). Prostaglandins (PGs) mediate the process of inflammation by causing erythema, vasodilatation, and pain. Aspirin (acetylsalicylic acid) irreversibly acetylates cyclooxygenase to permanently interfere with PG production for the life of the platelet or cell. All other NSAIDs reversibly interfere with the active site of cyclooxygenase and antagonize its activity. After cyclooxygenase inhibition, arachidonic acid may build up and be directed to leukotriene synthesis regulated by lipoxygenase. Some lipoxygenase inhibition by sodium meclofemate,[39] diclofenac,[40] and ketoprofen has been reported in vitro.[41] The clinical significance of this is unknown at present.

The antiinflammatory activity of NSAIDs extend beyond their ability to inhibit cyclooxygenase and lipoxygenase. Cell membrane–linked processes such as superoxide generation,[42] phospholipase C activity,[43] and oxidative phosphorylation[44] may be inhibited by the ability of NSAIDs to disrupt lipid membranes.[45] Inhibition of diacylglycerol production and alteration of membrane viscosity may also occur.[46]

The NSAIDs are categorized according to their molecular structure as outlined in Table 18–1 and are divided into either salicylates or nonsalicylate NSAIDs. The salicylates may be either acetylated or nonacetylated. The acetyl group is responsible for increased potency and toxicity of aspirin (acetylsalicylic acid) compared with the nonacetylated salicylates and nonsalicylate NSAIDs. The propionic acid derivatives, indole/indene acetic acid derivatives, hetroaryl acetic acid derivatives, arylacetic acid derivatives, and fenamic acid derivatives are nonsalicylate NSAIDs. Enolic acid, pyranocarboxylic acid, and naphthalkone are also nonsalicylates, with only one agent in each group (piroxicam, etodolac, and nabumetone) currently approved by the Food and Drug Administration in the United States.

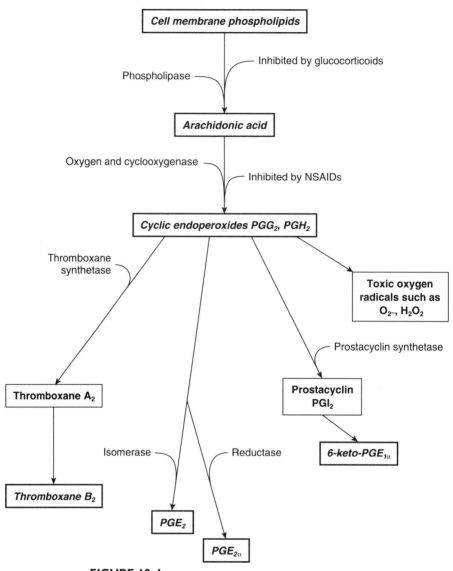

FIGURE 18–1
Cyclooxygenase pathway for arachidonic acid metabolism.

Differences in the half-lives of the NSAIDs do not correlate with their molecular structures and are important to recognize. The NSAIDs with a long half-life include naproxen, phenylbutazone, sulindac, diflunisal, piroxicam, and nabumetone. The longer half-life allows the agent more time to equilibrate between the plasma and synovial fluid and ranges from 12 to 24 hours. Piroxicam has an average half-life of 38 hours but has been reported to last for up to 158 hours.[47] The short-acting NSAIDs include indomethacin, ibuprofen, fenoprofen, ketoprofen, tolmetin, meclofenamate, diclofenac, etodolac, flurbiprofen, and ketorolac. The half-lives of these agents range between 1 and 8 hours. When there is concern about the toxicity of NSAIDs in elderly patients or those with pre-existing conditions, the short-acting agents are recommended.

All NSAIDs are metabolized in the liver by either hydroxylation, carboxylation, or glucuronidation and are excreted in the urine. In some patients with renal insufficiency, the inactive metabolites may be resynthesized or converted back into their active compounds. Indomethacin and sulindac, both indole acetic acid derivatives, undergo enterohepatic circulation and should be used with caution in patients with liver and cholestatic disease. As a general rule, there is more than 95% protein

TABLE 18–1
Chemical Classification and Product Names of Most Available Nonsteroidal Antiinflammatory Drugs

Acidic Agents
Arylcarboxylic acids

Salicylic acids:	Acetylated: acetylsalicylic acid (aspirin)
	Nonacetylated: diflunisal (Dolobid)
	Choline magnesium trisalicylate (Trilisate)
	Salsalate (Disalcid)
	Sodium salicylate
Anthranilic acids:	Mefenamic acid
	Meclofenamic acid (Meclomen)

Arylalkanoic acids

Arylacetic acids:	Diclofenac (Voltaren)
Arylpropionic acids:	Ibuprofen (Motrin, Advil Nuprin), flurbiprofen (Ansaid), ketoprofen (Orudis)
	Fenoprofen (Nalfon)
	Tiaprofenic acid (Surgam)
	Naproxen (Naprosyn)
	Oxaprozin (Daypro)
Heteroarylacetic acids:	Tolmetin (Tolectin)
	Ketorolac triethylamine (Toradol)
Indole/indene acetic acids:	Indomethacin (Indocin)
	Sulindac (Clinoril)
	Etodolac (Lodine)

Enolic acids

Pyrazolidinediones:	Phenylbutazone (Butazoladin)
	Oxyphenbutazone, azapropazone
Oxicams:	Piroxicam (Feldene)

Nonacidic Agents

Naphthalkone:	Nabumetone (Relafen)

binding of NSAIDs to serum albumin; drugs or medical conditions that decrease the protein binding increase the percent of free drug, and this may increase toxicity. The prodrugs sulindac and nabumetone are converted to the active compounds after absorption. The prodrug effect may spare the gastrointestinal tract from some toxicity and be useful for those sensitive to gastrointestinal side effects.

The possibility that NSAIDs might alter the course of OA was first described in vitro by Annefeld and Fassbender in 1983.[48] NSAIDs may influence cartilage degradation, by either stimulation or inhibition of the extracellular matrix production. Annefeld et al.,[49] using a semiquantitative method, measured the ultrastructural changes in lapine chondrocytes induced by steroids and classified the changes as either stimulatory or inhibitory according to the semiqualitative changes in the endoplasmic reticulum, nucleus, and mitochondria of the cell. As investigators proceeded to evaluate

NSAIDs in this in vitro system, the concept grew that these agents were **chondroprotective** because some NSAIDs stimulated ultrastructural changes in the chondrocyte. It is preferable not to use this term because the protection of cartilage degradation by NSAIDs has not been determined or established. At the present time in our current state of knowledge, no clinical study documents the ability of NSAIDs to protect articular cartilage or slow the progression of OA. To determine if NSAIDs alter the degradation of articular cartilage in OA, a 10- to 15-year longitudinal study of patients with early OA would need to be done.

Not surprisingly, NSAIDs have had both a positive and a negative effect on cartilage metabolism in several different experimental systems. For example, tiaprofenic acid (an NSAID not available in the United States), was found to increase proteoglycan production in cartilage explants of patients with OA as well as to increase proteoglycan aggregate size and decrease aggregate fragments.[50] Alternatively, aspirin, fenoprofen, and ibuprofen inhibit proteoglycan synthesis in normal canine articular cartilage slices, whereas indomethacin and sulindac do not.[51-55] Although these data are intriguing, the clinical significance of this is yet to be determined. Caution must be exercised in the interpretation of the effects of medications of cartilage explant cultures. In vitro studies do not account for the mechanical stimulus of an active joint or the interaction of the chondrocyte with the extracellular matrix compartment. Furthermore, investigators have shown that there is marked variability in chondrocyte metabolism.[56,57]

Choosing a nonsteroidal agent in the treatment of osteoarthritis is not a simple task. Patient response is influenced by factors other than pain relief and is not predictable.[58] In choosing a NSAID, it is prudent to recommend, initially, the drug with the fewest side effects and if the patient has concurrent illnesses or is elderly, a trial of an NSAID with a *short* half-life (4 to 6 hours) is warranted, with close follow-up. The elderly are at increased risk for the development of toxicity because of the reduction in hepatic mass, blood flow, glomerular filtration rate, and lean mass and the increase in body fat.[59] These factors change the distribution, protein binding, metabolism, and excretion of the medication.

NSAIDs have interactions with commonly used drugs that must be evaluated for each patient and condition. The most common and potentially serious interaction is between NSAIDs and warfarin. NSAIDs may effect the metabolism of s-warfarin, cause an increase in the prothrombin time, and potentiate a bleeding diathesis.[60] NSAIDs will displace warfarin from binding to serum proteins and produce an increase in free warfarin, resulting in an increased tendency to bleed. More important, NSAIDs themselves cause asymptomatic damage and bleeding in the gastrointestinal mucosa. This intestinal damage, coupled with an inhibition of thromboxane and decreased platelet aggregation ("plugging"), significantly increases the risk of gastrointestinal hemorrhage. On the basis of risk/benefit analysis, there is very little indication for the use of NSAIDs for the OA patient who is anticoagulated. We suggest the use of alternative medications, such as analgesics and corticosteroid injections, and very careful assessment of the need before NSAIDs are prescribed.

When one is considering analgesia and arthritis, it is important to consider pain to be a physiologic response. If an analgesic is effective, overuse of the joint may occur. The goals for the clinician and his or her patient are to decrease pain and improve well-being but to also avoid overuse and accelerated joint degeneration. In 1989 Rashad et al.[61] randomized 105 subjects with hip OA to treatment with either indomethacin or azapropazone (a weak prostaglandin inhibitor) and followed the progression of OA to determine the need for surgical arthroplasty. They reported that the azapropazone-treated subjects took 5 months longer than the indomethacin-treated group to reach the arthroplasty end point (15.6 versus 10.4 months) and had less radiographic progression of OA than the indomethacin group. This suggests that potent inhibitors of prostaglandin synthesis, such as indomethacin, may accelerate OA of the hip. Although the actual mechanism responsible for this effect is not determined, indomethacin may have created an "analgesic arthropathy" by effective pain relief and worsened the course of OA of the humoral head. These results suggest that analgesic compounds may have a role in the treatment of OA in patients who have pain out of proportion to the degree of inflammation or in whom the use of NSAIDs is contraindicated. Longitudinal studies are now underway to determine what role analgesic agents will have in the long-term treatment of OA.

Gastrointestinal Toxicity

Gastrointestinal (GI) toxicity is the most clinically significant side effect of NSAIDs. The mechanism by which NSAIDs damage the mucosa is complex. NSAIDs reduce mucosal defenses by the depletion of endogenous prostaglandins, decrease the magnitude of the mucus-bicarbonate barrier, disrupt the epithelial layer, reduce the surface hydrophobicity of epithelial cells, and diminish mucosal blood flow.[62] NSAID toxicity includes gastritis, esophagitis, mucosal erosions, peptic ulcers, GI perforation, GI hemorrhage, gut dysmotility, and dyspermeability. Toxicity may occur throughout the alimentary tract, but most commonly lesions are found near the prepyloric region and antrum of the stomach.[62] Esophagitis and duodenitis may develop and cause strictures.

The true incidence and risk of GI toxicity through use of NSAIDs is unknown. These lesions are often asymptomatic, making determination of incidence and relative risk impossible. GI toxicity caused by NSAIDs contributes to more than 70,000 hospitalizations and more than 7000 deaths annually in the United States alone.[63] Not all patients taking NSAIDs are at the same risk for the development of life-threatening events. Longitudinal data from the Arthritis, Rheumatism and Aging Medical Information System (ARAMIS) now permits the identification of several risk factors.[64] The relative risk of hospitalization for patients with rheumatoid arthritis taking NSAIDs is 5.2, compared with those who are not taking NSAIDs.[63] Major risk factors identified for GI toxicity include age, level of disability, previous history of NSAID-induced peptic ulcer disease, history of taking antiulcer medications, NSAID dose, and concomitant glucocorticoid use.[63] Gastrointestinal hemorrhage with NSAID use is a cause of increased morbidity and mortality in patients with rheumatoid arthritis and has been called "the second most deadly rheumatic disease."[63]

The evaluation of antiulcer agents for patients at increased risk of NSAID-related gastrointestinal hemorrhage is ongoing. No study to date has shown that a decrease in endoscopically recognized ulcers is related to a decrease in gastrointestinal hemorrhage, perforation, or death in patients who are taking NSAIDs. At present, the available antiulcer strategies include (1) the prevention of gastric acid secretion, (2) the neutralization of gastric acid, and (3) mucosal cytoprotection. Histamine (H_2)-receptor antagonists (cimetidine, ranitidine, famotidine) and ATPase inhibitors (omeprazole) reduce or prevent the secretion of gastric acid. Inorganic antacids, such as Maalox and Mylanta, neutralize gastric acids. Sucralfate (Carafate) and the prostaglandin analog misoprostol are cytoprotective agents.

Misoprostol (Cytotec) is a prostaglandin E_1 analog that supplies prostaglandin locally to the GI tract for protection. A large, randomized, double-blind, multicenter, placebo-controlled trial evaluated the protective effect of misoprostol on NSAID-related gastrointestinal ulcer formation.[65] The investigators described 638 "arthritis" patients receiving a variety of NSAIDs and followed them endoscopically at baseline and at 4, 8, and 12 weeks while they were taking misoprostol or placebo. The development of a duodenal or gastric ulcer was defined endoscopically as a circumscribed mucosal defect greater than or equal to 0.5 cm in diameter, with perceptible depth. By 12 weeks, 2 of 320 (0.6%) patients receiving 200 µg of misoprostol four times daily, compared with 15 of 323 (4.6%) patients receiving placebo, developed duodenal ulcers. Gastric ulceration developed in 6 of 320 (1.9%) patients taking misoprostol, compared with 25 of 323 (7.7%) patients taking placebo. The authors concluded that misoprostol lowered the frequency of duodenal and gastric ulcers. These results must be interpreted with caution, as we do not know the compliance rate with NSAIDs, NSAID dose, or prednisone use and dose. Further, we do not know the clinical significance of these asymptomatic endoscopically determined ulcerations. Misoprostol did cause diarrhea in 32.3% of the patients and 17.9% of the controls. If GI symptoms from misoprostol cause patients to skip their nonsteroidal medication, the beneficial effect observed may be from erratic or noncompliant NSAID use, rather than from misoprostol cytoprotection.

Two previous studies using endoscopic evaluation compared misoprostol with placebo,[66] and misoprostol with sucralfate in the prevention of NSAID-induced ulcers[67]; both concluded that misoprostol was superior for protection from gastric ulcers in patients receiving NSAIDs. In the first study of 420 patients, after 3 months 12.3% of patients receiving placebo, 4.2% of patients receiving 100 µg of misoprostol four times a day, and 0.7% of those receiving 200 µg of misoprostol four times a day developed new gastric ulcers.[66] Of 253 patients available for analysis in the second study, a NSAID-induced ulcer developed in 1.6% of the patients receiving misoprostol compared with 16% of the patients receiving sucralfate.[67] The only inclusion criteria for these two studies were abdominal pain and NSAID use. Although these results are intriguing and potentially important, NSAID ulcers are often asymptomatic and may not progress. The clinical significance of these results is not yet determined.

Finally, in two published controlled trials, ranitidine has been shown to be effective in decreasing duodenal ulcer formation associated with NSAIDs but relatively ineffective against gastric ulceration.[68,69] Therefore, in a review of the totality of experience with cytoprotective agents, misoprostol may be considered for use in patients at increased risk of morbidity and mortality from GI toxicity; side effects and cost will limit its use even in this group of subjects.

Renal Toxicity

Prostacyclin and prostaglandins contribute to the maintenance of renal hemodynamics under normal and adverse conditions. Nonsteroidal medications, by inhibiting PG production, may decrease glomerular filtration and cause renal insufficiency. Those persons at higher risk for renal toxicity have previous impairment of renal function, diabetes, hypertension, atherosclerosis, or congestive heart failure, and are hypovolemic or hypoalbuminemic[70]; these phenomena are due to a decrease in renin release, decreased renal blood flow, and decreased tubular transport. Interstitial nephritis and proteinuria, not uncommon with NSAID usage, are the result of local T-lymphocyte activation and infiltration and are reversible with removal of the offending NSAID.[71] Fenoprofen, indomethacin, naproxen, and tolmetin are the agents most commonly associated with interstitial nephritis.[72] Papillary necrosis is unusual and most likely related to marked renal medullary ischemia from chronic inhibition of prostaglandins.[73]

Some investigators suggest that sulindac may spare renal function. In a study comparing renal PG synthesis in normal women taking sulindac, indomethacin, or placebo, decreased renal excretion of prostaglandin E_2, prostaglandin F_{2a}, and 6-keto prostaglandin F_{1a} was noted with use of indomethacin as compared with sulindac and placebo.[74] It is suggested that sulindac and its metabolite, sulindac sulfone, are renally inactive similar to placebo and do not inhibit renal prostaglandin H synthetase (cyclooxygenase). The active metabolite of sulindac, sulindac sulfide, is converted to sulindac sulfone within the kidneys before excretion. Therefore sulindac may spare the renal vasculature from PG inhibition and subsequently decrease nephrotoxicity. Although decreased renal toxicity was shown in this one study, other investigators have not reproduced these findings.[75,76] Many clinicians and scientists now conclude that sulindac does not decrease the risk of renal toxicity.

Hepatic Side Effects

Abnormal liver function may occur with NSAID use and is usually manifested as a mild to moderate chemical hepatitis, which is reversible with removal of the offending agent. Rarely, hepatic dysfunction progresses to hyperbilirubinemia and hepatic necrosis.[77] A recent meta-analysis found elevations in serum glutamic oxaloacetic transaminase (SGOT) to be related to baseline SGOT levels, diclofenac use in patients with OA, aspirin use in patients with rheumatoid arthritis, duration of treatment, and daily dose of medication.[78] Factors such as other medications, disease duration, and sex did not contribute to SGOT elevations. The majority of SGOT elevations for the patients were minimal and were not related to clinical hepatitis. There is additional evidence showing advanced age, polypharmaceuticals, high doses of NSAIDs, decreased renal function, and prolonged treatment to be risk factors for NSAID-related hepatotoxicity.[77] *Phenylbutazone has been a causal factor in a number of fatalities from hepatocellular injury and cannot be recommended for routine use.*[79]

Cutaneous and Hypersensitivity Side Effects

Nonsteroidal antiinflammatory agents may cause a morbilliform rash, urticaria, photosensitivity, vesiculobullous changes, vasculitis, serum sickness, exfoliative dermatitis, erythema multiforme/Stevens-Johnson syndrome, and toxic epidermal necrolysis.[80] The American Academy of Dermatology reports increased skin reactions with piroxicam, sulindac, and meclofenamate.[81] Severe reactions have occurred with phenylbutazone and oxyphenylbutazone. If an allergic skin reaction occurs, the medication should be discontinued. If the patient requires the use of an NSAID and the adverse reaction was limited to the skin, another agent may be used *but should be from a different class.* NSAIDs from one class react similarly to other agents from the same class and should not be given to persons who have a previous history of a reaction.

Hypersensitivity reactions characterized by urticaria, laryngospasm, bronchospasm, angioedema, and anaphylaxis may occur in persons with nasal polyps, asthma, and vasomotor rhinitis.[82] With the inhibition of cyclooxygenase, prostaglandin precursors are shunted away from the bronchodilating regulatory prostaglandins and toward leukotriene formation. An excess of a leukotriene product such as leukotriene B_4 (LTB$_4$, the slow-reacting substance of anaphylaxis), is responsible for the bronchospasm and anaphylaxis of this syndrome. *Under these circumstances, patients with this syndrome should avoid aspirin and all NSAIDs completely.*

Hematologic Side Effects

Rarely, blood dyscrasias occur with the use of NSAIDs. Aplastic anemia, hemolytic anemia, neutropenia, agranulocytosis, and thrombocytopenia have been reported. Phenylbutazone and oxyphenbutazone are most strongly associated with these adverse effects, and these two agents should not be used for OA.[83]

Neutropenia is associated with the use of NSAIDs. A population-based case control study was performed with Medicaid claims from six states.[84] Cases were noted involving hospitalized patients with neutropenia. For each case, four controls were randomly chosen and matched for age, sex, state, and year. The frequency of exposure to NSAIDs within 30 days of hospitalization was compared with the frequency in the control cases. The odds ratio for the development of neutropenia was 4.2. No single class of medication was associated with increased risk because of the low incidence of neutropenia and the inability to evaluate individual drugs. A previous study found that for those taking NSAIDs, the incidence rate of neutropenia was 45 cases per million per year, and for agranulocytosis it was 7.2 cases per million per year.[85] The low incidence rate and relative risk of 4.2 suggest that 145 cases of neutropenia and 23 cases of agranulocytosis would occur for every million people taking NSAIDs for a year.[84]

Both aspirin and NSAIDs result in a bleeding tendency by blocking the synthesis of thromboxane A_2 in platelets. Nonaspirin NSAIDs reversibly bind to and inhibit cyclooxygenase for the life of the platelet; the antithrombotic effect is reversed when NSAID is metabolized or excreted. On the other hand, aspirin permanently inactivates cyclooxygenase. For approximately 1 week after aspirin is taken, inhibition of thromboxane exists. Therefore the bleeding abnormality persists for the life of the platelet, even after the discontinuation of aspirin. It is recommended that aspirin and other NSAIDs be discontinued before a surgical procedure to avoid the risk of excessive bleeding. There are no established standards for the minimum time necessary under these circumstances. One to 2 days for short-half-life NSAIDs and 7 to 10 days for aspirin and long-half-life NSAIDs should be sufficient.

Central Nervous System Side Effects

NSAIDs are associated with central nervous system (CNS) side effects because they are lipophilic and easily diffuse across the blood-brain barrier. Aspirin may cause reversible tinnitus and hearing loss that may guide therapy in young persons.[86] Other side effects include altered moods, confusion, insomnia, depression, paranoia, headaches, lightheadedness, and drowsiness. These central effects are most prominent with indomethacin, but are noticed with all NSAIDs. Aseptic meningitis has been reported with ibuprofen, indomethacin, sulindac, and tolmetin, but it is uncommon.[87] Salicylate overdose with serum levels of 250 mg/L or greater can cause confusion, hallucinations, agitation, seizures, and coma and may be fatal if not diagnosed and treated appropriately.

Pregnancy

Nonsteroidal antiinflammatory agents are not recommended for use in pregnancy, since their safety has not been established. They are designated category B, meaning that reproduction studies performed in rats, rabbits, and mice at doses up to six times the human dose have revealed no evidence of impaired fertility or harm to the fetus due to the drug.[88] Unfortunately, animal reproduction studies are not always predictive of human response. Therefore the drug should not be used during pregnancy for any condition unless clearly needed. Because OA and pregnancy will not often occur together, the chances that this issue will become a clinical problem is extremely remote. In addition, the patency of the ductus arteriosus is dependent on prostaglandins, so that NSAID use may cause premature closure in the fetus. Use of NSAIDs during late pregnancy should be avoided. In animal models and lactating mothers, some NSAIDs are found excreted in milk.[88]

INTRAARTICULAR GLUCOCORTICOIDS

In 1951 hydrocortisone become available for intraarticular injection and was employed for the treatment of OA. The rationale for its use as an antiinflammatory agent in OA can be considered similar to that for NSAID use (discussed above). Systemic glucocorticoid treatment is not recommended, as the beneficial effects are minimal or negligible and the side effects of prolonged use are significant. It is thought that glucocorticoids reduce joint inflammation by decreasing the production of the enzyme phospholipase A_2 leading to diminished production of prostaglandin and leukotriene.

Glucocorticoids have many biologic effects in the human body. They effect leukocyte movement, change leukocyte function, and alter humoral factors.[89] They have been noted to have a greater effect on leukocyte movement and cell-mediated inflammation than on leukocyte function and humoral processes. Saxne et al.[90] compared the use of intraarticular glucocorticoids with placebo, and found a reduction of interleukin-1 and some protease enzymes involved in cartilage degradation. In addition, corticosteroids may reduce synovial vascular permeability and inhibit angiogenesis.[91,92] These factors help suppress intraarticular inflammation.

A possible protective effect of intraarticular corticosteroids has been noted in experimentally induced osteoarthritis. In 1985, Williams and Brandt[93] found a dose-dependent protective effect of triamcinolone hexacetonide in chemically (iodoacetate) induced articular damage in the guinea pig model of OA. Also, in the anterior cruciate ligament resection model of OA in Pond-Nuki dogs, intraarticular triamcinolone hexacetonide or oral prednisone at 0.25 mg/kg/d decreased femoral cartilage erosions and significantly reduced osteophyte size compared with untreated or placebo-treated controls.[94] No controlled or comprehensive study exists assessing the long-term results of corticosteroid injections on the history of osteoarthritis in ambulatory patients.

Intraarticular corticosteroid use should be considered palliative and temporary (short-lived). It is used in single or multiple joints that are not responsive to other therapies or in patients who cannot tolerate NSAIDs. It has been used to facilitate rehabilitation, to aid patients undergoing physical therapy, to decrease effusions, and to prevent stretching and laxity of the capsule and ligaments. Most authors describe favorable results with intraarticular corticosteroids in OA, although little scientific data exist from blinded, placebo-controlled trials. The size of the joint, the volume of effusion, the type and dose of corticosteroid preparation, the injection technique, and the severity of synovitis are factors that influence the efficacy of intraarticular injections (Table 18–2). Contraindications to glucocorticoid articular injection include the presence or suspicion of a skin or joint infection, bacteremia, and recent trauma to neighboring structures.

Side effects of glucocorticoid injection include skin, articular, and systemic infection; postinjection flare; crystal-induced synovitis; cutaneous atrophy; and fat necrosis. Repeated corticosteroid use may induce "analgesic arthropathy," whereby a decrease or absence of pain may allow overuse of the joint and a more rapid deterioration.[95] Rarely, there may be some systemic absorption of corticosteroids from the joint that may result in fluid retention, hyperglycemia, and hypertension. We recommend no more than two injections per joint per year in routine cases. Each intraarticular injection for weight-bearing joints should be followed by a short period of rest (recommended time period, from 1 to 7 days). An occasional patient may appear to need up to three or four injections in a single joint during 1 year; this situation will be exceedingly unusual and should force the clinician to rethink the whole treatment plan for that patient. For example, is there another reason for the pa-

---

TABLE 18–2

Recommended Drug, Dose, and Volume for Intraarticular Joint Injection

JOINT	GENERIC GLUCOCORTICOID	TRADEMARK NAME	DOSE	VOLUME	NEEDLE SIZE
PIP	Triamcinolone acetonide	Kenalog-40	40 mg/ml	0.1 ml (4 mg)	27-30 G
DIP	Triamcinolone acetonide	Kenalog-40	40 mg/ml	0.1 ml (4 mg)	27-30 G
CMC	Triamcinolone acetonide	Kenalog-40	40 mg/ml	0.1 ml (4 mg)	27-30 G
Knee	Triamcinolone hexacetonide	Aristospan	20 mg/ml	1.0 ml of steroid and 1–2 ml of 1% lidocaine	19-22 G

PIP: Proximal interphalangeal joint. DIP: Distal interphalangeal joint. CMC: Carpal metacarpal joint.

tient's symptoms or a different cause for the problem? Finally, repeated injections into the same joint seem to lose efficacy over time; reasons for this well-known clinical phenomenon are not known. For an in-depth discussion, the reader is referred to Kelley et al. (reference 141), Chapters 41 (Aspirin and Salicylates), 43 (NSAIDs), and 48 (Corticosteroids).

JOINT LAVAGE

Improvement in the symptoms of osteoarthritis was observed by many investigators after arthroscopy of the knee. Interestingly, reduction of knee pain was noted when the joint was only lavaged and arthroscopic surgery was not performed. Some investigators suggest that this improvement is due to a washout effect of inflammatory mediators in the joint, and others believe that mechanically stretching of the joint capsule is responsible for the relief of pain.

Saline lavage of the arthritic knee may be performed with arthroscopic visualization and guidance or with a needle and syringe. Recently, two investigational groups—Chang et al.[96] and Ike et al.[97]—have shown that closed-joint lavage may be beneficial in a subgroup of patients with OA. In the study by Chang et al., 32 persons with osteoarthritis of the knee were randomized to arthroscopic surgery or closed-needle joint lavage. The patients were compared at baseline and at 3 and 12 months by standard clinical outcome measures. After 1 year, 58% of all subjects who underwent joint lavage reported clinical improvement compared with 44% of all subjects who underwent arthroscopy. For the subgroup that underwent arthroscopic surgery, predictors for successful outcome included meniscal tears of the anterior two thirds of the medial meniscus and any lateral meniscal tear. In this study, no clinical signs or symptoms (i.e., McMurray's sign, locking, or giving way of the knee) predicted the presence or absence of meniscal disease. Unfortunately, predictors for success of the lavage remain unknown, as intraarticular features of patients randomized to the lavage group were unknown. Of interest, the cost of arthroscopy was significantly higher than the cost of closed-needle lavage, but other post-procedure costs were not significantly different between the two groups.

Ike et al. evaluated tidal irrigation in the treatment of patients with refractory OA of the knee.[97] They randomized 77 patients from seven centers to receive physical therapy with or without tidal knee irrigation. They found statistically significant differences after 4 weeks of follow-up. The lavage group had decreased stiffness, recall stiffness, and knee tenderness compared with the control group using physical therapy. The interpretation of their short-term results is limited because there was no placebo or sham-irrigation group in this study. However, it does suggest that lavage of the joint may provide short-term improvement in flares of pain and inflammation in osteoarthritis.

ARTHROSCOPY

Osteoarthritis of the knee is characterized by the breakdown, softening, fragmentation and erosion of partial- or full-thickness articular cartilage. Arthroscopy aids in the inspection of the supporting structures of the joint. With arthroscopy, underlying subchondral bone and varying degrees of synovitis among the capsule may be visualized. Along the articular surfaces, osteophytes often develop and may be seen. Partial or complete tears of the anterior cruciate ligament and the posterior cruciate ligament can be seen, as well as the meniscal cartilage. Arthroscopy often provides an earlier method of establishing the diagnosis of OA in the absence of radiographic findings and may identify other contributing factors to the patient's symptom complex. Arthroscopy may be helpful in the therapy of OA in the interval before joint replacement is required, although carefully controlled longitudinal studies must be done to confirm this suspicion.

With the aid of specialized instruments, the arthroscopist is able to remove or repair meniscal tears, to remove loose bodies, and to shave the articular cartilage and synovium. These procedures may relieve symptoms, improve range of motion, and prolong the use of the osteoarthritic joint. Although pain is decreased and range of motion is improved with the removal of loose bodies and meniscal tears, the long-term outcome of arthroscopic debridement of the articular damage in the presence of OA is not yet known.

Arthroscopic surgery may be performed as a temporizing measure to postpone or delay partial or total knee replacement, although proof for this is lacking. Several studies report some reduction of pain after a tear in the anterior two thirds of the medial meniscus and a tear in the lateral meniscus are repaired.[96] However, the long-term consequence of meniscal debridement as well as the progression of joint degeneration is just beginning to be studied. For example, Chang et al.[96] reported that 1 year after closed knee lavage or arthroscopic debridement, more patients had improvement with saline lavage than with arthroscopy.[96] These results suggest that patient selection for arthroscopic surgery is critical and may not be justified for every patient with non-end-stage OA of the knee. Success rates for arthroscopic debridement have varied between 50% and 67%, depending on the age of the patient, the degree of arthritis, the activity level of the patient, the anatomic abnormality, and the length of patient follow-up.[98,99]

Arthroscopy in osteoarthritis of the hip, ankle, shoulder, wrist, and elbow is presently being used for both diagnostic and therapeutic procedures. Arthroscopy is available for both rheumatologists and orthopedists to perform in their offices because newer fiber optics have permitted the development of arthroscopes 1.6 mm in diameter. Office arthroscopy of the knee allows for both diagnosis and guided articular saline lavage. More experienced arthroscopists can perform more complex therapeutic procedures. The patient remains awake (local and intraarticular anesthetic is used), and the diagnosis is known immediately. It may provide a less expensive, less invasive, and equally diagnostic tool for both orthopedists and rheumatologists to use in diagnosis of early osteoarthritis and internal derangements. Studies comparing the diagnostic capabilities of the needle arthroscope are now under way.[100,101]

ARTHROPLASTY

Generally, when joint pain and swelling develop in patients with osteoarthritis, damage to the articular cartilage is irreversible. Many patients have a period of time when analgesic or antiinflammatory medications control their pain enough to let them perform most of their activities of daily living. Eventually, medical therapy is less effective, and patients with OA of the knee or hip will require joint replacement. Pain and disability are the key factors involved in the timing of the arthroplasty. When the patient is at or approaching an unacceptable level of pain or function, the operation is indicated.

Good medical and psychological health, in addition to cooperation with postoperative care, is mandatory for surgical success. Active infection, poor medical health, morbid obesity, neurologic abnormalities, and muscular abnormalities are relative contraindications for surgery.

There are a wide variety of surgical alternatives for the arthritic patient. The hip and knee are the most commonly replaced joints, as involvement of these joints greatly affects the patients daily activities. Unfortunately, artificial joints have a limited lifetime; prostheses last from 8 to 15 years for both the hip and the knee, depending on the type of artificial joint used. Because of the limited lifetime of the artificial joint, some physicians delay arthroplasty in order to avoid repeated joint replacements. A significant amount of research is devoted to developing prostheses with a longer lifetime. Predictors of failure of prostheses include an imperfect surgical fit, a high level of physical activity and obesity.[102]

An osteotomy, which literally means "a cut in the bone," allows for correction of varus or valgus alignment in younger patients with unicompartmental disease of the knee. This procedure is performed on the motivated patient who is able to participate in intensive physical therapy. If the surgical outcome is satisfactory, it may delay the need for a total joint replacement for up to 10 years.[102] Total joint replacement is reserved for those who have bicompartmental or tricompartmental joint disease and may not benefit from osteotomy. An indepth discussion of the types of orthopedic procedures, materials, and options is beyond the scope of this section, but these are discussed in recent reviews.[102]

REHABILITATION

Rehabilitation is essential for the prevention of joint destruction, restoration of joint function after damage has occurred, and maintenance of joint function. Rehabilitation helps the patient reach his or her maximum potential. An individualized program is developed to meet the needs of every patient. This includes occupational therapy, physical therapy, vocational counseling, and social work services. Rehabilitation is limited by the extent of arthritis, motor and neurologic skills, and the patient's own motivation.

The first goal for a patient with symptomatic OA of a joint is to reduce, control, and prevent pain. The second goal is to preserve the patient's functional level and prevent further pain, weakness, and disability. Energy conservation, in the form of maximizing function and decreasing muscle fatigue, is necessary for success. Adaptive equipment or substitutive devices are employed to compensate for lost function as needed. Education and guidance must be available to the patients, as they need to develop coping strategies, which are important factors in the rehabilitative program.

Applications of superficial heat, deep heat, ultrasound, and cold packs can enhance stretch and decrease pain, muscle spasm, and stiffness.[103,104] These can be used separately or in combination. More controversial is the use of transcutaneous electrical nerve stimulation (TENS) devices, acupuncture, articular stimulation, and laser therapy.[105,106] Although these methods are not used routinely and have not been studied in a scientific manner, many patients attest to their satisfactory results. Patients with OA who cannot tolerate medical therapy for OA may have significant pain relief with any or all of these modalities. More detailed descriptions of these modalities for the treatment of OA are available in several recent reviews[107,108] and in Kelley et al. (reference 141), Chapter 102.

INVESTIGATIONAL AGENTS

Proteoglycans and Glycosaminoglycans

Several biologic agents are being evaluated for therapy in OA. Nonsulfated and sulfated polysaccharides (glycosaminoglycans) may be complexed with polypeptides and called proteoglycans. These materials are extracted from animal or plant sources and are used experimentally for their viscoelastic properties. They are administered by intraarticular or intramuscular injection and are summarized in Table 18–3.

Studies of cartilage explants show a variety of responses to proteoglycans and glycosaminoglycans. Arteparon, a glycosaminoglycan extract of bovine lung and trachea (see Table 18–3), has been shown to inhibit crude preparations of serine proteases, neutral proteases, elastases, cathepsin B, and hyaluronidase in a wide variety of tissue culture systems.[109–112] Rumalon, an extract of bovine cartilage and bone marrow, stimulates $^{35}SO_4$, ^3H-proline, and ^{14}C-glucosamine incorporation into normal and osteoarthritic cartilage.[112,113] Cartrofen (SP54 or sodium pentosan sulfate) is an extract of beech hemicellulose and has been shown to inhibit hyaluronidase, elastase, and other lysosomal enzymes in cultured synovial cells and to increase the production of hyaluronic acid.[112] Animal models of osteoarthritis have shown that intramuscular injection of cartrofen inhibits cartilage elastase and proteoglycan degradation without changing the morphology or histology of cartilage and synovium.[112] Ru-

---

TABLE 18–3
Summary of Investigational Biological Compounds for the Treatment of Osteoarthritis

PROTEOGLYCAN GAG	SIZE (DALTONS)	SOURCE	COMPONENT
Arteparon	2,000–16,000	Bovine lung Trachea	Semisynthetic mixture of oversulfated GAG Principal GAG-chondroitan-sulfate
Cartrofen (SP54, sodium pentosan sulfate)	6,000	Beech hemicellulose	Semisynthetic polysaccharide (1>4) linked β-D-xylopyranose
Rumalon	10^5– (2×10^6)	Bovine extract of bone marrow and cartilage	GAG-peptide–associated complex
Hyaluronan (Hylan G-F)	500,000 (2×10^6)	Rooster comb Human umbilical cord	Repeating polysaccharide units consisting of N-acetyl-glucosamine and glucuronic acid

GAG: Glycosaminoglycan.

malon and arteparon, given by intraarticular and intramuscular injection in animals, have been shown to decrease cartilage degeneration, femoral ulceration, and progression of existing erosions.[112]

Clinical trials with arteparon, cartrofen and rumalon are limited because of the presence of adverse effects. Arteparon has been reported to cause bleeding due to a heparinoid anticoagulant-like effect; it is also antigenic and has been associated with anaphylaxis.[114] Rumalon lacks the anticoagulant effect but is also antigenic and has the potential to induce anaphylaxis. Cartrofen and hyaluronic acid (hyaluronic acid will be discussed below) are glycosaminoglycans and lack the antigenic protein constituent in order to eliminate this potential side effect. For all these agents, the current available extraction techniques lack reproducibility despite standardization.

Hyaluronan

Hyaluronic acid or hyaluronan is the major nonsulfated glycosaminoglycan component of synovial fluid and cartilage. It has been extracted from rooster combs for veterinary/medical use. Intraarticular injection of hyaluronan has been used in race horses with osteoarthritis since the 1970s in an attempt to limit glucocorticoid steroid injections. The material is viscous but does not act effectively as an intraarticular lubricant because its half-life is less than 24 hours. It may provide a local antiinflammatory effect or may stimulate cartilage and synovial metabolism.

The earliest studies of hyaluronan were performed in the meniscectomized sheep model of early OA. Five intraarticular injections of hyaluronan were found to decrease "lameness" of the sheep but also increase radiographically defined osteophytes.[115] Despite this, hyaluronan has been shown to reduce pain and improve joint mobility.[116] A positive effect was noted after five weekly intraarticular injections in several clinical trials in Japan.[117,118]

Two preliminary reports on the efficacy and safety of intraarticular hyaluronic acid (Hylan G-F, Synvisc) have been reported.[119,120] Both studies are randomized, double-blind, multicenter trials of Hylan G-F in patients with osteoarthritis of the knee. Moreland et al.[119] evaluated three weekly intraarticular injections of Hylan G-F in 104 patients after a 4-week washout period from NSAIDs and glucocorticoids. All patients who received one treatment (three weekly injections) showed statistically significant improvement in several clinical parameters compared with controls (sham injection). In those who had two treatments (two courses of three weekly treatments), there was also significant improvement in pain parameters from baseline. Furthermore, two treatments were found to be superior to one treatment after 26 weeks ($p < 0.05$). In the second study, Adams et al.[120] studied the safety and efficacy of three weekly injections of Hylan G-F 20 alone and in combination with continuous NSAID treatment. The groups were divided as follows: (1) NSAID continuation and three weekly injections of Hylan, (2) NSAID continuation and three weekly "sham" injections, and (3) NSAID discontinuation at baseline and three weekly injections of Hylan. At 12 and 26 weeks, the three groups studied showed significant improvement in pain parameters from baseline, except that NSAIDs alone were ineffective for rest pain and lateral tenderness. The patients who received the Hylan injections with or without NSAID therapy had a statistically significant better result than the group that received continuous NSAID therapy alone ($p < 0.05$). Local, transient pain and swelling occurred with 1% of 400 injections in the former study and with a few of the 238 injections in the latter. No adverse systemic effects were observed. In these two preliminary studies, three weekly intraarticular injections of Hylan were safe and effective. Further follow-up is needed to determine the long-term efficacy of this interesting substance.

The connection between hyaluronan and pain relief is not well understood. High-molecular-weight hyaluronan (1.9×10^6 daltons) is able to inhibit leukocyte chemotaxis, while having no effect on the production of free radicals in vitro.[121,122] Some investigators postulate that hyaluronate may localize in the extracellular matrix around the synoviocytes and stimulate biosynthetic activity.[121,122] This might improve the viscosity and elasticity of the cartilage. Hyaluronan may physically bind to and entrap noxious substances in synovial fluid to protect the intraarticular cells from their effects.[122] When injected into animals and human beings, hyaluronan has a half-life of less than 48 hours.

In postulating a mechanism of action of hyaluronan, one must account for the clinical benefit of material with a short intraarticular half-life.

Hyaluronan is presently approved in Japan, Canada, Italy, and Sweden for intraarticular injections in patients with OA. Various countries, including the United States, are presently involved in multicenter clinical trials of this and similar agents.

Intraarticular Morphine

Intraarticular morphine has been used for analgesia after arthroscopic knee surgery. Morphine may produce an antinociceptive effect by interacting with local opioid receptors in inflamed peripheral tissue. In a recent postarthroscopy study of knee pain, Stein et al.[123] compared intraarticular and intravenous morphine for patients in pain management. Pain was measured by visual analog scales (VAS), numerical rating scales, and the McGill pain questionnaire.[124] In their study of 78 patients, they found that the group with intraarticular morphine had equal or better reduction of pain than a group using intravenous morphine that was eradicated with the opiate antagonist naloxone. In this way, intraarticular morphine or other opioid receptor agonists may be considered in the future for patients with OA and for short-term relief of pain.

Intraarticular NSAIDs

Tenidap is a novel antiinflammatory drug in development for treatment of inflammatory arthritis and osteoarthritis. It has been shown to decrease intraarticular production of interleukin-1 and -6,[125] and decrease the interleukin-1 receptor production by chondrocytes in vitro.[126] Intraarticular tenidap has recently been compared with placebo in a small, short-term, open trial of 25 arthritis patients with knee effusions.[127] The authors found after 1 week that the use of tenidap had decreased the synovial fluid leukocyte count and improved the physician's global assessment score compared with the use of placebo. This may be an option for the delivery of NSAIDs in the future in those unable to tolerate oral therapy.

Chemical Synovectomy

Osmic acid (osmium tetraoxide) has been used intraarticularly in Scandinavia and Europe since the 1950s to induce a chemical synovectomy. It has been used with lidocaine and glucocorticoids to chemically alter or damage the synovium and decrease painful effusions. Most studies have been performed on patients with chronic, recurrent effusions from osteoarthritis and hemophilic hemarthroses.[128,129] This modality may be both painful and dangerous; it has not been studied in the United States, as there are other, less caustic ways to produce a synovectomy.

Radionuclide Synovectomy

Radioisotopes, such as radioactive gold (^{198}Au), yttrium (^{90}Y), erbium (^{169}Eb), dysprosium ferrous hydroxide (^{165}Dy-FHMA), and colloidal chromic phosphate (^{32}P-$CrPO_4$), have been used by various investigators to cause "radiosynovectomy."[130–134] Local injection of these materials in persons with rheumatoid arthritis and chronic knee effusions causes the synovium to atrophy. Studies with these radioisotopes were performed in the 1970s and 1980s but have fallen out of favor because of concerns with radionuclides and their carcinogenic effects after systemic absorption.

Superoxide Dismutase Inhibition

The inflammatory process of osteoarthritis involves free radical formation. Modification of superoxide and hydroxyl free radicals may dampen the inflammatory reaction. In vitro, free radicals degrade hyaluronic acid, collagen, and proteoglycans and inhibit the metabolism of chondrocytes.[135] Superoxide dismutase (SOD) catalyzes the formation of peroxide from free radicals, decreasing their serum concentration. Injections of orgotein, a protein extract of bovine liver with SOD activity, have been used in the treatment of race horses with inflammatory and traumatic arthritis.[136] In rabbits with osteoarthritis, no difference has been observed between the SOD-treated animals and controls.[137]

Several controlled clinical trials have been performed. Gammer and Broback[138] found no adverse effects of intraarticular orgotein (8 or 16 mg injected every 2 weeks for 6 weeks) when compared with methylprednisolone acetate. In 36 patients with osteoarthritis of the knee, they found a lessening of knee pain after 6 weeks, but only those who had a 16 mg injection of orgotein had a sustained improvement after 6 months.

In a more recent study, 139 patients with OA of the knee were randomized to receive placebo or one of three doses of orgotein.[139] After a flare of OA, intraarticular SOD decreased pain, improved global assessment, improved knee function, and was well tolerated. Comparison of a weekly intraarticular dose regimen of 8 mg for 4 weeks, 16 mg for 2 weeks, or one 32 mg injection showed that 16 mg/wk for 2 weeks was the most effective in pain relief. Adverse effects were infrequent and consisted of skin rash and pruritus. Discomfort was noted at the injection site, and posttreatment SOD-specific antibodies (IgG) were detected in 57% of the patients. No association between the presence of SOD antibodies, adverse effect, or clinical efficacy was noted. Further studies are under way with this product.

Electromagnetic Radiation

The final investigational modality to discuss in the management of OA is electromagnetic radiation. This has been applied locally to the knee in the form of pulsed electromagnetic fields (PEMF). Uncontrolled observations show 70% to 80% improvement of symptoms in more than 800 patients with "painful rheumatic conditions."[140] A double-blinded, controlled pilot study evaluated 27 patients with primary OA of the knee or hip under treatment with PEMF.[140] Trock et al.[140] used 18 half-hour, low-frequency pulsed waves over 1 month and 1 month later noted 23% to 61% clinical improvement with electromagnetic radiation compared with 2% to 18% improvement in the placebo group. Although this is an interesting finding, more studies are required to confirm these findings and to better define the response.

RECOMMENDATIONS FOR MANAGEMENT OF OSTEOARTHRITIS

Effective management of osteoarthritis rests on the establishment of an accurate diagnosis (Table 18–4). One must rule out other conditions that can mimic OA, including chronic mycobacterial or fungal infection, certain systemic diseases, osteonecrosis syndromes, and cancer in nearby structures. An in-depth discussion of the differential diagnosis of patients

TABLE 18–4
Differential Diagnosis of Hand Pain, Hip Pain, and Chronic Knee Pain in the OA Setting

Commonly Encountered Conditions that Mimic OA of the Hand
1. Reflex sympathetic dystrophy
2. Tendonitis syndrome, including de Quervain's disease
3. Radiculopathy from cervical spine
4. Nerve entrapment syndrome
5. Other joint and bone diseases: rheumatoid arthritis, psoriatic arthritis, sarcoid, CPPD deposition disease, urate gout

Hip Diseases Other than OA
1. Seronegative spondyloarthropathies
   a. Reiter's disease
   b. Ankylosing spondylitis
   c. Psoriatic arthritis
2. Rheumatoid arthritis
3. Avascular necrosis of femoral head
4. Congenital/developmental hip dysplasias
5. CPPD deposition disease
6. Metastatic tumor, insufficiency fracture, Paget's disease

Other Causes of Chronic Knee Pain
1. CPPD deposition disease
2. Chronic infection (mycobacterial, fungal)
3. Urate gout
4. Osteonecrosis
5. Rheumatoid arthritis
6. Seronegative spondyloarthropathies
   a. Ankylosing spondylitis
   b. Psoriatic arthritis
   c. Reiter's disease
7. Loose body, meniscal, or ligamental tear
8. Hypertrophic osteoarthropathy (HOA)

with acute and chronic monoarthritis and polyarthritis is found in Kelley et al. (reference 141), Chapters 22 and 23. Further, we recommend physical and occupational therapy for all of our patients to strengthen the supporting muscles and to provide protection of the joint. For persons who are functionally disabled, we recommend the early use of appropriate assistive devices. In the obese patient, weight reduction is strongly advised.

We encourage a symptomatic and regional approach to therapy in patients with OA (Figs. 18–2 to 18–4). On initial evaluation, we focus on the patient's quality of life and specifically we focus further on inflammatory and nonin-

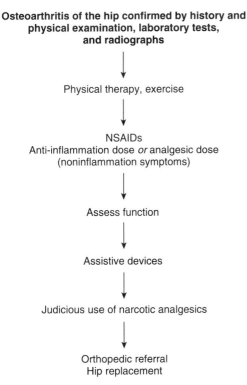

Osteoarthritis of the hands confirmed by history, physical examination, and radiographs

↓

Occupational therapy and local heat or cold or both

↓

Acetaminophen as needed for pain and discomfort

↓

Low-dose NSAID as needed for pain and discomfort

↓

Glucocorticoid injection for isolated cyst or inflammation of the joint or both

↓

For signs of inflammation: anti-inflammatory doses of NSAIDs if not contraindicated

↓

For instability, subluxation, or intractable pain and loss of function, recommend orthopedic consultation for possible joint fusion or arthroplasty

FIGURE 18–2
Guidelines for the treatment of OA of the hand.

Osteoarthritis of the hip confirmed by history and physical examination, laboratory tests, and radiographs

↓

Physical therapy, exercise

↓

NSAIDs
Anti-inflammation dose *or* analgesic dose (noninflammation symptoms)

↓

Assess function

↓

Assistive devices

↓

Judicious use of narcotic analgesics

↓

Orthopedic referral
Hip replacement

FIGURE 18–3
Stepwise outline for the treatment of OA of the hip.

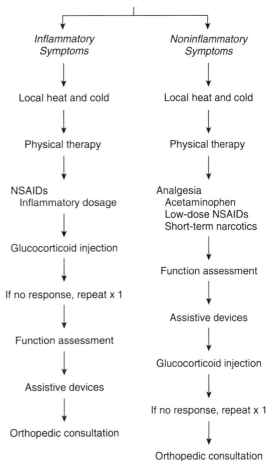

Osteoarthritis of the knee confirmed by history, physical examination, laboratory tests, and radiographs

Inflammatory Symptoms | *Noninflammatory Symptoms*

Inflammatory Symptoms:

↓

Local heat and cold

↓

Physical therapy

↓

NSAIDs
Inflammatory dosage

↓

Glucocorticoid injection

↓

If no response, repeat x 1

↓

Function assessment

↓

Assistive devices

↓

Orthopedic consultation

Noninflammatory Symptoms:

↓

Local heat and cold

↓

Physical therapy

↓

Analgesia
Acetaminophen
Low-dose NSAIDs
Short-term narcotics

↓

Function assessment

↓

Assistive devices

↓

Glucocorticoid injection

↓

If no response, repeat x 1

↓

Orthopedic consultation

FIGURE 18–4
Suggestions for the treatment of OA of the knee.

flammatory (or mechanical) signs and symptoms. Morning stiffness, joint swelling, erythema, warmth, and joint stiffness after sitting or resting for a period of time (known as the "gel phenomenon") are attributed to mild but definite inflammation of the joint or "synovitis." This is because the capillary network that supplies blood to the synovium is responsible for the production of synovial fluid. Inflammation increases the blood supply to the joint, which results in increased production of synovial fluid. In inflammatory arthritis, the increase in the volume of fluid within each joint produces swelling, stiffness, and "gelling." These patients often have improvement in their symptoms after activity as the mechanical pumping action of the joints and muscles reverses this process and decreases the volume of fluid within the joint. On the other hand, mechanical joint pain often occurs while and after the patient uses the joint. For example, mechanical pain in the hip and knee occurs when the patient is climbing up and down stairs or after an extended walk. It occurs at the end of the day rather than on awaking. However, structural and mechanical joint abnormalities often lead to secondary inflammation within the joint, so the distinction between inflammatory and noninflammatory joint pain is, in reality, less defined and not always easily demonstrated.

In the patient with OA, if inflammatory findings predominate, we concentrate on antiinflammatory medications such as the NSAIDs and glucocorticoid injections. For the patient with more mechanical symptoms, we advocate rest, analgesia, assistive devices, muscle strengthening, occupational therapy, and physical therapy.

The Hand

Persons with primary OA of the hand will have involvement of the first carpal metacarpal (CMC) joint, the proximal interphalangeal (PIP) joint, and the distal interphalangeal (DIP) joint. Osteophytes may cause a decrease in the range of motion of the fingers and may be painful. For single, isolated mechanical DIP, PIP, and CMC joint involvement, acetaminophen or low-dose NSAID and occupational therapy are recommended. For a single joint of the hand that has signs of inflammation, we use a 27- to 30-gauge needle and inject a small volume of concentrated triamcinolone acetonide into the joint (Table 18–2). Intraarticular cysts may occur, producing a subcutaneous nodule, and cause local symptoms. If an intraarticular cyst has formed and is symptomatic, we carefully isolate it, aspirate the joint fluid, and inject it similarly. If three or more joints are involved, and the patient has mechanical, noninflammatory symptoms, we recommend analgesics and occupational therapy. If a similar number of joints are involved with inflammatory symptoms, we consider the use of daily antiinflammatory dose NSAIDs after assessing the risk of NSAID-associated toxicities. For grossly unstable and painful joints (the first CMC or interphalangeal joints with OA), we consider arthroplasties, joint fusion or replacement. This is recommended only if the patient has suffered substantial functional loss of the hand accompanied by considerable pain that is poorly managed with glucocorticoid injections,

oral medications, physical therapy, and assistive devices (Fig. 18–2). We do not recommend this type of surgery for cosmesis only.

The first CMC joint of the thumb is always a major therapeutic challenge because of the marked functional impairment produced by loss of pinch and grasp. Consultation with a hand occupational therapy specialist in the early stages will be useful. Careful consideration should be given to an integrated program consisting of judicious use of specialized splints, intraarticular injections, joint-protection methods, assistive devices, and reorganization of the work and recreation environment. For the surgical approach to OA of the hand, the reader is referred to Kelley et al. (reference 141), Chapter 104.

The Hip

Osteoarthritis of the hip is a major problem for the patient because the hip is a weight-bearing joint. In general, weight-bearing joints create a disproportionate amount of pain and disability in those affected. In patients with isolated OA of the hip, we assess their symptoms (mechanical or inflammatory) and functional status. Similar to the approach used for OA of the hand, we recommend NSAIDs in antiinflammatory doses for inflammatory symptoms and rest, physical therapy, and analgesia for noninflammatory symptoms (Fig. 18–3). For those patients who are more than 20% above their ideal body weight, we strongly recommend weight loss and refer them to a dietitian. To avoid abnormal stress on the knees and the contralateral hip, we take precautions to assure the proper use of appropriate assistive devices when needed. If the patient's symptoms do not improve or worsen, and the range of motion greatly limits the patient's ability to function, we consider a referral to the orthopedist for joint replacement. We do not routinely inject the hip with glucocorticoids, except diagnostically to differentiate the hip pain from knee and back pain when the pain is poorly defined and when knee and back disease are also present. If injection of the hip is considered necessary, we recommend fluoroscope or computerized tomographic guidance. An in-depth approach to hip disease is discussed in Kelley et al. (reference 141), Chapter 108.

The Knee

Osteoarthritis of the knee is a common rheumatologic problem that is associated with pain and functional disability. Here again we treat patients who have inflammatory symptoms with antiinflammatory therapies and patients who have mechanical symptoms with analgesics, rest, assistive devices, and physical therapy (Fig. 18–4). We focus our initial examination on the presence or absence of inflammation and on the specific compartment involved. The knee is composed of three compartments, the patellofemoral compartment, the medial tibiofemoral compartment, and the lateral tibiofemoral compartment. For isolated patellofemoral compartment involvement, we use analgesics and recommend physical therapy and joint protection. If inflammation is present, we add NSAIDs in antiinflammatory doses or inject the knee with a glucocorticoid (see Table 18–2). For persons with medial and/or lateral compartment mechanical pain, we recommend conservative management with rest, physical therapy, assistive devices, and analgesics. We initially use NSAIDs for treatment of the inflammatory symptoms of the medial and lateral compartments of the knee. This is followed by a trial of intraarticular glucocorticoids and may be repeated. An occasional patient may develop a symptomatic synovial effusion or a popliteal (Baker's) cyst. This may require aspiration to decrease the intraarticular pressure. The direct connection between the popliteal cyst and the patellofemoral joint provides safe and easy access to the joint space for aspiration and injection and communication to the popliteal space for therapeutic benefit. If the patient's knee symptoms persist or become worse, or if clicking, locking, and falling occur, further diagnostic testing is required. Magnetic resonance scanning or diagnostic arthroscopy may be used. Some patients with progressive OA of the knee rapidly experience a significant loss of function. We will refer patients for surgical consultation when they have intractable pain, have an unstable knee, or have lost the function of the knee. Figures 18–1 to 18–4 are provided to guide the generalist in the work-up and management of OA. The surgical approach to the knee is outlined in Kelley et al. (reference 141), Chapter 109.

FOR THE FUTURE

Our goal is to detect the onset of OA at a stage where the disease is reversible. Earlier diagnoses will be obtained with the advent of needle arthroscopy, higher-resolution magnetic resonance imaging, and recognition of serologic markers of disease. Currently, patients from our clinic are involved in many ongoing studies involving both diagnostic and therapeutic interventions for osteoarthritis. Novel therapeutic modalities now under study in the treatment of OA include compounds that inhibit enzymatic breakdown of cartilage at an early, possibly reversible, stage of OA, cartilage transplantation, and orthopedic devices with improved longevity.

As the population ages and the proportion of elderly persons grows, so does the prevalence of OA. We need to have a better understanding of the pathogenesis of early OA in order to develop preventive measures and better therapeutic options for patients with this disease. The therapeutic options we have discussed provide an exciting and more optimistic future for those with osteoarthritis.

REFERENCES

1. National Center for Health Statistics. Prevalence of osteoarthritis in adults by age, sex, race, and geographic area: United States 1960–1962. Washington DC: Government Printing Office. Vital and Health Statistics, No. 15, Series 11, 1966.
2. Howell DS. Etiopathogenesis of osteoarthritis. In: Moskowitz RW, Howell DS, Goldberg VM, et al., eds. Osteoarthritis: diagnosis and management. Philadelphia: WB Saunders, 1984:129.
3. Howell DS, Treadwell DV, Tripple SB. Etiopathogenesis of osteoarthritis. In: Moskowitz RW, Howell DS, Goldberg VM, et al., eds. Osteoarthritis: diagnosis and medical/surgical management. 2nd ed. Philadelphia: WB Saunders, 1992:233.
4. Wolff J, Maquet P, Furlong R, trans. The law of bone remodeling, 1892. Berlin: Springer-Verlag, 1986.
5. Telhas H, Lindberg L. A method of inducing osteoarthritic changes in rabbit's knees. Clin Ortho 1972;86:66.
6. Buckwalter JA, Rosenberg LC, Hunzker EB. Articular cartilage: composition, structure, response to injury and methods of facilitating repair. In: Ewing JW, ed. Articular cartilage and knee joint function: basic science of arthroscopy. New York: Raven, 1990:19.
7. Mankin HJ, Brandt KD, Shulman LE. Workshop on etiopathogenesis of osteoarthritis. J Rheumatol 1986;13:1127.
8. Buchanan WW, Park WM. Primary generalized osteoarthritis: definition and uniformity. J Rheumatol 1983;10:4.
9. Kellgren JH, Lawrence JS, Bier F. Genetic factors in generalized osteoarthrosis. Ann Rheum Dis 1963;22:237.
10. Cooke TD. Pathogenetic mechanisms in polyarticular osteoarthritis. Clin Rheum Dis 1985; 11:203.

11. Knowlton RG, Katzenstein PL, Moskowitz RW, et al. Genetic linkage of a polymorphism in the type II procollagen gene (COL2A1) to primary osteoarthritis associated with mild chondrodysplasia. N Engl J Med 1990;322:526.

12. Ehlich GE. Erosive inflammatory and primary generalized osteoarthritis. In: Moskowitz RW, Howell DS, Goldberg VM, Mankin HK, eds. Osteoarthritis: diagnosis and management. Philadelphia: WB Saunders, 1992:329.

13. Mankin HJ. The reaction of articular cartilage to injury and osteoarthritis. N Engl J Med 1990;291:1285.

14. Martel-Pelletier J, Pelletier JP, Malemud CJ. Activation of neutral metalloproteinase in human osteoarthritic knee cartilage: evidence for degradation in the core protein of sulphated proteoglycan. Ann Rheum Dis 1988;47:801.

15. Tyler JA. Chondrocyte-mediated depletion of articular cartilage proteoglycans in vitro. Biochem J 1985;225:493.

16. Sandy JD, Nearne PJ, Boynton RE, et al. Catabolism of aggrecan in cartilage explants: identification of a major cleavage site within the interglobular domain. J Biol Chem 1981; 266:8683.

17. Pelletier JP, Martel-Pelletier J, Altman RD, et al. Collagenolytic activity and collagen matrix breakdown of the articular cartilage in the Pond-Nuki dog model of osteoarthritis. Arthritis Rheum 1983;26:866.

18. Proceedings of the Symposium on Osteoarthritis. Proteases: their involvement in osteoarthritis. J Rheumatol 1987;106(suppl):1.

19. Dean DD. Proteinase-mediated cartilage degradation in osteoarthritis. Semin Arthritis Rheum 1991;20(suppl):2.

20. Pelletier JP, Rougley P, DiBattista JA, et al. Are cytokines involved in osteoarthritic pathophysiology. Semin Arthritis Rheum 1991;20(suppl): 63.

21. Pelletier JP, Martel-Pelletier J, Howell DS, et al. Collagenase and collagenolytic activity in human osteoarthritic cartilage. Arthritis Rheum 1983;26:63.

22. Sapolsky AI, Malemud CJ, Norby DP, et al. Neutral proteinases from articular chondrocytes in culture. 2. Metal-dependent latent neutral proteoglycanase and inhibitory activity. Biochem Biophys Acta 1981;658:138.

23. Martel-Pelletier J, Pelletier JP, Cloutier JM, et al. Neutral protease capable of proteoglycan digesting activity in osteoarthritic and normal human articular cartilage. Arthritis Rheum 1984;27:305.

24. Pelletier JP, Martel-Pelletier J, Cloutier JM, et al. Proteoglycan-degrading acid metalloprotease activity in human osteoarthritic cartilage, and the effect of intraarticular steroid injections. Arthritis Rheum 1987;19:541.

25. Dean DD, Martel-Pelletier J, Pelletier JP, et al. Evidence for metalloproteinase and metalloprotease inhibitor (TIMP) imbalance in human osteoarthritic cartilage. J Clin Invest 1989;84:678.

26. Dean DD, Woessner JF Jr. Extracts of human articular cartilage contain an inhibitor of tissue metalloproteinases. Biochem J 1984;218:277.

27. Felson DT, Zhang Y, Anthony JM, Naimark A, Anderson JJ. Weight loss reduces the risk for symptomatic knee osteoarthritis in women. Ann Intern Med 1992;116:535.

28. Batchlor EE, Paulus HE. Principles of drug therapy. In: Moskowitz RW, Howell DS, Goldberg VN, Mankin HJ, eds. Osteoarthritis: diagnosis and management. 2nd ed. Philadelphia: WB Saunders, 1992:465.

29. Fife RS, Brandt KD. Other approaches to therapy. In: Moskowitz RW, Howell DS, Goldberg VN, Mankin HJ, eds. Osteoarthritis: diagnosis and management. 2nd ed. Philadelphia: WB Saunders, 1992:511.

30. Thonar EJ-MA, Shinmei M, Lohmander LS. Body fluid markers of cartilage changes in osteoarthritis. Med Clin North Am 1993;19:635.

31. Koch-Weser J. Drug therapy: acetaminophen. N Engl J Med 1979;295:1297.

32. Doyle DV, Dieppe PA, Scott J, Huskisson EC. An articular index for the assessment of osteoarthritis. Ann Rheum Dis 1981;40:75.

33. Parr G, Darekar B, Fletcher A, Bulpitt AJ. Joint pain and quality of life: results of a randomised trial. Br J Clin Pharmacol 1989;27:235.

34. Stamp J, Rhind V, Haslock I. A comparison of nefopam and flurbiprofen in the treatment of osteoarthrosis. Br J Clin Pract 1989;43:24.

35. Bradley JD, Brandt KD, Katz BP, Kalasinski LA, Ryan SI. A comparison of an antiinflammatory dose of ibuprofen, an analgesic dose of ibuprofen, and acetaminophen in the treatment of patients with osteoarthritis of the knee. N Engl J Med 1991;325:87.

36. Fries JF, Spitz PW, Young DY. The dimensions of health outcomes: the health assessment questionnaire, disability and pain scales. J Rheumatol 1982;9:789.

37. Williams HJ, Ward JR, Egger MJ, et al. Comparison of naproxen and acetaminophen in a two-year study of treatment of osteoarthritis of the knee. Arthritis Rheum 1993;36:1196.

38. Lim RKS, Guzman F, Rodger DW et al. Site of action on narcotic and non-narcotic analgesics determined by blocking bradykinin-evoked visceral pain. Arch Int Pharmacodyn Ther 1964; 152:25.

39. Boctor AM, Eickholt M, Puglsley TA. Meclofenamate sodium is an inhibitor of both the 5-lipoxygenase and cyclooxygenase pathways of the arachidonic acid cascade in vitro. Prostaglandins Leukot Med 1986;23:229.

40. Ku EC, Lee W, Koathari HV, Kimble EF, Liauw L, Tjan J. The effects of diclofenac on arachidonic acid metabolism. Semin Arthritis Rheum 1985;15:36.

41. Abramason S, Edelson H, Kaplan H, et al. The neutrophil in rheumatoid arthritis: its role and the inhibition of its activation by non-steroidal antiinflammatory drugs. Semin Arthritis Rheum 1983;13(suppl 1):148.

42. Biemond P, Swaak AJ, Peners JM, Beindroff CM, Koster JF. Superoxide production by polymorphonuclear leukocytes in rheumatoid arthritis and osteoarthritis. In vivo inhibition by anti-rheumatic drug piroxicam due to interference with activation of the NADPH-oxidase. Ann Rheum Dis 1986;45:249.

43. Bomalaski JS, Hirata F, Clark MA. Aspirin inhibits phospholipase C. Biochem Biophys Res Commun 1986;139:115.

44. Minta JO, Williams MD. Some non-steroidal antiinflammatory drugs inhibit the generation of superoxide anions by activated polymorphs by blocking ligand-receptor interactions. J Rheumatol 1985;12:751.

45. Abrahamson SB, Weismann G. The mechanism of action of nonsteroidal antiinflammatory drugs. Arthritis Rheum 1989;32:1.

46. Hochberg M. NSAIDs: mechanism and pathways of action. Hosp Pract 1989;24:185.

47. Hobbs DC, Twomey T. Piroxicam pharmacokinetics in man: aspirin and antacid interaction studies. J Clin Pharmacol 1979;19:270.

48. Annefeld M. The chondrocyte—the living element of articular cartilage. In: Articular cartilage and osteoarthrosis. Bern: Hans Huber, 1983:30.

49. Annefeld M. A new test method for the standardized evaluation of changes in the ultrastructure of chondrocytes. Int J Tissue React 1985;7:273.

50. Muir H, Carney SL, Hall LG. Effects of tiaprofenic acid and other nonsteroidal antiinflammatory drugs on proteoglycan metabolism in articular cartilage explant. Drugs 1988;35 (suppl 1):15.

51. Palmoski M, Brandt KD. In vivo effect of aspirin on canine osteoarthritic cartilage. Arthritis Rheum 1989;48:619.

52. Doherty M. "Chondroprotection" by nonsteroidal anti-inflammatory drugs. Ann Rheum Dis 1989;48:619.

53. Ghosh P. Anti-rheumatic drugs and cartilage. Clin Rheumatol 1988;2:309.

54. Herman JH, Appel AM, Hess EV. Modulation of cartilage destruction by select non-steroidal antiinflammatory drugs: in vitro effect on the synthesis and activity of catabolism-inducing cytokines produced by osteoarthritis and rheumatoid synovial fluid. Arthritis Rheum 1987;30:257.

55. McKenzie LS, Horsburgh BA, Ghosh P, Taylor TKF. Effect of antiinflammatory drugs on sulfated glycosaminoglycan synthesis in aged human articular cartilage. Ann Rheum Disease 1979;35:487.

56. Verbruggen G, Malfait AM, Veys EM, et al. Proteoglycan metabolism in isolated chondrocytes from human cartilage and short term tissue cultured human articular cartilage. Clin Exp Rheum 1989;7:13.

57. Morales TI, Hascall VC. Factors involved in the regulation of proteoglycan metabolism in articular cartilage. Arthritis Rheum 1989;32:1197.

58. Joyce CRB. Patient cooperation and the sensitivity of clinical trials. J Chron Dis 1962;15:1025.

59. Ouslander JG. Drug therapy in the elderly. Ann Intern Med 1981;95:711.

60. Vebeeck RK. Pharmacologic drug interactions with NSAIDs. Clin Pharmacokinet 1990;19:44.

61. Rashad S, Hemingway A, Rainsford K, et al. Effect of non-steroidal antiinflammatory drugs on the course of osteoarthritis. Lancet 1989;2:519.

62. Shorrack CJ, Rees WDW. Mechanism of gastric damage by nonsteroidal antiinflammatory drugs. Scand J Rheumatol 1989;78(suppl):5.

63. Fries JF. Non-steroidal gastropathy: the second most deadly rheumatic disease? The epidemiology and risk appraisal. J Rheumatol 1991;18 (suppl 28):6.

64. Fries JF, McShane DJ. ARAMIS (American Rheumatism Association Medical Information System). West J Med 1986;145:798.

65. Graham DY, White RH, Moreland LW, et al. Duodenal and gastric ulcer prevention with misoprostol in arthritis patients taking NSAIDs. Ann Intern Med 1993;119:257.

66. Roth SH. Misoprostol in the prevention of NSAID-induced gastric ulcers: a multicenter, double-blind, placebo controlled trial. J Rheumatol 1990;17:(suppl 20):20.

67. Agrawal NM, Roth SH, Graham DY, et al. Misoprostol compared with sucralfate in the prevention of NSAID induced gastric ulcer: a randomized, controlled trial. Ann Intern Med 1991;115:195.

68. Robinson MG Jr, Griffin JW, Bowers J, et al. Effect of ranitidine on gastroduodenal mucosal damage induced by NSAIDs. Dig Dis Sci 1989;34:424.

69. Ehsanullah RS, Page MC, Tidesley G, Wood JR. Prevention of gastroduodenal damage induced by NSAIDs: controlled trial of ranitidine. Br Med J 1988;297:1017.

70. Clements PJ, Paulus HE. Non-steroidal antiinflammatory drugs. In: Kelley WN, Harris EH, Ruddy S, Sledge CB, eds. Textbook of rheumatology. 4th ed. Philadelphia: WB Saunders, 1993:707.

71. Blackshear JL, Napier JS, Davidman M, Stillman MT. Renal complication of non-steroidal antiinflammatory drugs: identification and monitoring those at risk. Semin Arthritis Rheum 1985;14:163.

72. Abraham PA, Keane WF. Glomerular and interstitial disease induced by nonsteroidal antiinflammatory drugs. Am J Nephrol 1984;4:1.

73. DiBona GF. Prostaglandins and nonsteroidal antiinflammatory drugs: effects on renal hemodynamics. Am J Med 1986;80(suppl 1A):127.

74. Sedor JR, Williams SL, et al. Effects of sulindac and indomethacin on renal prostaglandin synthesis. Clin Pharmacol Ther 1984;36:85.

75. Berg KJ, Talseth T. Acute renal effects of sulindac and indomethacin in chronic renal failure. Clin Pharmacol Ther 1985;37:447.

76. Whelton A, Stout RL, Spilman PS, Klossen DK. Renal effects of ibuprofen, piroxicam and sulindac in patients with asymptomatic renal failure. Ann Intern Med 1990;112:568.

77. Katz LM, Love PY. Hepatic dysfunction in association with non-steroidal antiinflammatory drugs. In: Famey JP, Paulus HE, eds. Nonsteroidal antiinflammatory drugs: subpopulation therapy and drug delivery systems. New York: Marcel Dekker, 1991.

78. Furst DE, Anderson W. Differential effects of diclofenac and aspirin on serum glutamic oxaloacetic transaminase elevations in patients with rheumatoid arthritis and osteoarthritis. Arthritis Rheum 1993;36:804.

79. Benjamin SB, Isha KG, Zimmerman HJ, Grushka A. Phenylbutazone liver injury: a clinical pathologic survey of 23 cases and review of the literature. Hepatology 1981;1:255.

80. O'Brien WM, Bagby GF. Rare adverse reactions to NSAIDs. J Rheumatol 1985;12:13.

81. Stern RS, Bigby M. An expanded profile of cutaneous reactions to NSAIDs. JAMA 1984;52:1433.

82. Szczeklik A. Antipyretic analgesics and the allergic patient. Am J Med 1983; 75:82.

83. Inman WHW. Study of fatal bone marrow depression with special reference to phenylbutazone and oxyphenbutazone. Br Med J 1977;1:1500.

84. Storm BL, Carson JL, Schinnar R, et al. NSAIDs and neutropenia. Arch Intern Med 1993;153:2119.

85. Storm BL, Carson JL, Schinnar R, Snyder ES, Shaw M. Descriptive epidemiology of agranulocytosis. Arch Intern Med 1992;152:1495.

86. Day RO, Graham GG, Bieri D, et al. Concentration response relationships for salicylate induced ototoxicity in normal volunteers. Br J Clin Pharmacol 1988;28:695.

87. Sylvia LM, Forlenza SW, Brocanick JM. Aseptic meningitis associated with naproxen. Drug Intell Clin Pharm 1988;22:339.

88. Physicians Desk Reference (PDR). 47th ed. Montvale, NJ: Medical Economics Data, 1993:1485.

89. Parrillo JE, Fauci AS. Mechanisms of glucocorticoid action on immune processes. Ann Rev Pharmacol Toxicol 1979;19:179.

90. Saxne T, Heinegard D. Wollheim FA. Therapeutic effects on cartilage metabolism in arthritis as measured by release of proteoglycan structures into the synovial fluid. Ann Rheum Dis 1986;45:491.

91. Ebert RH, Barclay WR. Changes in connective tissue reaction induced by cortisone. Ann Intern Med 1952;37:506.

92. Folkman J, Ingber DE. Angiostatic steroids. In: Schleimer RP, Claman HN, Oronsky A, eds. Anti-inflammatory steroid action: basic and clinical aspects. San Diego: Academic Press, 1989.

93. Williams JM, Brandt KD. Triamcinolone hexacetonide protects against fibrillation and osteophyte formation following chemically induced articular cartilage damage. Arthritis Rheum 1985;28:1267.

94. Pelletier J-P, Martel-Pelletier J. Protective effects of corticosteroids on cartilage lesions and osteophyte formation in the Pond-Nuki dog model of osteoarthritis. Arthritis Rheum 1989;32:181.

95. Miller WT, Restifo RA. Steroid arthropathy. Radiology 1966;86:652.

96. Chang RW, Falconer J, et al. A randomized, controlled trial of arthroscopic surgery versus closed needle joint lavage for patients with osteoarthritis of the knee. Arthritis Rheum 1993;36:289.

97. Ike RW, Arnold WJ, et al. Tidal irrigation versus conservative medical management in patients with osteoarthritis of the knee. J Rheumatol 1992;19:772.

98. Richards RN, Lonergan RP. Arthroscopic surgery for the relief of pain in the osteoarthritic knee. Orthopedics 1984;7:1705.

99. Timoney JM, Kneisl JS, Barrack RL, Alexander H. Arthroscopy in the osteoarthritic knee: long term follow-up. Orthop Rev 1990;19:371.

100. Ike RW, O'Rourke K. Detection of intraarticular abnormalities in osteoarthritis of the knee: a pilot study comparing needle arthroscopy with standard arthroscopy. Arthritis Rheum 1993;36:1353.

101. Gramas D, Lane N, Antounian F. Needle arthroscopy: our preliminary experience. Arthritis Rheum 1993;37:S164.

102. Sledge CB, Poss R. Preface: orthopedic surgery and degenerative arthritis. Rheum Dis Clin North Am 1988;14:xi.

103. Feibel A, Fast A. Deep heating of joints: a reconsideration. Arch Phys Med Rehabil 1976;57:513.

104. Hashish I, Harvey W, Harris M. Anti-inflammatory effects of ultrasound therapy: evidence for a major placebo effect. Br J Rheumatol 1986;25:277.

105. Magura G, Aladjemoff L, Tannebaum J, Magwa A. Treatment of pain by TENs. Acta Anesthiol Scand 1978;22:589.

106. Gaw AC, Chang LW, Shaw LC. Efficacy of acupuncture in osteoarthritis pain: a controlled double-blind study. N Engl J Med 1975;293:275.

107. Cosgrove JL, Nicholass JJ, Barwak J, et al. The effects of a treatment team on a special unit. Am J Phys Med Rehabil 1988;67:253.

108. Nicholas JJ. Rehabilitation of patients with rheumatic disease. In: Kelley WN, Harris EH, Ruddy S, Sledge CB, eds. Textbook of rheumatology. 4th ed. Philadelphia: WB Saunders, 1993:1728.

109. Stevens RW, Sutherland J, Ghosh P. Human serum and synovial fluid hyaluronidase. Biochem Pharmacol 1976;25:1507.

110. Mikulikova D, Trnavsky K. Influence of a glycosaminoglycan (arteparon) on lysosomal enzyme release from human polymorphonuclear leukocytes. Z Rheumatol 1982;41:50.

111. Menninger H, Burkhadt, Roske W, et al. Lysosomal elastase: effect on mechanical and biochemical properties of normal cartilage inhibited by polysulfated glycosaminoglycans and binding to chondrocytes. Rheumatol Int 1981; 1:73.

112. Burkhardt D, Ghosh P. Laboratory evaluation of anti-arthritic drugs as potential chondroprotective agents. Semin Arthritis Rheum 1987; 17(suppl):3.

113. Adam M, Musilova J, Krabcova M, et al. Effect of cartilage bone marrow extract on the metabolism of collagen in osteoarthritis cartilage. Pharmacology 1980;21:53.

114. Fischer AM, Merton RE, Marsh NA, et al. A comparison of pentosan polysulfate and heparin II: effects of subcutaneous injection. Thromb Haemost 1982;47:109.

115. Ghosh P, Read R, Armstrong S, Wilson D, Marshall R, McNair P. The effects of intraarticular administration of hyaluronan in a model of early osteoarthritis in sheep. I. Gait analysis and radiological and morphological studies. Semin Arthritis Rheum 1993;22(suppl 1):18.

116. Peyron JG. Intraarticular hyaluronan injections in the treatment of osteoarthritis: state of the art review. J Rheumatol 1993;20(suppl 39):10.

117. Oshima Y, Intraarticular injection therapy of high molecular weight sodium hyaluronate on osteoarthritis of the knee joint: phase II clinical study. Jpn Pharmacol Ther 1983;11:2253.

118. Honma T. Clinical effects of high molecular weight sodium hyaluronate (ARTZ) injected into osteoarthritis knee joints. Jpn Pharmacol Ther 1989;17:5057.

119. Moreland LW, Arnold WJ, Saway A, Savory C, Sikes D. Efficacy and safety of intra-articular Hylan G-F (Synvisc), a viscoelastic derivative of hyaluronan, in patients with osteoarthritis of the knee. Arthritis Rheum 1993;37: S165.

120. Adams ME, Atkinson M, Lussler AJ, et al. Comparison of intra-articular Hylan G-F (Synvisc), a viscoelastic derivative of hyaluronan and continuous NSAID therapy, in patients with osteoarthritis of the knee. Arthritis Rheum 1993;37:S165.

121. Balazs EA, Denlinger JL. Viscosupplementation: a new concept in the treatment of osteoarthritis. J Rheumatol 1993;20(suppl 39):3.

122. Adams ME. An analysis of clinical studies of the use of cross-linked hyaluronan, Hylan, in the treatment of osteoarthritis. J Rheumatol 1993;20(suppl 39):16.

123. Stein C, Comisel K, Haimerl E, et al. Analgesic effect of intraarticular morphine after arthroscopic knee surgery. N Engl J Med 1991;325: 1123.

124. Stein C, Mendl G. The German counterpart to the McGill Pain Questionnaire. Pain 1988;32: 251.

125. Otterness IG, Bliven ML, Downs JT, Natoloi EJ, Hanson DC. Inhibition of interleukin-1 synthesis by tenidap: a new drug for arthritis. Cytokine 1991;3:277.

126. Littman BH, Weinblatt ME, Wall BA, Freundlich B, Stack C, and the Intraarticular Tenidap Investigators Group. Arthritis Rheum 1991;34:S341.

127. Pelletier J-P, McMollum R, DiBattista J, Loose LD, Cloutier J-M, Martel-Pelletier J. Regulation of human normal and osteoarthritic chondrocyte interleukin-1 receptor by antirheumatic drugs. Arthritis Rheum 1993;36:1517.

128. Anttinen J, Oka M. Intraarticular triamcinolone hexacetonide and osmic acid in persistent synovitis of the knee. Scand J Rheum 1975;4: 125.

129. Nissila M. Absence of increased frequency of degenerative joint changes after osmic acid injection. Scand J Rheum 1978;7:84.

130. Bridgman JF, Bruckner F, Eisen V, et al. Irradiation of the synovium in the treatment of rheumatoid arthritis. Q J Med 1973;42:357.

131. Yates DB, Scott JT, Ramsay N. Double-blind trial of yttrium-90 for chronic inflammatory synovitis of the knee. Ann Rheum Dis 1977; 36:481.

132. Ruotsi A, Hypen M. Rekonen A, Oka A. Erbium-[169] versus triamcinolone hexacetonide in the treatment of rheumatoid finger joints. Ann Rheum Disease 1979;38:45.

133. Sledge CB, Suckerman JD, Zalutsk MR, et al. Treatment of rheumatoid synovitis of the knee with intraarticular injection of dysprosium-[165] ferric hydroxide macroaggregates. Arthritis Rheum 1986;29:153.

134. Onetti CM, Gutierriz E, Hilba E, et al. Synoviorthesis with ^{32}P-colloidal chromic phosphate in rheumatoid arthritis. J Rheum 1982;9:229.

135. Monboisse JC, Poulin G, Braquet P, et al. Effect of oxy-radicals on several types of collagen. Int J Tissue React 1984;6:385.

136. Decker WE, Edmundson AH, Hill HE, et al. Local administration of orgotein in horses. Mod Vet Pract 1974;55:773.

137. Rosner IA, Goldberg VM, Getzy L, Moskowitz RW. A trial of intraarticular orgotein a superoxide dismutase in experimentally induced osteoarthritis. J Rheumatol 1980;7:24.

138. Gammer W, Broback L-G. Clinical comparison of orgotein and methylprednisolone acetate in the treatment of osteoarthritis of the knee joint. Scand J Rheumatol 1984;13:108.

139. McIlwain H, Silverfield JC, Cheatum DE, et al. Intra-articular orgotein in osteoarthritis of the knee: a placebo-controlled efficacy, safety, and dosage comparison. Am J Med 1989;87:295.

140. Trock DH, Bollet AJ, Dyer RH, Fielding LP, Miner WK, Markoll R. A double-blind trial of the clinical effects of pulsed electromagnetic fields in osteoarthritis. J Rheumatol 1993;20: 456.

141. Kelley WN, Harris EH, Ruddy S, Sledge CB, eds. Textbook of rheumatology. 4th ed. Philadelphia: WB Saunders, 1993.

19

UNCOMMON RHEUMATIC DISEASES

Gary R. Margolies

Gene V. Ball

The topics discussed in this chapter are uncommon disorders with poorly understood pathophysiology and etiology or manifestations that are so variable that finding adequate numbers of similar patients for study is not feasible. Thus treatment is not always satisfactory. This discussion will consider treatment for the general as well as the rheumatic aspects of Behçet's disease, sarcoidosis, amyloidosis, familial Mediterranean fever, relapsing polychondritis, and idiopathic hemochromatosis. For the majority of these disorders, drug therapies have not been shown to alter their natural history.

BEHÇET'S DISEASE

Behçet's disease (BD) is a chronic inflammatory disease of unknown cause. It was first described in 1937, when Turkish dermatologist Hulusi Behçet[1] reported two patients with a triad of aphthous ulceration of the mouth and genital tract and uveitis. It is now recognized that the gut, central and peripheral nervous systems, large blood vessels, and skin and joints may also be involved. Its prevalence in the United States is low, with estimates varying widely from 1 in 16,000 (Olmstead County, Minn.) to as low as 1 in 500,000.[2] A disease of young adults, it is much more common in Japan, East Asia, and the Eastern Mediterranean, where it is also likely to be more severe, particularly with respect to ocular disease. For example, Chajek and Fainaru[3] reported that BD caused blindness in eight of 41 Middle Eastern patients. Other clinical manifestations include relapsing arthritis, intestinal ulceration and perforation, venous thrombosis, erythema nodosum, and meningoencephalitis.

Whether BD is primarily a vasculitis remains unclear. Although small-vessel inflammation of the skin and retina are characteristic and increased circulating immune complexes have been reported in serum, immune complexes have not been well demonstrated within affected tissues. Hypercoagulability and increased neutrophil chemotaxis (as evidenced by the frequent demonstration of pathergy on skin testing) have also been noted.

An attractive hypothesis for the cause of BD maintains that the disorder is triggered in genetically susceptible persons by an aberrant immune reaction to one or more common environmental agents. The putative agents include streptococcal antigens, viruses, certain foods, and heavy metals.

Inasmuch as neither clinical nor laboratory features of BD are pathognomonic, diagnosis is based on the fulfillment of various clinical criteria. All of the many diagnostic schema require the presence of two, three, or four "major" criteria: (1) recurrent aphthous ulceration in the mouth, (2) ocular involvement (hypopyon, retinal vasculitis, iridocyclitis), (3) skin lesions, and (4) genital ulcers. A recent scheme requires recurring oral ulcers (minimum frequency of three times per year) plus at least two of the other three major criteria. In others the diagnosis is based on the presence of two major criteria in addition to two or more "minor" criteria (vascular thrombosis, gastrointestinal ulcers, epididymitis, and central nervous system lesions).

The clinical course of BD is variable. Its onset may be insidious, but its natural history tends to be one of recurrent attacks that last several weeks or longer. Life-threatening complications, such as meningoencephalitis and major venous and arterial thrombosis, are rare. These manifestations, as well as uveitis with the attendant risk of visual loss, constitute the most compelling basis for the use of cytotoxic and immunosuppressive drug therapy.

Arthritis occurs in a substantial minority of patients with BD. It is characteristically inflammatory, nondeforming, and monarticular and most commonly involves the knee, ankle, or wrist. Episodes generally last 2 to 8 weeks. Pseudopodagra (so-called goutlike attacks) and punched-out lesions of the first metatarsal head have been reported.

Treatment of BD is aimed at control of inflammation and thromboses. However, despite the obvious inflammatory component of BD, few prospective, controlled, or large trials have demonstrated a substantial or sustained benefit of any antiinflammatory pharmacologic approach. Nevertheless, there have been numerous case reports and small clinical trials pertaining to the use of colchicine, topical and systemic corticosteroids, cyclophosphamide, azathioprine, cyclosporine A, sulfasalazine, methotrexate, chlorambucil, thalidomide, and others.

Colchicine is a potent inhibitor of polymorphonuclear leukocyte chemotaxis, which, as mentioned above, has been observed to be accelerated in BD. Miyachi et al.[4] reported improvement of some or all of the mucocutaneous manifestations in five Japanese patients with BD who were given colchicine in a dose of 1.0 mg/d. Similarities with the acute attacks of gout make the idea of treating the arthritis of BD with colchicine also attractive, but results from a double-blind controlled trial showed improvement in arthralgia but no significant measurable change in arthritis.[5]

Corticosteroids, both topical and systemic, are widely used for symptomatic control of many of the minor as well as the more serious manifestations of BD. Once again, however, evidence is lacking that these agents have substantial impact on any of the major features. Dosage is empiric and tends to be proportionate to the severity of the manifestations. It is difficult to interpret the anecdotal reports of reduction of disease activity with the use of prednisone and other corticosteroids. Activity of arthritis and stomatitis is usually episodic,

and improvement is likely to be spontaneous in some, if not all, instances.

Immunomodulatory agents, including antifolates, alkylating agents, and cyclosporine A, have been given to small numbers of patients with chorioretinitis, uveitis, and central nervous system disease. O'Duffy et al.[6] described 21 patients with meningoencephalitis or uveitis treated with various drug regimens. Eight of nine patients studied retrospectively were believed to improve after receiving chlorambucil in a dose of 0.1 mg/kg/d for at least 3 months. This drug was thought to be superior to others, mainly systemic corticosteroids; however, Hamza[7] described two patients who developed solid malignant tumors after receiving chlorambucil for BD. Yazici et al.[8] prospectively studied Turkish men with BD who were given azathioprine in a dose of 2.5 mg/kg/d for 24 months in a randomized, placebo-controlled trial. Significantly fewer episodes of oral ulcers, arthritis, and hypopyon uveitis were reported in the group receiving azathioprine.

Low-dose cyclosporine A (less than 5 mg/kg/d) has been used by several groups for the treatment of uveitis and retinal vasculitis. Results are somewhat conflicting, but there is enough evidence of improvement to warrant further investigation of this drug, and some authors advocate its use for patients with substantial ocular involvement.

Methotrexate may also have a role in the treatment of BD. Jorrizo et al.[9] include two patients with BD in their series of patients with "unusual neutrophilic vascular reactions." In both patients treated with 15 to 20 mg of methotrexate weekly, the cutaneous lesions cleared. The favorable safety profile of low-dose methotrexate in patients with other rheumatologic conditions makes it a promising drug.

Systemically administered "tolerizing agents" have also been tried in the treatment of BD. Uveitis in one of our patients has been treated successfully with oral retinal protein S, given by investigators at the National Institutes of Health (personal communication) (Table 19–1).

Given the lack of data on drug therapy in BD, there can be no categorical recommendation for treatment. Because most episodes are self-limited, supportive therapy is warranted for mucocutaneous lesions and arthritis. It may be reasonable to try low-dose colchicine, prednisone, or weekly methotrexate for particularly

TABLE 19–1
Proposed Treatment Scheme for Behçet's Disease

INVOLVEMENT	DRUG/DOSAGE
Mucocutaneous lesions	Colchicine 0.6 mg b.i.d. or prednisone <15 mg/d
Arthritis (mild)	NSAIDs, prednisone, or
Arthritis (refractory or severe)	methotrexate, 10–20 mg/wk
Uveitis (anterior)	Azathioprine 2.5 mg/kg/d,
Uveitis (posterior)	cyclosporine A ≤5 mg/kg/d
Meningoencephalitis	High-dose corticosteroids ± chlorambucil 0.1 mg/kg/d

severe joint or oral involvement. Azathioprine may also prove useful in treating these problems as well as anterior uveitis.

Retinitis and central nervous system disease pose more difficult dilemmas as to when and how to treat, considering the ominous events that can ensue. Among conventional drugs, chlorambucil for meningoencephalitis and cyclosporine A for retinitis seem to show the most promise at present, although their use is by no means a standard to follow. Finally, all patients with thrombotic complications of BD should receive appropriate anticoagulation with heparin followed by warfarin. Long-term use of warfarin to prevent future thrombosis is a reasonable approach to the patient with known thrombotic events, although its role in the primary prevention of thrombosis in BD is untested.

AMYLOIDOSIS

Amyloidosis represents a group of diverse pathologic processes characterized by an accumulation of extracellular proteinaceous material. Classification of the various systemic amyloidoses is based on the structure of the amyloid protein component as well as the underlying cause. Prognosis, clinical features, and treatment schema vary according to amyloid type. Primary amyloidosis and amyloidosis associated with multiple myeloma are caused by deposition of an immunoglobulin light chain, designated AL amyloid. It has been observed that a substantial number of patients originally discovered to have primary amyloidosis later develop full features of multiple myeloma as well. Whether or not the two represent different stages of the same condition is an issue that is germane to decisions regarding treatment.

Secondary or reactive amyloidosis is typified by accumulation of the acute-phase reactant amyloid protein A (AA) as a rare complication of a number of long-standing inflammatory disorders, including tuberculosis, leprosy, rheumatoid arthritis, and ankylosing spondylitis. Secondary amyloidosis has been found in Europe in particular as a complication of juvenile chronic arthritis (juvenile rheumatoid arthritis and childhood ankylosing spondylitis).

Heredofamilial amyloidosis includes familial amyloid polyneuropathy, hereditary cerebral angiopathy, familial Mediterranean fever (FMF), and possibly Alzheimer's dementia. They are grouped together because they are hereditary; however, these disorders differ in their principal manifestations as well as in the amyloid component expressed.

Chronic hemodialysis-associated amyloidosis results from the accumulation of beta-2 microglobulin and is designated AH. There are other, nonsystemic forms of amyloidosis that will not be discussed here.

Manifestations of primary and secondary amyloidosis are thought to relate primarily to interference of amyloid substance with function of the involved organs. Renal deposition is common, causing proteinuria, which may result in nephrotic syndrome, or it may cause renal failure. Cardiac deposition, resulting in restrictive cardiomyopathy or conduction disturbance, is a major predictor of mortality. Other target organs are the liver, skin, and peripheral nerves.

Articular symptoms are most closely linked to multiple myeloma and hemodialysis-associated amyloidosis. In the latter, manifestations are usually limited to the bones and connective tissues. Myeloma-associated disease may be difficult to distinguish from nodular rheumatoid arthritis.

It is unclear whether direct tissue deposition alone is responsible for many or all of the manifestations observed. Inflammation, while critically linked to the generation of amyloid substance in secondary amyloidosis, is not thought to play a major role within the amyloid lesion itself. Thus there is little rationale for the use of adrenal corticosteroids in treatment of the manifestations.

Treatment strategies focus on the following three goals:

1. To improve or mitigate the underlying disorder
2. To prevent the expression and deposition of amyloid components
3. To remove amyloid deposits

To date, no therapy has been effective in causing regression of existing lesions. Therefore therapy is directed primarily to the underlying disorder.

Treatment of AL (Immunocyte-derived) Amyloidosis

Alkylating agents, usually melphalan combined with prednisone, have been the mainstay of medical treatment for multiple myeloma and are generally credited with prolonging survival in these patients. This regimen decreases the activity of the light chain secreting clone of plasma cells, and it has been used in the treatment of myeloma-associated AL disease. Because of a presumed similar etiology, primary AL disease has been treated with similar regimens. Gertz et al.[10] reported on 153 patients with biopsy-proven primary amyloidosis who were given melphalan and prednisone cycled every 6 weeks. Eighteen percent showed a clinical response, usually with decreasing proteinuria, and survival was longer in responders. Median survival was 14 months for nonresponders and 90 months for responders; however, 10 patients died of acute leukemia or myelodysplastic syndromes attributed to melphalan therapy.

Given the dismal prognosis of these patients, the risk of a late death due to leukemia would likely be preferable to early death with no treatment. Nevertheless, the uncertain benefit of this therapy and the real danger of inducing cancer warrants careful consideration and discussion before it is offered to any patient with primary amyloidosis.

Colchicine has also been used in the treatment of primary amyloidosis, as it may inhibit the deposition of amyloid. In 1985, Kyle et al.[11] described a randomized trial comparing colchicine with melphalan/prednisone in 101 patients with primary AL disease. Although there was no significant difference in survival between the two groups, in a subgroup of patients with cardiac involvement survival improved on a regimen of melphalan/prednisone.

Secondary Amyloidosis

Treatment of underlying inflammatory disease is the primary goal in all patients with secondary amyloidosis. Although successful antiinflammatory therapy may arrest or retard deposition, standard antiinflammatory agents are not likely to result in regression of amyloid deposits and have not been shown to reduce mortality or long-term complications. There are case reports of regression of proteinuria and arthropathy in patients with ankylosing spondylitis treated with colchicine.[12] Similar success with colchicine has been reported in patients with juvenile rheumatoid arthritis and reactive amyloidosis. Besides its antiinflammatory properties, colchicine may have the added advantage of directly inhibiting amyloid deposition. Thus colchicine is a reasonable agent to try in patients with reactive amyloidosis, particularly in those patients whose underlying inflammatory disease began in childhood.

Hemodialysis-Associated Amyloidosis

Hemodialysis-associated amyloidosis, the most recently described of the systemic amyloidoses, arises only after years of chronic hemodialysis treatment for end-stage renal disease. It is thought that inefficient clearance of beta-2 microglobulin by dialyzers over many years leads to the accumulation and subsequent deposition of amyloid. It has been postulated that the dialysis membrane itself influences amyloid deposition, although there are reports of beta-2 microglobulin amyloidosis occurring in longstanding nondialyzed uremic patients as well as patients undergoing long-term peritoneal dialysis.[13] Clinical manifestations are limited to arthropathy and chronic joint pain, punched-out lytic bone lesions, carpal tunnel syndrome, and trigger finger. At present, specific drug therapy has not been used. It should be mentioned that other, potentially more treatable causes of articular complaints, such as hyperparathyroidism, should be excluded in these patients. It has been shown that newer membranes of the high-flux type are more efficient at removing beta-2 microglobulin than are the older cuprophane dialyzers. In addition, renal transplantation has been observed to arrest the progression

TABLE 19–2
Treatment Recommendations for Systemic Amyloidosis

TYPE/MANIFESTATION	AGENT
AL	
Myeloma associated	Melphalan, 0.15 mg/kg/d for 7 days; prednisone 60 mg/d for 7 days, repeated every 6 weeks
Primary	Consider above regimen
	For patients who are unable/unwilling to take the above regimen, consider colchicine 0.6 mg b.i.d.
AA	
Infection-related	Treat infection appropriately
Ankylosis spondylitis or rheumatoid arthritis	Trial colchicine 0.6 mg PO b.i.d.
FMF	Begin colchicine 1.0 mg/d irrespective of size or age; increase up to 2.0 mg/d if attacks are not controlled

of hemodialysis-associated amyloidosis and has been reported to cause regression of carpal tunnel syndrome in some cases (Table 19–2).

FAMILIAL MEDITERRANEAN FEVER

The drug treatment of FMF has been successful. FMF is an autosomal recessive inflammatory disorder that occurs in people of Mediterranean and Armenian descent, particularly in Sephardic Jews who account for up to 60% of reported cases.[14] It is characterized by relapsing episodes of fever with peritonitis, pleuritis, or arthritis, and it also is known by the appropriate term *relapsing polyserositis*. The underlying genetic defect that leads to the expression of the disease is still unknown.

The arthritis of FMF is the presenting finding in a minority of patients, but it is present in three fourths of patients at some time in the course of the disease. Arthritis attacks are generally abrupt in onset, monarticular, and of less than 1 week in duration. The large joints are affected most often. Polyarthritis is present in a minority of patients. Synovial effusion is usually present, and synovial fluid white blood cell counts are characteristically very high, averaging more than 100,000/mm^3. A chronic form of arthritis occurs in a small percentage of patients with FMF.

Amyloidosis of the AA type is a dread complication of FMF. The amyloidosis is systemic and, most important, renal.

Colchicine was first used in 1972 to treat the acute manifestations of FMF, and within a year it was being used for low-dose long-term

therapy.[15,16] It was the first and, to date, is the only effective agent for FMF. Zemer et al.[17] followed 350 Israeli children with FMF who were treated with up to 2 mg of colchicine per day for 6 to 13 years. Ninety-five percent of the treated patients had improvement in their disease manifestations, and 64% had no further attacks. Most of the patients who did not respond completely had persistent or recurrent arthritis.

Peters et al.[18] reported on 85 FMF patients treated with 1.2 to 1.8 mg/d of colchicine for at least 3 years. Attacks of fever and pain were dramatically reduced in frequency, with approximately 45% of the patients having complete arrest of attacks.

Although a minority of patients treated with colchicine will continue to have attacks, the clear benefits seen in most patients have led to its accepted use in all FMF patients who tolerate the drug. Dosing of colchicine should begin at 0.5 to 1.0 mg/d irrespective of the patient's weight or age. The dose is titrated upward to 2 mg/d until episodes stop. There is no evidence that higher doses are any more effective for those patients who do not respond completely to 2 mg/d. The observed side effects of colchicine in patients with FMF have generally been mild and include diarrhea, nausea, and rash. In the series reported by Zemer et al.,[17] seven patients had more severe toxic reactions, including intractable diarrhea, angioneurotic edema, and leukopenia in one. All seven patients were successfully desensitized with progressive doses of colchicine and were subsequently able to continue treatment. The patient who had been leukopenic, a 7-year-old girl, was given 0.001 mg of colchicine orally; the dose was doubled daily for 10 days and then 0.5 mg was given daily for 3 months. Dosage was then increased to 1 mg/d over the next 3 months, and normal blood cell counts were maintained.[17]

Colchicine is not thought to be abortive for acute attacks, although patients who experience a prodrome such as transient abdominal or articular symptoms before a full-blown attack may be able to prevent the attack by taking an additional dose of colchicine. Patients with acute attacks of arthritis or serositis or those who have not responded to long-term colchicine are often given nonsteroidal antiinflammatory drugs (NSAIDs) as well as narcotic analgesics. Garcia-Gonzalez and Weisman[19] reported a patient with FMF who had recurring prolonged episodes of arthritis that were refractory to colchicine and NSAIDs as well as repeated injections of intraarticular corticosteroids.[19] This patient responded to a synovectomy.

There is further evidence that colchicine prevents amyloidosis in FMF. Amyloidosis develops histologically in 6% to 30% of patients with FMF, but clinical manifestations (i.e., renal disease) are substantially less frequent. Nevertheless, renal failure was the most frequent cause of early death in patients with FMF. However, long-term use of colchicine has been shown to prevent the development of amyloidosis as well as to arrest or slow the progression of amyloidosis in those patients in whom it was documented before the onset of colchicine therapy.

Should all patients, including young children, have lifelong treatment with colchicine? Despite the effectiveness of colchicine, concerns have been raised as to its effect on (1) normal growth and development, (2) female and male reproductive function, and (3) risk of neoplasia. To date, in both boys and girls treated with colchicine for FMF, normal height and weight curves were maintained. Observed reproductive problems are unusual. There were two infants with trisomy-21 out of 91 pregnancies followed up in patients with FMF who were treated with colchicine.[20] For this reason, amniocentesis has been recommended for all pregnancies in which one or both parents are being treated with colchicine. Small series have shown no association of colchicine use during pregnancy and adverse fetal outcome, but conclusive evidence for its complete safety in pregnancy is lacking. The in-

cidence of malignant neoplasms does not appear to be increased in those patients treated over a long term. However, the fact that colchicine is a cytotoxic agent and the relatively limited experience (less than 20 years) with the drug warrant further long-term follow-up studies in patients with FMF.

SARCOIDOSIS

Sarcoidosis is a chronic inflammatory disorder defined by the presence of noncaseating granulomas. Its cause is unknown, although clinical and pathologic similarities to other granulomatous diseases, including tuberculosis, have raised the question of an infectious or other environmental trigger. The most common sites of involvement are the lungs, skin, and eyes. Other areas that may be involved are the lymph nodes, heart, bones, central nervous system, and joints.

Rheumatic involvement in sarcoidosis is generally divided into two categories. The first consists of articular involvement during the acute presentation of the illness. The triad of arthritis, erythema nodosum, and hilar adenopathy make up Lofgren's syndrome, which may be accompanied by fever.[21] Arthritis arises most often in the knees and ankles. Although joints may be tender and swollen, maximal tenderness may be juxtaarticular; dactylitis has also been described. Symptoms tend to remit spontaneously over a period of several weeks.

The second category consists of synovitis that accompanies the slower-onset, more chronic, and systemic form of the disease. This process tends to be nondestructive, and symptoms are generally mild. In contrast to the acute form, chronic or recurrent sarcoid arthropathy is characterized by granulomas within the synovium.

The treatment of chronic sarcoidosis has revolved about controlling pulmonary disease, both for the relief of symptoms and for the prevention of impaired pulmonary function. Corticosteroids, generally given at low doses, are the agents used most frequently for controlling pulmonary symptoms, including cough and dyspnea. Higher doses of systemic corticosteroids are used to treat symptom flares and are also used in attempts to reverse worsening of pulmonary function. It remains unclear, however, whether the chronic administration of corticosteroids alters the outcome of chronic pulmonary sarcoid.

Skin and eye manifestations of sarcoidosis are also often treated with systemic as well as topical corticosteroids. Other agents have been used to reduce the toxicity of corticosteroids and to treat skin lesions that are refractory to corticosteroids. Several small studies have investigated the effectiveness of chloroquine and related 4-aminoquinolone drugs in cutaneous sarcoidosis; most have found these agents helpful, either alone or as an adjunct to corticosteroid therapy.[22-24] In a recent review of chloroquine for cutaneous sarcoid, Zic et al.[25] recommended using chloroquine, 250 mg twice a day for 14 days followed by 250 mg/d, for long-term suppression. The only randomized, blinded, placebo-controlled trial of chloroquine was done in 1967 on patients with lung disease and showed only transient improvement in the treatment group.[26]

The definitive treatment of refractory sarcoidosis has not been established. Numerous immunomodulating agents have been tried for systemic or pulmonary sarcoidosis. These include azathioprine, chlorambucil, methotrexate, and cyclosporine A. In 1990, Lower and Baughman[27] reported subjective and objective improvement in 12 of 14 patients with refractory pulmonary sarcoidosis who were treated with 10 mg weekly of oral methotrexate. These findings are encouraging, as previous investigations of methotrexate for sarcoidosis used substantially higher doses with more potential toxicity.

For the management of acute sarcoidosis with arthritis or periarthritis, no specific therapy other than analgesics or NSAIDs may be necessary, as spontaneous resolution is the most likely outcome. In fact, some argue that the acute form of sarcoidosis may represent a distinctly separate disease from the chronic, more insidious form. For chronic synovitis, low-dose systemic corticosteroids may be helpful when NSAIDs or analgesics fail. Inasmuch as the articular process is generally neither progressive nor destructive, treatment should be directed at symptom control that is acceptable to the patient. The efficacy of methotrexate or azathioprine has not been established; if either is used, it should be only for the rare patient with destructive or particularly recalcitrant arthropathy.

RELAPSING POLYCHONDRITIS

Relapsing polychondritis (RP) is an inflammatory disorder of unknown cause characterized by episodes of destruction of cartilage. The disease typically affects young adults but is also well described in both children and the elderly. RP often shares features with rheumatoid arthritis and other systemic inflammatory disorders or occurs in association with other diseases, and it is presumed to be an autoimmune disease. There may be a pathophysiologic role of antibodies to type II collagen, which have been isolated and characterized in some patients with RP.

Episodes of pain and erythema develop most commonly about the cartilage of the external ears, nose, larynx, trachea, and costochondral cartilages. Episodes last from days to weeks and may result in chronic degeneration and deformity of cartilaginous structures. Complications include loss of olfaction and hearing due to direct extension of destruction into the special sense structures. Scleritis and episcleritis occur frequently. Potentially life-threatening complications include airway compromise from tracheal collapse and aortic valve incompetence or rupture. Central nervous system findings resembling cerebral vasculitis have also been described.[28]

Articular involvement is variable but is present in a majority of patients. The arthropathy may resemble rheumatoid arthritis, although it is generally nonerosive.

Prednisone or other systemic corticosteroids constitute the principal therapy of RP. It is generally accepted that corticosteroids are effective both in aborting acute painful episodes of cartilage inflammation and in suppressing disease activity over a long period. Doses during initial attacks may range from 20 to 60 mg of prednisone daily, with tapering down to the lowest daily dose that prevents relapse. Episodes of acute airway embarrassment have been treated successfully with pulses of intravenous methylprednisolone or nebulized racemic ephedrine.[29,30] Whether corticosteroid therapy should be continued during clinically quiescent periods is not clear. There are several reports of aortic valve disease progressing despite control of other symptoms, and there is no convincing evidence that corticosteroids alter aortic valve dilatation.[31] The low prevalence of RP prevents studies of other drug therapies. Therefore therapy in patients who have developed resistance to corticosteroids or in those who would benefit from corticosteroid-sparing regimens is likely to remain empiric. Dapsone and colchicine have been tried in some patients, with improvement in symptoms; cyclosporine A has been reported to be successful as well.[32]

Ocular symptoms and signs may respond to immunomodulatory drugs other than prednisone. There are sporadic reports of successful treatment of scleritis with cyclophosphamide or azathioprine in patients with RP in whom oral corticosteroids failed.[33]

IDIOPATHIC HEMOCHROMATOSIS

Idiopathic hemochromatosis (IH) is an inherited disorder of iron metabolism that results in iron overload. The mode of inheritance is autosomal recessive, with a genotype frequency as high as one in 400 births. Demonstrable disease is less frequent, with manifestations occurring earlier and more often in men. Clinical manifestations relate to hepatic, cardiac, pancreatic endocrine, and gonadal dysfunction as well as arthritis.

Detectable joint involvement occurs in as many as 90% of patients with IH in whom clinical disease develops. The metacarpophalangeal joints, wrists, knees, and hips are involved most often. The arthropathy is often inflammatory and may be indistinguishable from the arthritis of calcium pyrophosphate dihydrate deposition; however, only one fifth of IH patients with joint involvement will have chondrocalcinosis demonstrated on plain radiograph.[34] The prevalence of overt arthritis increases with age and may be asymptomatic when the disease is discovered in other organs. It is not uncommon, however, for articular pain to be the initial presenting complaint. For this reason, we recommend that all patients with premature or atypical osteoarthritis-like findings, especially in the metacarpophalangeal joints, be screened for IH. Pronounced swelling accompanied by enlargement (caused by degenerative changes) of the second and third metacarpophalangeal joints will produce the "iron fist" of idiopathic hemochromatosis.

Diagnosis of IH is made by the demonstration of pathologic iron deposition in tissue in the absence of other conditions known to cause iron overload, such as thalassemia or conditions requiring repeated red blood cell transfusions. Diagnostic evaluation should begin with the determination of serum iron saturation or the serum ferritin level. If neither value is substantially elevated, IH can be excluded. When serum iron saturation is greater than 60% or the ferritin level is greater than 600 µg/L in a patient with suggestive symptoms, further evaluation is warranted. Definite diagnosis is made with liver biopsy, although newer techniques in magnetic resonance imaging may prove useful as a noninvasive method of demonstrating pathognomonic increased hepatic iron stores.

IH is treated with repeated therapeutic phlebotomy at any stage when excess iron stores are detected; 500 ml is removed weekly until a mild iron deficiency anemia develops. Maintenance phlebotomy at 2-month intervals is continued indefinitely, and patients should be monitored regularly to ensure that a mild iron deficient state exists. Removal of excess iron before it is deposited in target tissues prevents clinical manifestations of the disease. Iron removal will not likely result in substantial improvement of IH arthropathy. Thus therapy is generally preventive of further end-organ damage. The treatment of established arthropathy is similar to the treatment of osteoarthritis and calcium pyrophosphate dihydrate deposition.

REFERENCES

1. Behçet H. Uber rezidivierende, aphthose, durch ein Virus verursachte Gershwure am Mund, Auge und an den Genitalien. Derm Wschr 1937;105: 1152.
2. Shimizu T, Ehrlich GE, Inaba G. Behçet's disease (Behçet's syndrome). Semin Arthritis Rheum 1979;8:223.
3. Chajek T, Fainaru M. Behçet's disease: report of 41 cases and a review of the literature. Medicine 1975;54:179.
4. Miyachi Y, Taniguchi S, Ozaki M, et al. Colchicine in the treatment of the cutaneous manifestations of Behçet's disease. Br J Dermatol 1981; 104:67.
5. Yurdakul S, Yazici H, Tuzun Y, et al. The arthritis of Behçet's disease: a prospective study. Ann Rheum Dis 1983;42:505.
6. O'Duffy JD, Robertson D, Goldstein N. Chlorambucil in the treatment of uveitis and meningoencephalitis of Behçet's disease. Am J Med 1984;76:75.
7. Hamza M. Cancer complicating Behçet's disease treated with chlorambucil [Letter]. Am J Med 1984;76:789.

8. Yazici H, Pazarli H, Barnes C, et al. A controlled trial of azathioprine in Behçet's syndrome. N Engl J Med 1990;322:281.

9. Jorizzo JL, White WL, Wise CM, et al. Low-dose weekly methotrexate for unusual neutrophilic vascular reactions: cutaneous polyarteritis nodosa and Behçet's disease. J Am Acad Dermatol 1991;24:973.

10. Gertz MA, Kyle RA, Greipp PR. Response rates and survival in primary systemic amyloidosis. Blood 1991;77:257.

11. Kyle RA, Greipp PR, Garton JP, et al. Primary systemic amyloidosis: comparison of melphalan/prednisone versus colchicine. Am J Med 1985; 79:708.

12. Escalante A, Ehresmann GR, Quismorio FP Jr. Brief report: regression of reactive systemic amyloidosis due to ankylosing spondylitis following the administration of colchicine. Arthritis Rheum 1991;34:920.

13. Thielemans C, Dratwa M, Bergman P, et al. Continuous ambulatory peritoneal dialysis vs hemodialysis: a lesser risk of amyloidosis. Nephrol Dial Transplant 1988;3:291.

14. Sohar E, Gafni J, Pras M, et al. Familial Mediterranean fever: a survey of 470 cases and review of the literature. Am J Med 1967;43:227.

15. Goldfinger SE. Colchicine for familial Mediterranean fever. N Engl J Med 1972;287:1302.

16. Zemer D, Revach M, Pras M, et al. A controlled trial of colchicine in preventing attacks of familial Mediterranean fever. N Engl J Med 1974; 291:932.

17. Zemer D, Livneh A, Danon YL, et al. Long-term colchicine treatment in children with familial Mediterranean fever. Arthritis Rheum 1991;34: 973.

18. Peters R, Lehman T, Schwabe A. Colchicine use for familial Mediterranean fever. West J Med 1983;138:43.

19. Garcia-Gonzalez A, Weisman MH. The arthritis of familial Mediterranean fever. Semin Arthritis Rheum 1992;22(3):139.

20. Hansteen IL. Colchicine and chromosomal aberrations. Lancet 1969;2:744.

21. Lofgren S. Primary pulmonary sarcoidosis. I. Early signs and symptoms. Acta Med Scand 1953;145: 424.

22. Brodhagan H, Gilg I. Hydroxychloroquine in the treatment of sarcoidosis. In: Turiaf J, Chabot J, eds. La Sarcoidose: rapports de la IV conference international. Paris: Mason et Cie, 1967:764.

23. Johns CJ, Schonfel SA, Scott PP, et al. Longitudinal study of chronic sarcoidosis with low-dose maintenance corticosteroid therapy: outcome and complications. Ann N Y Acad Sci 1986; 465:702.

24. Jones E, Callen JP. Hydroxychloroquine is effective therapy for control of cutaneous sarcoidal granulomas. J Am Acad Dermatol 1990; 23:487.

25. Zic JA, Horowitz DH, Arzubiaga C, et al. Treatment of cutaneous sarcoidosis with chloroquine. Arch Dermatol 1991;127:1035.

26. Krasnitz A. Chloroquine therapy in pulmonary sarcoidosis. N Y State J Med 1967;67:1729.

27. Lower EE, Baughman RP. The use of low dose methotrexate in refractory sarcoidosis. Am J Med Sci 1990;299(3):153.

28. Stewart SS, Ashizawa T, Dudley AW Jr, et al. Cerebral vasculitis in relapsing polychondritis. Neurology 1988;38:150.

29. Lipnick RN, Fink CW. Acute airway obstruction in relapsing polychondritis: treatment with pulse methylprednisolone. J Rheumatol 1991;18:98.

30. Nebulized racemic ephedrine in the treatment of acute exacerbation of laryngeal relapsing polychondritis. J Laryngol Otol 1992;106:63.

31. McAdam LP, O'Hanlan MA, Bluestone R, et al. Relapsing polychondritis: prospective study of 23 patients and a review of the literature [Review]. Medicine 1976;55:193.

32. Svenson KLG, Homdahl R, Klareskog L, et al. Cyclosporine A treatment in a case of relapsing polychondritis. Scand J Rheumatol 1984;13:329.

33. Hoang-Xaun T, Foster CS, Rice BA. Scleritis in relapsing polychondritis: response to therapy. Ophthalmology 1990;97:892.

34. Huaux JP, Geubel A, Koch MC, et al. The arthritis of hemochromatosis: a review of 25 cases with special reference to chondrocalcinosis, and a comparison with patients with primary hyperparathyroidism and controls. Clin Rheumatol 1986;5:317.

INFECTIOUS AGENT ARTHRITIS

Mitchell F. Fung
James S. Louie

The effective treatment of an infectious arthritis begins with a prompt and specific diagnosis, followed by therapies that aid in the destruction of the offending microorganism and removal of the detritus, which impairs the host defenses and damages the tissues. Of equal importance are the processes that monitor the effectiveness of these therapies. A knowledge of the host and its defenses, the microorganism, and the factors that mediate these interactions may change the perception that ". . . despite newer, more potent antibiotics and more effective techniques of joint drainage, the morbidity and mortality from bacterial arthritis has not significantly decreased in the past two decades."[1] Accordingly, we will review the tenets of specific diagnosis, discuss the choices of antibiotics for empiric and specific therapy, and outline the procedures that are useful in the sequential evaluation of outcome for both acute and chronic forms of arthritis induced by infectious agents.

EARLY AND SPECIFIC DIAGNOSIS

A monarthritis, or any arthritis with fever, positions infectious arthritis at the top of the differential diagnosis. Less typical presentations occur when the host is either very young or very old, has significant comorbid diseases, or takes drugs that alter the inflammatory and immune responses. Prompt diagnosis demands the recovery of synovial fluid or synovial tissue for the specific identification of the infectious agent by appropriate culture. When preexisting arthritis or problematic joints with unique anatomic relationships are affected, immediate collaboration with a radiologist to outline the affected structures and with an orthopedist to facilitate aspiration or biopsy is warranted. It is also worth emphasizing that in virtually all cases of infectious agent outbursts, the offending organism gets into the joint via the bloodstream; blood cultures are part of the diagnostic work-up in all patients. It is axiomatic that a diligent search for the source of the septicemia should be undertaken immediately.

A *tentative* identification is derived from the Gram stain of any bacteria within the cells recovered from the synovial fluid. Gram stain preparations are more easily viewed when the cells are concentrated and dispersed by means of a cytocentrifuge. Organisms should be visible in 60% of nongonococcal bacterial arthritis.

The *specific* identification of the offending microorganisms traditionally depends on the culture and growth on supportive media. Many bacteria require special attention to maximize growth in media. Thus, when gonococcal arthritis is suspected, synovial fluid should be cultured on chocolate agar and transported quickly to the laboratory for incubation in 5% to 7% CO_2. When Lyme disease is suspected, the fluid should be cultured in Barbour-Stoenner-Kelly (BSK) media (Sigma B3528) and incubated at 33° C to recover *Borrelia burgdorferi*. Even with typical infections, inoculation of larger volumes of synovial fluid into blood culture bottles may enhance the 90% recovery rate reported for nongonococcal bacterial infections.

A new molecular technique to identify pathogens that are difficult to culture uses the polymerase chain reaction (PCR) to amplify small quantities of specific bacterial DNA. Two different primers of oligonucleotides are selected to encompass a DNA sequence that codes for a characteristic bacterial protein. When these specific primers, nucleotides, and a polymerase are added to synovial fluid samples with bacterial DNA, a process occurs within a thermocycler which sequentially changes the temperature to dissociate the double strands of the bacterial DNA (~96°), anneal the primers to the single strands of bacterial DNA (~56°), and fill in the intervening nucleotides between the primers (~72°). This process constructs sufficient copies of the specific DNA fragment for identification by Southern blot. With this technique, *Neisseria gonorrhoeae, Borrelia burgdorferi,* and other bacteria have been identified in synovial fluid, and *Mycobacterium tuberculosis* and the actinomycete producing Whipple's disease have been identified in biopsies of synovial tissue.[2–4] More recently, it has been possible to identify the genes that encode for antibiotic resistance in some bacteria. The sensitivity of this molecular method of identification requires great care in the collection and assay procedures to prevent contamination and false-positives.

SELECTION OF ANTIBIOTICS

Because rapid destruction of cartilage and joint may ensue in acute bacterial joint infections, antibiotics should be instituted by an intravenous route immediately after synovial fluid and other clinical fluids and tissue have been recovered and processed for culture or PCR. An increasing array of antibiotics of different classes are available (Table 20–1). The clinical setting, the age of the host, local patterns of bacterial resistance, and a careful review of the Gram stains of the synovial fluid all influence the empiric choice of antibiotics (Table 20–2). As described by Goldenberg,[1] unique clinical settings raise the suspicions of specific infections, as when intravenous drug users present with *Pseudomonas aeruginosa* in the sternoclavicular joint, or when the patient with rheumatoid arthritis is infected with *Staphylococcus aureus* in a pannus-laden joint. Interestingly, the age of the host confers a spectrum of different infections, which may disseminate to the joint tissue. Neonates and young children are prone to develop septic arthritis as a result of upper respiratory infections of *Haemophilus*

influenzae. Young adults demonstrate *S. aureus, Streptococcus pneumoniae,* or *N. gonorrhoeae* associated with skin, lung, or venereal infections, and the elderly are susceptible to gram-negative bacilli attendant to genitourinary and gastrointestinal infections. In addition, because patterns of bacterial resistance differ in each locality, the experience of your local hospital microbiology laboratory may influence the initial choices of antibiotics.

Gram stains of bacteria within synovial fluid cells modulate this empiric decision for antibiotics. *Gram positive cocci* suggest *Staphylococcus* or *Streptococcus* species. Since most *S. aureus* organisms produce a β-lactamase, empiric coverage calls for a β-lactamase–resistant penicillin. Nafcillin or oxacillin is given four times a day; cefazolin is given three times a day and is less expensive, and ceftriaxone is given only once a day, offering a greater convenience. The antibacterial activity of the β-lactam antibiotics, the penicillins and the cephalosporins, is dependent on their ability to penetrate the bacterial cell wall through protein-lined channels called porins, resist inactivation by bacterial enzymes (β-lactamases), and bind and inactivate the penicillin-binding proteins (PBPs) (Fig. 20–1). Staphylococci often elaborate β-lactamases as exoenzymes, hydrolyzing the cyclic amide bond of the β-lactam ring and inactivating the antibiotic (Fig. 20–2). The β-lactamase–resistant penicillins such as nafcillin have a bulky acyl side chain at the R position which prevents hydrolysis by steric hindrance. Another strategy that avoids hydrolysis uses a β-lactamase inhibitor, such as clavulanate or sulbactam, which acts as a suicide inhibitor to form the acyl intermediate with a β-lactamase–susceptible penicillin or cephalosporin. The treatment of gram-positive cocci identified from patients in a setting where *S. aureus* is resistant to methicillin (MRSA) and other β-lactamase–resistant penicillins will require vancomycin. These bacteria have developed chromosomal mutations, which have decreased the affinities of the penicillin-binding proteins for the antibiotics. Vancomycin succeeds by binding to a different cellular constituent to inhibit cell wall synthesis. Vancomycin also changes the bacterial wall permeability and impairs RNA synthesis. These multiple mechanisms may be responsible for the low frequency of resistance.

TABLE 20–1
Antibiotic Classification

GENERIC NAME	TRADE NAME	ADMINISTRATION ROUTES
Penicillins		
β-lactamase-susceptible, nonantipseudomonal		
Penicillin G		IV, IM, PO
Benzathine penicillin G	Bicillin	IM
Penicillin V (phenoxymethyl)	Pen Vee K	PO
Ampicillin	Amcill, Polycillin	IV, PO
Amoxicillin	Amoxil	PO
β-lactamase-susceptible, antipseudomonal		
Azlocillin	Azlin	IV
Mezlocillin	Mezlin	IV, IM
Piperacillin	Pipracil	IV
Ticarcillin	Ticar	IV, IM
Combination β-lactamase inhibitors and		
β-lactamase agents		
Amoxicillin plus clavulanate	Augmentin	PO
Ticarcillin plus clavulanate	Timentin	IV
Ampicillin plus sulbactam	Unasyn	IV, IM
Piperacillin plus tazobactam	Zosyn	IV
β-lactamase-resistant		
Cloxacillin	Tegopen	PO
Dicloxacillin	Dynapen, Pathocil	PO
Nafcillin	Unipen, Nafcil	IV
Oxacillin	Prostaphlin, Bactocil	IV, IM
Methicillin	Staphcillin, Celbenin	IV
Cephalosporins		
First generation		
Cefazolin	Ancef, Kefzol	IV, IM
Cephalothin	Keflin	IV, IM
Cephapirin	Cefadyl	IV, IM
Cephradine	Velosef, Anspor	IV, IM, PO
Cephalexin	Keflex	PO
Cefadroxil	Duricef, Ultracef	PO
Second generation		
Cefamandole	Mandol	IV, IM
Cefonicid	Monocid	IV, IM
Cefotetan	Cefotan	IV, IM
Cefoxitin	Mefoxin	IV, IM
Ceforanide	Precef	IV, IM
Cefmetazole	Zefazone	IV
Cefuroxime	Zinacef, Kefurox	IV, IM
Cefuroxime axetil	Ceftin	PO
Cefaclor	Ceclor	PO
Cefprozil	Cefzil	PO
Loracarbef	Lorabid	PO
Third generation		
Cefotaxime	Claforan	IV
Ceftizoxime	Cefizox	IV, IM
Ceftriaxone	Rocephin	IV, IM
Cefixime	Suprax	PO
Cefpodoxime proxetil	Vantin	PO

Continued on following page.

TABLE 20–1
Antibiotic Classification—*Continued*

GENERIC NAME	TRADE NAME	ADMINISTRATION ROUTES
Cephalosporins—*Continued*		
With good antipseudomonal activity		
Cefoperazone	Cefobid	IV
Cefsulodin	Cefomonil	IV
Ceftazidime	Fortaz, Tazicef, Tazidime	IV, IM
Aminoglycosides		
Amikacin	Amikin	IV, IM
Gentamicin	Garamycin	IV, IM
Netilmicin	Netromycin	IV, IM
Spectinomycin	Trobicin	IM
Streptomycin		IM
Tobramycin	Nebcin	IV, IM
Macrolides and Lincomycins		
Clindamycin	Cleocin	IV, IM, PO
Erythromycin		
base, stearate, estolate, ethyl succinate	E-mycin, Erythrocin, Ilosone, E.E.S.	PO
lactobionate, gluceptate		IV
Clarithromycin	Biaxin	PO
Azithromycin	Zithromax	PO
Tetracyclines		
Tetracycline, Oxytetracycline	Terramycin	IV, PO
Doxycycline	Vibramycin, Doryx, Vibra-tabs	IV, PO
Minocycline	Minocin	PO
Fluoroquinolones		
Ciprofloxacin	Cipro	IV, PO
Oflaxacin	Floxin	IV, PO
Lomefloxacin	Maxaquin	PO
Carbapenems		
Imipenem + Cilastatin	Primaxin	IV, IM
Monobactams		
Aztreonam	Azactam	IV
Chloramphenicol	Chloromycetin	IV, PO
Vancomycin	Vancocin, Vancoled	IV, PO
Trimethoprim-Sulfamethoxazole	Bactrim, Septra	IV, PO
Metronidazole	Flagyl, Metric 21, Protostat	IV, PO

Gram negative bacilli in a clinical situation suggestive of Enterobacteriaceae should be treated with a third-generation cephalosporin (e.g., ceftriaxone), or a quinolone (e.g., ciprofloxacin). The third-generation cephalosporins have complex additions at two positions (R1, R2) which confer a broad spectrum of activity against both gram-positive and gram-negative bacteria, with particular resistance to the β-lactamases located in the periplasmic space be-

TABLE 20–2
Antibiotic Therapy of Bacterial Arthritis Prior to Culture and Susceptibility Results

SYNOVIAL FLUID GRAM STAIN	PROBABLE PATHOGEN	THERAPEUTIC REGIMEN
Gram-positive cocci	*Staphylococcus aureus,* "methicillin"-susceptible *Staphylococcus epidermidis* *Streptococcus pneumoniae* *Streptococcus pyogenes* *Streptococcus agalactiae*	Nafcillin, 2 g q6h IV; *or* cefazolin, 1–2 g q8h IV or IM
	Staphylococcus aureus, "methicillin"-resistant	Vancomycin, 1 g q12h IV
Gram-negative cocci	*Neisseria gonorrhoeae*	Ceftriaxone* 1 g, IV, in a single daily dose
Gram-negative bacilli	Enterobacteriaceae	Ceftriaxone* 1 g, IV, in a single daily dose; *or* ticarcillin/clavulanic acid, 3.1 g q6h IV
	Pseudomonas aeruginosa	Ceftazidime 2 g q8h IV; *or* piperacillin† 4–5 g q6h IV, *plus* an aminoglycoside‡
Indeterminate		
Young adult	*N. gonorrhoeae*	As above
Older adult	Enterobacteriaceae	As above

*Ceftizoxime, ceftazidime, or cefotaxime may also be used.

†Azlocillin or mezlocillin may be substituted if they are equally active and less expensive.

‡Tobramycin, netilmicin, or amikacin should not be used unless the isolate is resistant to gentamicin but susceptible to an alternative (the dose of amikacin is three times higher than the other drugs); the doses of these aminoglycosides should be regulated according to assays of peak-trough concentrations in the blood.

Adapted from Parker RH. Septic arthritis. In: Hoeprich P, ed. Infectious diseases. 4th ed. Philadelphia: JB Lippincott, 1989:1380.

tween the inner and outer membranes of the gram-negative bacteria. In addition, the side chain may extend the half life and allow less frequent and more convenient dosing. Gram-negative bacilli in an immunocompromised host should receive antibiotic coverage for *Pseudomonas aeruginosa*. Again, a third-generation cephalosporin with antipseudomonal activity, such as ceftazidime, a quinolone, or an antipseudomonal extended-spectrum penicillin (e.g., piperacillin or mezlocillin) and an aminoglycoside may be selected.

Gram-negative cocci suggest neisserial infections. Because more than 5% of gonococci are resistant to penicillin, all infected patients should be given a third-generation cephalosporin, such

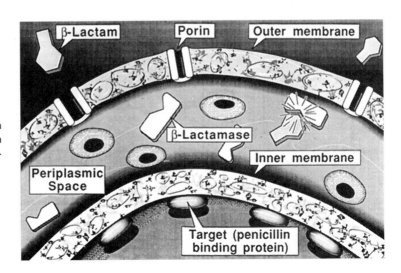

FIGURE 20–1
β-Lactam and β-lactamase activity in the gram-negative organism. (From Gentry LW. Bacterial resistance. Orthop Clin North Am 1991;22:381.)

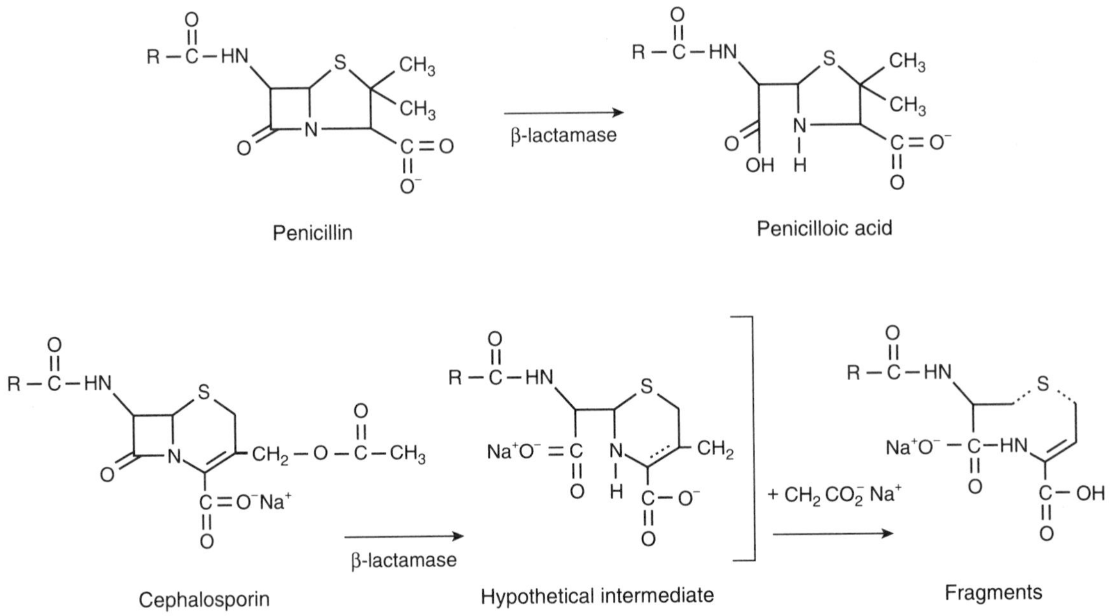

FIGURE 20–2
Hydrolysis of the β-lactam ring. (From Gentry LW. Bacterial resistance. Orthop Clin North Am 1991;22:381.)

as ceftriaxone, or a quinolone. Similarly, when *no bacteria are identified on Gram stain* from a young adult or an elderly person, a third-generation cephalosporin (e.g., ceftriaxone) provides coverage against the most likely offending organisms, *N. gonorrhoeae* and Enterobacteriaceae, respectively. In this situation, because *S. aureus* remains a major pathogen in all age groups, antistaphylococcal medications should be added until synovial fluid culture results are available to modify this empiric therapy. A patient given prior antibiotics will pose special difficulties; in this case empiric treatment will be definitive because culture results will not be available to guide therapy. The above-mentioned clinical situations will dictate the choice of drug.

When the culture and susceptibility results become available, the antibiotic regimen should be modified to a more specific spectrum on the basis of the antibiotic susceptibility profile of the offending organism and the clinical response (Table 20–3). Clinical laboratories use a variety of methods that correlate with standards promoted by the National Committee for Clinical Laboratory Standards (NCCLS). The minimal inhibitory concentration (MIC) is the lowest concentration of an antimicrobial that does not permit visible growth of the retrieved microorganism. Broth-dilution methods in test tubes (macro)

are read by eye, while automated microdilution techniques are read by optical scanner. The minimum bactericidal concentration (MBC) is defined by the concentration of an antibiotic that kills 99.9% of the initial inoculum of viable organisms after incubation for a fixed length of time under a given set of conditions read by serial dilutions in a pour plate. Timed-killed curves can be generated with both methods. The disk diffusion method records the diameter of a zone of inhibition of bacterial growth on agar around antibiotic-impregnated paper disks. The diameters of inhibited growth are reported to correlate inversely with MICs derived from broth microdilutions and are read as sensitive, intermediately sensitive, or resistant to the antibiotic tested.[5] The serum bactericidal test (SBT) is performed by diluting serum from a patient receiving antimicrobial therapy that is bactericidal to the infective microorganism. SBTs of >1:8 assure measurable bactericidal activity in the serum for at least three half-lives of the antibiotic being tested.[5] Practically, bactericidal tests are used only to follow endocarditis, although some have recommended the SBT to verify the effectiveness of antibiotics in the treatment of children with septic arthritis or osteomyelitis.

One should remain aware that these in vitro susceptibility tests show good but not absolute

TABLE 20–3
Antimicrobial Therapy of Septic Arthritis After Culture Results

PRIMARY ANTIMICROBIAL(S)	ALTERNATIVE	ORAL DRUG FOR COMPLETION
Staphylococcus aureus, "methicillin" susceptible		
Nafcillin	Cefazolin	Dicloxacillin
Oxacillin	Vancomycin	Cephalexin (cephradine or cefadroxil)
S. aureus, "methicillin"-resistant		
Vancomycin	Teichoplanin (not available)	Clindamycin or trimethoprim sulfa if susceptible
Streptococcus pyogenes or *pneumoniae*		
Penicillin G	Cefazolin	Penicillin V
		Cephalexin (cephradine or cefadroxil)
Neisseria gonorrhoeae, β-lactamase negative		
Penicillin G	Cefazolin	Amoxicillin
	Ampicillin	Tetracycline or doxycycline
N. gonorrhoeae, β-lactamase positive		
Ceftriaxone	Cefotaxime	Ciprofloxacin
	Ceftizoxime	Cefuroxime axetil
	Ciprofloxacin	Amoxicillin-clavulanic acid
Enterobacteriaceae	Ofloxacin	
Specific agent chosen according to in vitro susceptibility of isolate		
Pseudomonas aeruginosa		
Either piperacillin, azlocillin, mezlocillin, or ticarcillin plus an aminoglycoside	Ceftazidime ± aminoglycoside	Ciprofloxacin
Bacteroides fragilis		
Metronidazole	Clindamycin	Metronidazole
		Clindamycin
Peptococcus spp. and other anaerobes		
Clindamycin	Penicillin G	Clindamycin

Adapted from Parker RH. Septic arthritis. In: Hoeprich P, ed. Infectious diseases. 4th ed. Philadelphia: JB Lippincott, 1989:1381.

correlation with the in vivo activity of the antimicrobial. The predictive value of susceptibility testing which identifies bacterial resistance to an antibiotic is ~95% in most laboratories. Both chromosomal mutations and acquisition of new DNA from plasmids can result in the development of a wide variety of resistance mechanisms, including the elaboration of β-lactamases, which inactivate the β-lactam antibiotics, alteration of the antibiotic target by decreasing the efficiency of the penicillin-binding protein (PBP), restriction of the permeability of the bacteria to antibiotic, or bypass of the metabolic inhibition accorded by the antibiotic.[5] The predictive value of bacterial sensitivity to an antibiotic is only 80% to 85%, with most discrepancies related to β-lactam therapies for pseudomonads and enterococci.[5,6] Most laboratories know and adjust for the

poor reliability of sensitivities of *Pseudomonas* by the rapid-identification microtiter techniques, and of *Salmonella* by disk-diffusion methods. In addition, antibiotics that deter growth of pseudomonads in vitro may not be effective in vivo because of the high bacterial inoculum, low pH, and poor antibiotic penetration in the closed spaces of infected joints. Careful monitoring is essential for adjusting these clinical decisions.

There are no controlled studies on the optimal duration and route of antibiotic therapy for infectious arthritis. Accordingly, general experience recommends that prolonged treatment with intravenous antibiotics continues for at least 2 weeks, followed by a course of oral antibiotics for another 1 to 4 weeks, for nongonococcal infections. Because parenterally administered antibiotics achieve high concentrations in infected synovial fluid, intraarticular antibiotics are rarely necessary. All antibiotics, except erythromycin, attain synovial fluid concentrations that are much higher than the average MIC or MBC for most microorganisms.[7–9] More recently, efforts to administer intravenous antibiotics at home and to change early to oral antibiotics at two to three times the usual dose have been successful in children and in adults with less cost and better patient satisfaction.[10–14]

Relative contraindications to the use of some antibiotics occur in specific clinical situations. Patients with a history of penicillin allergy can be treated with clindamycin, vancomycin, or cephalosporins with caution. In patients who are pregnant, penicillins, cephalosporins, and erythromycin base can safely be used, but tetracycline, chloramphenicol, erythromycin estolate, aminoglycosides, quinolones, and sulfonamides should be avoided.

DOCUMENTING CLINICAL RESPONSE

All the clinical data that prompt and validate the diagnosis should be recorded and displayed in a sequential fashion to document the effectiveness of the treatment regimen (Table 20–4).

Clinically, in acute infectious arthritis, fever, and malaise as well as local joint tenderness and erythema should improve within 24 to 48 hours. Within 3 to 5 days, the synovial fluid volume and the white cell count should decrease by 30% to 50%, and the synovial fluid glucose should have increased to within 75% of normal. When the diagnosis of infectious arthritis is secure, lack of clinical improvement should prompt procedures to identify a sequestered infection that requires surgical drainage. When the diagnosis of septic arthritis is not secure, concomitant nonsteroidal antiinflammatory drugs (NSAIDs) should be avoided for 5 to 7 days, so that any clinical improvement is correctly attributed to the empiric antibiotic therapy. Concomitant use of NSAIDs with antibiotics cleared by the kidney, such as the aminoglycosides and vancomycin, requires monitoring of renal function and antibiotic drug levels.

Joints that are clinically difficult to evaluate or that have a complex anatomic structure, such as the hip or shoulder, may require imaging by radionuclide scanning, computed tomography (CT), or magnetic resonance imaging (MRI). Radionuclide scanning procedures are sensitive but not very specific, since all localize to infections

TABLE 20–4
Clinical Response

	DAY 0 DIAGNOSIS	DAY 1–4		DAY 5–7 [REVIEW DIAGNOSIS]		WEEK 1–2
Clinical						
Fever	Present	Afebrile:	GC	Afebrile:	NGC	
Joint	Inflamed	Improved:	GC	Improved:	NGC	Clinical cure
Laboratory						
SF volume	+++	++		±		± Postinfectious effusion
SF WBC	20,000–100,000: NGC 10,000–50,000: GC	↓ 30%–50%:	GC	↓ 30%–50%:	NGC	
SF culture [PCR]	+++	–				
Radiology						
[MRI, CT scan]	[Difficult arthrocentesis]			[Sequestered infection]		
Antibiotics	Empiric IV	Adjust per susceptibilities day 3: GC Change to oral: GC				Change to oral: NGC

[ ] = if atypical course, consider [ ]; GC = gonococcal arthritis; NGC = nongonococcal arthritis; SF = synovial fluid.

and to inflammatory foci of any cause, including the acute joints of rheumatoid, psoriatic, and other inflammatory arthritides. Technetium phosphate bone scans become abnormal within days of the onset of a bone infection, within minutes describing a "hot" area of increased vascular flow which persists for hours. Occasionally, a "cold" photodeficient area is noted initially. Gallium binds to transferrin, lactoferrin, and related receptors on leukocytes and other metabolically active cells within inflammatory loci. Thus gallium scans may identify infected bone when the bone scans are negative because of restricted blood flow from increased intramedullary pressure. Third, reinfusing Indium-labeled peripheral blood white cells can also outline foci of inflammation in bones, joints, and soft tissue.

Computed tomography (CT scan) identifies bony lesions early, particularly at a time when conventional radiographs may be difficult to interpret. MRI affords the early detection of fluid, loculations, and soft tissue abnormalities.[15,16] Most prefer the T-2 weighted images where the bone is dark and the fluid is white and the use of gadolinium, which localizes within inflamed tissue. Standard x-ray films at the time of initial diagnosis can provide information to rule out other possible diagnoses, such as fractures, but are not sensitive for following cartilage space loss or the development of osteomyelitis.

REMOVAL OF DETRITUS

Closed-needle aspiration should be the initial method of drainage in all cases of infectious arthritis in accessible joints. Aspiration with a large-bore needle is attempted daily for 5 days in joints such as the knee, wrist, ankle, and smaller joints when an effusion is clinically detectable.[17] Because closed needle drainage may not remove all the detritus, it is prudent to request an orthopedic consultation for consideration of drainage procedures early in the clinical course. Open surgical drainage of the hips and shoulders is generally preferred because complete drainage is difficult, particularly in children, whose anatomy predisposes to avascular necrosis.[1,18,19] Although not difficult to aspirate, the redundant spaces within the shoulder can allow for sequestered infection, especially if there is a delay in diagnosis. The multiple articulations of the wrist, including the intercarpal and radiocarpal joints, and the

sacroiliac and sternoclavicular joints are difficult to aspirate. In general, the more complex the anatomy, the presence of preexisting joint damage, and the longer the delay in the institution of therapy point toward an earlier use of open surgical drainage.

Arthroscopic surgery is the procedure of choice in accessible joints, such as the knee. Diagnostically, arthroscopy allows biopsies of the infected synovium to be performed under direct vision. Therapeutically, arthroscopy enables more effective removal of inflammatory debris by irrigation of all of the joint spaces, including the posterior compartment of the knee. The frequency of introducing bacteria into the joint during arthroscopy is less than 1%, particularly when the small-needle arthroscopes are used.[20] Compared to arthrotomy, arthroscopy also carries the advantage of decreased morbidity of the procedure (without the need for general anesthesia), improved joint mobility, and shorter hospital stays.[20]

If pain, fever, effusion, and synovial leukocytosis persist after needle aspiration or arthroscopic lavage, an open drainage procedure to explore and to debride loculations, adhesions, and bony sequestrum should be undertaken promptly. Open surgical drainage procedures are usually followed by a decreased range of motion in the affected joint, and this may be permanent.

INFECTIONS OF PROSTHETIC JOINTS

Prosthetic joint infections represent a special kind of bacterial arthritis. Early infections after joint replacement are usually caused by *Staphylococcus epidermidis, S. aureus,* or gram-negative bacilli. To decrease the risk of infection, attention must be given to improved surgical technique, laminar airflow environments, and the prophylactic use of antibiotics given 30 to 60 minutes before and continued for 1 to 2 days after surgery.[21] Cefazolin, 1 to 2 g given intravenously, is the recommended antistaphylococcal antibiotic. Intravenous vancomycin, 1 g, is used in hospitals with a high frequency of methicillin-resistant *S. aureus* (MRSA) or for patients who are allergic to penicillins or cephalosporins.[22] After premedication with diphenhydramine, vancomycin is given over a period of 60 minutes since rapid intravenous administration can induce hypotension, particularly during induction of anesthesia.[23] When patients with prosthetic joints undergo other surgical procedures in which bacteremia is likely to occur, antistaphylococcal antibiotics are recommended.

If an infection develops within the prosthetic site and continues despite antibiotic therapies, the usual recommendation is to remove the prosthesis, perform a wide surgical debridement, and administer antibiotics intravenously for 2 months and orally for a few months before attempting a second prosthetic joint placement. Serial joint aspirations to record the culture, volume, cell count, and glucose level will be more helpful than an erythrocyte sedimentation rate, x-rays, and scans. When cultures from the prosthetic site are sterile, a custom-made implant is often necessary to compensate for the deficient bone and soft tissues. The implant and cement are often soaked in antibiotics, and intravenous antibiotics are continued for another 4 to 6 weeks. This two-stage reimplantation protocol has eradicated infection in 95% of cases, with 65% good to excellent clinical results at an average of 4 year's follow-up.[24,25]

Actually, if an infection of the prosthesis is discovered early within the first weeks, antibiotics may suffice, particularly if the organism is gram positive and sensitive to the antibiotics. In most late infections, the prolonged immobility required for the reimplantation may be hazardous for those of advanced age with comorbid diseases, such as rheumatoid arthritis.[26] In some instances, it may be necessary to retain the infected prosthesis and to suppress the infection with continual antibiotics. In rare instances, amputation may be necessary. In an attempt to shorten the prolonged hospitalization and rehabilitation period, various antibiotics configured in a slow-release solid bead have been placed in the prosthetic site, but the efficacy of these procedures has not been rigorously assessed at this time.

JOINT REHABILITATION

The acute phase of infection mandates the use of protected rest with the joint in a functional anatomic position. Splints are often necessary. Passive range-of-motion exercises are initiated as soon as the acute stage of infection has subsided. Studies in animals suggest that continuous passive motion facilitates rehabilitation.[27]

To prevent muscle atrophy, isotonic or muscle-tightening exercises are initiated in the acute phase of the infection. Thus quadriceps-setting exercises are recommended for infections in the knee. As the joint pain resolves, the patient is instructed in a program of stretching, active range-of-motion exercises, and muscle strengthening at least twice each day. Some patients develop a postinfectious arthritis, which presents as a sterile, recurrent, inflammatory effusion, when resuming function.[28] This is attributed to sequestered bacterial products, such as antigenic bacterial cell wall components, exotoxins, or endotoxins. Differentiation from an incompletely treated infection or a superinfection may require repeated culture. NSAIDs may be helpful in these patients once infection is ruled out.

CHRONIC INFECTIOUS AGENT ARTHRITIS

Many pathogenic microorganisms are capable of circumventing host defenses by residing intracellularly. Infectious arthritis induced by these agents present less typically, particularly when they have progressed to more chronic phases. Because diagnosis is delayed by the slow growth in culture, PCR may find greater applicability. Antibiotics that attain effective intracellular concentrations are preferred, but susceptibility testing of these slower-growing organisms and the duration of therapy are not standardized. Furthermore, the clinical response is more prolonged, making the recommendations for removal of infected material and rehabilitation less precise. Continuing experience is necessary.

Mycobacterial Infections

The increase of pulmonary tuberculosis in the United States as a result of new immigration and immunocompromised disease states is expected to spawn greater recognition of bone and joint involvement, which occurs in 5% of patients infected with M. tuberculosis.[29–31] The two most common rheumatic manifestations are spinal tuberculosis, also known as Pott's disease, and peripheral tuberculous arthritis. Pott's disease is treated with the standard chemotherapy for pulmonary tuberculosis consisting of 9 months of INH, 5 mg/kg/d orally to a maximum 300 mg/d, and rifampin, 10 mg/kg/d orally to a maximum of 600 mg/d. Pyrazinamide (PZA), 25 mg/kg/d orally to a maximum dose of 2 g/d, is added for the first 2 months of the 9-month regimen.[32] If the spine is not stable and if neurologic involvement is anticipated, spinal fusion prevents vertebral collapse and neurologic sequelae in more than 93%.[33] Paravertebral cold abscesses respond to the chemotherapeutic regimen and generally do not require surgical drainage. Others recommend surgical excision of all tuberculous granulation tissue and disk material to facilitate greater access of chemotherapeutic agents to the area of infection.[34] Similarly, early peripheral arthritis responds to the chemotherapy regimen, but late lesions with sequestrum require surgical debridement.

Because multidrug-resistant tuberculosis is becoming more common, susceptibility testing is required on all isolates. For patients at increased risk, especially those who have received incomplete courses of therapy, empiric treatment requires four antituberculosis drugs, usually isoniazid (INH), ethambutol, rifampin, and PZA.

In most urban centers, any patient with tuberculosis that has disseminated to the joint or to other sites should be tested for human immunodeficiency virus (HIV). HIV patients coinfected with tuberculosis should receive the same regimens as HIV-negative patients, even though bacteremia and extrapulmonary involvement occur in the majority. If INH and rifampin are used without PZA, duration of treatment is extended from 9 to at least 12 months. Most therapeutic regimens are continued for 12 months after the culture becomes negative.[35]

Other mycobacterial infections that induce arthritis in the immunocompromised hosts include *Mycobacterium kansasii*, which responds to the same regimen outlined for *M. tuberculosis*, *Mycobacterium marinum*, which is treated with rifampin and ethambutol, and *Mycobacterium gastri*, which responds to streptomycin for 2 months combined with rifampin and ethambutol for 9 months.[36] *Mycobacterium avium-intracellulare* is treated with ethambutol, and various regimens, which include clarithromycin, cycloserine, rifampin or rifabutin, and amikacin.

Mycobacterium leprae infections reflect the importance of the immune status of the host in the expression of disease. Those with the tuberculoid form demonstrate a good cell-mediated response and a positive lepromin skin test. Those in the lepromatous state demonstrate an anergy of the cell-mediated immunity and a proliferation of *M. leprae* in the skin, nerves, and joints. The lepra bacillus is identified in synovial fluid cells by acid-fast stains in one third and in synovial tissue in one half.[37,38] Lepromatous leprosy is treated with rifampin, 600 mg at least once a month or even daily, dapsone, 100 mg/d, and clofazimine, 300 mg once a month and 50 mg daily, for a period of 2 years.[39] The erythema nodosum leprosum reaction that occurs with specific chemotherapy requires prednisone, 60 mg in divided doses, or thalidomide, 200 mg twice daily tapering to 50 to 100 mg at night.[38] With the chronic sequelae attendant to untreated disease, consultations with specialists in neurology, orthopedics, and physical medicine are required for the evaluation of nerve, bone, and functional impairment.

Fungal Arthritis

Traditionally, most fungal arthritis is treated with the polyene, amphotericin B (AMB), which binds to ergosterol and damages the fungal cell wall. AMB is given intravenously at a maximum dose of 1 mg/kg in 500 ml of dextrose and water over 2 to 4 hours daily or three times a week for a total of 2 to 2.5 g. Initially 1 mg is administered to test for acute toxicity and the dose is increased daily from an initial 10 to 20 mg/d. To forestall fever and severe chills, patients are premedicated with aspirin or acetaminophen, diphenhydramine, and/or hydrocortisone, 25 mg, administered within the infusion. Occasionally, narcotics such as meperidine, 50 mg, are required within the infusion to prevent rigors. Chronic toxicity in the kidneys and bone marrow requires monitoring of the blood urea nitrogen, creatinine, potassium, and magnesium levels and complete blood cell counts. If the serum creatinine approaches 2.5 mg/dl, the dose and frequency of AMB are attenuated. These toxicities and a variable efficacy have prompted the search for different formulations. AMB administered in lipid complexes or liposomes shows increased efficacy and decreased toxicity in experimentally produced fungal infections.[37,38] AMB is rarely given intraarticularly because of the induction of a chemical synovitis.

The azoles are broad-spectrum antifungal agents that inhibit fungal cytochrome P_{450}-dependent enzymes and the synthesis of membrane ergosterol. They are less toxic than AMB

TABLE 20–5
Fungal Arthritis

ORGANISM	PRIMARY ANTIFUNGAL	ALTERNATIVE
Coccidioides immitis	Amphotericin B	Fluconazole
	Liposomal amphotericin B	Itraconazole
		Amphotericin B—intraarticular
Candida species		
Localized	Fluconazole	Ketoconazole
Disseminated	Amphotericin B	Amphotericin B plus flucytosine
Histoplasma capsulatum		
Mild	Itraconazole	Fluconazole
Moderate-severe	Itraconazole or amphotericin B	
Blastomycosis		
Non-AIDS patients	Itraconazole	Amphotericin B
AIDS patients	Amphotericin B (?)	
Cryptococcus neoformans	Amphotericin B plus flucytosine	Fluconazole
Sporothrix schenckii	Amphotericin B	Amphotericin B—intraarticular

Dosing
Amphotericin B: 0.6 mg/kg/d IV × 7d then 0.8 mg/kg/qod IV. Start test dose 1 mg day 1, 10 mg day 2, 20 mg day 3, up to 50 mg/d. Adjust dose by renal function. Total dose = 2.5 g.
Fluconazole, itraconazole, and ketoconazole: 400 mg PO qd.
Flucytosine: 150 mg/kg/d in four divided doses.

and can be given orally. As a group, the imidazoles, miconazole and ketoconazole, are more toxic than the triazoles, fluconazole and itraconazole. Combinations of azoles with AMB may confer improved efficacy with decreased toxicities, but further studies are needed.[40] Inasmuch as the orally administered azoles require gastric acid for absorption, they should not be used in patients who are achlorhydric or who are taking antacids or H_2 blockers. Flucytosine, a competitive antimetabolite of uracil in the synthesis of yeast RNA, is used adjunctively with AMB because of early resistance. It is never used alone because rapid resistance develops. Other azoles, polypeptides, echinocandins, and nikkomycins represent new drugs that may also broaden antifungal therapeutic options. Current treatment recommendations for selected fungal arthritides follow (Table 20–5).

Treatment of coccidiodomycosis involves medical and surgical interventions. AMB produces cure rates of 50% to 70%, and relapses are frequent. Azoles may become the drugs of choice. Itraconazole and fluconazole (each at a dose of 400 mg by mouth daily) provide response rates similar to AMB against coccidioidomycosis arthritis. Ketoconazole suffers from limited efficacy and frequent relapses of infection.[41] Intraarticular AMB has been used successfully, despite the local toxicity. Synovectomy

to debride the joint and reduce the fungal burden alone does not effect a cure.[42–44] Improved outcome is obtained by combining synovectomy and debridement with intravenous AMB, and therefore this is the recommended treatment.[45]

The role of antifungal susceptibility testing remains to be standardized. Inconsistencies have been noted in monitoring the treatment of coccidioidomycoses as well as candidiasis.[40] Coccidioidomycosis complement-fixation titers of serum and/or synovial fluid may be prognostic and should be obtained every other month. Complement-fixation titers >1:16 at the completion of therapy are likely to result in clinical relapse but titers of <1:4 may persist for years.[46] Skeletal radiographs are not reliable markers for progress, inasmuch as abnormalities may persist for months after clinical and microbiologic cure.[43]

Isolated *Candida* arthritis responds to fluconazole or AMB, although the duration of therapy is not clear.[40] Open drainage is rarely necessary, except when there is hip involvement. If antifungal drugs are ineffective, synovectomy is an alternative.[47]

Histoplasmosis arthritis is uncommon. If the disease is severe, itraconazole, 400 mg/d orally for 6 months, represents the drug of choice in patients who do not have AIDS. Alternatively, a short course of AMB, up to 500 mg total, can be used. If severe systemic infection is present, a total dose of 2 g is needed.[48] NSAIDs and, less often, corticosteroids can be used against the arthritis associated with erythema nodosum.

Disseminated blastomycosis leads to death in 30% to 80% of cases. Treatment includes AMB or itraconazole. Because loculations are common, open drainage is often necessary.

Cryptococcal arthritis occurs in patients with impaired cell-mediated immunity, such as those with AIDS or lymphoreticular cancers or those receiving corticosteroids.[49] Treatment includes high-dose AMB with flucytosine for a period sufficient to yield conversion of cultures with minimal or no toxicity.[40] Surgical drainage and excision are often required for an adjacent osteomyelitis.

Sporothrix schenckii is the most reported cause of fungal arthritis. AMB for 12 weeks, combined with surgery, is the treatment of choice. Intraarticular AMB has been used successfully in a patient refractory to a full course of intravenous AMB.[50]

SUMMARY

Clinical awareness, prompt identification of the infectious agent and initiation of therapy, a considered choice of antibiotics, and continuing attention to the host factors, particularly the removal of pus, remain the primary determinants for the successful treatment of infectious arthritis. In the future, DNA hybridization techniques such as the PCR should increase the capabilities for specific diagnosis of infections by agents that are difficult to identify, particularly those that produce chronic arthritis. We hope that newer classes of antibiotics will retain their effectiveness in controlling bacterial growth in spite of increasing patterns of antimicrobial resistance.[51] Other methods of enhancing host defenses to complete bacterial killing may be forthcoming. For the present, effective care for this most treatable group of patients demands our continued vigilance.

ACKNOWLEDGMENTS

We acknowledge Drs. Scott Filler, Milton Louie, William Kim, Anne Hollister, and Jeffrey Phillips for their comments and contributions to this chapter.

REFERENCES

1. Goldenberg DL. Bacterial arthritis. In: Kelley WN, Harris ED, Ruddy S, Sledge CB, eds. Textbook of rheumatology. 4th ed. Philadelphia: WB Saunders, 1993:1449.
2. Liebling MR, Nishio MJ, Rodriguez A, Sigal LH, Louie JS. The polymerase chain reaction for the detection of *Borrelia burgdorferi* in human body fluids. Arthritis Rheum 1993;36:665.
3. Liebling MR, Arkfeld DG, Michelini GA, et al. Identification of *Neisseria gonorrhoeae* in synovial fluid using the polymerase chain reaction. Arthritis Rheum 1994;37:702.
4. Relman DA, Schmidt TM, MacDermott RP, et al. Identification of the uncultured bacillus of Whipple's disease. N Engl J Med 1992;327:293.
5. Stratton CW. In vitro testing: correlations between bacterial susceptibility, body fluid levels and effectiveness of antibacterial therapy. In: Lorian V. Antibiotics in laboratory medicine. 3rd ed. Baltimore: Williams & Wilkins, 1991:849.
6. Lorian V, Burns L. Predictive value of susceptibility tests for the outcome of antimicrobial therapy. J Antimicrob Chemother 1990;25:175.
7. Parker RH, Schmid FR. Antibacterial activity of synovial fluid during treatment of septic arthritis. Arthritis Rheum 1971;14:96.
8. Nelson JD. Antibiotic concentrations in septic joint effusions. N Engl J Med 1971;284:349.
9. Baciocco EA, Lies RL. Ampicillin and kanamycin concentrations in joint fluid. Clin Pharmacol Ther 1971;12:858.
10. Tetzlaff TR, McCracken GH, Nelson JD. Oral antibiotic therapy for skeletal infections of children. II. Therapy of osteomyelitis and supportative arthritis. J Pediatr 1978;92:485.
11. Prober CG, Yeager AS. Use of the serum bactericidal titer to assess the adequacy of oral antibiotic therapy in the treatment of acute hematogenous osteomyelitis. J Pediatr 1979;95:131.
12. Bryson YJ, Conner JD, LeClerc M, et al. Brief clinical and laboratory observation: high-dose oral dicloxacillin treatment of acute staphylococcal osteomyelitis in children. J Pediatr 1979;94:673.
13. Kolyvas E, Ahronheim G, Marks MI, et al. Oral antibiotic therapy of skeletal infections in children. Pediatrics 1980;65:867.
14. Black J, Hunt TL, Godley PJ, et al. Oral antimicrobial therapy for adults with osteomyelitis or septic arthritis. J Infect Dis 1987;155:968.
15. Resnick CS, Ammann AM, Walsh JW. Chronic septic arthritis of the adult hip: computed tomographic feature. Skeletal Radiol 1987;16:513.
16. Rosenberg D, Baskies AM, Deckers PJ. Pyogenic sacroiliitis: an absolute indication for computerized scanning. Clin Orthop 1984;184:128.
17. Goldenberg DL, Reed JI. Bacterial arthritis. N Engl J Med 1985;312:764.
18. Broy SB, Schmid FR. A comparison of medical drainage (needle aspiration) and surgical drainage (arthrotomy or arthroscopy) in the initial treatment of infected joints. Clin Rheum Dis 1986;12:501.

19. Bulmer JH. Septic arthritis of the hip in adults. J Bone Joint Surg 1966;48B:289.

20. Broy S, Stulberg SD, Schmid FR. The role of arthroscopy in the diagnosis and management of the septic joint. Clin Rheum Dis 1986;12:489.

21. Lidwell OM, Elson RA, Lowbury EJ, et al. Ultraclean air and antibiotics for prevention of postoperative infection: a multicenter study of 8052 joint replacement operations. Acta Orthop Scand 1987;58:4.

22. Antimicrobial prophylaxis in surgery. In: Abramowitz M, ed. Med Lett Drugs Ther 1993; 35:91.

23. Maki D, Bohn MJ, Stolz SM, et al. Comparative study of cefazolin, cefamandole, and vancomycin for surgical prophylaxis in cardiac and vascular operations. J Thorac Cardiovasc Surg 1992;104:1423.

24. Frymoyer JW, ed. Orthopedic knowledge update 4. American College of Orthopedic Surgeons, 1993.

25. Wilson MG, Kelley K, Thornhill TS. Infection as a complication of total knee replacement in arthroplasty: risk factors and treatment in sixty-seven cases. J Bone Joint Surg 1990;72A:878.

26. Gardner GC, Weisman MH. Pyarthrosis in patients with rheumatoid arthritis: a report of 13 cases and a review of the literature from the past 40 years. Am J Med 1990;88:503.

27. Salter RB, Bell RS, Keeley FW. The protective effect of continuous passive motion on living articular cartilage in acute septic arthritis: an experimental investigation in the rabbit. Clin Orthop 1981;159:223.

28. Goldenberg DL. "Post-infectious" arthritis: new look at an old concept with particular attention to disseminated gonococcal infection. Am J Med 1983;74:925.

29. Evanchick CC, Davis DE, Harrington TM. Tuberculosis of peripheral joints: an often missed diagnosis. J Rheumatol 1986;13:187.

30. Berney S, Goldstein M, Bishko F. Clinical and diagnostic features of tuberculous arthritis. Am J Med 1972;53:36.

31. Meier JL, Hoffman GS. Mycobacterial and fungal infections. In: Kelley WN, Harris ED, Ruddy S, Sledge CB, eds. Textbook of rheumatology. 4th ed. Philadelphia: WB Saunders, 1993:1467.

32. Sanford JP. Guide to antimicrobial therapy—1993. Dallas: Antimicrobial Therapy, Inc., 1993:1.

33. Chakirgill GS. Evaluation of anterior spinal fusion for treatment of vertebral tuberculosis. Orthopedics 1991;14:601.

34. Alarcon GS. Arthritis due to tuberculosis, fungal infections, and parasites. Curr Opin Rheumatol 1992;4:516.

35. Small PM, Schecter GF, Goodman PC, et al. Treatment of tuberculosis in patients with advanced human immunodeficiency virus infection. N Engl J Med 1991;324:289.

36. Perandones CE, Roncoroni AJ, Frega NS, et al. Mycobacterium gastri arthritis: a case report—septic arthritis due to *Mycobacterium gastri* in a patient with a renal transplant. J Rheumatol 1991;18:777.

37. Pernambuco JCA, Opromolla DUA, Tolentin MM, et al. Arthritis is lepromatous Hansen's disease [Abstract]. Int J Leprosy 1979;47:353.

38. Louie JS, Koransky JR, Cohen AH. Lepra cells in synovial fluid of a patient with erythema nodosum leprosum. New Engl J Med 1973;289:1410.

39. WHO Study Group. Chemotherapy of leprosy for control programs. WHO Technical Report 675. Geneva: WHO 1982.

40. Graybill JR. Future directions of antifungal chemotherapy. Clin Infect Dis 1992;14(suppl 1):170.

41. Lopez-Berestein G, Bodey GP, Fainstein V. Treatment of systemic fungal infections with liposomal amphotericin B. Arch Int Med 1989; 149:2533.

42. Bayer AS, Guze LB. Fungal arthritis. II. Coccidioidal synovitis: clinical, diagnostic, therapeutic, and prognostic considerations. Semin Arthritis Rheum 1979;8:200.

43. Winter WG Jr, Larson RK, Honeggar MM, et al. Coccidioidal arthritis and its treatment—1975. J Bone Joint Surg 1975;57A:1152.

44. Gillespie R. Treatment of cranial osteomyelitis from disseminated coccidioidomycosis. West J Med 1986;145:694.

45. Bried JM, Galgiani JN. Coccidioides immitis infections in bones and joints. Clin Orthop 1986; 211:235.

46. Koster FT, Galgiani JN. Coccidioidal arthritis. In: Espinoza L, ed. Infections in the rheumatic diseases. Orlando, Florida: Grune & Stratton, 1988:165.

47. Karsh J. Candida arthritis. In: Espinoza L, ed. Infections in the rheumatic diseases. Orlando, Florida: Grune & Stratton, 1988:189.

48. Goodwin RA, Loyd JE, Des Prez RM. Histoplasmosis in normal hosts. Medicine 1989;60:231.

49. Ricciardi DD, Sepkowitz DV, Berkowitz LB, et al. Cryptococcal arthritis in a patient with AIDS: case report and review of the literature. J Rheumatol 1986;13:455.

50. Downs NJ, Hinthorn DR, Mhatre VR, et al. Intraarticular amphotericin B treatment of *Sporothrix schenckii* arthritis. Arch Intern Med 1989; 149:954.

51. Davies J. Inactivation of antibiotics and the dissemination of resistance genes. Science 1994; 264:375.

21

LYME DISEASE

Nancy A. Shadick

Lyme disease is a tick-borne illness caused by the spirochete, *Borrelia burgdorferi,* which causes a multisystem disease of the skin, nervous system, heart, and joints.[1] Although the clinical picture may vary, the disease usually begins with erythema migrans accompanied by flu-like or meningitis-like symptoms. Weeks later meningitis, facial palsy, atrioventricular nodal block, or migratory musculoskeletal pain may develop, followed months to years later by episodes of oligoarticular arthritis, encephalopathy, polyneuropathy, or acrodermatitis.[2,3]

EPIDEMIOLOGY

Lyme disease is the most common vector-borne illness in the United States. Nearly 50,000 cases from the 48 contiguous states have been reported to the Centers for Disease Control since 1980.[4] The highest density of cases is found in three endemic areas: the Northeast (extending from Maryland to northern Massachusetts), the upper Midwest (including Wisconsin and Minnesota), and the Far West (including Northern California and Oregon).[5,6] Two members of the Ixodidae family, *Ixodes dammini* found in the Northeast and Midwest, and *Ixodes pacificus* found in the Far West are the most common vectors of Lyme disease in the United States.[7]

Endemic areas of Lyme disease are located worldwide and include Europe, China, Russia, and Japan.[8,9] Transmission is by ixodid ticks as well. The *Ixodes ricinus* tick has been known to cause erythema migrans in Europe since 1950.[10]

The clinical syndrome of Lyme disease was first described in Europe[11] in 1913. The first cases in the United States were identified in Cape Cod

in 1962 and Lyme, Connecticut, in 1965, but polymerase chain-reaction technology has identified *B. burgdorferi* in tick specimens as far back as 1940.[12–14] The recent increase in Lyme disease is thought to be partially due to the increase in the density and population of deer, the most common host of the adult *I. dammini* tick. Deforestation of much of the Northeast eliminated the conditions favorable for deer and deer ticks, but certain areas such as Long Island, New York, and certain islands off Cape Cod maintained their populations. As farming decreased and suburban metropolitan areas proliferated, deciduous forests returned along with the deer, creating ecologic conditions suitable for endemicity.

Competent reservoir hosts and tick vectors are necessary to maintain endemicity. A reservoir host must be frequently infected and capable of sustaining borrelial infection. A competent vector must, in turn, be able to receive and transmit infection from a competent reservoir host. In the Northeast, the white-footed mouse *(Peromyscus leucopus)* is the most important reservoir for the larval and nymphal tick and appears to be the means through which high rates of infectivity are maintained in endemic areas.[15] The *I. dammini* tick has a 2-year, three-stage life cycle (larva, nymph, and adult).[16] Both larval and nymph forms feed on the white-footed mouse or other small mammals. The nymphal tick, which feeds during the late spring and summer, most commonly transmits the disease to humans. The adult form transmits *B. burgdorferi* to humans during the late fall or winter when it feeds on larger mammals, such as deer, horses, cows, or dogs.

Infection with *B. burgdorferi* occurs by horizontal transmission.[17] Infected nymphal ticks transmit *B. burgdorferi* to the white-footed mouse, which then passes it on to larval ticks. Larvae then molt into nymphs and transmit infection to either other mice or humans. Between 20% and 80% of ticks may harbor the spirochete in endemic areas, but infection rates vary considerably within these endemic areas.[18] Dormant, infected ticks can sustain infection until the next season and, as adults, can transmit the spirochete while feeding on deer and/or humans.

In the Far West, the woodrat serves as reservoir host for Lyme disease, and the nonhuman-biting tick, *Ixodes neotomae*, is the rodent- and rabbit-feeding vector responsible for maintaining infection. *I. pacificus*, which mostly feeds on lizards, is responsible for the transmission to humans. When no lizards are available, *I. pacificus* will feed on small mammals and, at a relatively low rate (1%), transmits *B. burgdorferi* to humans.[19] Other vectors, *Ixodes scapularis* and *Amblyomma americanum,* are likely vectors in the southeast United States and Texas, respectively.

BIOLOGY OF *BORRELIA BURGDORFERI*

The causative agent of Lyme disease was first isolated from *I. dammini* ticks captured on Shelter Island, New York.[1] The organism is a member of the phylum spirochete, which has a spiral-shaped body with 7 to 11 flagella arranged along an axial filament that lies between the outer and inner membranes of the cell.[20] Four to seven linear and circular plasmids, two of which encode for the organism's outer surface lipoproteins 31 kD OspA and 34 kD OspB, are found in the spirochete.[21] Both OspA and OspB are transcribed from an operon located on a linear plasmid. The expression of these proteins varies between isolates and will sometimes lose pathogenicity through multiple passages in culture.[22] Other immunologically important peptides include the 41 kD flagellar protein, which bears resemblance to other spirochetes, the 60 kD, 66 kD, and 83 kD heat shock proteins, and the low-molecular-weight proteins between 18 and 25 kD.

The organism grows very slowly, dividing every 12 to 24 hours in vitro and more slowly in vivo. It is grown in Barbour-Stoenner-Kelly medium at 33° and has now been cultured from blood, skin, and spinal and joint fluid.[23] Spirochetes are extracellular organisms, although studies have demonstrated that *B. burgdorferi* can live inside phagocytes.[24] (For more detail on pathogenesis, the reader is referred to Kelley et al., Lyme Disease, reference 102.)

DIAGNOSIS

The diagnosis of Lyme disease is made clinically with supportive serologic and epidemiologic data. A history of a tick bite in an area with known Lyme disease and erythema migrans are the most important data in diagnosing Lyme disease. The risk of developing Lyme disease after a tick bite in an endemic area is low (approximately 5% in one study).[25] Because culture or direct visualization of *B. burgdorferi* in tissue is difficult, infection can rarely be proved. In early Lyme disease 53% of patients have an elevated erythrocyte sedimentation rate (ESR), 19% have liver function test abnormalities, and 12% have a hematocrit value less than 37%, but these tests are nonspecific.[26] Erythema migrans, a red patch at the site of the tick bite that clears centrally and expands over a period of days to weeks to form a large, round lesion, usually more than 5 cm in diameter, is pathognomonic for Lyme disease. The lesions can be pleomorphic, however. Not all necessarily have central clearing; some may be vesiculated, and "satellite" lesions can be observed. Nearly one third of the patients with Lyme disease do not have erythema migrans.[27] In this case, a flulike syndrome with fever, headache, shaking chills, arthralgias, or lymphadenopathy after a tick bite may provide a clue to the diagnosis. A small percentage of patients may have asymptomatic infection with *B. burgdorferi*. In the United States, the frequency of asymptomatic infection in endemic areas ranges between 3% and 5%.[13] The Centers for Disease Control national surveillance case definition is weighted heavily toward serologic confirmation, and late manifestations cannot be the sole basis for clinical diagnosis.[28]

Antibody Tests

Early in the course of infection, T lymphocytes proliferate preferentially to *B. burgdorferi* antigens.[29] Approximately 3 to 6 weeks after infection a specific IgM response becomes detectable.[30] A specific IgG response appears anywhere from 6 to 8 weeks but may not peak until months later and can remain elevated indefinitely. The IgG response expands over time to novel *B. burgdorferi* antigens supporting the theory that live spirochetes persist throughout the course of Lyme disease.[31]

The two most commonly used methods for detecting antibodies to *B. burgdorferi* are the enzyme-linked immunosorbent assay (ELISA) and the indirect immunofluorescent assay (IFA), both of which use sonicated homogenates of the whole organism.[30] Because of its greater sensitivity and specificity, the ELISA is preferred over the IFA. Serologic testing remains unstandardized, and results vary between laboratories. False-positive serologic results are seen with a number of other diseases, including syphilis, relapsing fever, Rocky Mountain spotted fever, infectious mononucleosis, autoimmune disease, and neurologic illnesses such as amyotrophic lateral sclerosis.[30,32] Even a borderline positive rheumatoid factor or antinuclear antibody can result in a false-positive Lyme ELISA titer. The prevalence of false-positive results ranges from 5% to 10% in the United States.[33]

False-negative serologic findings occur, particularly in early infection and in cases in which antibiotic treatment early in the disease may attenuate the specific antibody response.[30] Serum samples during the acute illness are negative in most patients by standard ELISA. By antibody capture immunoassay (ELISA capture) to IgM, 90% of patients will have a detectable IgM response.[34] IgG, IgM, and IgA capture enzyme immunoassay decreases nonspecific binding to cross-reactive epitopes by adsorption of the test serum with *Escherichia coli* and thus is able to detect small increases in *B. burgdorferi*–specific antibody compared with total antibody. Both indirect ELISA and ELISA capture assays can be used to measure intrathecal antibody production to *B. burgdorferi*, the most specific diagnostic test for neurologic Lyme.[35] Increased cerebrospinal fluid (CSF) serum ratios of specific IgG and IgA provide evidence for active central nervous system (CNS) infection in early and late neuroborreliosis. The antibody capture immunoassay is currently available only from a few specialty laboratories.[34]

Western Blot Analysis

Western blot techniques, though unstandardized, are a promising adjunct to the serologic diagnosis of Lyme disease. Expansion of the immunoglobulin G response to novel *B. burgdorferi* polypeptides occurs over time[31] and includes immune reactivity to a 31 kD OspA, a 34 kD OspB, and a 23 kD OspC outer surface protein. The 41 kD flagellar protein shares homology with other spirochetes, and the 58, 66 and 74 kD heat shock proteins share homology with other heat shock proteins in the *E. coli* family, making these polypeptides less specific for Lyme disease.[36] The 31 kD (OspA) and 34 kD (OspB) reactivity is found in persons with prolonged episodes of arthritis.[37] The functions of the 21, 28, and 93 kD proteins, which are more specific for Lyme disease, are not known. Requiring 5 of 10 IgG bands after the first weeks of infection (18, 21, 28, 30, 39, 41, 45, 58, 66, 93) had a sensitivity of 83% and a specificity of 95% in one prospective analysis.[38] The Western blot's utility is primarily in confirming exposure in the presence of a borderline ELISA titer, a presumed false-positive result, or in following the specific immune response over time. This technique has become increasingly available but is limited by variability in interpretation and performance of the assay.

Diagnostic Tests Under Investigation

The T cell proliferative assay may be useful in diagnosing early disease or seronegative disease but is costly, labor-intensive, and not widely available.[29] Further, its clinical utility has not been documented. Healthy controls may have a T cell proliferative response to *B. burgdorferi*. Urinary antigen excretion has been documented in infected humans and mice with active Lyme disease, but is currently a research tool.[39] Polymerase chain reaction (PCR) is a highly sensitive technique that amplifies *B. burgdorferi* DNA. It has been used to identify *B. burgdorferi* DNA in patients' tissues and to test ticks for infectivity.[40] PCR is a difficult test to perform with a high rate of contamination. There also have been few studies demonstrating its clinical utility. A recent report, however, demonstrated that PCR testing can detect *B. burgdorferi* DNA in synovial fluid and that the test may be helpful in elucidating whether prolonged arthritis after antibiotic therapy is due to active infection or an autoimmune reaction that persists after eradication of the spirochete.[41]

One should test for Lyme disease initially with ELISA or ELISA capture assay for IgM or

IgG, followed by a Western blot analysis if a borderline titer or a false-positive is suspected. Work-up of neurologic Lyme disease should include analysis of the CSF for IgG, IgA, or IgM antibody.

CLINICAL MANIFESTATIONS AND TREATMENT RECOMMENDATIONS (TABLE 21–1)

In Vitro and In Vivo Studies

Results of in vitro antimicrobial studies of 18 agents demonstrate that *B. burgdorferi* is susceptible to the action of tetracyclines, semisynthetic penicillins, macrolides, and second- and third-generation cephalosporins. *B. burgdorferi* was noted to be moderately sensitive to penicillin G and resistant to chloramphenicol, aminoglycosides, trimethoprim-sulfamethoxazole, quinolones, and rifampin.[42] Cefuroxime demonstrated a higher minimum bactericidal concentration (MBC) in vitro (1.0 µg/ml) than ceftriaxone (0.08 µg/ml) or erythromycin (0.32 µg/ml), but the MBC was similar to that of amoxicillin (0.8 µg/ml) and doxycycline (1.6 µg/ml). *B. burgdorferi* was less susceptible to tetracycline (3.2 µg/ml) and penicillin G (6.4 µg/ml). Penicillin G, which demonstrated a high MBC in vitro, had weak protective activ-

TABLE 21–1
Treatment Recommendations

SYSTEM	REGIMEN
Early infection* (local or disseminated)	
Adults	Doxycycline 100 mg orally bid for 10–30 d[†]
	Amoxicillin 500 mg orally tid for 10–30 d[†]
	Cefuroxime axetil 500 mg orally bid for 20 d[†]
Children (ages 8 or less)	Amoxicillin 250 mg orally tid or 20 mg/kg/d in divided doses for 10–30 d[†]
	Alternative in case of allergy to penicillin:
	Erythromycin[‡] 250 mg orally tid or 30 mg/kg/d in divided doses for 10–30 d[†]
Arthritis* (intermittent or chronic)	Doxycycline 100 mg orally bid for 30 d
	Amoxicillin and probenecid, 500 mg of each qid orally for 30 d
	Ceftriaxone 2 g IV once a day for 14–30 d
	Penicillin G 20 million IU in 6 divided doses for 14–30 d
Neurologic abnormalities*	
Early or late	Ceftriaxone 2 g IV once daily for 14–30 d[§]
	Cefotaxime 2 g IV tid for 14–30 d[§]
	Penicillin G 20 million IU in 6 divided doses daily for 14–30 d[§]
	Alternatives in case of allergy to penicillin or cephalosporin
Early	Doxycycline 200 mg orally bid for 30 d
Early or late	Vancomycin[‡] 1 g bid for 14–30 d
Facial palsy alone	Oral regimens may be adequate
Cardiac abnormalities	
First-degree AV block (PR interval <0.3 s)	Oral regimens, as for early infection
High-degree AV block	Parenteral regimens, as for neurologic abnormalities
Acrodermatitis	Oral regimens for 1 month are usually adequate
Pregnancy	
Localized, early disease	Amoxicillin 500 mg tid for 21 d
All other manifestations	Ceftriaxone 2 g IV once a day for 14–30 d
	Penicillin G 20 million IU IV in 6 divided doses for 14–30 d

*Treatment failures have occurred with any of the regimens given. Re-treatment may be necessary.
†The duration of therapy is based on clinical response.
‡These antibiotics have not yet been tested systematically for this indication in Lyme disease.
§For early neurologic abnormalities, 2 weeks of therapy is generally adequate. The appropriate duration of therapy is not yet clear for patients with late neurologic abnormalities, and 4 weeks of therapy may be preferable.
Reprinted by permission from Steere AC. Lyme disease. N Engl J Med 1989;321:587. Copyright 1989, Massachusetts Medical Society.

ity in a Syrian hamster model; it binds to *B. burgdorferi* immediately but remains sensitive to β-lactamase for only 4 to 7 days.[43]

With the exception of erythromycin, the in vivo findings in the Syrian hamster models paralleled the in vitro studies. Three antibiotics with similar MBCs in vitro—cefuroxime, doxycycline, and amoxicillin—demonstrated comparable activities in preventing borreliosis in the hamster model. The in vivo activity of cefotaxime improved when the treatment schedule was modified from once a day to three times a day for 5 days. Penicillin G, when given at a high dosage of 150 mg/kg, showed a similar improvement when given more frequently.[42]

The in vivo and in vitro susceptibilities of *B. burgdorferi* to azithromycin, clarithromycin, and vancomycin have also been investigated. In one study, *B. burgdorferi* was more susceptible to azithromycin (MBC 0.04 mg/L) than erythromycin (MBC 0.16 mg/L) and tetracycline (MBC 1.6 mg/L). Azithromycin was more effective than tetracycline and erythromycin in vivo in eliminating infection from the hamster model.[44] Tissue concentrations exceeding the MBC were present for 24 hours after the last dosage. Clarithromycin was effective in vivo against *B. burgdorferi*–induced arthritis in the hamster, being more than 1 log stronger than tetracycline.[45] *B. burgdorferi* has in vivo and in vitro susceptibility to vancomycin. Vancomycin, a glycopeptide antibiotic not previously known to be active against spirochetes, demonstrates synergy with penicillin at one fourth the minimum inhibitory concentration (MIC) of each drug.[46] *B. burgdorferi* was shown to be susceptible in vitro to roxithromycin, a new semisynthetic macrolide, but treatment with the drug failed in five of nine animals in a gerbil model. Roxithromycin, therefore, is not recommended for treatment of Lyme disease.[47]

Early Lyme Disease

Acute, localized disease consisting of erythema migrans, with or without flulike symptoms, can be treated with oral antibiotics, although untreated erythema migrans will resolve on its own (median duration of eruption, 28 days). Steere et al.[48] reported that penicillin or tetracycline was associated with a more rapid resolution of erythema migrans than no therapy. And, in another study, tetracycline was com-

pared with phenoxymethylpenicillin and erythromycin at doses of 250 mg four times daily for 10 days and was found to be more effective in preventing major late manifestations, such as meningoencephalitis, myocarditis, or recurrent attacks of arthritis.[49] However, with all three antibiotic agents, half of the patients experienced symptoms of headache, musculoskeletal pain, fatigue, and lethargy at 1 year of follow-up.

Treatment failures with penicillin and tetracycline have been reported[50] and have led to longer durations of therapy and to the use of other tetracyclines and β-lactam drugs. In a trial comparing amoxicillin/probenecid, 500 mg three times daily, with doxycycline, 100 mg twice a day, for 21 days, there was a 100% response rate and protection against major sequelae; 15% of the patients, however, had fatigue and arthralgias for 3 months after taking the antibiotics.[51] In a study of 198 patients with erythema migrans,[52] 2 g/d of oral penicillin V or tetracycline for 10 days produced a response. In another study of higher doses of oral penicillin V (1 million units three times a day) for 12 days compared with ceftriaxone 1 g intramuscularly per day for only 5 days, ceftriaxone was superior in preventing minor symptoms in 19 patients who had two or more symptoms before therapy.[53]

Doxycycline, 100 mg twice daily, has replaced tetracycline as a recommended agent for early localized Lyme disease because of its better gastrointestinal absorption, longer half-life, and superior CNS penetration. Amoxicillin is recommended over penicillin because of its better in vitro activity against *B. burgdorferi*. The recommended duration of therapy is 10 to 21 days.

Penicillin allergy, which can occur in 1% to 10% of the general population, can have significant morbidity.[54] Tetracyclines are contraindicated in pregnancy and during lactation and are associated with photosensitivity reactions during the summer months, a time when early[55] Lyme disease is commonly detected. Erythromycin is the usual alternative agent prescribed, although it is less effective in treating erythema migrans and in preventing late manifestations. The need for alternative therapies for early Lyme disease has led to clinical studies of newer and related antibiotics.

Azithromycin, an analog of erythromycin, is an azalide antibiotic with greater in vivo activity against *B. burgdorferi* in the hamster model.[43] In addition azithromycin has a longer half-life, better tissue penetration, and less gastrointestinal intolerance.[55] In a recent pilot study, azithromycin for 5 days (500 mg on the first day followed by 250 mg once a day thereafter) was compared with amoxicillin/probenecid, 500 mg three times a day for 10 days, and doxycycline, 100 mg twice a day for 10 days. Three of 16 patients who were receiving azithromycin developed mild diarrhea, but no patient required that the drug be discontinued. Of six patients receiving amoxicillin/probenecid who developed a drug eruption, four required discontinuation of the drug. The three antibiotic regimens appeared equally effective in treating early Lyme disease at the end of 6 months. However, the study size was too small for definite conclusions.[56]

Cefuroxime, a second-generation cephalosporin, has good in vitro and in vivo activity against *B. burgdorferi* in a Syrian hamster model.[43] In a prospective, blinded multicenter clinical trial comparing cefuroxime axetil (an oral form of cefuroxime), 500 mg twice a day, with doxycycline, 100 mg three times a day, for 20 days, the two regimens appeared equally effective in treating Lyme disease and preventing late Lyme disease at 1 year of follow-up. Doxycycline was associated with more photosensitive reactions (15% versus 0%) and cefuroxime with more diarrhea (21% versus 7%).[57]

Our current recommendation for the treatment of early Lyme disease is oral doxycycline (100 mg twice daily) or amoxicillin (500 mg three times daily). The optimal duration of therapy is unknown, and the treatment duration is based on clinical response. We recommend 3 weeks of therapy.

Meningitis or Meningoencephalitis

The most common acute neurologic manifestation of disseminated Lyme disease is meningitis.[26] The meningitis is self-limited, but antibiotic treatment shortens its duration.[49] There is both clinical and experimental evidence of early invasion of the central nervous system by *B. burgdorferi*. Headache and meningismus are found in 64% of patients with symptoms of early Lyme disease.[26] Garcia-Monco et al.,[58] in a study of Lyme disease in Lewis rats, demonstrated changes in blood-brain barrier permeability within 12 hours of inoculation. Concomitant with these changes, white blood cells and spirochetes were found in the CSF within 24 hours of inoculation. Using frozen CSF serum samples from patients with erythema migrans and early neurologic symptoms (but no antibody of *B. burgdorferi* in the serum or CSF), the investigators found spirochetal antigens by immunoblot in three of five samples.[58] The study suggests that *B. burgdorferi* may be found in the CNS early in the course of acute, disseminated disease.

Persons with suspected neurologic Lyme disease should have a spinal tap to confirm meningeal inflammation with lymphocytic pleocytosis and an elevated CSF protein. Selective concentration of CSF antibody should by confirmed by sending off simultaneous serum and CSF samples. Most patients with meningitis have evidence of locally synthesized IgG, IgM, and/or IgA antibody to *B. burgdorferi* in the CSF, but among American patients with late neurologic abnormalities selective concentration of specific antibody is less common and typically consists of only the IgG or IgA isotype.[35]

A third-generation cephalosporin is the agent of choice for the treatment of meningitis or meningoencephalitis. Cephalosporins have an overall safe and efficacious profile for a variety of infections.[59] They may be used as therapy for patients with penicillin allergy, although they share certain structural similarities with penicillin and up to 15% of the patients may have both penicillin and cephalosporin allergy. Ceftriaxone and cefotaxime can be given once or twice daily; they have an excellent in vitro activity against *B. burgdorferi* and good CSF penetration. Ceftriaxone[60] and cefotaxime[61,62] appear superior to benzylpenicillin for neurologic Lyme disease. In one small randomized study, 2 g of parenteral ceftriaxone for 14 days had a better response rate than 20 million units of penicillin for 10 days in the treatment of late neurologic findings.[60] The duration of effective therapy ranges from 2 to 4 weeks.

A single case report noted the efficacy of chloramphenicol, 1 g intravenously every 6 hours for 10 days, in the treatment of neurologic Lyme disease,[63] and one report notes success with tetracycline for Lyme meningitis.[64] Doxycycline has been used in nine patients with neurologic Lyme disease, 100 mg twice daily or intravenously for 14 days.

Lyme disease can produce a subtle encephalopathy with deficits in verbal memory and concentration.[65] A positive serum serologic finding and intrathecal production of IgG can assist in diagnosing the disease. Both parenteral ceftriaxone and penicillin have been reported to be effective therapy, although the optimum dosage and duration of therapy have not been established.

Our current recommendation for the treatment of neurologic manifestations of Lyme disease is a 14- to 30-day course of 2 g of parenteral ceftriaxone. Early meningitis can usually be treated with 14 days of therapy, while encephalitis and later neurologic manifestations may require a 30-day course. Effective alternate parenteral therapies are cefotaxime or penicillin. In the case of a penicillin allergy, doxycycline, 200 mg twice daily for 30 days, or vancomycin, 1 g intravenously for 14 to 30 days, can be used. In the case of a treatment failure, re-treatment may be necessary.

Bell's Palsy

Facial nerve paralysis is the most common cranial nerve abnormality in Lyme disease; it is found in up to 5% of untreated cases.[26] With or without antibiotics, it will usually resolve within 2 months, so the primary reason for treating Bell's palsy is to shorten its course and prevent late manifestations. We recommend that an isolated seventh nerve palsy without concurrent CSF inflammatory changes be treated with oral amoxicillin (500 mg three times daily) or doxycycline (100 mg twice daily) for 21 to 30 days. With concurrent meningitis or radiculoneuritis, parenteral therapy with ceftriaxone (2 g daily) is recommended.

Peripheral Neuropathy

Peripheral neuropathy in Lyme disease occurs in acute and chronic forms. In the acute form, an early, severe but spontaneously resolving axonal radiculoneuropathy is often associated with meningitis or cranial neuritis. The chronic form appears later in the course of disease, sometimes along with acrodermatitis, and is clinically and electrophysiologically milder.[66] This form resolves slowly with antibiotic therapy. Lyme radiculoneuritis or polyneuropathy presents with numbness, paresthesias, or burning pain in an extremity, often followed by sensory loss, hyporeflexia, or weakness.[65] Nerve-conduction studies reveal mild to moderate reduction in motor and sensory conduction velocities. To date, no intraneural *B. burgdorferi* have been demonstrated in biopsy specimens.

Lyme neuropathy is antibiotic responsive, with improvement demonstrable both clinically and electrophysiologically. In a series of 25 patients with chronic peripheral neuropathy from Lyme disease, neuropathic symptoms began a median of 8 months after erythema migrans. Roughly one half of the patients had symmetric nonpainful paresthesias, and the others had asymmetric radicular pain. Both groups had denervation of paraspinal and limb muscles, but 6 months after treatment with intravenous ceftriaxone 76% were improved. In general, the clinical response is not as dramatic as in meningitis, reflecting slow recovery from axonal injury.[66] The intravenous antibiotic regimens used for the treatment of meningitis are recommended for the treatment of Lyme peripheral neuropathy.

Our current recommendation for the treatment of Lyme neuropathy is parenteral ceftriaxone, 2 g daily for 14 to 30 days. Parenteral penicillin G, 20 million units in divided doses, is an effective alternative. Oral doxycycline, 100 mg twice daily for 30 days, can be used as an alternative, although experience with this drug is limited.

Lyme Carditis

Lyme carditis, present in approximately 8% of untreated persons with Lyme disease,[67] typically consists of varying degrees of atrioventricular block, but myopericarditis, mild congestive heart failure, and tachyarrythmias have been reported. Common presenting symptoms consist of fatigue or light-headedness, palpitations, syncope, or exertional dyspnea. Spirochete-like structures have been demonstrated in cardiac tissue,[68–70] and *B. burgdorferi* was cultured from the myocardium in a patient with dilated cardiomyopathy. One fatality from cardiac complications associated with Lyme disease occurred in a patient with concurrent babesiosis who had pancarditis and spirochetes in myocardial tissue.[69]

Although Lyme carditis has been treated successfully with oral antibiotics,[71] intravenous antibiotics are currently recommended in all cases of Lyme carditis, save the most benign form (PR interval of less than 0.30 second). Antimicrobial therapy has been reported successful in improving the ejection fraction of patients with dilated cardiomyopathy from Lyme disease.[72,73] There is a relationship between duration of infection and improvement in left ventricular function, with improvement unlikely after more than 6 months of symptoms. Both intravenous benzylpenicillin[71] and ceftriaxone[74] for 2 weeks resolve carditis. Although the optimum duration of therapy has not been established, 2 to 3 weeks of intravenous penicillin or ceftriaxone appears sufficient. Lyme carditis frequently requires hospitalization with cardiac monitoring and placement of a temporary pacemaker for bradyarrhythmias. Although Lyme carditis is usually self-limited, there are case reports of complete heart block[68,75] and persistent first-degree block following infection.

We currently recommend 2 g intravenous ceftriaxone for 14 days for the treatment of Lyme carditis. Oral antibiotic therapies with doxycycline, 100 mg twice daily, or amoxicillin, 500 mg three times daily, can be given for 10 to 21 days if the PR interval is less than 0.30 second.

Arthritis

Sixty percent of untreated Lyme disease patients will develop arthritis. Common manifestations include migratory musculoskeletal pain in the early stages of disease, sometimes followed by intermittent oligoarticular asymmetric arthritis, particularly of the knee. Without treatment, persons with Lyme arthritis improve at a rate of 10% per year.[76] Eleven percent of persons in one study who had untreated arthritis developed chronic synovitis.[76] Erosive synovitis, cartilage loss, cysts, and enthesopathy have been reported.[77] A subgroup of persons with chronic arthritis were found to have DR2 and DR4 phenotypes more frequently than other phenotypes.[77a] The presence of DR4 was associated with a lack of response to antibiotic therapy, suggesting that *B. burgdorferi* may trigger an autoimmune response independent of the organism's viability. Patients with DR4 specificity developed strong immunoglobulin G responses to both OspA and OspB near the beginning of prolonged episodes of arthritis, from 5 months to 7 years after disease onset in one report.[37]

During acute arthritis, laboratory abnormalities include a mild peripheral leukocytosis and an elevated ESR. Synovial fluid characteristics include a leukocytosis ranging from 500 cells/mm³ to 110,000 cells/mm³, mostly polymorphonuclear leukocytes, an elevated protein level, but a normal glucose value.[67,76] In one study, 10 days of intravenous benzylpenicillin treatment cured 55% of cases with Lyme arthritis, whereas intramuscular benzathine penicillin each week for 3 weeks cured only 35% of the cases.[78] In a randomized study, intravenous ceftriaxone was compared with intravenous penicillin for the treatment of persistent and remitting arthritis. At 3 months of follow-up, two of seven penicillin-treated patients improved, compared with 17 of 18 ceftriaxone-treated patients.[60] Oral treatment with amoxicillin/probenecid or doxycycline successfully treats most cases of Lyme arthritis, although these regimens may not have adequate central nervous system penetration to treat concomitant neuroborreliosis.[79]

It may take up to 3 months for a response to antibiotics to appear. Intraarticular corticosteroid injections should be avoided, since this may prolong synovitis. Refractory chronic Lyme arthritis with early joint damage may be treated with hydroxychloroquine or synovectomy.[78]

Our current recommendation for the treatment of Lyme arthritis is 2 g of parenteral ceftriaxone for 2 to 4 weeks, although oral doxycycline, 100 mg twice daily, or amoxicillin and probenecid, 500 mg four times daily, for 30 days can be used. Treatment failure occurs with any regimen, and re-treatment may be necessary.

Tick Bite Prophylaxis

Treating patients for Lyme disease after an *I. dammini* tick bite remains a controversial subject despite recent studies on the risks and benefits of empirical therapy.[25,80,81] *Ixodes* ticks must feed for a minimum of 24 hours to transmit *B. burgdorferi*, at which time their risk of transmission is only 5%. After a tick has fed for 2 days the risk of transmission increases to 50%, and almost all infected ticks will have transmitted the spirochete to their host after more than 4 days of attachment.[82] Nymphal *Ixodes* ticks measure roughly 1.5 mm and transmit pathogens to human hosts more frequently than larvae or adult forms.[82,83] Larvae are rarely infected and adults, which are 5 mm in length, are generally large enough to be removed before *B. burgdorferi* can be transmitted. Since adults feed mostly in the winter and nymphs mostly in the spring, nymphal bites are most likely to result in Lyme disease.

Some investigators have proposed the use of the scutal index (measuring the chest/scutum: abdomen ratio) to approximate the amount of engorgement, and therefore feeding time, which can estimate the risk of *B. burgdorferi* transmission.[84] To the untrained eye, however, this is a difficult and unreliable measure. Still others[82] have proposed that replete nymphal *Ixodes* ticks can be detected when the branches of the tick's gut cannot be readily distinguished by means of a hand lens.

Whether to provide prophylaxis against Lyme disease after a tick bite was systematically studied in a recent cost-effectiveness analysis by Magid et al.[80] The model incorporated the outcomes' cost and cost-effectiveness of three alternatives to treat patients bitten by *Ixodes* ticks in areas of endemic Lyme disease: empirically treating all patients with 2 weeks of doxycycline, treating only patients in whom erythema migrans develops, or treating only patients with erythema migrans or a positive serologic test for Lyme disease 1 month after exposure. Empirical treatment of patients with tick bites was indicated when the probability of *B. burgdorferi* infection after a tick bite was 0.036 or higher. The authors stated that treatment may be preferred when the probability of infection ranges from 0.01 to 0.035 but is not recommended for a probability of infection lower than 0.01. Two studies reported that *B. burgdorferi* transfer occurs in approximately 10% of persons bitten by infected ticks.[26,85] The authors suggested that empiric therapy, therefore, is not warranted in areas where the prevalence of tick infection is less than 10%, since the product prevalence would be equal to 0.001.

This decision model was confirmed by a recent controlled trial of antimicrobial prophylaxis for Lyme disease after deer tick bites in an endemic area of Connecticut.[81] The study compared a treatment arm of amoxicillin, 250 mg four times a day for 10 days, with a placebo arm for the development of symptoms of Lyme disease. The area's proportion of infected nymphal ticks was 12%, which resulted in a 1.2% infection rate. Although there were two cases of erythema migrans in the placebo arm, there were no cases of late Lyme disease. The

---

TABLE 21–2
Guidelines for Tick Prevention

When living in or traveling to a known endemic area:
1. Wear long-sleeved shirts.
2. Tuck long pants into socks or boots.
3. Wear light-colored clothing so that ticks can be easily spotted.
4. Stay on hiking paths; avoid brush.
5. Search exposed skin every 4 hours when outside.
6. Once inside, check your skin, particularly skin folds.

---

authors concluded that routine prophylactic therapy for tick bites in such an endemic area of Lyme disease was not indicated, since the risk of Lyme disease among persons with a recognized deer tick bite was low. The 1.2% infection rate falls at the lower end of the discretionary range of treatment according to the cost-effectiveness model of Magid et al.[80] and confirms their findings.

The decision to treat a tick bite should be made on an individualized basis, as the anxiety associated with watching and waiting for symptoms often drives the physician and patient toward prophylactic therapy. This is especially true in the pregnant patient, in whom risking possible dissemination of the spirochete to the fetus can be an unacceptable alternative. Empiric treatment can also be justified in a patient in whom disseminated disease would be of dire consequence. Currently, the most effective means of preventing Lyme disease is to practice tick bite control measures, such as wearing protective clothing, avoiding tick-infested areas, and checking for ticks after potential exposure if living in or traveling to endemic areas (Table 21–2).

No data exist on the optimal dose or duration of prophylactic therapy. If empirical therapy is chosen, we recommend oral doxycycline, 100 mg twice daily, or amoxicillin, 250 mg three times daily, for 10 days.

TREATING THE PREGNANT PATIENT

Transplacental transmission of *B. burgdorferi* has been documented with Dieterle's silver stain in three infants, both from mothers with untreated or inadequately treated Lyme disease contracted in the first trimester. Two died shortly after birth, one of a congenital cardiac malformation[86] and the other of encephalitis[87]; the third infant was stillborn.[88] In a retrospective review of 19 women with Lyme disease contracted in all three trimesters, five adverse outcomes were reported, including syndactyly, cortical blindness, intrauterine fetal death, prematurity, and hyperbilirubinemia and rash.[89] Thirteen of these patients had received appropriate antibiotic therapy. In one review of pregnant women with Lyme disease, no deaths or abnormalities were reported, although two deliveries were premature.[90] In another study, 10 pregnancies complicated by localized Lyme disease that was treated had no adverse outcomes, and in six samples no IgM antibody existed to suggest intrauterine infection.[91]

We recommend the treatment of all manifestations other than early, localized Lyme disease with parenteral therapy—either ceftriaxone, 2 g daily, or penicillin G, 20 million units daily in divided doses, for 14 to 30 days. Doxycycline is contraindicated in pregnancy because of its potential toxic effects on the fetus; therefore erythema migrans should be treated with 21 days of oral amoxicillin (500 mg three times daily).

THE POST-LYME SYNDROME

A 2- to 4-week course of intravenous therapy for disseminated Lyme disease is usually curative, although in some cases resolution of symptoms may be delayed for 6 to 8 months. Whether a "post-Lyme syndrome" exists is controversial. Dinerman and Steere[92] have described fibromyalgia following Lyme disease in 8% of their cohort (15 patients), which was not responsive to antibiotics. Fatigue, arthralgias, and memory complaints can persist after treatment; in one series, up to 30% of the patients reported persistent complaints, such as myalgias, arthralgias, persistent fatigue, and attention and concentration difficulties, despite a lack of objective abnormalities to suggest active infection.[93] In some cases, residual morbidity from disseminated infection is present; in others, fibromyalgia or the chronic fatigue syndrome has occurred.

No data exist to support the hypothesis that patients with Lyme disease benefit from prolonged antibiotic treatment. Indeed, long-term intravenous antibiotic therapy can be associated with significant morbidity. In one series, 25 patients who had received intravenous ceftriaxone for close to 6 months developed biliary disease; 14 of them required cholecystectomy.[94] Twenty-two patients developed a total of 29 bloodstream infections. In an extreme case, one patient with suspected seronegative Lyme disease was treated with 3 weeks of intravenous ceftriaxone and developed granulocytopenia, fever, hepatitis, and *Clostridium difficile* diarrhea.[95]

Diagnostic serologic testing for Lyme disease remains imperfect and unstandardized, and false-positive findings occur.[33] Several investigators have reported a high rate of misdiagnosis among patients with Lyme seropositivity and complaints of fatigue, arthralgias, and memory difficulties who were evaluated at a Lyme disease referral center.[96–98] Every effort should be made to document objective abnormalities before embarking on a course of treatment for presumed Lyme disease (Fig. 21–1). A recent cost-effectiveness analysis examined the consequences of treating patients with parenteral antibiotic therapy who had chronic fatigue, myalgia, and a positive serologic test for Lyme disease but lacked classic manifestations.[99] According to the model, it would cost $86,221 for each true positive case treated and 29 cases of drug toxicity would occur. Only when patients would be willing to pay $3485 to eliminate anxiety about not treating possible true Lyme disease would the model's strategy break even. For most patients with a positive Lyme titer and only nonspecific symptoms, the risks and costs of empirical parenteral antibiotic therapy exceed the benefits.

FUTURE DIRECTIONS

Work on a *B. burgdorferi* vaccine is promising. The outer surface proteins (Osp), lipoproteins that are B cell and T cell immunogens in human infection, are protective against Lyme disease in rabbits, mice, and hamsters.[100,101] Immunization with recombinant flagellar protein, however, provides no protection against *B. burgdorferi*. Mice immunized with recombinant OspA were protected against *B. burgdorferi* by means of syringe and tick inoculation.[102] Phase I trials of recombinant OspA lipoprotein in humans have begun.

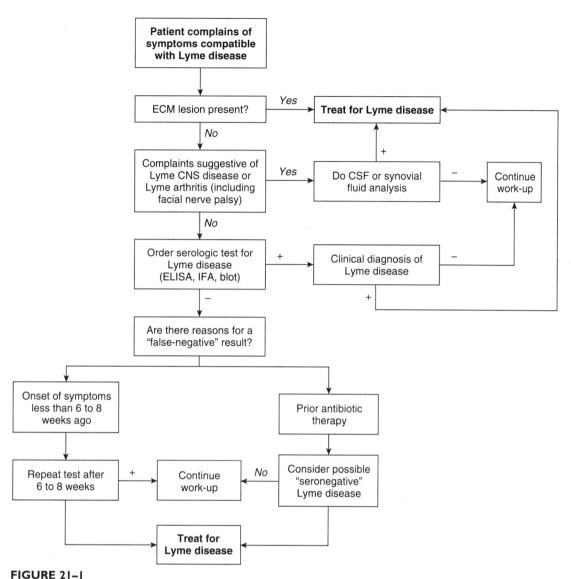

FIGURE 21–1

Diagnostic work-up for Lyme disease. (Reproduced from Sigal LH. Current recommendations for the treatment of Lyme disease. Drugs 1992;43[5]:683–99.)

Lyme disease remains a public health problem. Persons at risk need to be educated about prevention and signs and symptoms of Lyme disease. Early recognition and treatment of erythema migrans and neurologic symptoms can prevent later morbidity.

REFERENCES

1. Burgdorfer W, Barbour AG, Hayes SF, et al. Lyme disease—a tick borne spirochetosis. Science 1982;216:1317.
2. Steere AC, Broderick TF, Malawista SE. Erythema chronicum migrans and Lyme arthritis: the enlarging clinical spectrum. Ann Intern Med 1977;86:685.
3. Steere AC. Lyme disease. N Engl J Med 1989; 321:586.
4. Dennis DT, Ettestad PJ, Campbell GL, et al. National surveillance of Lyme disease in the United States. Presented at the VI International Conference on Lyme Borreliosis. Bologna, Italy, June 1994.
5. Tsai TF, Bailey RE, Moore PM. National surveillance of Lyme disease. 1987–1988. Conn Med 1992;53:324.
6. Ciesielski CA, Markowitz LE, Horsley R, et al. The geographic distribution of Lyme disease in the United States. Ann NY Acad Sci 1988;539: 283.

7. Anderson JF. Epizootiology of *Borrelia* in *Ixodes* tick vectors and reservoir hosts. Rev Infect Dis 1989;2:S1451.

8. Stanek G, Pletschette M, Flamm H, et al. European Lyme borreliosis. Ann NY Acad Sci 1988;539:274.

9. Dekonenko EJ, Steere AC, Berardi VP, et al. Lyme borreliosis in the Soviet Union: a cooperative US-USSR report. J Infect Dis 1988;1258:748.

10. Hellerstrom S. Erythema chronicum migrans afzelius with meningitis. Acta Derm Venereol 1951;31:227.

11. Afzelius A. Erythema chronicum migrans. Acta Derm Venereol 1921;2:120.

12. Steere AC, Malawista SE, Snydman DR, et al. Lyme arthritis: an epidemic of oligoarticular arthritis in children and adults in three Connecticut communities. Arthritis Rheum 1977;20:7.

13. Steere AC, Taylor E, Wilson ML, et al. Longitudinal assessment of the clinical and epidemiologic feature of Lyme disease in a defined population. J Infect Dis 1986;154:295.

14. Persing DH, Telford SR, Rys PN, et al. Detection of *Borrelia burgdorferi* DNA in museum specimens of *Ixodes dammini* ticks. Science 1990;249:1420.

15. Levine JF, Wilson ML, Spielman A. Mice as reservoirs of the Lyme disease spirochete. Am J Trop Med Hyg 1985;34:355.

16. Spielman A, Wilson ML, Levine JF, et al. Ecology of *Ixodes dammini*–borne babesiosis and Lyme disease. Ann Rev Entomol 1985;30:439.

17. Burgdorfer W. Vector/host relationships of the Lyme disease spirochete, *Borrelia burgdorferi*. Rheum Dis Clin North Am 1989;15:775.

18. Burgdorfer W, Hayes SF, Benach JL. Development of *Borrelia burgdorferi* in *Ixodid* tick vectors. Ann NY Acad Sci 1988;539:172.

19. Brown RN, Lane RS. Lyme disease in California: a Novel enzootic transmission cycle of *Borrelia burgdorferi*. Science 1992;256:1439.

20. Barbour AG, Hayes SF. Biology of *Borrelia* species. Microbiol Rev 1986;50:381.

21. Howe TR, Mayer LW, Barbour AG. A single recombinant plasmid expressing two major outer surface proteins of the Lyme disease spirochete. Science 1985;227:645.

22. Barbour AG, Heiland RA, Howe TR. Heterogeneity of major proteins in Lyme disease borreliae: a molecular analysis of North American European isolate. J Infect Dis 1985;152:478.

23. Barbour AG. Isolation and cultivation of Lyme disease spirochetes. Yale J Biol Med 1984;57:521.

24. Georgilis K, Steere AC, Klempner MS. Infectivity of *Borrelia burgdorferi* correlates with resistance to elimination by phagocytic cells. J Infect Dis 1991;163:150.

25. Costello CM, Steere AC, Pinkerton RE, Feder HM. A prospective study of tick bites in an endemic area for Lyme disease. J Infect Dis 1987;155:1322.

26. Steere AC, Bartenhagen NH, Craft JE, et al. The early clinical manifestations of Lyme disease. Ann Intern Med 1983;99:76.

27. Malane MS, Grant-Kels JM, Feder HM, Luger S. Diagnosis of Lyme disease based on dermatologic manifestations. Ann Intern Med 1991;114(6):490.

28. Epidemiology Section, State of Connecticut Department of Health Services. Lyme disease in Connecticut. Conn Epidemiol 1990;10:9.

29. Dattwyler RJ, Volkman DJ, Luft BJ, et al. Seronegative Lyme disease: dissociation of the specific T and B lymphocyte responses to *Borrelia burgdorferi*. N Engl J Med 1988;319:1441.

30. Craft JE, Grodzicki RL, Steere AC. The antibody response in Lyme disease: evaluation of diagnostic tests. J Infect Dis 1984;149:789.

31. Craft JE, Fischer DK, Shimamoto GT, et al. Antigens of *Borrelia burgdorferi* recognized during Lyme disease: appearance of a new IgM response and expansion of the IgG response late in the illness. J Clin Invest 1988;78:934.

32. Magnarelli LA, Miller JN, Anderson JF, Rivere GR. Cross-reactivity of nonspecific treponemal antibody in serologic tests for Lyme disease. J Clin Microbiol 1990;28:1276.

33. Schwartz BS, Goldstein MD, Ribeiro JMC, Schulze TL, Shaheid SI. Antibody testing in Lyme disease: a comparison of results in four laboratories. JAMA 1989;262:3431.

34. Berardi VP, Weeks KE, Steere AC. Serodiagnosis of early Lyme disease: analysis of IgM and IgG antibody responses by using an antibody-capture enzyme immunoassay. J Infect Dis 1988;158:754.

35. Steere AC, Berardi, Weeks KA, et al. Evaluation of the intrathecal antibody response to *Borrelia burgdorferi* as a diagnostic test for Lyme neuroborreliosis. J Infect Dis 1990;161:1203.

36. Hansen K, Bangsborg JM, FJordvang H, et al. Immunochemical characterization of an isolation of the gene for a *Borrelia burgdorferi* immunodominant 60 kD antigen common to a wide range of bacteria. Infect Immun 1988;56:2047.

37. Kalish RA, Leong JM, Steere AC. Association of treatment-resistant chronic Lyme arthritis with HLA DR4 and antibody reactivity to OspA and OspB of *Borrelia burgdorferi*. Infect Immun 1993;61(7):2774.

38. Dressler F, Whalen JA, Reinhardt, Steere AC. Western blotting in the serodiagnosis of Lyme disease. J Infect Dis 1993;167:392.

39. Hyde RW, Johnson RC, White TJ, Shelburne CE. Detection of antigens in urine of mice and humans infected with *Borrelia burgdorferi*, etiologic agent of Lyme disease. J Clin Microbiol 1989;27:58.

40. Persing DH, Telford SR, Spielman A, Barthold SW. Detection of *Borrelia burgdorferi* infection in *Ixodes dammini* ticks with the polymerase chain reaction. J Clin Microbiol 1990;28:566.

41. Nocton JJ, Dressler F, Rutledge BJ, et al. Detection of *Borrelia burgdorferi* by polymerase chain reaction in synovial fluid from patients with Lyme arthritis. N Engl J Med 1994;330:229.
42. Johnson RC, Kodner C, Coleman L. In vitro and in vivo susceptibility of *Borrelia burgdorferi*. V International Conference on Lyme Borreliosis 1992:A3.
43. Johnson RC, Kodner CB, Jurkovich PJ, Collins JJ. Comparative in vitro and in vivo susceptibilities of the Lyme disease spirochete *Borrelia burgdorferi* to cefuroxime and other antimicrobial agents. Antimicrob Agents Chemother 1990;34(11):2133.
44. Johnson RC, Kodner C, Russell M, Girard D. In vitro and in vivo susceptibility of *Borrelia burgdorferi* to azithromycin. J Antimicrob Chemother 1990:SA33.
45. Alder J, Mitten M, Jarvis K, et al. Efficacy of clarithromycin for treatment of experimental Lyme disease in vivo. Antimicrob Agents Chemother 1993;37(6):1329.
46. Dever LL, Jorgensen JH, Barbour AG. In vitro activity of vancomycin against the spirochete *Borrelia burgdorferi*. Antimicrob Agents Chemother 1993;37(5):1115.
47. Hansen K, Hovmark A, Lebech AM, et al. Roxithromycin in Lyme borreliosis: discrepant results of an in vitro and in vivo animal susceptibility study and a clinical trial in patients with erythema migrans. Acta Derm Venereol 1992;72(4):297.
48. Steere AC, Malawista SE, Newman JH, et al. Antibiotic therapy in Lyme disease. Ann Intern Med 1980;193:1.
49. Steere AC, Hutchinson GJ, Rahn DW, et al. Treatment of the early manifestation of Lyme disease. Ann Intern Med 1983;99:22.
50. Dattwyler RJ, Halperin JJ. Failure of tetracycline therapy in early Lyme disease. Arthritis Rheum 1987;30:442.
51. Dattwyler DJ, Halperin JJ, Volkman DJ, Luft BJ. Treatment of late Lyme borreliosis—randomized comparison of ceftriaxone and penicillin. Lancet 1988;1:1191.
52. Asbrink E, Hovmark A. Early and late cutaneous manifestations in *Ixodes*-borne borreliosis. Ann NY Acad Sci 1988;539:4.
53. Weber K. Lymphocytic meningoradiculitis of Bannwarth and erythema migrans disease. J Neurol 1984;231:281.
54. Green CR, Rosenblum A. Report of the penicillin study group–American Academy of Allergy. J Allergy Clin Immunol 1971;48:331.
55. Standiford HC. Tetracyclines and chloramphenicol. In: Mandell GL, Douglas RG, Bennett JE, eds. Principals and practice of infectious diseases. 3rd ed. New York: Churchill Livingstone, 1990:284.
56. Massarotti EM, Luger SW, Rahn DW, et al. Treatment of early Lyme disease. Am J Med 1992;92:396.
57. Nadelman RB, Luger SW, Frank E, et al. Comparison of cefuroxime axetil and doxycycline in the treatment of early Lyme disease. Ann Intern Med 1992;117(4):273.
58. Garcia-Monco JC, Villar BF, Alen JC, et al. *Borrelia burgdorferi* in the central nervous system: experimental and clinical evidence for early invasion. J Infect Dis 1990;161:1187.
59. Donowitz GR, Mandell GL. Cephalosporins. In: Mandell GL, Douglas RG, Bennett JE, eds. Principals and practice of infectious diseases. 3rd ed. New York: Churchill Livingstone, 1990:246.
60. Dattwyler RJ, Halperin JJ, Volkman DJ, et al. Treatment of late Lyme borreliosis—randomized comparison of ceftriaxone and penicillin. Lancet 1988;1:1191.
61. Bojar M, Hercogova J, Valesova M, Jirous J. Cefotaxime in the treatment of Lyme borreliosis. Presented at the Fourth European Congress of Clinical Microbiology in Nice, France, 1989.
62. Pfister HW, Preac-Mursic V, Wilske B, et al. Randomized comparison of ceftriaxone and cefotaxime in Lyme neuroborreliosis. J Infect Dis 1991;163:311.
63. Diringer MN, Halper JJ, Dattwyler RJ. Lyme meningoencephalitis: report of a severe, penicillin-resistant case. Arthritis Rheum 1987;30:705.
64. Dotevall L, Alestig K, Hanner P, et al. The use of doxycycline in nervous system *Borrelia burgdorferi* infection. Scand J Infect Dis 1988;S53:74.
65. Logigian EL, Kaplan REF, Steere AC. Chronic neurologic manifestations of Lyme disease. N Engl J Med 1990;323:1438.
66. Logigian EL, Steere AC. Clinical and electrophysiologic findings in chronic neuropathy of Lyme disease. Neurology 1992;42(2):303.
67. Steere AC, Broderick TF, Malawista SE. Erythema chronicum migrans and Lyme arthritis: epidemiologic evidence for a tick vector. Am J Epidemiol 1978;108(4):312.
68. de Koning J, Hoogkaamp-Korstanje JAA, van der Line MR, et al. Demonstration of spirochete in cardiac biopsies of patients with Lyme disease. J Infect Dis 1989;160:150.
69. Stanek F, Klein J, Bittner R, Glogar D. Isolation of *Borrelia burgdorferi* from the myocardium of a patient with longstanding cardiomyopathy. N Engl J Med 1990;322:249.
70. Marcus LC, Steere AC, Duray PH, et al. Fatal pancarditis in a patient with coexistent Lyme disease and babesiosis: demonstration of spirochete in the myocardium. Ann Intern Med 1985;103:374.
71. McAlister HF, Klementowicz PT, Andrews C, et al. Lyme carditis: an important cause of reversible heart block. Ann Intern Med 1989;110:339.
72. Gasser R, Dusleag J, Fruhwald F, et al. Early antimicrobial treatment of dilated cardiomyopathy associated with *Borrelia burgdorferi*. Lancet 1992;340:982.
73. Vegsundvag J, Nordeide J, Reikvam A, Jenum P. Late cardiac manifestation of infection with

Borrelia burgdorferi (Lyme disease). BMJ 1993; 307:173.

74. Blaauw AA, van der Linden SJ, Kuiper J. Lyme carditis in the Netherlands. Ann Intern Med 1989;111:261.

75. Artigao R, Torres G, Guerrero A, et al. Irreversible complete heart block in Lyme disease. Am J Med 1991;90:531.

76. Steere AC, Schoen RT, Taylor E, et al. The clinical evolution of Lyme arthritis. Ann Intern Med 1987;107:725.

77. Lawson JP, Steere AC. Lyme arthritis: radiologic findings. Radiology 1985;154:37.

77a. Steere AC, Dwyer E, Winchester R. Association of chronic arthritis with HLA DR4 and HLA DR2 alleles. N Engl J Med 1990;323: 219.

78. Steere AC, Malawista SE, Craft JE, et al. International symposium on Lyme disease. Yale J Biol Med 1984;57:445.

79. Steere AC, Levin RE, Molloy PJ, et al. Antibiotic treatment of Lyme arthritis. Arthritis Rheum 1993;36(9):S40.

80. Magid D, Schwartz B, Craft J, et al. Prevention of Lyme disease after tick bites—a cost-effectiveness analysis. N Engl J Med 1992;327:534.

81. Shapiro ED, Gerber MA, Holabird NB, et al. A controlled trial of antimicrobial prophylaxis for Lyme disease after deer tick bites. N Engl J Med 1992;327:1769.

82. Matuschka FR, Spielman A. Risk of infection from and treatment of Lyme disease. Lancet 1993;342:529.

83. Matuschka RE, Fischer P, Heiler M, et al. Stage-associated risk of transmission of the Lyme disease spirochete by European *Ixodes* ticks. Parasitol Res 1992;78:695.

84. Falco RC, Fish D, Piesman J. Duration of *Ixodes dammini* attachment to humans. Presented at V International Conference on Lyme Borreliosis 1992.

85. Falco RC, Fish D. A survey of tick bites acquired in a Lyme disease endemic area in southern New York State. Ann NY Acad Sci 1988;539:456.

86. Schlesinger PA, Duray PH, Burke BA, et al. Maternal-fetal transmission of the Lyme disease spirochete *Borrelia burgdorferi*. Ann Intern Med 1985;103:67.

87. Weber K, Bratzke JH, Neubert U, et al. *Borrelia burgdorferi* in a newborn despite oral penicillin for Lyme borreliosis during pregnancy. Pediatr Infect Dis 1988;7:286.

88. MacDonald AB, Benach JL, Burgdorfer W. Stillbirth following maternal Lyme disease. N Y State J Med 1987;87:615.

89. Markowitz LE, Steere AC, Benach JL, et al. Lyme disease during pregnancy. JAMA 1986; 255:3394.

90. Luger SW. Active Lyme borreliosis in pregnancy: outcome of six cases with Stage 1, Stage 2 and Stage 3 disease. IV International Conference on Lyme Borreliosis. Stockholm 1990.

91. Sigal LH. Therapy for Lyme disease. Drugs 1992;43(5):683.

92. Dinerman H, Steere AC. Lyme disease associated with fibromyalgia. Ann Intern Med 1992;117:281.

93. Shadick NA, Phillips CB, Larson MG, et al. Chronic sequelae of Lyme disease. Arthritis Rheum 1991;34(9):S114.

94. Genese C, Finelli L, Parkin W, Spitalny KC. Ceftriaxone-associated biliary complications of treatment of suspected disseminated Lyme disease—New Jersey. 1990–1992. MMWR 1993; 42:39.

95. Nadelman RB, Arlin Z, Wormser GP. Life-threatening complication of empiric ceftriaxone therapy for 'seronegative Lyme disease.' South Med J 1991;84(10):1263.

96. Sigal LH. Summary of the first 100 patients seen at a Lyme disease referral center. Am J Med 1990;117:281.

97. Hsu V, Patella SJ, Sigal LH. Chronic Lyme disease as the incorrect diagnosis in patients with fibromyalgia. Arthritis Rheum 1993;36(11):1493.

98. Steere AC, Taylor E, McHugh GL, Logigian EL. The overdiagnosis of Lyme disease. JAMA 1993;269:1812.

99. Lightfoot RW, Luft BJ, Rahn DW, et al. Empiric parenteral antibiotic treatment of patients with fibromyalgia and fatigue and a positive serologic result for Lyme disease: a cost-effectiveness analysis. Ann Intern Med 1993;119: 503.

100. Milch LJ, Barbour AG. Analysis of North American and European isolates of *Borrelia burgdorferi* with antiserum and to a recombinant antigen. J Infect Dis 1989;160:351.

101. Fikrig E, Barthold SW, Kantor FS, Flavell RA. Protection of mice against the Lyme disease agent by immunizing with recombinant Osp A. Science 1990;250:553.

102. Kelley WN, Harris ED, Ruddy S, Sledge CB, eds. Textbook of rheumatology. 4th ed. Philadelphia: WB Saunders, 1993.

OSTEOPOROSIS AND RHEUMATIC DISORDERS

Meryl S. LeBoff
John P. Wade

Osteoporosis, a decreased quantity of bone with superimposed fractures, is a major public health problem that results in a vertebral fracture in one third of women by the age of 65 and/or a hip fracture in one third of women and one sixth of men by the age of 90. Osteoporosis causes an estimated 1.5 million fractures annually in the United States at a cost of approximately $10 billion. With the aging of society and a rise in age-related and unexplained fractures, it is estimated that the number of fractures and the cost will increase severalfold by the beginning of the twenty-first century.[1] Strategies to prevent bone loss in patients at risk of osteoporosis may have a substantial impact on reducing the anticipated fractures and health care costs.

The skeleton is composed of 20% of the more metabolically active trabecular bone located in the spine, epiphyses, and pelvis and 80% of cortical bone concentrated in the appendicular skeleton. Bone mass is normally maintained by the tight coupling of bone resorption by osteoclasts and bone formation by osteoblasts. Peak bone mass is achieved after puberty to the third decade; thereafter there are decreases in bone mass with age in both sexes. In women, there is a superimposed menopausal acceleration of bone loss. In the course of a lifetime, women lose approximately 50% of the bone in the spine and proximal femur and 30% of the bone in the appendicular skeleton; men lose approximately two thirds of these amounts.[1,2] Bone loss, therefore, is a universal component of aging.

Osteoporosis in rheumatic patients is of particular concern because bone loss may result from the disease process and from the medications used to control inflammation. Decreased bone mass, combined with an increased tendency of persons with musculoskeletal disease to fall, may also increase the risk of fracture. This chapter will focus on the diagnosis and treatment of osteoporosis in general and in patients with systemic rheumatic disorders and on the skeletal effects of corticosteroids and other drugs used to treat rheumatic diseases.

OSTEOPOROTIC RISK FACTORS AND SECONDARY CAUSES OF BONE LOSS AND OSTEOPOROSIS

There are several nutritional, reproductive, and lifestyle factors that may increase the risk of osteoporosis, including inadequate calcium intake, gonadal deficiencies, decreased body mass index and fat, inactivity, excessive alcohol intake, and cigarette smoking. Recent data show strong genetic determinants of bone mass.[3] The identification of a vitamin D receptor allele associated with a decreased bone mass may make it possible to direct treatments to children or adolescents whose genotype may predispose them to an increased risk of osteoporosis.[4,5]

Although osteoporosis is a heterogeneous disorder, it develops as a consequence of a net increase in bone resorption, insufficient bone formation, or both. Hypercortisolism in Cushing's syndrome can often produce osteoporosis, and administration of exogenous corticosteroids is the most common secondary cause of bone loss.[6] Hyperthyroidism increases bone turnover;

TABLE 22–1
Causes of Osteoporosis/Osteopenia

Primary osteoporosis: Juvenile osteoporosis, idiopathic osteoporosis, postmenopausal osteoporosis, involutional osteoporosis

Endocrine abnormalities: Corticosteroid excess, thyrotoxicosis, hypogonadism, primary hyperparathyroidism, prolactinomas, hypercalciuria

Process affecting the marrow: Multiple myeloma, leukemia, lymphoma, anemias—sickle cell disease, thalassemia minor

Immobilization:

Gastrointestinal diseases: Postgastrectomy, primary biliary or alcoholic cirrhosis

Drugs: Anticonvulsants, heparin, methotrexate, corticosteroids, excess thyroid hormone, GnRH agonist, lithium, cyclosporin A

Connective tissue disorders: Osteogenesis imperfecta, scurvy, homocystinuria, Ehlers-Danlos syndrome

Rheumatologic disorders: Ankylosing spondylitis, rheumatoid arthritis

Modified from LeBoff MS, Fuleihan El-Hajj G, Brown E. Osteoporosis and Paget's disease of bone. In: Branch WT, ed. Office practice of medicine. Philadelphia: WB Saunders, 1994:700.

supraphysiologic doses of thyroid hormone may cause bone loss,[7] even though concentrations of thyroid hormone may be within the normal range and the thyroid-stimulating hormone (TSH) level is suppressed. Amenorrhea and hypogonadism from use of GnRH agonists[8] or cytotoxic drugs, anorexia nervosa,[9] or hyperprolactinemia and testosterone deficiency[10] in men may be associated with bone loss. Table 22–1 lists some of the other secondary causes of osteopenia and osteoporosis.[11]

BONE DENSITOMETRY

The advances in bone densitometry and the development of the newer technique of dual x-ray absorptiometry (DXA) make it possible to precisely and rapidly quantify the amount of bone in the relevant fracture sites of the spine, proximal femur, forearm, and total body with minimal radiation exposure (e.g., 3 to 6 mrads each and 0.5 mrad for total body). The bone mineral density (BMD) in a patient is compared with that of (1) young normal controls to assess whether there is a decrease in BMD from peak bone mass (T score) and (2) age-matched controls to determine whether the bone density is reduced relative to age-matched controls (Z score, Fig. 22–1). Recent prospective studies

show that in subjects more than 60 years of age, a 1 SD decrement in BMD compared with age-adjusted controls is associated with a 1.3 to 2.8 increase in relative risk of fracture.[12,13] A reduced bone density of the proximal femur, moreover, is more predictive of increased risk of a hip fracture than is a bone density determination at an alternative site.

The indications for bone densitometry established by the Scientific Advisory Board of the National Osteoporosis Foundation and now incorporated into the Health Care Financing Administration policy include bone density measurements: (1) Measurements are made in estrogen-deficient women with menopause or amenorrhea to determine whether hormone replacement therapy or an alternate therapy is indicated to protect the skeleton. Here a bone density cutoff of 1 SD below young normals (T score) is used to define increased risk of subsequent bone loss. Although the cardioprotective effects of combined estrogen and progesterone therapy[14] may subsequently justify the use of this therapy in women with little risk of osteoporosis, universal hormone replacement therapy is not generally advocated. Bone density measurements are also made (2) in corticosteroid-treated patients to ascertain whether therapy should be modified; (3) in subjects with vertebral abnormalities or radiologic findings of osteopenia; (4) in patients with primary hyperparathyroidism, to diagnose a low bone mass in order to determine those at risk of osteoporosis who might benefit from parathyroidectomy; and (5) in patients with secondary hyperparathyroidism to assess which patients might benefit from therapeutic intervention(s). Bone densitometry is also useful in assessing the therapeutic efficacy of a given treatment for the purpose of appropriate modifications in therapy if necessary. In normal premenopausal women use of bone densitometry for screening purposes is not cost-effective.

OSTEOPOROSIS IN RHEUMATOID ARTHRITIS (RA)

RA is associated with development of periarticular and generalized osteopenia and increased incidence of fractures, which, in turn, may add substantially to the disability already associated with RA. Investigations using bone densitometry in patients with long-standing RA show significant decrements in BMD of the proximal femur,

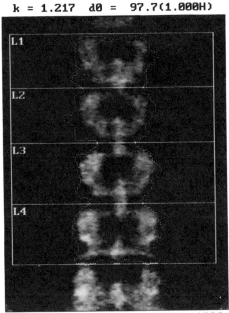

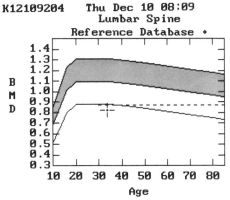

k = 1.217 d0 = 97.7(1.000H)

·Mar 28 11:13 1994 [119 x 138]
Hologic QDR-1000/W (S/N 886)
Lumbar Spine V4.59

K12109204   Thu Dec 10 08:09
Lumbar Spine
Reference Database ◆

BMD(L1-L4) = 0.813 g/cm^2

Region	BMD	T(30.0)		Z	
L1	0.798	-1.91	79%	-1.91	79%
L2	0.828	-2.42	76%	-2.42	76%
L3	0.795	-2.80	72%	-2.80	72%
L4	0.830	-2.87	72%	-2.87	72%
L1-L4	0.813	-2.52	75%	-2.52	75%

◆ Age and sex matched
T = peak bone mass
Z = age matched   TK   11/04/91

FIGURE 22–1

Bone density of the lumbar spine (L1 to L4) in a 33-year-old man treated with corticosteroids, as measured by DXA. Note the marked reduction in bone density that is 2.52 standard deviations below peak bone mass (T score) and 2.52 standard deviations below age-matched controls (Z score).

the lumbar spine, and the appendicular sites ranging from ~5% to 25%.[15–19] Consistent with these findings is evidence of increased trabecular bone loss in iliac crest biopsies in women with RA.[20] Although the reports of circulating levels of sex corticosteroids in women with RA are conflicting, recent data showed reduced levels of the major adrenal androgen precursor to estrogen, dehydroepiandrosterone sulfate (DHEAS), in postmenopausal women with RA compared with control subjects, possibly a consequence of chronic illness and an alteration in the hypothalamic-pituitary-adrenal axis and suppression of the immune system.[21,22] These low adrenal androgen levels are of potential importance because, in addition to being precursors of estrone, androgens are protective to bone. Sambrook et al.,[23] moreover, recently showed a positive correlation between DHEAS levels and longitudinal changes in femoral neck bone density in postmenopausal women with RA.

Other factors postulated to contribute to the decreased BMD and osteoporotic fractures in RA include inactivity, corticosteroid therapy,

and enhanced inflammatory process with elevated mediators of bone resorption.[3,16,18,24,25] Longitudinal studies in ambulatory RA have failed to show accelerated generalized bone loss of the spine early in the course of the disease, although loss in the distal radius was increased, indicating a localized periarticular bone loss.[26] These findings suggest that the more generalized osteopenia of the spine and femur might occur later with a reduction in physical activity and possibly secondary to the use of corticosteroids. Physical activity correlates with bone density measurements[3] and is an important determinant of osteoporosis in RA; recent studies, moreover, show that disease activity, disease duration, and functional disability affect bone loss.[27]

Early studies in patients with RA indicated that the accelerated bone loss was due to corticosteroid administration.[16,28] Corticosteroids are associated with osteoporosis in an estimated 30% to 50% of subjects.[6] Consistent with these deleterious effects of corticosteroids on bone are the observations of Dykman et al.,[28] who showed that large cumulative doses of corticosteroids in patients with rheumatic diseases increased both trabecular bone loss in the forearm and the risk of skeletal fractures. Als et al.[29] observed decreased bone density in corticosteroid-treated premenopausal women with RA, which correlated with the duration of therapy and the cumulative dose. A recent randomized control trial by Laan et al.[30] showed early bone loss in the spine in a group of rheumatoid patients treated for up to 20 weeks with prednisone (mean dose 7.5 mg), which was partially reversible with discontinuation of therapy. Reid et al.,[31] however, showed that although patients with RA who are treated with corticosteroids undergo an early reduction in bone density, patients on long-term corticosteroid therapy have less bone loss than patients treated with calcium supplements or antiinflammatory drugs, including nonsteroidal antiinflammatory drugs (NSAIDs), penicillamine, and gold. A large cross-sectional study of 195 patients with rheumatoid arthritis suggested that bone loss in patients with RA was more evident in the proximal femur than in the spine[32]; cumulative corticosteroid dose and disability were significantly correlated with bone density. Patients who had discontinued corticosteroid therapy, however, had bone densities similar to those of patients who had never used corticosteroids. Other data indicate that postmenopausal women with RA taking long-term low-dose corticosteroids or groups of premenopausal and postmenopausal women taking low doses of prednisone do not have an additional decrease in bone density compared with non-corticosteroid-treated subjects with RA.[16,26,28,29,33] The lack of an adverse effect of low-dose corticosteroids on bone mass in postmenopausal women with RA probably results from suppression of the active inflammatory process and cytokines and/or improved function and increased physical activity. Corticosteroids may, therefore, produce an early loss of bone, but this bone loss may be attenuated over time by better control of the disease process, increased ambulation, and physical activity.

RHEUMATOID ARTHRITIS: POTENTIAL MEDIATORS OF BONE LOSS

The release of inflammatory cytokines or other local factors from the macrophages, fibroblasts, and T cells present in rheumatoid synovium may also contribute to the increased bone loss in RA.[34,35] The following are potential mediators of bone loss in rheumatoid arthritis: (1) interleukin-1, interleukin-6; (2) tumor necrosis factor; (3) heparin; and (4) prostaglandins. There are significant elevations of interleukin (IL)-1, which stimulates osteoclast formation and bone resorption in the blood and synovial fluid in patients with RA.[34,36,37] Elevations of tumor necrosis factor (TNF) alpha in the blood and synovial fluid[18,38] and high concentrations of IL-6 in the synovium,[18,37,39] both of which can increase bone resorption and stimulate osteoclast formation, may also contribute to the development of osteoporosis in patients with RA. In addition, release of mast cell heparin in patients with RA may accelerate bone loss. The mechanisms underlying the effects of heparin on skeletal metabolism have not been fully elucidated, although heparin promotes PTH-mediated bone loss and may increase bone collagen metabolism.[40] Lastly, large amounts of prostaglandins are produced in the rheumatoid synovium, and high concentrations of prostaglandins, in particular prostaglandin E_2 (PGE_2), enhance bone resorption.[41]

BONE METABOLISM IN RHEUMATOID ARTHRITIS

To assess whether the skeletal changes in patients with RA represent more generalized abnormalities in mineral metabolism, investigators have examined indices of skeletal homeostasis. Normally there is an inverse relationship between changes in calcium concentrations and parathyroid hormone (PTH) secretion so that a small decrease in the ionized calcium concentration augments PTH release, with the attendant renal conservation of calcium, mobilization of calcium from bone, and activation of 25-hydroxyvitamin D to 1,25-dihydroxyvitamin D, which in turn stimulates intestinal calcium absorption. The reduced serum calcium levels in patients with RA reported in early studies probably represent decreased calcium-binding proteins from chronic disease and not a reduction in ionized calcium concentrations, although the latter were not measured.[42] Moreover, in patients with RA, levels of PTH and vitamin D metabolites are generally similar to those in controls, thus indicating no abnormality in calcium metabolism.[43] Urinary hydroxyproline and pyridinoline concentrations, markers of bone resorption, are normal or elevated in patients with RA, although the increased hydroxyproline in this setting may reflect activation of components of the complement system or cartilaginous destruction.[44–46] Serum osteocalcin, a noncollagenous, calcium-binding protein produced by osteoblast, is an index of bone formation. Studies show decreased, normal, or increased serum osteocalcin levels in patients with RA, which suggest suppressed, normal, or increased bone turnover, respectively.[43,47]

CORTICOSTEROIDS AND OSTEOPOROSIS

The importance of corticosteroids in treating a variety of rheumatic conditions such as RA, polymyalgia rheumatica, giant cell arthritis, connective tissue disease (systemic lupus erythematosis, mixed connective tissue disease, polymyositis, and overlap syndromes), and vasculitis is well established.[48] The concern over bone loss is one of the limiting factors in making treatment decisions about the dose and duration of corticosteroid administration. Dykman et al.[28] observed, in a group of rheumatic patients, that the risk of bone loss or associated fracture risk is determined by the cumulative corticosteroid dose, age greater than 50, and/or menopausal status. Corticosteroids impair intestinal calcium absorption, increase urinary calcium excretion, and decrease bone formation in association with enhanced bone resorption.[6,49–53] In addition, corticosteroids reduce sex hormone production indirectly by reducing endogenous ACTH levels and adrenal androgen production and directly through gonadal effects.[6,21,54] Use of corticosteroids is associated with increased fractures at the predominantly trabecular sites of the vertebrae and ribs.[55] Although in vitro studies have shown both stimulation and inhibition of bone resorption following corticosteroid exposure,[56,57] parathyroidectomized rats exposed to corticosteroids do not display enhanced bone loss, which suggests that the bone resorption in this setting may be mediated by parathyroid hormone.[58] However, patients treated with corticosteroids have had significantly elevated PTH levels or values indistinguishable from those of normal control subjects.[49,59] Although doses of prednisone ≥15 mg/d impair intestinal calcium absorption,[50] low doses of prednisone (range, 2.5 to 10 mg/d) in patients with RA do not affect levels of para-

thyroid hormone levels[33] as measured by the immunoradiometric assay for intact hormone.[60] Although earlier studies indicated that corticosteroids interfere with the activation of vitamin D to 25-hydroxyvitamin D as well as 1,25-dihydroxyvitamin D, more recent data show that corticosteroids do not interfere with the metabolism of vitamin D but may negatively influence calcium-transport mechanisms in the bowel mucosae. Corticosteroids reduce serum osteocalcin levels in a dose-dependent relationship, thereby indicating suppression of bone formation.[41,53,61] Alternate-day glucocorticoid regimens, while they may not decrease intestinal calcium absorption and stimulate parathyroid hormone release, do not prevent bone loss in adults.[62]

Other drugs used to treat RA may also have an effect on mineral metabolism. NSAIDs, gold, and penicillamine do not appear to prevent osteopenia in RA,[31] although the effects of nonsteroidal drugs on bone loss are conflicting. It is possible that some NSAIDs that inhibit prostaglandin synthesis may play a role in retarding the progressive bone loss in patients with high endogenous prostaglandin production such as occurs in RA. Methotrexate in high doses used to treat childhood leukemia is associated with osteoporotic fractures.[63] In a preliminary cross-sectional study, low doses of methotrexate used for the treatment of RA did not reduce bone mass, although prospective, randomized studies are warranted.[64] Recent data show that the immunosuppressant drug cyclosporin A is effective in the treatment of RA. Cyclosporin A produces a time- and dose-dependent bone loss in rodent models, and therapy with both cyclosporin and prednisone is associated with osteoporosis in transplant recipients,[65–67] raising the possibility that use of this drug in patients with RA may accelerate the development of osteoporosis. Alternative agents, such as azathioprine or cyclophosphamide, do not produce osteoporosis, but these agents are associated with an increased risk of cancer. Corticosteroid-induced osteoporosis, therefore, is likely to continue to be a problem in the future.

BONE LOSS IN SYSTEMIC LUPUS ERYTHEMATOSUS

The importance of bone loss in patients with systemic lupus erythematosus cannot be overemphasized. Patients are often young women taking high doses of prednisone for prolonged periods of time who may have associated renal disease and/or premature ovarian failure as a result of immunosuppressive or alkylating therapy.[68] On the basis of studies in patients with cancer, daily oral cyclophosphamide for 6 to 48 months is associated with the development of amenorrhea in 50% to 70% of women. Regimens that use pulse cyclophosphamide for shorter periods of time may minimize the risk of ovarian toxicity.[69] There is a risk of lupus flares with pregnancy, and some investigators have therefore raised concerns about instituting hormone replacement therapy in postmenopausal women. Further studies of hormone replacement therapy in patients with lupus are needed.

BONE LOSS IN OSTEOARTHRITIS

Osteoarthritis (OA) is the most common musculoskeletal disorder treated by the rheumatologist. The osteophyte formation in OA may factitiously elevate bone density measurements of the spine without affecting the proximal femur sites, making it difficult to assess bone density in the lumbar spine.[70] Hannan et al.[71] demonstrated that proximal femur bone density was higher in women with mild OA of the knee than in subjects with no OA, although patients with advanced OA of the knee had bone density similar to that of control subjects. The association of increased body weight with OA may partly explain this higher bone mass. Patients with OA typically develop age-related bone loss.[16] Degenerative arthritis of the axial skeleton and lower extremities results in decreased levels of function. The common occurrence of these two age-related disorders should be considered in the management of these patients.[70,71]

BONE LOSS IN POLYMYALGIA RHEUMATICA

Osteopenia in patients with polymyalgia rheumatica is not generally found to be a problem, although the bone loss has not been widely studied.[72] Persons with polymyalgia rheumatica are generally physically active soon after initiation of treatment. Although some patients with polymyalgia rheumatica may have associated low-grade peripheral synovitis, they lack

significant joint involvement and are likely to participate in day-to-day weight-bearing activities. The initial dose of prednisone used to treat patients with polymyalgia rheumatica and the duration of therapy are widely variable. Frequently the clinician will try therapy with NSAIDs before the initiation of prednisone therapy, which may facilitate a shorter duration of treatment with prednisone. Occasionally symptoms are controlled without corticosteroids. In some instances, prolonged intermediate doses of prednisone are required and significant bone loss might be expected.

BONE LOSS IN ANKYLOSING SPONDYLITIS

Ankylosing spondylitis is also associated with the development of osteoporosis. Typically, patients with ankylosing spondylitis have low back pain, starting in the teenage years, that consists of persistent pain and morning stiffness. Eventually, the inflammatory symptoms and pain may subside, but patients have residual decreased range in the axial skeleton and are less active. Because this disorder is often associated with peripheral arthritis, particularly of the large joints of the lower extremities including the hips, there may be a further decrease in weight-bearing activity. Eventually, total joint arthroplasty may further limit physical activity and weight-bearing exercises.

Will et al.[73] showed a reduction in bone density in both the spine and the proximal femur in men with mild ankylosing spondylitis compared with age-matched controls; this suggests a primary early loss of bone, even in physically active patients with minimal biochemical or radiologic evidence of ankylosing spondylitis.[73] Evaluation of testicular function in 22 males with ankylosing spondylitis[74] showed increased luteinizing hormone levels and deficient testicular reserve that may contribute to the development of osteoporosis. An atypical osteomalacia diagnosed by histologic criteria has also been documented in four men with ankylosing spondylitis who had no alterations in calcium or PTH levels.[75]

In patients with chronic ankylosing spondylitis, the most significant complication of concern is spinal fracture.[76] The fracture potential increases in the cervical, thoracic, and lumbar regions because of the ankylosed spine. Minor trauma is the most common cause of fracture in these persons. Serious complications include complete and incomplete spinal cord lesions and development of other associated neurologic deficits. Radiographic visualization of the fracture site may be difficult because of the extensive syndesmophyte formation. The use of a radionuclide bone scan, tomography, or a CT scan may help to visualize the fracture radiographically. The importance of osteopenia in the fracture potential is not known. Nevertheless, active intervention with agents that reduce bone loss should be considered in these patients.

EVALUATION OF A PATIENT WITH BONE LOSS OR OSTEOPOROSIS

The physical examination and laboratory evaluation of a patient with reduced bone mass or osteoporosis are directed at excluding secondary causes of bone loss. Laboratory tests include the measurement of serum calcium, phosphorus, and alkaline phosphatase levels and liver tests; a complete blood count; serum and possibly urinary protein electrophoresis; measurement of a sensitive TSH level; 25(OH) vitamin D, urinary calcium, and creatinine levels; and in some instances tests of gonadal function and serum PTH concentrations. Additional specific tests to rule out endocrinologic or neoplastic processes and a possible bone biopsy (after a double tetracycline label) should be considered in patients in whom there is a question of osteomalacia without biochemical changes to support the diagnosis; in patients with severe bone loss; and in those in whom primary osteoporosis is uncommon, such as children, premenopausal women, men less than 60 years of age, and blacks. Reversal of the underlying cause of osteoporosis may yield substantial improvements in bone mass.

STRATEGIES FOR THE PREVENTION AND TREATMENT OF OSTEOPOROSIS

The goals of therapy for osteoporosis include the reduction of risk factors for bone loss, avoidance of prolonged immobilization, conservative management of pain, and an attempt to halt the disease progression by decreasing bone resorption and increasing bone formation. A regular weight-bearing program that includes endurance, resistance exercises, or both[35] may produce a modest increase in bone mass.

Calcium

Data confirming the efficacy of increased intakes of calcium in decreasing bone loss are controversial. Recent data show that the benefit from calcium depends on the years since menopause, customary calcium intake, and age. Prospective studies show that calcium supplementation is ineffective or minimally effective in preventing bone loss in women within 5 years of menopause, when estrogen deficiency has a predominant influence on bone loss.[77] Supplemental calcium is beneficial in late-postmenopausal women with low calcium intakes (<400 mg daily). In prepubertal children calcium intakes of ~1600 mg daily increase bone density at different sites approximately 3% to 5%, which may ultimately confer an increased peak bone mass.[78]

On the basis of calcium balance studies, premenopausal women require 1000 mg and postmenopausal women require 1500 mg of elemental calcium per day to prevent a negative calcium balance.[79] These calcium intakes are generally safe, unless a patient has an underlying disorder of calcium homeostasis. Dairy products are the dietary source that have the greatest amount of calcium. An 8 ounce glass of milk contains ~300 mg of elemental calcium, and several calcium-supplemented orange juices with comparable amounts of calcium are now available. Calcium carbonate, the most widely used calcium salt, contains 40% of elemental calcium. Each tablet of EX Tums, for example, contains 300 mg of elemental calcium, and Oscal 500 and a new Tums each have 500 mg of elemental calcium. Calcium carbonate should be taken with food because patients with achlorhydria are unable to absorb this calcium salt well on an empty stomach.[80] Adverse effects of calcium carbonate may include constipation. Calcium citrate contains 24% elemental calcium; this calcium salt is a more bioavailable calcium preparation than calcium carbonate, and it may be taken fasting.[81]

Estrogen

Estrogen therapy in postmenopausal women prevents bone loss and decreases the risk of fracture by 50%, possibly through direct interaction with estrogen receptors on bone cells[82,83] or a reduction in cytokines that stimulate bone resorption (e.g., IL-1, IL-6).[84–86] In women with no contraindications to its use, hormone replacement therapy is the treatment of choice to prevent or treat osteoporosis.[87] Estrogen is effective many years after menopause when considerable bone loss has occurred, but this therapy should be continued for 7 years or more to reduce the risk of hip fractures in older women.[88,89] On the basis of data from several observational studies, estrogen therapy reduces the risk of cardiovascular disease, the leading cause of death in postmenopausal women, by ~50%. Estrogen therapy decreases total cholesterol and low-density lipoprotein concentrations and raises high-density lipoprotein levels. The cardioprotective effect of estrogens is mediated, in part, by changes in lipoprotein profiles and by several other mechanisms, such as possible antioxidant and direct vascular effects.

Estrogen is administered in a sequential or continuous regimen with a progestin to diminish the risk of endometrial hyperplasia or carcinoma. Oral estrogen/progesterone regimens often used include (1) 0.625 mg conjugated estrogen daily, with 10 mg of medroxyprogesterone added on days 1 to 13 of each month in a sequential regimen, or (2) 0.625 mg conjugated estrogen daily, with 2.5 or 5 mg of medroxyprogesterone in a daily continuous hormone replacement regimen. Unlike the sequential hormone replacement regimen that usually produces regular monthly withdrawal bleeding, daily continuous hormone replacement induces atrophy of the endometrium so that ≥80% of women are amenorrheic at 1 year; in the first 6 months of this latter regimen, however, ≤45% of women may develop irregular bleeding.[90,91] According to the guidelines of the American College of Obstetrics and Gynecology,[92] endometrial biopsies are not routinely necessary unless a woman has had irregular bleeding, is overweight before starting hormone replacement therapy, or develops unexpected or severe vaginal bleeding concurrent with the hormone therapy. In women who have had a hysterectomy, estrogen is administered alone. Because of the possibility of a slight increase in the risk of breast cancer with estrogen use, regular breast examinations and annual mammography should be performed according to the guidelines of the American Cancer Society. Contraindications to estrogen therapy are breast or endometrial cancer and active thrombolytic or liver disease (see other guidelines in reference 92). Transdermal estrogens, which, unlike oral estrogens, do not affect serum-binding proteins or clotting factors, also prevent bone loss but produce less beneficial effects on lipoproteins. Studies in postmenopausal patients with breast cancer show that Tamoxifen, an estrogen antagonist that has estrogen agonist-like effects on bone, clotting factors, and the endometrium, prevents bone loss.[93] New drugs that are estrogen antagonists for breast tissue and endometrium but have estrogen-like effects on bone are under investigation (e.g., Raloxifen).[94]

Calcitonin

Calcitonin is a 32-amino acid peptide produced by the parafollicular cells of the thyroid, which inhibits bone resorption through its direct effects on osteoclasts that have high affinity calcitonin receptors. Calcitonin is approved by the Food and Drug Administration (FDA) for the treatment of osteoporosis. Parenteral calcitonin (100 IU every other day or daily) will generally maintain BMD or produce an increment in bone mass that is greatest in subjects with high-turnover osteoporosis.[95,96] Adverse effects of calcitonin include nausea in ~10% to 15% of patients, flushing, inflammation at the injection site, and rhinorrhea (nasal calcitonin). There may also be a beneficial analgesic effect. There may be a plateau effect after 18 to 26 months of therapy, possibly a result of refilling in remodeling space and/or downregulation of calcitonin receptors. Studies in postmenopausal women with osteoporosis show that use of a calcitonin nasal spray (200 IU daily) for 12 months prevents bone loss in the spine and forearm.[97] Nasal calcitonin is also effective in preventing bone loss in early-postmenopausal women.[52,98] Prospective, randomized, placebo-controlled investigations are in progress to assess the effects of different doses of nasal calcitonin in preventing bone loss and fractures; this mode of therapy is associated with fewer adverse effects.

Bisphosphonates

Bisphosphonates are pyrophosphate analogs that are absorbed onto the hydroxyapatite of bone and inhibit bone resorption; these compounds have a sustained effect because of their long half-life in bone. Etidronate, administered intermittently to older osteoporotic women, produced a 5% increase in bone density of the spine and a 50% reduction in vertebral fractures at 2 years.[99] Although this reduction in fractures was not significant at 3 years, vertebral fractures were significantly decreased in a subgroup of women at very high risk of fracture; an open-label follow-up is in progress.[32,100] Adverse effects of etidronate include mild gastrointestinal symptoms and, at high doses, impaired mineralization of bone. Clinical trials of many new bisphosphonates, which are more potent inhibitors of bone resorption without affecting bone formation (at doses used clinically), are under way to assess their effects on bone density and fractures.

Sodium Fluoride

Sodium fluoride stimulates bone formation and produces large increments in BMD. Adverse effects of fluoride occur in up to ~40% of subjects and include gastrointestinal irritation and a lower-extremity pain syndrome with stress fractures. A slow-release fluoride preparation is associated with fewer adverse effects.[101] In prospective, controlled studies of high doses of sodium fluoride for the treatment of osteoporosis (75 mg/d), vertebral fractures did not significantly decrease and nonvertebral fractures increased despite an increase in bone density.[102] Recent data show that a slow-release fluoride preparation is associated with fewer adverse effects and a significant reduction in vertebral fractures; use of fluoride therapy, however, should be restricted to investigative protocols.

1,25(OH)₂ Vitamin D

Use of $1,25(OH)_2$ vitamin D may enhance calcium absorption and bone formation (at pharmacologic doses). Although some studies show that administration of $1,25(OH)_2$ vitamin D for osteoporosis is ineffective in maintaining bone mass, high doses of $1,25(OH)_2$ vitamin D produced some increase in bone density.[103] A reduction in fractures in some studies with $1,25(OH)_2$ vitamin D therapy[104] may result from reversal of mild vitamin D deficiency. $1,25(OH)_2$ vitamin D has a narrow margin of safety, with potential risks of hypercalcemia and hypercalciuria. In elderly nursing home patients with low or low-normal vitamin D levels, vitamin D (800 units) with calcium (1.2 g) decreased hip fractures by 43%.[105] Thus, even in the elderly, treatment interventions may have a major impact in reducing fractures. In the absence of vitamin D insufficiency, however, most treatment regimens should ensure adequate intake with physiologic doses of vitamin D (400 IU/d in a multivitamin).

Parathyroid Hormone

Low doses of parenteral PTH (1–34, the active amino terminus) given with calcitriol increased trabecular bone in the spine[106] but may cause small losses of cortical bone. Future directions in the treatment of osteoporosis may include use of anabolic growth factors or other approaches that may stimulate bone formation.

Because existing therapeutic interventions for established osteoporosis generally only partially reverse bone loss, preventive strategies to optimize skeletal mass, such as reduction of risk factors for bone loss, identification and treatment of patients at risk of bone loss (according to bone density criteria or possibly genetic tools), adequate calcium and vitamin D nutrition, and a regular weight-bearing exercises program, are important.

It is imperative to identify and treat underlying secondary causes of osteoporosis. Our approach to the treatment of postmenopausal women with osteoporosis is to use hormone replacement therapy as the gold standard for therapy because of the combined benefit on the risk of cardiovascular disease and osteoporosis. The ongoing prospective randomized Women's Health Initiative will assess the effects of combined daily continuous estrogen and progesterone therapy on cardiovascular disease, fractures, and breast and uterine cancers. Physicians should, therefore, cautiously evaluate the risk-benefit ratio for hormone replacement therapy in a given patient. Patient compliance with hormone replacement therapy is, however, only ~30%, and at present there is not widespread acceptance of this mode of therapy in postmenopausal women. Alternative treatment strategies at present include use of calcitonin injections or intermittent etidronate, although the latter is not FDA approved for the treatment of osteoporosis. We are concerned about the long retention time of etidronate in bone and therefore are cautious about using this drug in premenopausal or early-postmenopausal women and withhold use of this agent in patients with vitamin D insufficiency. In a postmenopausal woman with a history of breast cancer, Tamoxifen therapy may preserve trabecular bone, although at present we advocate uterine surveillance in these women because of the small increased risk of uterine cancer. The availability of bone densitometry makes it feasible to ensure a therapeutic response to these treatment strategies so that in patients who do not maintain or increase bone mass alternative approaches may be implemented. Therapies that hold promise for the near future include nasal calcitonin, more potent bisphosphonates, and new estrogen agonists on bone and the cardiovascular system that act as estrogen antagonists on the uterus and breast.

STRATEGIES TO PREVENT OR TREAT CORTICOSTEROID-INDUCED BONE LOSS

Osteoporosis is a well-documented sequela of corticosteroid therapy.[6] Studies in patients with Cushing's syndrome show that correction of the hypercortisolism may produce an increase of up to ~20% in bone mass over 2 years.[107] A reduction in corticosteroid dose may, furthermore, produce a reversal of bone loss in some instances.[30] Strategies to prevent bone loss in all patients should therefore include use of the lowest corticosteroid dose possible and prophylactic therapy in corticosteroid-treated patients at risk of bone loss.[108] The goals of therapy in corticosteroid-treated osteoporosis include an attempt to reverse the bone loss (Table 22–2). Despite the severity of the bone loss in some corticosteroid-treated patients (~5% to 20% bone loss over 1 to 2 years), there are few prospective, randomized controlled investigations that examine therapeutic interventions in these patients. A prophylactic graduated exercise program, as is clinically feasible, may prevent the bone loss that results from immobilization and inactivity. In patients who are taking corticosteroids, calcium (1000 mg daily) inhibits bone resorption and decreases bone loss.[81] Thus patients should be advised to maintain an adequate calcium intake as discussed above for osteoporosis. Hahn et al.[51] showed in rheumatic patients taking corticoste-

---

TABLE 22–2

Therapy of Corticosteroid-induced Bone Loss or Osteoporosis

Attempt to stop disease progression and increase bone density in all patients

1. Reduce corticosteroid dose or discontinue therapy if feasible
2. Exercise against gravity
3. Maintain adequate calcium intake
4. Hydrochlorothiazide (if urinary calcium ≥4 mg/kg/d)
5. Vitamin D or 25-hydroxyvitamin D (monitoring serum and urinary calcium levels)
6. Estrogens/progesterone in postmenopausal women, testosterone when indicated in men
7. Calcitonin
8. Bisphosphonates

No FDA-approved treatments.

---

roids that vitamin D (50,000 units two to three times weekly) and 25-hydroxyvitamin D (~40 μg/d), each with 500 mg of elemental calcium, increased intestinal calcium absorption, suppressed PTH release, and had beneficial effects on bone density (~8% and ~16% increments, respectively).[51] It was found that $1,25(OH)_2$ vitamin D was ineffective in corticosteroid-induced osteoporosis.[59] In a recent study, however, calcium and $1,25(OH)_2$ vitamin D, with or without calcitonin, reduced vertebral bone loss in corticosteroid-treated subjects, although calcitonin therapy had a sustained effect during the second year when the other treatments were stopped.[109] Because of the negative calcium balance resulting from corticosteroid therapy, vitamin D supplementation (vitamin D, 50,000 units once weekly) to raise the patient's 25-hydroxyvitamin D level to the upper range of normal may offset the negative calcium balance; careful monitoring of the serum and urinary calcium levels is necessary to minimize the risk of vitamin D intoxication. In a corticosteroid-treated patient who has an elevated urinary calcium level (≥4 mg/kg/d), possibly as a consequence of corticosteroid therapy or who develops hypercalciuria coincident with vitamin D treatment, hydrochlorothiazide therapy (25 to 50 mg two times daily) with sodium restriction is effective in reducing urinary calcium excretion.[108,110] In the absence of corticosteroid therapy, hydrochlorothiazide is associated with a higher bone density at multiple sites[111] and a reduction in the risk of hip fractures.[112] In a retrospective study, estrogen and progesterone therapy prevented bone loss in corticosteroid-treated postmenopausal women[6]; prospective randomized controlled studies of the effects of hormone replacement therapy on corticosteroid-induced bone loss are warranted. In patients with RA not treated with corticosteroids, a recent prospective, placebo-controlled study showed that estrogen replacement increased bone density in both the spine and the proximal femur.[113] In another study, however, in patients with RA, some of whom were treated with corticosteroids, hormone replacement therapy prevented bone loss in the spine but not in the proximal femur site.[23] In men with testosterone deficiency resulting from corticosteroid therapy, treatment with parenteral testosterone or a new transdermal testosterone preparation may have beneficial effects on bone.

The presence of enhanced bone resorption in corticosteroid-treated subjects has led investigators to examine the effects of calcitonin, an osteoclast inhibitor, on BMD in a variety of patients with rheumatic diseases. Ringe and Welzel[114] showed that parenteral calcitonin (100 units every other day) produced a small increase in bone density in the forearm in patients with rheumatic diseases, whereas bone density declined in the control group. Several recent studies, including preliminary data from a large multicenter placebo-controlled trial, show that calcitonin maintains bone mass or produces a small increment in bone in patients taking moderate doses of corticosteroids.[115–117] Low doses of nasal calcitonin (200 units for 1 month, then 100 units daily) prevented bone loss at 1 year in patients with RA not treated with corticosteroids, although a 1.8% bone loss noted in the second year of therapy was significantly less than that in the control group.[118] Use of antiresorptive bisphosphonates may also prove beneficial in the treatment of corticosteroid-induced bone loss. In patients undergoing long-term corticosteroid therapy, a prospective placebo-controlled study of oral pamidronate (APD, or 3-amino-1-hydroxypropylidene-1, 1-bisphosphonate) and calcium produced an ~20% increment in lumbar spine bone density over 1 year,[119] with subsequent stable bone densities. The preliminary controlled study by Adachi et al.[120] showed that intermittent cyclical therapy with etidronate also prevented corticosteroid-induced bone loss; additional prospective, controlled studies of the effects of bisphosphonates

in the treatment of corticosteroid-induced osteoporosis are warranted.

Unlike the antiresorptive drugs discussed above, fluoride stimulates bone formation. Rickers et al.,[121] in a prospective randomized short-term trial, were unable to demonstrate an effect of calcium, fluoride, and vitamin D in preventing corticosteroid-induced bone loss at a trabecular and a cortical site in the forearm over a 24-week interval. Meunier et al.,[122] however, in a 2-year study, observed a 63% increment in trabecular bone on histomorphometric analysis of iliac crest biopsies in corticosteroid-treated patients consistent with an anabolic effect of fluoride on trabecular bone in this group of patients; long-term, randomized controlled studies demonstrating a beneficial effect of fluoride on the reduction fractures would be necessary to establish a role for this therapy in the treatment of corticosteroid-induced bone loss.

In summary, in corticosteroid-treated patients, an initial approach is to select the lowest corticosteroid dose possible to treat the underlying process; alternatives to corticosteroid therapy for the rheumatic process may be considered in patients with accelerated bone loss. Because not all patients treated with corticosteroids develop osteoporosis, we obtain a bone density determination at baseline and within 1 year in patients starting long-term ($\geq$ 3 months) corticosteroid therapy ($\geq$ 5 to 7.5 mg daily) so that therapy may be instituted to protect the skeleton; furthermore, bone densitometry is used to assess the skeletal response to a treatment intervention so that modifications in therapy may be instituted. In a patient with osteopenia or osteoporosis, other secondary causes of bone loss are vigorously pursued and treated. At present there are no FDA-approved therapies for corticosteroid-induced bone loss. To minimize the corticosteroid-induced negative calcium balance, our approach is to provide adequate calcium intake (1000 mg for premenopausal women and 1500 mg for postmenopausal women) and vitamin D or supraphysiologic doses of vitamin D (e.g., 50,000 units vitamin D once weekly or bimonthly) to maintain the 25-hydroxyvitamin D level in the *upper* normal range with careful monitoring of the serum calcium and urinary calcium concentrations to prevent the development of hypercalcemia, hypercalciuria, or nephrolithiasis. Hydrochlorothiazide therapy (25 mg twice daily) will reduce the hypercalciuria associated with corticosteroid therapy or concurrent calcium or vitamin D therapy. Provided there are no contraindications, as discussed above, we use gonadal steroid replacement in both the prevention and the treatment of corticosteroid-induced bone loss in postmenopausal women or hypogonadal men. Alternatively, calcitonin or bisphosphonate therapy may have beneficial effects in corticosteroid-treated patients with evidence of increased risk of fracture or a reduced bone mass or fractures, although we tend not to use etidronate in younger patients because of a theoretic concern about the very long half-life in bone. Data from the prospective effects of calcitonin and new bisphosphonates on bone loss in corticosteroid-treated subjects should be forthcoming in the near future. If a patient treated with corticosteroids continues to lose bone or develops fractures while on a given intervention to protect bone mass, we assess the need for further diagnostic evaluation for concurrent secondary causes of bone loss and consider alternate treatment options. Finally, if the prednisolone derivative, deflazacort, which appears to have fewer effects on bone metabolism than prednisone[120,123,124] at comparable antiinflammatory doses, has less effect on bone loss, as some studies have suggested, use of this corticosteroid or other bone-sparing corticosteroid analogs may mitigate against the development of or reduce the severity of corticosteroid-induced osteoporosis.

REFERENCES

1. Riggs BL, Melton LJ III. The prevention and treatment of osteoporosis. N Engl J Med 1992; 327:620.
2. Riggs BL, Wahner HW, Dunn WL, Mazess RB, Offord KP, Melton LJ. Differential changes in bone mineral density of the appendicular and axial skeleton with aging: relationship to spinal osteoporosis. J Clin Invest 1981;67:328.
3. Sambrook PN, Eisman JA, Champion GD, Yeates MG, Pocock NA, Eberl S. Determinants of axial bone loss in rheumatoid arthritis. Arthritis Rheum 1987;30:721.
4. Morrison NA, Qi JC, Tokita A, et al. Prediction of bone density from vitamin D receptor alleles. Nature 1994;367:284.
5. Mundy GR. Boning up on genes. Nature 1994; 367:216.
6. Lukert BP, Raisz LG. Glucocorticoid-induced osteoporosis: pathogenesis and management. Ann Intern Med 1990;112:352.
7. Ross DS, Neer RM, Ridgway EC. Subclinical hyperthyroidism and reduced bone density as a possible result of prolonged suppression of the pituitary-thyroid axis with L-thyroxine. Am J Med 1987;82:1167.
8. Friedman AJ, Daly M, Juneau-Norcross M, et al. A prospective, randomized trial of gonadotropin releasing-hormone agonist plus estrogen-progestin add-back regimens for women with leiomyomata uteri. J Clin Endocrinol Metab 1993;76:1439.
9. Rigotti NA, Neer RM, Skates SJ, Herzog DB, Nussbaum SR. The clinical course of osteoporosis in anorexia nervosa: a longitudinal study of cortical bone mass. JAMA 1991;265:1133.
10. Finkelstein JS, Klibanski A, Neer RM, Greenspan SL, Rosenthal DI, Crowley WF Jr. Osteoporosis in men with idiopathic hypogonadotropic hypogonadism. Ann Intern Med 1987; 106:354.
11. LeBoff MS, Fuleihan El-Hajj G, Brown E. Osteoporosis and Paget's disease of bone. In: Branch WT, ed. Office practice of medicine. Philadelphia: WB Saunders, 1994:700.
12. Cummings SR, Black DM, Nevitt MC, et al. Bone density at various sites for prediction of hip fractures: the study of osteoporotic fractures research group. Lancet 1993;341(8837):72.
13. Melton LJ, Atkinson EJ, O'Fallon WM, Wahner HW, Riggs BL. Long-term fracture prediction by bone mineral assessed at different skeletal sites. J Bone Miner Res 1993;8(10):1227.
14. Stampfer MJ, Colditz GA, Willett WC, et al. Postmenopausal estrogen therapy and cardiovascular disease. Ten year follow-up from the Nurses' Health Study. N Engl J Med 1991;325: 756.
15. Sambrook PN, Ansell BM, Foster S, Gumpel JM, Hesp R, Reeve J. Bone turnover in early rheumatoid arthritis. 2. Longitudinal bone density studies. Ann Rheum Dis 1985;44:580.
16. Reid DM, Kennedy NSJ, Smith MA, Tothill P, Nuki G. Total body calcium in rheumatoid arthritis: effects of disease activity and corticosteroid treatment. Br Med J 1982;285:330.
17. Caldwell JR, Furst DE. The efficacy and safety of low-dose corticosteroids for rheumatoid arthritis. Semin Arthritis Rheum 1991;21:1.
18. Miossec P, Briolay J, Dechanet J, Wijdenes J, Martinez-Valdez H, Banchereau J. Inhibition of the production of proinflammatory cytokines and immunoglobulins by interleukin-4 in an ex vivo model of rheumatoid synovitis. Arthritis Rheum 1992;35:874.
19. Hooyman JR, Melton LJ III, Nelson AM, O'Fallon WM, Riggs BL. Fractures after rheumatoid arthritis. Arthritis Rheum 1984;27: 1353.
20. Mellish RWL, O'Sullivan MM, Garrahan NJ, Compston JE. Iliac crest trabecular bone mass and structure in patients with non-steroid treated rheumatoid arthritis. Ann Rheum Dis 1987;46:830.
21. Sambrook PN, Eisman JA, Champion GD, Pocock NA. Sex hormone status and osteoporosis in postmenopausal women with rheumatoid arthritis. Arthritis Rheum 1988;31:973.

22. Parker LN, Levin ER, Lifrak ET. Evidence for adrenocortical adaptation to severe illness. J Clin Endocrinol Metab 1985;60:947.
23. Sambrook P, Birmingham J, Champion D, et al. Postmenopausal bone loss in rheumatoid arthritis: effect of estrogens and androgens. J Rheumatol 1992; 19:357.
24. Avioli LV. Osteoporosis in rheumatoid arthritis [Editorial]. Arthritis Rheum 1987;30:830.
25. Harris ED Jr. Rheumatoid arthritis: pathophysiology and implications for therapy. N Engl J Med 1990;322:1277.
26. Sambrook PN, Eisman JA, Yeates MG, Pocock NA, Eberl S, Champion GD. Osteoporosis in rheumatoid arthritis: safety of low dose corticosteroids. Ann Rheum Dis 1986;45:950.
27. Laan RFJM, Buijs WCAM, Verbeek ALM, et al. Bone mineral density in patients with recent onset rheumatoid arthritis: influence of disease activity and functional capacity. Ann Rheum Dis 1993;52:21.
28. Dykman TR, Gluck OS, Murphy WA, Hahn TJ, Hahn BH. Evaluation of factors associated with glucocorticoid-induced osteopenia in patients with rheumatic diseases. Arthritis Rheum 1985;28:361.
29. Als OS, Gotfredsen A, Christiansen C. The effect of glucocorticoids on bone mass in rheumatoid arthritis patients: influence of menopausal state. Arthritis Rheum 1985;28:369.
30. Laan, RFJM, van Riel PLCM, van de Putte LBA, van Erning LJThO, van t Hof MA, Lemmens JAM. Low-dose prednisone induces rapid reversible axial bone loss in patients with rheumatoid arthritis. Ann Intern Med 1993; 119:963.
31. Reid DM, Kennedy NSJ, Smith MA, et al. Bone loss in rheumatoid arthritis and primary generalized osteoarthrosis: effects of corticosteroids, suppressive antirheumatic drugs and calcium supplements. Br J Rheumatol 1986;25:253.
32. Hall GM, Spector ID, Griffin AJ, Jawad ASM, Hall ML, Doyle DV. The effect of rheumatoid arthritis and steroid therapy on bone density in postmenopausal women. Arthritis Rheum 1993;36:1510.
33. LeBoff MS, Wade JP, Mackowiak S, El-Hajj Fuleihan G, Zangari M, Liang M. Low dose steroids do not have adverse effects on bone density or indices of mineral metabolism in postmenopausal women with rheumatoid arthritis. Clin Res 1989;37:354A.
34. Sambrook PN, Reeve J. Bone disease in rheumatoid arthritis [Editorial]. Clin Sci 1988;74:225.
35. Dalsky GP, Stocke KS, Ehsani AA, Slatopolsky E, Lee WC. Weight-bearing exercise training and lumbar bone mineral content in postmenopausal women. Ann Intern Med 1988;108:824.
36. Wood DD, Ihrie, EJ, Dinarello CA, Cohen PL. Isolation of an interleukin-1-like factor from human joint effusions. Arthritis Rheum 1983; 26:975.
37. Firestein GS, Alvaro-Garcia J, Maki R. Quantitative analysis of cytokine gene expression in rheumatoid arthritis. J Immunol 1990;144:3347.
38. Saxne T, Palladino MA, Heinegard D, Talal N, Wollheim FA. Detection of tumor necrosis factor-alpha but not TNF-beta in rheumatoid arthritis synovial fluid and serum. Arthritis Rheum 1988;31:1041.
39. Guerne PA, Zuraw BL, Vaughan JH, Carson DA, Lotz M. Synovium as a source of interleukin-6 in vitro. J Clin Invest 1989;83:585.
40. Goldhaber P. Heparin enhancement of factors stimulating bone resorption in tissue culture. Science 1965;147:407.
41. Raisz LG, Kream BE. Regulation of bone formation. N Engl J Med 1983;309:83.
42. Scott DL, Farr M, Hawkins CF, Wilkinson R, Bold AM. Serum calcium levels in rheumatoid arthritis. Ann Rheum Dis 1981;40:580.
43. Weisman MH, Orth RW, Catherwood BD, Manolagas SC, Deftos LJ. Measures of bone loss in rheumatoid arthritis. Arch Intern Med 1986;146:701.
44. Als OS, Christiansen C, Hellesen C. Prevalence of decreased bone mass in rheumatoid arthritis: relation to anti-inflammatory treatment. Clin Rheumatol 1984;3:201.
45. Mbuyi JM, Dequeker J, Teblick M, Merlevede M. Relevance of urinary excretion of alcian blue glucosamino-glycans complexes and hydroxyproline to disease activity in rheumatoid arthritis. J Rheumatol 1982;9:579.
46. Reid KB, Lowe DM, Porter RR. Isolation and characterization of Clq., a subcomponent of the first component of complement, from human and rabbit sera. Biochem J 1972;130:749.
47. Gevers G, Devos P, et al. Increased levels of osteocalciin (serum bone Gla-protein) in rheumatoid arthritis. J Bone Miner Res 1986;25:260.
48. NIH Conference. Glucocorticoid therapy for immune-mediated diseases: basic and clinical correlates. Arch Intern Med 1993;119:1198.
49. Dempster DW. Bone histomorphometry in glucocorticoid-induced osteoporosis. J Bone Miner Res 1989;4:137.
50. Klein RG, Arnaud SB, Gallagher JC, Deluca HF, Riggs BL. Intestinal calcium absorption in exogenous hypercortisolism: role of 25-hydroxyvitamin D and corticosteroid dose. J Clin Invest 1977;60:253.
51. Hahn TJ, Halstead LR, Teitelbaum SL, Hahn BL. Altered mineral metabolism glucocorticoid-induced osteopenia: effect of 25-hydroxyvitamin D administration. J Clin Invest 1979; 64:655.
52. Gennari C, Agnusdei D, Montagnani M, Gonnelli S, Civitelli R. An effective regimen of intranasal salmon calcitonin in early postmenopausal bone loss. Calcif Tissue Int 1992; 50:381.
53. Canalis E. Effect of glucocorticoids on Type I collagen synthesis, alkaline phosphatase activ-

ity, and deoxyribonucleic acid content in cultured rat calvariae. Endocrinology 1983;112: 931.

54. Rosen H, Jamed ML, Barkan AL. Dexamethasone suppresses gonadotropin-releasing hormone (GnRH) secretion and has direct pituitary effects in male rats: differential regulation of GnRH receptor and gonadotropin responses to GnRH. Endocrinology 1988;122:2873.

55. Adinoff AD, Hollister JR. Steroid-induced fractures and bone loss in patients with asthma. N Engl J Med 1983;309:265.

56. Reid IR, Katz JM, Ibbertson HK, Gray DH. The effects of hydrocortisone, parathyroid hormone, and the bisphosphonate APD, on bone resorption in neonatal mouse calvaria. Calcif Tissue Int 1986;38:38.

57. Stern PH. Inhibition by steroids of parathyroid hormone-induced 45Ca release from embryonic rat bone in vitro. J Pharmacol Exp Ther 1969;168:211.

58. Jee WSS, Park HZ, Roberts WE, Kenner GH. Corticosteroid and bone. Am J Anat 1970;129: 477.

59. Dykman TR, Haralson KM, Gluck OS, et al. Effect of oral 1,25 dihydroxyvitamin D and calcium on glucocorticoid-induced osteopenia in patients with rheumatic diseases. Arthritis Rheum 1984;27:1336.

60. Nussbaum SR, Zahradnik RJ, Lavigne JR, et al. Highly sensitive two-site immunoradiometric assay of parathyrin, and its clinical utility in evaluating patients with hypercalcemia. Clin Chem 1987;33:1364.

61. Reid IR, Chapman GE, Fraser TR, et al. Low serum osteocalcin levels in glucocorticoid-treated asthmatics. J Clin Endocrinol Metab 1986;62:379.

62. Gluck OS, Murphy WA, Hahn TJ, Hahn B. Bone loss in adults receiving alternate day glucocorticoid therapy. Arthritis Rheum 1981;24: 892.

63. Ragab AH, Frech RS, Vietti TJ. Osteoporotic fractures secondary to methotrexate therapy of acute leukemia in remission. Cancer 1970;25: 580.

64. Katz JN, LeBoff MS, Wade JP, Brown EM, Liang MH. Effect of methotrexate on bone density and calcium homeostasis in rheumatoid arthritis. Clin Res 1989;37:509A.

65. Movsowitz C, Epstein S, Fallon M, Ismail F, Thomas S. Cyclosporin-A in vivo produces severe osteopenia in the rat: effect of dose and duration of administration. Endocrinology 1988;123:2571.

66. Aubia J, Masramon J. Bone histology in renal transplant patients receiving cyclosporin. Lancet 1988;1:1048.

67. Rich GM, Mudge GH, Laffel GL, LeBoff MS. Cyclosporine A and prednisone-associated osteoporosis in heart transplant recipients. J Heart Lung Transplant 1992;11:950.

68. Boumpas DT, Austin HA III, Vaughan EM, Yarboro CH, Klippel JH, Balow JE. Risk for sustained amenorrhea in patients with systemic lupus erythematosus receiving intermittent pulse cyclophosphamide therapy. Ann Intern Med 1993;119:366.

69. Steinberg AD, Steinberg SC. Long-term preservation of renal function in patients with lupus nephritis receiving treatment that includes cyclophosphamide versus those treated with prednisone alone. Arthritis Rheum 1991;34:945.

70. Cooper C, Cook PL, Osmond C, Fisher L, Cawley MID. Osteoarthritis of the hip and osteoporosis of the proximal femur. Ann Rheum Dis 1991;50:540.

71. Hannan MT, Anderson JJ, Zhang Y, Levy D, Felson DT. Bone mineral density and knee osteoarthritis in elderly men and women: the Framingham study. Arthritis Rheum 1993;36: 1671.

72. Reid DM, Nicoll JJ, Smith MA, Higgin B, Tothill P, Nuki G. Corticosteroids and bone mass in asthma: comparisons with rheumatoid arthritis and polymyalgia rheumatica. Br Med J (Clin Res Ed) 1986;293:1463.

73. Will R, Palmer R, Bhalla AK, Ring F. Osteoporosis in early ankylosing spondylitis: a primary pathological event? Lancet 1989;1:1483.

74. Tapia-Serrano R, Jiminez-Balderas FJ, Murrieta S, Bravo-Gatica C, Guerra R, Mintz G. Testicular function in active ankylosing spondylitis: therapeutic response to human chronic gonadotropin. J Rheumatol 1991;18:841.

75. Nelson AM, Riggs BL, Jowsey JO. Atypical axial osteomalacia. Arthritis Rheum 1978;21: 715.

76. Hunter T, Dubo HI. Spinal fractures complicating ankylosing spondylitis. A longterm follow-up study. Arthritis Rheum 1983;26:751.

77. Dawson-Hughes B, Dallal GE, Krall EA, Sadowski L, Sahyoun N, Tannenbaum S. A controlled trial of the effect of calcium supplementation on bone density in postmenopausal women. N Engl J Med 1990;323:878.

78. Johnston CC Jr, Miller JZ, Selmenda CW, et al. Calcium supplementation and increases in bone mineral density in children. N Engl J Med 1992;327:82.

79. Heaney RP, Recker RR, Saville PD. Menopausal changes in calcium balance performance. J Lab Clin Med 1978;92:953.

80. Recker RR. Calcium absorption and achlorhydria. N Engl J Med 1985;313:70.

81. Reid IR, Ibbertson HK. Calcium supplements in the prevention of steroid-induced osteoporosis. Am J Clin Nutr 1986;44:287.

82. Eriksen EF, Colvard DS, Berg NG, et al. Evidence of estrogen receptors in normal human osteoblast-like cells. Science 1988;241:84.

83. Komm BS, Terpening CM, Benz DJ, et al. Estrogen binding, receptor mRNA, and biologic response in osteoblast-like osteosarcoma cells. Science 1988;241:81.

84. Manolagas SC, Jilka RL. Cytokines, hematopoiesis, osteoclastogenesis, and estrogens [Editorial]. Calcif Tissue Int 1992;50:199.

85. Pacifici R, Rifas L, McCracken R, et al. Ovarian steroid treatment blocks a postmenopausal increase in blood monocyte interleukin 1 release. Proc Natl Acad Sci USA 1989;86:2398.

86. Pacifici R. Is there a causal role for IL-1 in postmenopausal bone loss? Calcif Tissue Int 1992;50:295.

87. American College of Physicians. Guidelines for counselling postmenopausal women about preventative hormone therapy. Ann Intern Med 1992;117:1038.

88. Felson DT, Zhang Y, Hannan MT, Kiel DP, Wilson WF, Anderson JJ. The effect of postmenopausal estrogen therapy on bone density in elderly women. N Engl J Med 1993;329:1141.

89. Lindsay R, Tohme JF. Estrogen treatment of patients with established postmenopausal osteoporosis. Obstet Gynecol 1990;76:290.

90. Weinstein L, Bewtra C, Gallagher JC. Evaluation of a continuous combined low-dose regimen of estrogen-progestin for treatment of the menopausal patient. Am J Obstet Gynecol 1990;162:1534.

91. Gibbons WE, Judd HL, Moyer D, et al. Evaluation of sequential versus estrogen/progestin replacement therapy on uterine bleeding patterns and endometrial histology. Multiuniversity National Upjohn Study Collaborative. Soc Gynecologic Invest 1991; [Abstract].

92. American College of OB-GYN. Hormone replacement therapy: a review of the recent guidelines of the American College of Obstetrics and Gynecology regarding hormone replacement therapy. ACOG Technical Bull 1992;166:1.

93. Love RR, Mazess RB, Barden HS, et al. Effects of tamoxifen on bone mineral density in postmenopausal women with breast cancer. N Engl J Med 1992;326:852.

94. Black LJ, Sato M, Rowley ER, et al. Raloxifene (LY139481 HCl) prevents bone loss and reduces serum cholesterol without causing uterine hypertrophy in ovariectomized rats. J Clin Invest 1994;93(1):63.

95. Gruber HE, Ivey JL, Baylink DJ, et al. Long-term calcitonin therapy in postmenopausal osteoporosis. Metabolism 1984;33:295.

96. Gennari C, Chierichetti SM, Bigazzi S, Fusi L, Gonnelli S, Terrarra R, Zacchei F. Comparative effects on bone mineral content of calcium and calcium plus salmon calcitonin given in two different regimens in postmenopausal osteoporosis. Curr Ther Res 1985;38:455.

97. Overgaard K, Riis BJ, Christiansen C, Podenphant J, Johansen JS. Nasal calcitonin for treatment of established osteoporosis. Clin Endocrinol 1989;30:435.

98. Overgaard K, Riis BJ, Christiansen C, Hansen MA. Effect of calcitonin given intranasally on early postmenopausal bone loss. Br Med J 1990;299:477.

99. Watts NB, Harris ST, Genant HK, et al. Intermittent cyclical etidronate treatment of postmenopausal osteoporosis. N Engl J Med 1990;323:73.

100. Harris ST, Watts NB, Jackson RD, et al. Four-year study of intermittent cyclic etidronate treatment of postmenopausal osteoporosis: three years of blinded therapy followed by one year of open therapy. Am J Med 1993;95:557.

101. Pak CYC, Sakhaee K, Zerwekh JE, Parcel C, Peterson R, Johnson K. Safe and effective treatment of osteoporosis with intermittent slow release sodium fluoride; augmentation of vertebral bone mass and inhibition of fractures. J Clin Endocrinol Metab 1989;68:150.

102. Riggs BL, Hodgson SF, O'Fallon WM. Effect of fluoride treatment on the fracture rate in postmenopausal women with osteoporosis. N Engl J Med 1990;322:802.

103. Gallagher JC, Goldgar O. Treatment of postmenopausal osteoporosis with high doses of synthetic calcitriol. Ann Intern Med 1990;113:649.

104. Tilyard MW, Spears GF, Thompson J, Dovey S. Treatment of postmenopausal osteoporosis with calcitriol or calcium. N Engl J Med 1992;326:356.

105. Chapuy MC, Arlot ME, Duboeuf F, et al. Vitamin D3 and calcium to prevent hip fractures in elderly women. N Engl J Med 1992;327:1637.

106. Slovik DM, Rosenthal DI, Doppelt SH, et al. Restoration of spinal bone in osteoporotic men by treatment with human parathyroid hormone (1–34) and 1,25-dihydroxyvitamin D. J Bone Miner Res 1986;4:377.

107. Pocock NA, Eisman JA, Dunstan CR, Evans RA, Thomas DH, Huq NL. Recovery from steroid-induced osteoporosis. Ann Intern Med 1987;107:319.

108. Hahn TJ. Steroid and drug induced osteopenia. In: Favus MJ, ed. Primer of the metabolic diseases and disorders of mineral metabolism. American Society of Bone Mineral Research, 1993:250.

109. Sambrook P, Birmingham J, Kelly P, et al. Prevention of corticosteroid osteoporosis: a comparison of calcium, calcitriol, and calcitonin. N Engl J Med 1993;328:1747.

110. Adams JS, Wahl TO, Lukert BP. Effects of hydrochlorothiazide and dietary sodium restriction on calcium metabolism in corticosteroid treated patients. Metabolism 1981;30:217.

111. Wasnich RD, Benfante RJ, Yano K, Heilbrun L, Vogel JM. Thiazide effect on the mineral content of bone. N Engl J Med 1983;309:344.

112. Ray A, Downey W, Griffin MR, Melton LJ III. Long-term use of thiazide diuretics and risk of hip fracture. Lancet 1989;1:687.

113. Van den Brink HR, Lems WF, Ven Everdingen AA, Bijlsma JW. Adjuvant oestrogen treatment increases bone mineral density in postmenopausal women with rheumatoid arthritis. Ann Rheum Dis 1993;52:302.

114. Ringe JD, Welzel D. Salmon calcitonin in the therapy of corticoid-induced osteoporosis. Eur J Clin Pharmacol 1987;33:35.

115. Pasero GP, Gennari C, Dimunno O, Agnusdei D, Montagnani M. Prevention of glucocorticoid-induced osteopenia by calcitonin. In: Pecile A, ed. Calcitonin. Amsterdam: Excerpta Medica, 1984:315.

116. Luengo M, Picado C, Del Rio L, Guanabens N, Montserrat JM, Setoain J. Treatment of steroid-induced osteopenia with calcitonin in corticosteroid dependent asthma. Am Rev Respir Dis 1990;142:104.

117. Montemurro L, Schiraldi G, Fraioli P, Tosi G, Riboldi A, Rizzato G. Prevention of corticosteroid-induced osteoporosis with salmon calcitonin in sarcoid patients. Calcif Tissue Int 1991;49:71.

118. Sileghem A, Geusens P, Dequeker J. Intranasal calcitonin for the prevention of bone erosion and bone loss in rheumatoid arthritis. Ann Rheum Dis 1992;51(6):761.

119. Reid IR, King AR, Alexander CJ, Ibbertson HK. Prevention of steroid-induced osteoporosis with (3-amino-1-hydroxypropylindene)-1, 1-bisphosphonate (APD). Lancet 1988;1:143.

120. Adachi JD, Bensen WG, Bianchi F, et al. Intermittent cyclical etidronate therapy (ICT) prevents corticosteroid-induced bone loss. Fourth International Symposium on Osteoporosis and Consensus Development Conference, Hong Kong [Abstract], 1993.

121. Rickers H, Deding A, Christiansen C, Rodbro P, Naestoft J. Corticosteroid-induced osteopenia and vitamin D metabolism: effect of vitamin D2, calcium, phosphate, and sodium fluoride administration. Clin Endocrinol 1982;16: 490.

122. Meunier PJ, Briancon D, Chavassieu P, et al. Treatment with fluoride: bone histomorphometric findings. In Christiansen C, Johansen JS, Riis BJ, eds. Osteoporosis. Viborg, Denmark: Norhaven AG, 1987:824.

123. Gennari C, Imbimbo B, Montagnani M, Bernini M, Nardi P, Avioli LV. Effects of prednisone and deflazacort on mineral metabolism and parathyroid hormone activity in humans. Calcif Tissue Int 1984;36:245.

124. Montecucco C, Caporali R, Caprotti P, Caprotti M, Notario A. Sex hormones and bone metabolism in postmenopausal rheumatoid arthritis treated with two different glucocorticoids. J Rheumatol 1992;19:1895.

INDEX

Note: Page numbers in *italics* refer to illustrations; page numbers followed by t refer to tables.

ISBN 0-7216-5382-0

90038

9 780721 653822